PEDIATRIC EMERGENCY MEDICINE

Editors

Gary R. Strange, M.D., F.A.C.E.P.

Head, Department of Emergency Medicine
University of Illinois College of Medicine
Professor of Emergency Medicine
University of Illinois at Chicago
Chicago, Illinois

William R. Ahrens, M.D.

Assitant Professor of Clinical Emergency Medicine
Adjunct Assistant Professor of Pediatrics
University of Illinois at Chicago
Director, Pediatric Emergency Services
University of Illinois Hospital
Chicago, Illinois

Robert W. Schafermeyer, M.D., F.A.C.E.P., F.A.A.P.

Associate Chairman, Department of Emergency Medicine
Department of Emergency, Carolinas Medical Center
Clinical Professor of Emergency Medicine and Pediatrics
University of North Carolina at Charlotte School of Medicine
Charlotte, North Carolina

William C. Toepper, M.D., F.A.C.E.P., F.A.A.P.

Director, Pediatric Emergency Medicine Education
Illinois Masonic Medical Center
Clinical Assistant Professor of Emergency Medicine
University of Illinois at Chicago
Chicago, Illinois

PEDIATRIC EMERGENCY MEDICINE

A COMPREHENSIVE STUDY GUIDE

COMPANION HANDBOOK

American College of Emergency Physicians

Gary R. Strange, M.D., F.A.C.E.P.
William R. Ahrens, M.D.
Robert W. Schafermeyer, M.D., F.A.C.E.P., F.A.A.P.
William C. Toepper, M.D., F.A.C.E.P., F.A.A.P.

McGraw-Hill
Health Professions Division
New York St. Louis San Francisco Auckland Bogotá
Caracas Lisbon London Madrid Mexico City Milan Montreal
New Delhi San Juan Singapore Sydney Tokyo Toronto

McGraw-Hill

*A Division of The **McGraw·Hill** Companies*

PEDIATRIC EMERGENCY MEDICINE:
A Comprehensive Study Guide
COMPANION HANDBOOK

1234567890 DOCDOC 998

ISBN 0-07-062008-3

This book was set in Times Roman by Bi-Comp, Inc.
The editors were John Dolan and Muza Navrozov.
The production supervisor was Richard C. Ruzycka.
The cover was designed by Marsha Cohen/Parallelogram.
The index was prepared by Alexandra Nickerson.
R. R. Donnelley & Sons Company was printer and binder.

This book was printed on recycled, acid-free paper.

Library of Congress Cataloging-in-Publication Data

Pediatric emergency medicine : a comprehensive study guide :
companion handbook / American College of Emergency Physicians ;
Gary R. Strange...[et al.].
p. cm.
Includes bibliographical references and index.
ISBN 0-07-062008-3
1. Pediatric emergencies—Handbooks, manuals, etc. I. Strange,
Gary R., date. II. American College of Emergency Physicians.
[DNLM: 1. Emergencies—in infancy & childhood handbooks.
2. Pediatrics handbooks. WS 39 P3713 1999]
RJ370.P4524 1999
618.92′0025—dc21
DNLM/DLC
for Library of Congress

CONTENTS

CONTRIBUTORS

Thomas Abrunzó, M.D., M.S., M.P.H., F.A.A.P., F.A.C.E.P.
Clinical Associate Professor of Pediatrics, University of South Florida College of Medicine, St. Joseph's Hospital, Tampa, Florida [66, 67]

Susan Aguila-Mangahas, M.D.
Fellow, Division of General and Emergency Pediatrics, University of Illinois at Chicago, Chicago, Illinois [48]

Steven E. Aks, D.O.
Clinical Assistant Professor of Emergency Medicine, University of Illinois at Chicago, Consultant, Toxicon Consortium, Chicago, Illinois [81, 88, 90, 91, 94, 103]

Yona Amitai, M.D.
Department of Pediatrics, Hadassah Hospital, Mt. Scopus, Jerusalem, Israel [96]

David A. Arai, M.D.
Assistant Clinical Professor, Department of Emergency Medicine, Baylor University Medical Center, Dallas, Texas [118]

Joilo Barbosa, M.D.
Resident, Internal Medicine and Emergency Medicine, University of Illinois at Chicago, Chicago, Illinois [30, 32]

Roger Barkin, M.D., M.P.H., F.A.A.P., F.A.C.E.P.
Vice President for Pediatric and Newborn Programs, Professor of Surgery, Department of Emergency Medicine, University of Colorado Health Sciences Center, Denver, Colorado [60]

Brian A. Bates, M.D.
Clinical Assistant Professor of Pediatrics, University of Texas, San Antonio, Director, Children's Emergency Center, Women's and Children's Hospital, San Antonio, Texas [5, 7]

The numbers in brackets refer to chapter(s) authored or co-authored by the contributor.

Elizabeth E. Baumann, M.D.

Instructor in Pediatrics, Section of Pediatric Endocrinology, Department of Pediatrics, University of Chicago and Wyler Children's Hospital, Chicago, Illinois [53, 54, 55]

Ken Bizovi, M.D.

Clinical Instructor of Emergency Medicine, University of Illinois at Chicago, Consultant, Toxicon Consortium, Chicago, Illinois [83]

Ira J. Blumen, M.D.

Assistant Professor of Medicine, Section of Emergency Medicine, Medical Director, University of Chicago Aeromedical Network, Pritzker School of Medicine/University of Chicago, Chicago, Illinois [117, 118]

Mary Jo A. Bowman, M.D.

Assistant Professor of Clinical Pediatrics, Emergency Department, Children's Hospital, Ohio State University College of Medicine, Columbus, Ohio [109, 110, 111]

Richard M. Cantor, M.D., F.A.A.P., F.A.C.E.P., A.A.C.T.

Medical Director, Central New York Poison Control Center, Department of Emergency Medicine, SUNY University Hospital, Assistant Professor of Emergency Medicine and Pediatrics, State University of New York at Syracuse, Syracuse, New York [22]

Mary Ann Cooper, M.D., F.A.C.E.P.

Associate Professor of Emergency Medicine, University of Illinois at Chicago, Chicago, Illinois [116]

Stephen A. Colucciello, M.D., F.A.C.E.P.

Director of Clinical Services and Trauma Coordinator, Department of Emergency Medicine, Carolinas Medical Center, Clinical Assistant Professor of Emergency Medicine, University of North Carolina, Chapel Hill, Instructor of Paramedic Education, Central Piedmont Community College, Charlotte, North Carolina [14, 15]

Kathleen Connors, M.D.

Department of Emergency Medicine, State University of New York Health Science Center, Assistant Professor of Emergency Medicine, SUNY Health Science Center at Syracuse, Syracuse, New York [23, 24, 25, 26, 27, 28]

Michael Cowan, M.D.

Fellow, Division of Pediatric Emergency Medicine, Department of Pediatrics, University of Texas Southwestern Medical Center at Dallas, Dallas, Texas [2]

Timothy Erickson, M.D., F.A.C.E.P., A.A.C.T.

Assistant Professor of Emergency Medicine, University of Illinois at Chicago, Director, Toxicology Fellowship, Toxicon Consortium, Chicago, Illinois [78, 80, 92, 97, 99, 101, 105, 109, 110]

Susan Fuchs, M.D., F.A.A.P.

Associate Professor of Pediatrics, University of Pittsburgh, Attending Physician, Pediatric Emergency Medicine, Children's Hospital of Pittsburgh, Pittsburgh, Pennsylvania [33, 34, 35, 36, 37, 38, 39, 40, 41, 42]

Marianne Gausche, M.D., F.A.C.E.P.

Associate Professor of Medicine, UCLA School of Medicine, Los Angeles, California, Director, Emergency Medical Services, Department of Emergency Medicine, Harbor-UCLA Medical Center, Torrance, California [58, 59]

Michael J. Gerardi, M.D., F.A.C.E.P., F.A.A.P.

Director, Pediatric Emergency Services, St. Barnabas Medical Center, Livingston, New York, Clinical Assistant Professor of Medicine, UMDNJ-Robert Wood Johnson Medical School, New Brunswick, New Jersey [8]

Colin Goto, M.D.

Fellow, Division of Pediatric Emergency Medicine, University of Texas Southwestern Medical Center at Dallas, Dallas, Texas [5, 6]

John W. Graneto, D.O., M.Ed., F.C.O.E.P., F.A.C.O.P.

Assistant Professor of Pediatrics and Emergency Medicine, Chicago College of Osteopathic Medicine of Midwestern University, Downers Grove, Illinois, Director, Pediatric Services and Pediatric Residency Program Director, Chicago Osteopathic Hospital and Medical Center, Chicago, Illinois [50]

Michael Green, M.D.

Chief Resident, Department of Emergency Medicine, University of Illinois at Chicago, Chicago, Illinois [95]

Russell H. Greenfield, M.D., F.A.C.E.P.

Director, Emergency Department, Presbyterian Matthews Hospital, Matthews, North Carolina [16, 17, 18, 19, 20]

Leon Gussow, M.D.

Attending Physician, Department of Emergency Medicine, Cook County Hospital, Consultant, Toxicon Consortium, Chicago, Illinois [79, 107]

Suchinta Hakim, M.D., F.A.A.P., F.A.C.E.P.

Assistant Clinical Professor of Emergency Medicine, Loyola University College of Medicine, Chicago, Illinois [43]

Brenda N. Hayakawa, M.D., F.A.A.P., F.R.C.P.C.

Department of Emergency Medicine, Royal Columbian Hospital, Westminster, British Columbia, Canada [74]

Bruce E. Herman, M.D.

Assistant Professor of Pediatrics, Department of Emergency Medicine, Primary Children's Medical Center, University of Utah School of Medicine, Salt Lake City, Utah [109, 110, 111]

Donald Scott Hill, M.D.

Resident, Emergency Medicine, Department of Emergency Medicine, University of Illinois at Chicago, Chicago, Illinois [113]

Daniel Hryhorczuk, M.D., M.P.H.

Great Lakes Center for Occupational and Environmental Safety and Health, University of Illinois at Chicago, Director, Toxicon Consortium, Chief, Section of Clinical Toxicology, Cook County Hospital, Chicago, Illinois [96]

Will Ignatoff

Medical Student, Department of Emergency Medicine, University of Illinois at Chicago, Chicago, Illinois [105]

David M. Jaffe, M.D., F.A.A.P.

Director, Division of Emergency Medicine, St. Louis Children's Hospital, Associate Professor of Pediatrics, Washington University School of Medicine, St. Louis, Missouri [10]

Shabnam Jain, M.D.

Assistant Professor of Pediatrics, Section of Emergency Medicine, Grady Memorial Hospital, Emory University School of Medicine, Atlanta, Georgia [45, 46]

Paula Kienberger Jaudes, M.D.
Associate Professor of Clinical Pediatrics, Chief, Section of Chronic Diseases, Pritzker School of Medicine/University of Chicago, Executive Vice-President, LaRabida Children's Hospital and Research Center, Chicago, Illinois [119]

Katherine M. Konzen, M.D., M.P.H.
Assistant Professor of Pediatrics, Mayo Medical Center, Rochester, Minnesota [68]

Jane E. Kramer, M.D.
Director, Pediatric Emergency Services, Rush Presbyterian St. Lukes Medical Center, Assistant Professor of Pediatrics, Rush Medical College, Chicago, Illinois [70, 71, 72, 73]

Anne Krantz, M.D.
Division of Occupational Medicine, Cook County Hospital, Consultant, Toxicon Consortium, Chicago, Illinois [89]

Jerrold Leikin, M.D.
Associate Professor of Medicine, Rush Medical College, Medical Director, Rush Poison Control Center, Chicago, Illinois [82, 84, 91, 102]

Jeffrey J. Leinen, M.D.
Section of Emergency Medicine, Department of Medicine, Pritzker School of Medicine/University of Chicago, Chicago, Illinois [117]

Steven Lelyveld, M.D., F.A.C.E.P., F.A.A.P.
Associate Professor of Clinical Pediatrics and Medicine, Chief, Section of Pediatric Emergency Medicine, Pritzker School of Medicine/University of Chicago, Chicago, Illinois [44, 47]

Marshall Lewis, M.D.
Chief Resident, Department of Pediatrics, University of Illinois at Chicago, Chicago, Illinois [57]

Jordan D. Lipton, M.D.
Emergency Department, Pinnacle Emergency Consultants, Gaston Memorial Hospital, Gastonia, North Carolina [21]

Wendy Ann Lucid, M.D.

Director and Section Chief, Pediatric Emergency Services, Good Samaritan Regional Medical Center, Phoenix, Arizona [11, 12, 13]

Mark Mackey, M.D.

Assistant Professor of Emergency Medicine, University of Illinois at Chicago, Chicago, Illinois [56]

Diana Mayer, M.D.

Assistant Professor of Pediatrics, Department of Pediatrics, University of Illinois at Chicago, Chicago, Illinois [75, 76, 77]

Bonnie McManus, M.D.

Toxicology Fellow, Department of Emergency Medicine, University of Illinois at Chicago, Consultant, Toxicon Consortium, Chicago, Illinois [87, 93]

Arlene Mrozowski, D.O.

Attending Physician, Department of Emergency Medicine, St. Vincent's Medical Center, Bridgeport, Connecticut [52]

Thomas T. Mydler, M.D.

Assistant Professor of Pediatrics, Division of Pediatric Emergency Medicine, University of Texas Southwestern Medical Center at Dallas, Dallas, Texas [6]

Frank P. Paloucek, Pharm. D.

Assistant Professor of Pharmacy Practice, Adjunct Assistant Professor of Emergency Medicine, University of Illinois at Chicago, Chicago, Illinois [106]

Barbara Pawel, M.D.

Clinical Assistant Professor of Pediatrics, Department of Emergency Medicine, UMDNJ-Robert Wood Johnson Medical School, New Brunswick, New Jersey [114]

Elizabeth C. Powell, M.D.

Assistant Professor of Pediatrics, Northwestern University School of Medicine, Attending Physician, Division of Pediatric Emergency Medicine, Children's Memorial Hospital, Chicago, Illinois [49]

Patricia Primm, M.D.

Assistant Professor of Pediatrics, University of Texas Southwestern Medical Center at Dallas, Dallas, Texas [4]

Kimberly S. Quayle, M.D.

Division of Emergency Medicine, St. Louis Children's Hospital, Instructor in Pediatrics, Washington University School of Medicine, St. Louis, Missouri [9]

Rebecca Reamy Lynn, M.D.

Fellow, Division of Pediatric Emergency Medicine, Department of Pediatrics, University of Texas Southwestern Medical Center at Dallas, Dallas, Texas [4]

Sally Reynolds, M.D.

Assistant Professor of Pediatrics, Northwestern University School of Medicine, Attending Physician, Division of Pediatric Emergency Medicine, Children's Memorial Hospital, Chicago, Illinois [49]

T. J. Rittenberry, M.D., F.A.C.E.P.

Clinical Assistant Professor of Emergency Medicine, Assistant Residency Director, Department of Emergency Medicine, University of Illinois at Chicago, Chicago, Illinois [95, 98]

Jaime Rivas, M.D.

Chief Resident, Department of Emergency Medicine, University of Illinois at Chicago, Chicago, Illinois [98]

Simon Ros, M.D.

Associate Professor, Department of Pediatrics, Loyola University Medical Center, Maywood, Illinois [112]

Julia A. Rosekrans, M.D., F.A.C.E.P., F.A.A.P.

Head, Section of Pediatric Emergency Services, Director, Pediatric Residency, Department of Pediatrics, Mayo Medical Center, Consultant in Pediatric and Adolescent Medicine, Mayo Graduate School of Medicine, Rochester, Minnesota [61, 62, 63, 64, 65]

Robert L. Rosenfield, M.D.

Professor of Pediatrics and Medicine, Head, Section of Pediatric Endocrinology, Wyler Children's Hospital, Pritzker School of Medicine/University of Chicago, Chicago, Illinois [53, 54, 55]

John P. Rudzinski, M.D.

Vice Chairman, Department of Emergency Medicine, Rockford Memorial Hospital, Clinical Associate Professor of Surgery, University of Illinois at Rockford, Rockford, Illinois [56]

John P. Santamaria, M.D., F.A.C.E.P., F.A.A.P.

Director, Pediatric Emergency Services, Director, Wound and Hyperbaric Center, St. Joseph's Hospital, Clinical Assistant Professor of Pediatrics, University of South Florida School of Medicine Tampa, Florida [66, 67]

Elizabeth Schwarz, M.D.

Institute for Juvenile Research, Department of Child Psychiatry, University of Illinois at Chicago, Chicago, Illinois [120]

Susan M. Scott, M.D.

Fellow, Division of Pediatric Emergency Medicine, University of Texas Southwestern Medical Center at Dallas, Dallas, Texas [1, 3]

Kimberly Sing, M.D.

Fellow in Toxicology, Toxicon Consortium, University of Illinois at Chicago, Chicago, Illinois [104]

Jonathan Singer, M.D.

Professor of Pediatrics and Emergency Medicine, Department of Emergency Medicine, Wright State University School of Medicine, Dayton, Ohio [51]

David F. Soglin, M.D.

Assistant Professor of Pediatrics, Rush Medical College, Director of Pediatric Education, Cook County Children's Hospital, Chicago, Illinois [70, 71, 72, 73]

Gary R. Strange, M.D., F.A.C.E.P.

Head, Department of Emergency Medicine, University of Illinois College of Medicine, Professor of Emergency Medicine, University of Illinois at Chicago, Chicago, Illinois [108, 113, 115, 116]

Todd Brian Taylor, M.D., F.A.C.E.P.

Emergency Physician, Good Samaritan Regional Medical Center, Phoenix, Arizona [11, 12, 13]

William C. Toepper, M.D., F.A.C.E.P., F.A.A.P.
Director, Pediatric Emergency Medicine Education, Illinois Masonic Medical Center, Clinical Assistant Professor of Emergency Medicine, University of Illinois at Chicago, Chicago, Illinois [29, 30, 31, 32]

David A. Townes, M.D.
Resident, Emergency Medicine, University of Illinois College of Medicine, University of Illinois Hospital, Chicago, Illinois [108]

Timothy Turnbull, M.D.
Assistant Professor of Emergency Medicine, University of Illinois at Chicago, Chicago, Illinois [86]

Michael Van Rooyen, M.D.
Assistant Chief of Emergency Service, University of Illinois Hospital, Assistant Professor of Emergency Medicine, University of Illinois at Chicago, Chicago, Illinois [69]

Robert A. Wiebe, M.D.
Professor of Pediatrics, Chief, Division of Pediatric Emergency Medicine, University of Texas Southwestern Medical Center at Dallas, Dallas, Texas [1, 3]

Dean Wolanyk, M.D.
Attending Physician, Department of Emergency Medicine, Rockford Memorial Hospital, Assistant Clinical Professor of Medicine and Surgery, University of Illinois at Rockford, Rockford, Illinois [56]

Matthew Wols, M.D.
Resident in Emergency Medicine, Department of Emergency Medicine, University of Illinois at Chicago, Chicago, Illinois [43]

Tom Wright, M.D.
Fellow in Child Psychiatry, Department of Child Psychiatry, University of Illinois at Chicago, Chicago, Illinois [120]

Michelle Zell-Kanter, Pharm. D.
Toxicon Consortium, University of Illinois at Chicago, Chicago, Illinois [85, 97, 100]

PREFACE

This handbook accompanies the first edition of our text *Pediatric Emergency Medicine: A Comprehensive Study Guide.* The purpose of the handbook is to provide an on-the-spot summary of the clinical problem for the student, resident, or clinician. The handbook does not replace the text. Rather, it addresses the need for a more portable reference for its audience.

Because the handbook was developed after the text, we were able to update some of the material and references. In particular, the chapters on congestive and inflammatory diseases of the heart and immunoprophylaxis have recent updates included (see, e.g., Appendixes A and B). For the most part, though, the handbook is a condensation of the fuller text and serves as a good introduction to pediatric EM. Readers looking for a more in-depth analysis should consult *Pediatric Emergency Medicine: A Comprehensive Study Guide.*

As we are now preparing material for the next edition of the book, we welcome reader's comments on the text and handbook. It is our intention that both books evolve in response to the changes in pediatric emergency medicine and to the needs of our readers.

THE EDITORS

PREFACE

PEDIATRIC EMERGENCY MEDICINE

Section I
Resuscitation

1 Introduction

Susan M. Scott / Robert A. Wiebe

Cardiopulmonary arrest in the pediatric population differs from that in adults in its etiology, physiology, and emotional aspects. The establishment of separate techniques and protocols for both pediatric basic and advanced life support has acknowledged these differences.

Cardiac arrest in the adult is usually a primary event that results from a sudden dysrhythmia. The pediatric cardiac arrest usually results from deterioration of an underlying medical problem. Decreased tissue perfusion, hypoxia, and acidosis generally precede cardiac arrest. The antecedent period of deterioration results in significant end-organ damage and makes the restoration of spontaneous circulation difficult.

There are no nationwide statistics to indicate the incidence of cardiac arrest in the pediatric population. From 45 to 70 percent of pediatric cardiac arrests occur in infants less than one year of age. Many of these patients have an underlying illness. In infants and young children, sudden infant death syndrome and respiratory diseases are the leading etiologies of cardiorespiratory arrest. After one year of age, trauma becomes a leading cause of pediatric death.

PROGNOSIS

Many studies have evaluated the outcome of pediatric cardiopulmonary arrest (Table 1-1). These reports are difficult to interpret, since they vary in respect to the population reviewed, whether the arrest occurred in or out of the hospital, the presence of prehospital CPR, and the etiology of the arrest itself. Isolated respiratory arrests have a much better resuscitation success rate, long-term survival, and neurologic outcome than cardiac arrests. Other outcome indicators include the initial pH, duration of the resuscitation, and the number of doses of epinephrine used during the resuscitation. Two studies have found no long-term survivors in patients who received more than two standard doses of epineph-

TABLE 1-1 Outcome Studies of Pediatric Cardiopulmonary Resuscitation

Author	Population	Outcome
Ehrlich, 1974	In hospital	78% initial survival 47% discharged
Friesen et al., 1982	In and out of hospital	18% initial survival 9% discharged
Eisenberg et al., 1983	Out of hospital	6% discharged
Lewis et al., 1983	In and out of hospital	25% mortality for respiratory alone 87% mortality for cardiorespiratory
Ludwig et al., 1983	In and out of hospital	In hospital, 65% long-term survival Out of hospital, 29% long-term survival
Torphy et al., 1984	Out of hospital	33% initial survival
Wark, 1984	Out of hospital	66% initial survival 42% discharged
Applebaum, 1985	Out of hospital	No long-term survivors
Gillis et al., 1986	In hospital	17% overall long-term survivors 44% long-term survival for respiratory arrest alone 9% long-term survival for cardiopulmonary arrest
Nichols, 1986	In and out of hospital	57% overall initial survival 38% overall long-term survival 23% survival out of hospital 44% survival in hospital
O'Rourke, 1986	Out of hospital	21% long-term survival
Tsai and Kallsen, 1987	Out of hospital	No survivors
Fiser and Wrape, 1987	In and out of hospital	39% initial survival 22% discharged
Zaritsky et al., 1987	In and out of hospital	34% discharged

rine. This may indirectly reflect the severity of the hypoxia, ischemia, and acidosis, which render the heart refractory to treatment. Future efforts to improve outcome in pediatric CPR should be directed toward preventive care, early recognition of shock and respiratory failure, improved prehospital care, and increased public knowledge of basic life support skills.

For a more detailed discussion, see Scott SM, Wiebe RA: Introduction, chap. 1, p. 1, in *Pediatric Emergency Medicine: A Comprehensive Study Guide.*

2 Respiratory Failure

Michael Cowan / Thomas Abromo

Respiratory failure occurs when the exchange of oxygen and carbon dioxide across the alveolar-capillary network becomes inadequate. It can result from pulmonary pathology, or it may be the end result of disease involving other organ systems. Respiratory failure is usually preceded by a period of respiratory insufficiency, characterized clinically by increased work of breathing and by hypoxia and hypercarbia.

ANATOMY AND PHYSIOLOGY

Young infants are obligate nose breathers, and obstruction of the nasal passages can produce respiratory difficulty. The upper airway in infants and young children is narrow and therefore susceptible to obstruction from congenital anomalies, foreign bodies, and infections. The chest wall is highly elastic and collapsible, and the chest wall musculature is poorly developed. The lower airways are vulnerable to mucus plugging and ventilation-perfusion mismatch. Limited alveolar space makes the infant dependent on increasing the respiratory rate to augment minute ventilation. Increased muscle exertion can result in muscle fatigue and respiratory failure because of infants' limited metabolic reserve.

History

A patient in respiratory distress will usually present with a history of trouble breathing. Parents of infants may note coughing or rapid, noisy breathing. Difficulty in bottle-feeding is an important indication of respiratory compromise in infants. In older children, wheezing or decreased physical activity may be the presenting complaints. Infants with a history of significant prematurity may have bronchopulmonary dysplasia, a syndrome characterized by varying degrees of hypoxia, hypercarbia, reactive airway disease, and susceptibility to respiratory infections. Infants with a history of sweating while bottle-feeding may have undiagnosed congestive heart failure. A patient with a history of a chronic cough or a history of multiple pneumonia may have an underlying disorder such as reactive airway disease, cystic fibrosis, or a retained foreign body. Respiratory symptoms can also be due to systemic disorders such as tachypnea accompanied diabetic ketoacidosis or sepsis.

Physical Examination

Mental status is the first factor to evaluate. Infants and young children with mild respiratory difficulty will have normal mental status. Patients with more severe disease become irritable or anxious, and can appear restless. Young infants in severe distress will often not make eye contact and usually will not bottle-feed. Incipient respiratory failure is heralded by extreme agitation, and finally by lethargy or somnolence.

Respiratory rate is a sensitive indicator of pulmonary status. It is important to realize that normal respiratory rate varies with age. Virtually all infants and children with respiratory distress will be tachypneic, and persistent tachypnea almost always indicates respiratory distress.

Visual inspection of the chest wall may reveal retractions, which signify the use of accessory muscles of respiration. Retractions are seen in the supraclavicular and subcostal areas. In more severe cases, nasal flaring is seen. Retractions imply a significant degree of respiratory distress.

Listening to grossly audible breath sounds will help to localize the pathology. Stridor, a high-pitched sound that can be heard on both inspiration and expiration, indicates upper airway pathology. Grossly audible wheezing usually indicates obstruction at the level of the lower airways. Lower airway disease resulting in alveolar collapse can be associated with grunting, which is caused by premature closure of the glottis during expiration. Grunting increases airway pressure and can preserve functional residual capacity. It is most often seen in infants and always indicates severe respiratory distress, whether from primary lung disease or from a systemic illness such as sepsis.

Auscultation of the chest supplements the information gained from general observation of the patient. The first factor to assess is air exchange. Breath sounds are then evaluated for specific findings, such as wheezing, rales, rhonchi, or localized areas of diminution. In patients with isolated tachypnea and no positive auscultatory findings, consider a metabolic process such as sepsis or metabolic acidosis.

Laboratory Studies

Laboratory studies are useful in assessing the degree of respiratory compromise. Measurement of oxygen saturation via percutaneous pulse oximetry allows rapid assessment of a patient's oxygen status. The slope of the oxygen-hemoglobin dissociation curve is such that patients with marginal oxygen saturations may have significant hypoxemia. Pulse oximetry is unreliable in patients with low perfusion states, carbon monoxide toxicity, and methemoglobinemia.

In patients with moderate to severe respiratory distress, an arterial blood gas may be necessary. Strictly defined, respiratory failure is signified by an arterial oxygen tension (Pa_{O_2}) less than 60 mmHg despite supplemental inhaled oxygen of 60%, or an arterial carbon dioxide tension greater than 60 mmHg. However, a patient who does not meet strict criteria for respiratory failure may develop muscle fatigue such that the work of breathing cannot be sustained. Conversely, a patient with severe underlying lung disease may be well adjusted to chronic hypercarbia.

Indications for Assisted Ventilation

The most common indication for assisted ventilation in a pediatric patient in respiratory distress is progressive muscle fatigue. This emphasizes the need for serial examination in the patient in respiratory distress. Decreasing P_{O_2} or rising P_{CO_2} in spite of aggressive therapy may indicate the need for assisted ventilation, but must be viewed by the context of the patient's clinical status.

Establishing the Airway

The airway of the pediatric patient can be more difficult to manage than that of the adult. The large, prominent occiput of the young infant can force the head into flexion, occluding the airway. The oral cavity of the infant or young child is small, and the tongue is relatively large. The epiglottis is larger, longer, and less rigid than in adults, and the vocal cords are more anterior. Up to the age of about 8 years, the subglottic ring or the cricoid cartilage is the most narrow part of the airway.

Ventilatory assistance begins with establishing a patent airway. Try to open the airway with a jaw-thrust maneuver by placing two or three fingers under the angle of the mandible and lifting the jaw upward and outward. If a cervical injury is not a consideration, place the child in the sniffing position, with the head slightly extended and the neck slightly flexed. Do not overextend the head, as this may cause airway obstruction.

An oropharyngeal airway can bypass obstruction from a posteriorly displaced tongue, which is especially common in unconscious patients. The appropriate oral airway spans the distance from the central incisors to the angle of the mandible. However, oral airways are inappropriate for conscious patients, in whom they can produce vomiting. In awake patients, a nasopharyngeal airway is useful for bypassing the tongue. The diameter of the nasopharyngeal airway should approximate that of the patient's nostril.

Providing Ventilation

Initial ventilation is provided by the bag-valve-mask (BVM) technique. A transparent mask should fit snugly from the bridge of the nose to the prominence of the symphysis of the mandible. Circular masks with seals are more effective than triangular masks in infants and small children. The mask is held in place with the thumb and forefinger of the hand, while the remaining fingers lift the jaw to maintain a patent airway and establish a seal.

Two types of bags that are commonly available are the anesthesia bag and the self-inflating bag. The anesthesia bag is collapsible and refills by the constant inflow of oxygen. When used correctly, anesthesia bags deliver a very high concentration of oxygen, avoid excessive airway pressure, and assure a tight seal. However, using the anesthesia bag requires a significant amount of expertise.

The self-inflating bag requires less training and usually provides adequate ventilation. To deliver an inspired oxygen content of 60% to 90%, it must come equipped with a reservoir and be used with an oxygen flow rate of 10 to 15 L/min. Self-inflating bags usually have a pop-off valve to regulate maximum inspiratory pressure. In resuscitations, the valve is bypassed, since many patients need high inspiratory pressures to provide adequate oxygenation and ventilation. In patients with normal lung compliance, the valve can prevent complications of barotrauma, such as pneumothorax. Self-inflating bags come in three sizes: 250 mL for neonates, 450 mL for infants and young children, and 1000 mL for adults. Infants are ventilated at a rate of 20 to 30 breaths per minute and older children at 16 to 20 breaths per minute.

During assisted ventilation, air is forced into the stomach and gastric distension can occur, impeding ventilation and inducing regurgitation and aspiration of gastric contents. Gentle cricoid pressure, the Sellick maneuver, can reduce gastric distension and prevent aspiration until a nasogastric tube is placed. Nasogastric suction can eliminate gastric distension.

Advanced Airway Management

In most situations that require BVM ventilation, insertion of an endotracheal tube is necessary. In spontaneously breathing patients, 3 to 5 min of 100% oxygen delivered by a nonrebreather mask provides the patient with 3 to 4 min of adequate oxygenation even in the face of apnea. In patients receiving assisted ventilation, minimizing the time of bagging is important in reducing the possibility of aspiration. In this situation, several breaths with 100% oxygen provide an adequate reservior of oxygen.

After preoxygenation, the head is placed in the sniffing position to align the oral, pharyngeal, and laryngeal vectors. A towel placed under the shoulders may assist in alignment. The mouth is opened and any debris removed from the airway by suctioning. The laryngoscope blade is inserted into the right corner of the mouth, and the tongue is swept to the left. For infants and young children, a straight blade is preferred (Table 2-1). The epiglottis is elevated, and the endotracheal tube is inserted between the vocal cords. During laryngoscopy, the Sellick maneuver is performed to reduce the risk of aspiration. This maneuver can also aid in visualizing the anteriorly displaced vocal cords of infants and small children.

TABLE 2-1 Endotracheal Tube Size and Length and Size of Laryngoscope Blades[a] by Age

Endoctracheal tubes	
Newborn	3.0 uncuffed
Newborn–6 months	3.5 uncuffed
6–18 months	3.5–4.0 uncuffed
18 months–3 years	4.0–4.5 uncuffed
3–5 years	4.5 uncuffed
5–6 years	5.0 uncuffed
6–8 years	5.5–6.0 uncuffed
8–10 years	6.0 cuffed
10–12 years	6.0–6.5 cuffed
12–14 years	6.5–7.0 cuffed
Laryngoscope blades	
<2.5 kg	0 straight
0–3 months	1.0 straight
3 months–3 years	1.5 straight
3 years–12 years	2.0 (straight or curved)
Adolescent	3.0 (straight or curved)

[a] Tube size = (16 + age)/4 = internal diameter of endotracheal tube or patient's fifth digit.

Depth can be calculated by taking the internal diameter and multiplying by 3.

During intubation, heart rate and oxygen saturation are continuously monitored.

With a well-positioned endotracheal tube of proper size (see Table 8.4), an audible air leak is heard when ventilation is applied at a pressure of 15 to 20 cmH_2O. If no air leak is audible, the tube is too tight. If the air leak is too large, ventilation will be inadequate.

Correct endotracheal tube placement is confirmed clinically by observing adequate chest wall expansion and auscultating bilateral breath sounds. Asymmetric breath sounds imply that the tube is in either the right or left mainstem bronchus. The right mainstem bronchus is more likely to be intubated, and breath sounds are heard louder on the right side. This situation is corrected by slowly withdrawing the tube until equal breath sounds are heard. If unilateral breath sounds persist despite withdrawal of the tube, a pneumothorax is possible.

End-tidal carbon dioxide is the partial pressure of carbon dioxide at the end of an exhaled breath. This can be measured by colorimetry and is useful in confirming a tracheal, as opposed to esophageal, intubation. In an esophageal intubation, the colorimeter fails to detect the presence of carbon dioxide, which is normally present in expired air.

A chest x-ray will confirm optimal tube placement, which is signified by the tip being midway between the carina and the vocal cords.

Mechanical Ventilation

The two major types of mechanical ventilators are pressure ventilators and volume ventilators. Both assist the patient by delivering compressed gases with positive pressure.

A volume ventilator delivers a preset volume of gas during each mechanical inspiration. This type of ventilator compensates for all changes in resistance. The danger of volume ventilators is that they generate high airway pressures, which can result in barotrauma. Currently, they are used for children and older infants. The usual tidal volume in an infant or child is 12 to 15 mL/kg. The rate depends on the patient's age and the clinical condition.

Pressure ventilators terminate inspiration when a preset pressure is reached and therefore avoid excessive inflating pressures. They do not compensate for changes in lung compliance and deliver a variable amount of gas with each breath. Currently, pressure ventilators are used predominantly in neonates and young infants.

Both volume and pressure ventilators have the ability to provide positive end-expiratory pressure (PEEP), which is especially important in situations in which there is decreased lung compliance.

The major side effect of excessive PEEP is decreased venous return to the right side of the heart and decreased cardiac output. In the emergency department setting, PEEP is usually set at 3 to 5 cmH_2O.

For a more detailed discussion, see Cowan M, Abramo T: Respiratory failure, chap. 2, p. 4, in *Pediatric Emergency Medicine: A Comprehensive Study Guide.*

3 Shock

Susan M. Scott / Robert A. Wiebe

INTRODUCTION

Shock results from insufficient delivery of nutrients and inadequate removal of the waste products at a cellular level, resulting in tissue hypoxia and altered acid-base status. The clinical manifestations of shock result from cell dysfunction and the compensatory mechanisms activated to preserve metabolic integrity.

Shock can be compensated, decompensated, or irreversible. In compensated shock, blood pressure and tissue perfusion are maintained. In decompensated shock, inadequate organ perfusion can result in severe metabolic derangement. In irreversible shock, cell death occurs. Aggressive management in the early stages of shock is vital to avoid the cascade from tissue hypoxia to multiple organ failure and cell death.

Clinically, shock is categorized as hypovolemic, septic, distributive, or cardiogenic. While each category has specific etiologies and varies in presentation, there is considerable overlap clinically and biochemically, especially in the more advanced stages.

PATHOPHYSIOLOGY

Shock affects all organ systems. Hypoperfusion of the brain, hypoxia, and metabolic abnormalities cause mental status changes. Myocardial dysfunction and loss of vascular tone and integrity occur. Increased work of breathing can lead to muscle fatigue and respiratory failure. Decreased renal perfusion results in oliguria and, in severe cases, acute tubular necrosis. Shunting of blood away from the splanchnic circulation leaves the intestine vulnerable to ischemic injury. Decreased clearance of microaggregates impairs microcirculatory flow. Activation of the coagulation cascade can produce disseminated intravascular coagulation. Many of the systemic manifestations of shock result from chemical mediators that are released in response to tissue hypoxia. In this sense, shock behaves as an acute systemic inflammatory disease.

Hypovolemic Shock

Hypovolemic shock occurs secondary to a decrease in circulating intravascular volume. Common causes in the pediatric age group include severe gastroenteritis, acute hemorrhage, and fluid loss secondary to severe burns.

The decreased intravascular volume results in decreased cardiac preload, decreased stroke volume, and ultimately decreased cardiac output and impaired peripheral perfusion. Compensatory mechanisms include increases in heart rate, myocardial contractility, and systemic vascular resistance. The kidney's retention of sodium and water increases. With acute volume losses of 10 to 15 percent, the compensatory mechanisms can usually maintain tissue perfusion. With volume losses greater than 25 percent, decompensated shock will occur unless aggressive resuscitation is instituted.

Septic Shock

Sepsis is an inflammatory response to invading microorganisms and the toxins they produce. Clinically, there are alterations in temperature, heart rate, respiratory rate, and the white blood cell count. If the inflammatory response progresses, septic shock develops, characterized by the abnormal distribution of blood throughout the circulatory system.

In early septic shock, there is normal or high cardiac output and a wide pulse pressure. Systemic vascular resistance is decreased, the pulses are bounding, and the extremities are pink and warm. The patient usually has a normal mental status but is tachypneic. The late or decompensated phase is characterized by cardiac dysfunction and poor peripheral perfusion. Mental status is usually impaired, and the extremities are cool, with diminished or absent pulses.

Distributive Shock

Distributive shock is characterized by the maldistribution of normal intravascular volume. Causes of distributive shock include anaphylaxis and neurogenic or spinal shock.

Anaphylactic shock is characterized by profound vasodilatation and increased vascular permeability. Anaphylaxis is initiated by the interaction of an antigen with cell-bound IgE. Increased capillary permeability results in the loss of intravascular fluid into the interstitium.

Neurogenic shock is characterized by hypotension secondary to a loss of sympathetic cardiovascular tone, with pooling of blood in the vascular bed. Etiologies of neurogenic shock include total transection of the spinal cord, brainstem injuries, and, rarely, isolated intracranial injuries.

Cardiogenic Shock

Cardiogenic shock results when the heart fails to deliver sufficient nutrients to the rest of the body as a result of primary cardiac dysfunction. In infants and children, cardiogenic shock most commonly results from dysrhythmias, such as supraventricular tachycardia, or congenital heart lesions that obstruct the left ventricular outflow tract. In either case, inadequate output provokes compensatory mechanisms similar to those provoked by other forms of shock.

RECOGNITION

Recognition of shock in its early stages is of paramount importance. In infants and young children, early phases of shock are notoriously difficult to detect, in part because compensatory mechanisms are able to preserve blood flow to vital organs until late in the disease process.

History

The history of present illness can provide information that may increase the index of suspicion for shock. Profuse vomiting or diarrhea, polyuria, or trauma-related blood loss suggest hypovolemic shock. Septic shock is usually associated with a febrile illness and is especially common in young infants and immunosuppressed patients. Cardiogenic shock is often preceded by symptoms of congestive heart failure but can present in a fulminant form in young infants with undiagnosed congenital heart disease. Anaphylactic shock should be suspected in a hypotensive patient with any manifestation of an acute allergic reaction. Neurogenic shock is possible in any patient with an acute spinal cord injury, but should be diagnosed with great caution in the presence of head trauma and altered mental status, where hemorrhage is the most likely cause of shock.

Physical Examination

A careful physical examination is the key to the early diagnosis of shock. The first and easiest factor to assess is the patient's mental status. Irritability or lethargy can imply central nervous system dysfunction secondary to hypoperfusion. Young infants and children rely on tachycardia as the primary compensatory mechanism to protect cardiac output, and a markedly increased heart rate accompanies most cases of shock. Tachypnea is also present, as the lungs attempt to compensate for the metabolic acidosis derived from anaerobic metabolism. Peripheral pulses may appear diminished by palpation, although blood pressure may remain within normal limits. Capillary refill may be prolonged to more than 2 s, and the extremities may feel cool or appear mottled. In early septic shock, the opposite may be true, with bounding pulses and warm extremities. Infants and young children can maintain normal blood pressure until very late in the course of shock.

Laboratory Data

In cases of hemorrhagic shock, hemoglobin and hematocrit can confirm the presence of blood loss, but shortly after the event they are usually normal or only slightly decreased and are not reliable indicators of the degree of hemorrhage. An elevated white blood cell count can support the presence of a bacterial infection in a patient with suspected septic shock, but it is neither sensitive nor specific enough to certify the diagnosis. Neutropenia in a child suspected to be in septic shock suggests an overwhelming bacterial infection. Thrombocytopenia suggests the possibility of disseminated intravascular coagulation.

Elevation of the blood urea nitrogen and serum creatinine imply prerenal azotemia. Evaluation of serum electrolytes may reveal an anion gap acidosis. Blood sugar should be measured to rule out hypoglycemia and to exclude the possibility of diabetic ketoacidosis. Hypocalcemia is common in shock and can negatively affect many physiologic functions.

The arterial blood gas is a sensitive measure of the overall metabolic state of the patient. While respiratory alkalosis is common in the early stages of shock, the presence of metabolic acidosis implies significantly impaired perfusion.

TREATMENT

The primary goal for the management of the patient in shock is the restoration of perfusion and oxygenation. The first step in management is to provide adequate oxygen delivery. Assessment of the adequacy of the airway and ventilation is performed while administering 100% oxygen. Intubation and assisted ventilation is indicated in cases of fulminant shock and when acidosis is not immediately corrected with volume resuscitation. This is particularly important in managing septic and cardiogenic shock. Early intubation will protect the airway, and ventilatory support will remove the work of breathing and improve metabolic balance.

After establishment of oxygenation and ventilation, treatment includes rapid fluid replacement to establish effective intravascular volume. Fluid resuscitation begins with the infusion of isotonic crystalloid, either lactated Ringer's solution or normal saline. The initial fluid bolus is 20 mL/kg, which, in an unstable patient, is administered as quickly as possible. The hemodynamic status is then reassessed by evaluating improvement in mental status, heart rate, and peripheral perfusion. If improvement is not apparent, an additional 20 mL/kg is administered, and the patient is reassessed. The vast majority of patients in hypovolemic shock will respond to 40 mL/kg if ongoing fluid losses have been stopped. If an additional 20 mL/kg is required, the patient is a candidate for invasive monitoring, and a cause for shock other than simple hypovolemia must be considered.

Septic shock causes increased capillary permeability, which results in leakage of intravascular fluid into the interstitium. Whether the hydrating solution should be crystalloid or colloid is controversial. Crystalloid may lead to the development of pulmonary edema by lowering intravascular oncotic pressure. Colloid may better maintain oncotic pressure but can eventually leak into the interstitium owing to the significant loss of vascular integrity. The resuscitation of septic shock may require the use of both crystalloid and colloid to restore adequate perfusion.

Pressor Agents

Several drugs are available as adjunctive agents in the treatment of shock when fluid resuscitation alone is not sufficient to stabilize the cardiovascular system. Inotropic agents increase myocardial contractility, while chronotropic agents increase heart rate. Table 3-1 reviews the tissue effects produced by stimulation of these adrenergic receptors.

The most widely used group of pressor agents is the sympathomimetic amines. These drugs include the endogeneous catecholamines, epinephrine, norepinephrine, and dopamine, and the synthetic catecholamines, dobutamine and isoproterenol.

The choice of pressors for managing shock remains controversial. Table 3-2 provides a summary of pressor agents commonly used to manage pediatric patients in shock.

TABLE 3-1 Adrenergic Receptors

Receptors	Tissue effect
Alpha	Peripheral vasodilatation Dilatation of the iris Intestinal smooth muscle relaxation Increased bladder and intestinal spincter tone
$Beta_1$	Increased heart rate Improved myocardial contractility
$Beta_2$	Peripheral vasodilatation Bronchodilatation Bladder, uterine, and intestinal smooth muscle relaxation

Epinephrine is produced in the adrenal medulla and is secreted during times of stress. At lower doses, it has a predominantly inotropic effect. As the dose increases, alpha effects begin to predominate, causing increased vascular resistance. Epinephrine is used in shock with hypotension and poor perfusion. Some prefer its use in septic shock because of the possible depletion of endogenous catecholamines which may occur in sepsis. It has also been shown to increase renal blood flow when used with low-dose dopamine.

Norephinephrine is produced in the adrenal medulla and produces profound vasoconstriction because of its alpha effect. It is used primarily in profound hypotension refractory to volume expansion and other vasoactive agents. Its profound effect on systemic vascular resistance has been helpful in the treatment of septic shock.

Dopamine is an endogenous catecholamine with cardiac beta-adrenergic effects, peripheral alpha-adrenergic effects, and renal dopaminergic effects. Low-dose dopamine causes vasodilatation of the afferent renal arteries, resulting in increased renal blood flow. In moderate doses, the effect is primarily inotropic, and in high doses, the alpha effect predominates and there is peripheral vasoconstriction. Poor response to dopamine has been seen in septic shock. Common adverse effects of dopamine include hypoperfusion of the myocardium with resulting ischemia and tachydysrhythmias.

Dobutamine is a synthetic catecholamine with $beta_1$ cardiac and $beta_2$ peripheral effects that result in enhanced myocardial contractility and decreased systemic vascular resistance. Dobutamine is useful in the treatment of myocardial dysfunction associated with shock, since it enhances myocardial contractility, decreases

TABLE 3-2 Inotropic Agents Sympathomimetic Amines

Agents	Receptor	Dose	Clinical effects and considerations
Dobutamine	Beta	1–20 μg/kg/min	Enhances myocardial contractility. Useful in cardiac decompensation seen in shock states
Dopamine	Alpha beta	1–20 μg/kg/min	Improves renal blood flow in low doses (approx. 4 μg/kg/min) Improves myocardial contractility as dose increases Alpha effect in high doses Poor response sometimes seen in septic shock Useful in low doses in combination with other inotropes
Epinephrine	Alpha beta	0.05–1.0 μg/kg/min	Low-dose beta effect High-dose alpha effect Useful in septic shock Useful in combination with low-dose dopamine
Isoproterenol	Beta	0.05–0.5 μg/kg/min	Refractory bradycardia with hypotension Associated with tachydysrhythmia and myocardial ischemia
Norepinephrine	Alpha	0.05–1.0 μg/kg/min	Profound alpha effect Refractory hypotension

afterload, and increases preload. Higher doses may have significant chronotropic effect and dysrhythmic potential.

Isoproterenol is a synthetic catecholamine with $beta_1$ and $beta_2$ activity. It increases heart rate and myocardial contractility and decreases systemic vascular resistance. It is used primarily in the treatment of bradycardia and hypotension associated with heart block. It is associated with myocardial ischemia and tachydysrhythmias.

Amrinone is a phosphodiesterase inhibitor, most commonly used as an adjunct to the sympathomimetics in efforts to improve myocardial function. Because of its significant effect on systemic vascular resistance, it is used with caution in patients with hypotension.

HEMOGLOBIN REPLACEMENT

When hemorrhage is the cause of shock, early administration of packed red blood cells should be considered. Type O negative is used when immediate replacement is needed to prevent death. Type-specific blood is preferred when the demand is somewhat less urgent, and fully crossmatched blood is used when the condition of the patient permits a delay of 30 min or more. Boluses of packed red blood cells (5 to 10 mL/kg) may be provided by rapid infusion, with careful assessment between boluses. It is important to provide warmed blood and to watch closely for acidemia, hypocalcemia, hyperkalemia, and hypothermia.

MANAGEMENT OF UNDERLYING CONDITIONS

Early recongition and treatment of the underlying condition is an important part of comprehensive shock management. The patient with septic shock needs appropriate antibiotics. Diagnostic studies, such as lumbar puncture, should be deferred until the patient is stable. With hypovolemic shock, attention must be directed to assessing ongoing losses from hemorrhage or from the gastrointestinal tract. Cardiogenic shock may require pharmacologic therapy to reduce afterload or surgical intervention to correct a life-threatening obstruction (Sec. IV). Anaphylactic shock will require epinephrine, elimination of the offending cause, and antihistamines. Glucocorticoids may prevent or lessen delayed reactions.

For a more detailed discussion, see Scott SM, Wiebe RA: Shock, chap. 3, p. 10, in *Pediatric Emergency Medicine: A Comprehensive Study Guide.*

4 Cardiopulmonary Resuscitation

Patricia A. Primm / Rebecca Reamy Lynn

Pediatric cardiopulmonary resuscitation (CPR) differs from CPR in the adult. Primary cardiac arrest is rare in children. Rather, there is a respiratory arrest that leads to hypoxemia and acidosis, and culminates in a bradycardic or asystolic arrest. Inevitably, by the time asystole occurs, severe damage to the brain, kidney, and gastrointestinal tract has occurred. Survival in children from a cardiac arrest is dismal, and most who do survive have significant neurological impairment (Chap. 1).

PEDIATRIC BASIC LIFE SUPPORT

Pediatric basic life support (PBLS) provides artificial oxygenation and ventilation. It is extremely important for infants and children, in whom the etiology of arrest is primarily respiratory.

The Sequence

Basic CPR technique assumes that one rescuer is present in a prehospital setting. The sequence below is followed in the delivery of PBLS when one provider is present:

- Determine unresponsiveness
- Open the airway
- Provide rescue breathing
- Assess pulse
- Provide chest compressions for 1 min
- Notify emergency medical services (EMS)
- Resume rescue breathing and chest compressions
- Reassess pulse.

This sequence emphasizes the importance of quickly restoring ventilation.

Determine Unresponsiveness

The rescuer quickly determines the level of consciousness by tapping the child and speaking loudly. If alone, the rescuer shouts for help. In cases of suspected neck injury, the cervical spine is immobilized. If an assistant is available, he or she can maintain in-line traction while CPR is performed.

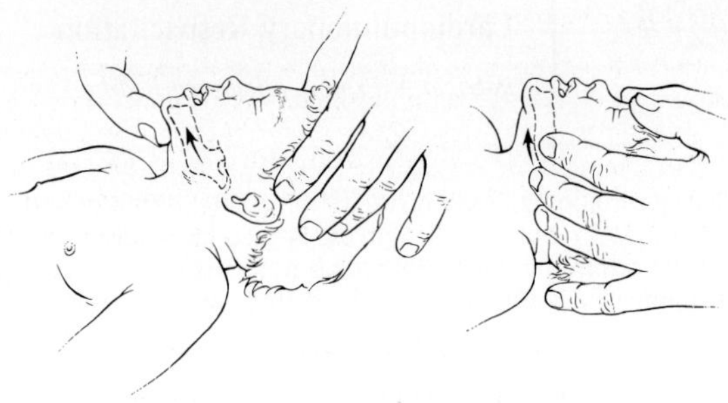

FIG. 4-1 *A*. To open the airway: Place one hand on the patient's forehead and tilt head back into a neutral or slightly extended position. Use the index finger of the other hand to lift the patient's mandible upward and outward. *B*. To open the airway while maintaining cervical spine stabilization, place two or three fingers under each side of the lower jaw angle and lift the jaw upward and outward. Maintain the neck in a neutral position manually to prevent cranial cervical motion.

Open the Airway

Establishing an airway is essential and may result in the resumption of spontaneous respirations. Infants and small children are especially vulnerable to obstruction of the airway from collapse of the relatively large tongue against the posterior pharynx.

The airway is opened by the head-tilt, chin-lift maneuver (Fig. 4-1*A*). If a neck injury is possible, use the jaw-thrust maneuver with in-line cervical stabilization (Fig. 4-1*B*).

Provide Rescue Breathing

If no spontaneous respirations are present, rescue breathing is begun. In an infant, the rescuer places his or her mouth or mouth-to-mask device over the infant's nose and mouth. In a child, the rescuer makes a mouth-to-mouth seal, pinching off the child's nose with the thumb and forefinger. Two slow (1- to 1.5-s) breaths are provided to the patient with the rescuer pausing to take a breath between the two rescue breaths. The correct volume will cause the chest to rise. If the airway appears obstructed, the head-tilt chin-lift is repositioned and another rescue breath is attempted. If rescue breathing again fails, foreign-body ingestion should be suspected.

Foreign-Body Aspiration

Foreign-body aspiration is likely in infants and children who have experienced a sudden onset of respiratory distress associated with coughing, gagging, or stridor. The rescuer should do not intervene as long as the patient has spontaneous coughing, has adequate ventilation, and can phonate. He or she should intervene if the cough becomes ineffective, there is increasing respiratory difficulty, or the patient loses consciousness.

Foreign Body in the Airway of an Infant

In the conscious or unconscious infant with airway obstruction from a foreign body, a combination of back blows and chest thrusts is used to clear the obstruction. The infant is straddled face down over the rescuer's forearm and supported on the rescuer's thigh, with the head lower than the trunk. Five back blows are delivered between the infant's scapulae, using the heel of the hand. After the back blows, the infant is turned face up, and five chest thrusts are delivered over the midsternum. The foreign body is removed if it is visualized. Blind finger sweeps should not be used. If the infant is unconscious, rescue breathing should be attempted. If the airway remains obstructed, the series of back blows, chest thrusts, and rescue breathing is repeated until the object is removed.

Foreign Body in the Airway of a Child

In the conscious child with airway obstruction from a foreign body, a series of five Heimlich maneuvers is performed. These consist of five subdiaphragmatic abdominal thrusts. The rescuer stands behind the victim, with his or her arms under the patient's axillae and wrapped around the patient's chest. The thumb side of one fist is placed against the patient's abdomen, above the umbilicus and below the xiphoid, and is grasped with the other hand. Five quick upward thrusts are administered as separate, distinct maneuvers.

The unconscious child is placed on the back on a flat surface. The rescuer kneels beside the child and straddles the child's hips. The heel of one hand is placed above the umbilicus and below the xiphoid and grasped with the other hand. A quick upward thrust is administered and repeated five times, if necessary. If the foreign body is visualized, it is removed. In necessary, rescue breathing is initiated. If the airway remains obstructed, an additional five abdominal thrusts are administered.

Assess the Pulse

After opening the airway and initiating rescue breathing, the rescuer checks for the presence of a pulse. In infants, a pulse is best felt over the brachial or femoral arteries. In children, the carotid pulse is easily palpated. If no pulse is present, the rescuer initiates chest compressions in coordination with rescue breathing.

Chest Compressions

Chest compressions establish some circulation to vital organs. They may be more effective in children than in adults. The mechanism that produces blood flow during compressions is under investigation. To perform chest compressions, place the patient on a firm, flat surface. In infants, the area of compression is the lower one-third of the sternum, or one finger width below the intermammary line (Fig. 4-2*A*). Using two fingers, the rescuer compresses the chest to a depth of one-third to one-half the depth of the chest, which corresponds to a depth of 1/2 to 1 in.

In children, the heel of the hand is placed two finger widths above the lower edge of the xiphoid (Fig. 4-2*B*). The chest is compressed one-third to one-half of its anteroposterior diameter, or 1 to 1.5 in. The chest is allowed to return to a resting position between compressions, but the hand is not removed. For infants and children up to 8 years of age, the rate of compressions is 100 per minute. At the end of every fifth compression, a 1- to 1.5-s pause is allowed for ventilation.

The patient is reassessed for the development of a pulse or spontaneous respirations after 20 cycles of compressions and ventilations (approximately 1 min) and every few minutes thereafter.

Notify Emergency Medical Services

The EMS system is activated after 1 min of rescue support. If the rescuer is unable to activate the system, CPR continues until help arrives or the rescuer becomes exhausted.

Complications of Basic Life Support

Complications of BLS in pediatric patients are similar to those in adults. These include gastric distension, lung contusion, pneumothorax, fractured ribs, liver laceration, and damage to other organs. In children, gastric distension can result in respiratory compromise.

PEDIATRIC ADVANCED LIFE SUPPORT

This chapter focuses on resuscitation and support of the cardiovascular system during cardiac arrest (Fig. 4-3).

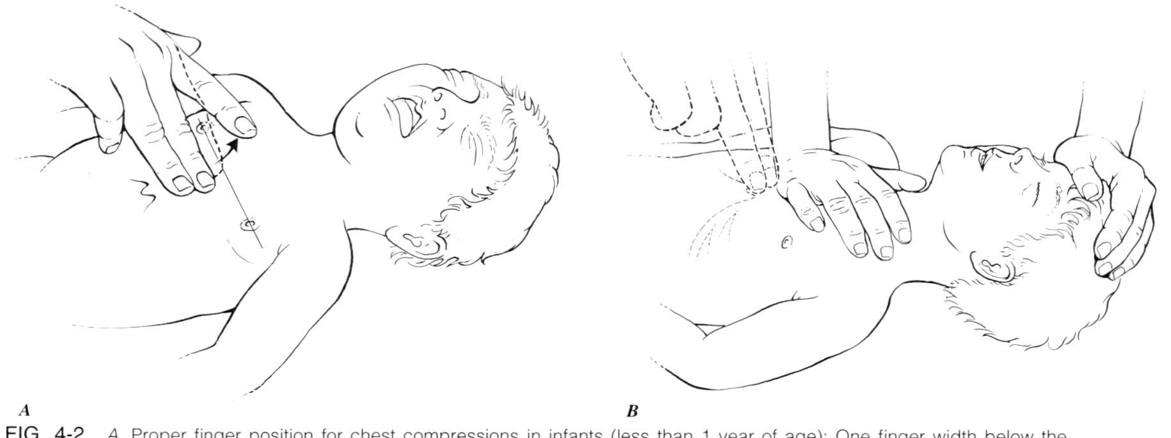

FIG. 4-2 *A*. Proper finger position for chest compressions in infants (less than 1 year of age): One finger width below the intermammary line, use two fingers to perform compressions. *B*. Proper finger position for chest compressions in children (from 1 to 8 years of age): Two finger widths above xiphoid, use the heel of one hand to perform compressions.

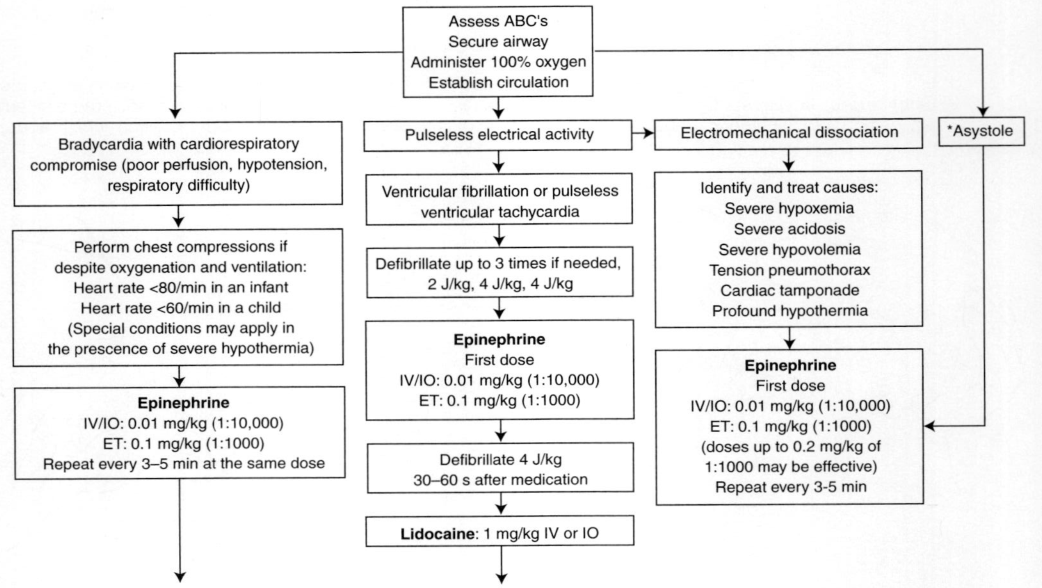

Assess ABC's
Secure airway
Administer 100% oxygen
Establish circulation
Bradycardia with cardiorespiratory compromise (poor perfusion, hypotension, respiratory difficulty)
Perform chest compressions if despite oxygenation and ventilation:
Heart rate <80/min in an infant
Heart rate <60/min in a child
(Special conditions may apply in the prescence of severe hypothermia)
Epinephrine
IV/IO: 0.01 mg/kg (1:10,000)
ET: 0.1 mg/kg (1:1000)
Repeat every 3–5 min at the same dose
Pulseless electrical activity
Ventricular fibrillation or pulseless ventricular tachycardia
Defibrillate up to 3 times if needed, 2 J/kg, 4 J/kg, 4 J/kg
Epinephrine
First dose
IV/IO: 0.01 mg/kg (1:10,000)
ET: 0.1 mg/kg (1:1000)
Defibrillate 4 J/kg
30–60 s after medication
Lidocaine: 1 mg/kg IV or IO
Electromechanical dissociation
Identify and treat causes:
Severe hypoxemia
Severe acidosis
Severe hypovolemia
Tension pneumothorax
Cardiac tamponade
Profound hypothermia
Epinephrine
First dose
IV/IO: 0.01 mg/kg (1:10,000)
ET: 0.1 mg/kg (1:1000)
(doses up to 0.2 mg/kg of 1:1000 may be effective)
Repeat every 3-5 min
*Asystole

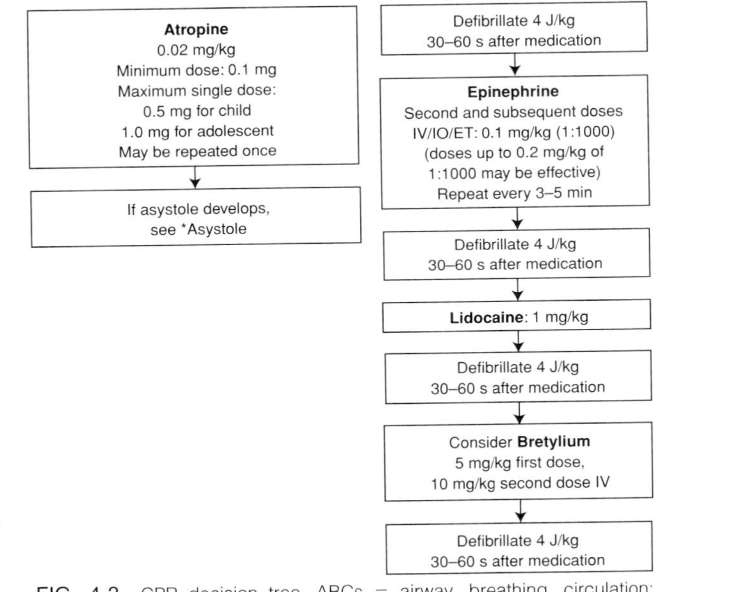

FIG. 4-3 CPR decision tree. ABCs = airway, breathing, circulation; ET = endotracheal; IO = intraosseous; IV = intravenous.

Oxygen

Since most pediatric patients suffer hypoxic-ischemic arrests, oxygen is the first and most essential drug administered during a pediatric resuscitation. It should supersede attempts to deliver intravenous medication and, except in extremely rare circumstances, defibrillation or cardioversion. The majority of pediatric patients who survive a cardiopulmonary arrest with good neurologic outcome will do so with ventilation with 100% oxygen alone. It is delivered by bag-valve-mask until an artificial airway is secured.

Delivery of Fluids and Medications

It is often difficult to obtain peripheral venous access in an infant or young child, especially when the patient is extremely dehydrated or in full cardiopulmonary collapse. Pending venous access, medications that can be delivered via the endotracheal tube include epinephrine, atropine, lidocaine, and naloxone. However, recent studies have cast doubt on the reliability of absorption of endotracheally administered epinephrine in the arrest situation. Since epinephrine is the primary pharmacologic adjunct used in pediatric advanced life support (PALS), it is essential that intravenous access be obtained in a timely fashion.

Venous Access

In the event that peripheral venous access is not immediately successful, access is established by cannulating a central vein or inserting an intraosseous catheter. A protocol limiting attempts at establishing a peripheral line can hasten the attainment of venous access via an intraosseous or central line.

In infants and small children, the two preferred sites for central venous catheterization are the right internal jugular and the femoral veins. In emergent situations, catheterization of the subclavian vein is associated with a high rate of complications. If a femoral venous catheter is used, the tip is inserted to a level above the diaphragm.

Intraosseous (IO) lines are relatively easily to place, and virtually every drug required in an acute resuscitation can be delivered by this route. The optimal site of insertion for an IO line is the proximal tibia. Alternatively, the distal tibia or distal femur can be used.

Contraindications to the use of an IO line include osteogenesis imperfecta and osteopetrosis. An ipsilateral fracture is also a contraindication.

Reported complications of IO insertion include iatrogenic fracture, tissue necrosis from extravasation of fluid and medication, compartment syndrome, and osteomyelitis.

Fluid Therapy

Reestablishing effective intravascular volume is essential in patients with cardiovascular collapse secondary to severe dehydration or massive acute blood loss. Volume expansion is attained by administering isotonic crystalloid in the form of normal saline or Ringer's lactate. Alternatively, a colloid solution such as 5% albumin is used.

In children in cardiopulmonary arrest who do not respond to oxygenation and ventilation, a fluid bolus of 10 to 20 mL/kg may provide sufficient circulating volume to aid in the restoration of a perfusing rhythm. For a more detailed discussion of fluid therapy, see Chap. 3.

Pharmacologic Therapy

While the emphasis in the adult arrest is on providing rapid defibrillation and managing acute arrhythmias, both defibrillation and pharmacologic therapy are adjuncts to adequate oxygenation and ventilation in pediatric arrests (Table 4-1).

Epinephrine

Epinephrine is the most important agent used in pediatric resuscitation. It is the drug of choice for asystole and bradycardia both with and without a pulse, the most common dysrhythmias encountered in pediatric resuscitation.

Epinephrine is an endogenous catecholamine with both beta- and alpha-stimulating properties. In an arrest situation, alpha-mediated vasoconstriction probably plays the most important role.

The initial dose of epinephrine recommended for asystolic or pulseless arrest is 0.01 mg/kg of 1:10,000 solution administered intravenously or intraosseously. Second and subsequent doses are 0.1 mg/kg of 1/1000 solution. Second doses are administered 3 to 5 min after the first and 3 to 5 min thereafter. Doses as high as 0.2 mg/kg may be effective.

In the event that intravenous or intraosseous access is delayed, epinephrine is administered intratracheally at a dose of 0.1 mg/kg of a 1/1000 solution. This can be diluted in 2 to 3 mL of normal saline and administered via a suction catheter placed through the distal tip of the endotracheal tube. The recommended dose reflects the erratic absorption of epinephrine from the lungs.

If a perfusing rhythm is restored, an epinephrine infusion is

TABLE 4-1 Drugs Used in Pediatric Advanced Life Support

Drug	Dose	Remarks
Adenosine	0.05 to 0.2 mg/kg Maximum single dose: 12 mg	Rapid IV bolus
Atropine sulfate	0.02 mg/kg per dose	Minimum dose: 0.1 mg Maximum single dose: 0.5 mg in child, 1.0 mg in adolescent
Bretylium	5 mg/kg; may be increased to 10 mg/kg	Rapid IV
Calcium chloride 10%	20 mg/kg; may be increased	Slowly IV
Epinephrine For bradycardia	IV/IO: 0.01 mg/kg (1 : 10,000) ET: 0.1 mg/kg (1 : 1000)	Be aware of effective dose of preservatives administered (if preservatives are present in epinephrine preparation) when high doses are used

For asystolic or pulseless arrest	First dose: IV/IO: 0.01 mg/kg (1 : 10,000) ET: 0.1 mg/kg (1 : 1000) Doses as high as 0.2 mg/kg may be effective Subsequent doses: IV/IO/ET: 0.1 mg/kg (1 : 1000) Doses as high as 0.2 mg/kg may be effective	Be aware of effective dose of preservative administered (if preservatives are present in epinephrine preparation) when high doses are used
Lidocaine	1 mg/kg per dose	
Sodium bicarbonate	1 meq/kg per dose or 0.3 × kg × base deficit	Infuse slowly and only if ventilation is adequate

Abbreviations: IV indicates intravenous route; IO, intraosseous route; and ET, endoctracheal route.

Drug	Dose, μg/kg/min	Dilution in 100 mL, D5W, mg/kg	IV Infusion rate, μg/kg/min
Dopamine	2–20	6	1 mL/h = 1
Dobutamine	5–20	6	1 mL/h = 1
Epinephrine	0.01–2.0	0.6	1 mL/h = 0.1
Lidocaine	20–50	6	1 mL/h = 1

useful in maintaining blood pressure until cardiovascular stability is achieved. Especially in infants, it may be preferable to dopamine. At low doses (<3 μg/kg/min), beta-adrenergic action predominates. At higher doses, alpha-mediated vasoconstriction is predominant.

Atropine Sulfate

Atropine sulfate is a parasympatholytic drug that accelerates sinus and atrial pacemakers and increases atrioventricular conduction. It is less useful in the treatment of bradycardia in pediatric patients than in adults, where bradycardia is often secondary to atrioventricular (AV) block. In infants and children, epinephrine is the primary pharmacologic therapy for symptomatic bradycardia, except in the unusual setting of AV block bradycardia, where atropine is the drug of choice. Atropine is also indicated in vagally induced bradycardia during intubation. It is often administered prophylactically prior to intubation.

The recommended dose of atropine is 0.02 mg/kg with a minimum dose of 0.1 mg in infants and a maximum dose of 0.5 mg in a child or 1 mg in an adolescent. The minimum recommended dose reflects the propensity for atropine to cause a paradoxical bradycardia if not given in a vagolytic dose. The endotracheal dose is the same as the intravenous and intraosseous dose.

Sodium Bicarbonate

Sodium bicarbonate has been used as a buffer for the metabolic acidosis that usually accompanies arrest states. Currently, there are no data to support the use of sodium bicarbonate in an arrest situation. The exception to this is a hyperkalemic arrest. In patients resuscitated from cardiac arrest with ongoing metabolic acidosis, the role of therapy with sodium bicarbonate is under investigation.

Complications of therapy with sodium bicarbonate include hypernatremia, hyperosmolality, and metabolic alkalosis, which can impede delivery of oxygen to the tissues by shifting the oxygen-hemoglobin dissociation curve to the left.

Calcium

Calcium is necessary in myocardial excitation-contraction coupling and has a positive inotropic effect, but it may impair cardiac relaxation. Ionized hypocalcemia is common in prolonged arrests; however, the administration of calcium has not been shown to improve the outcome. Likewise, calcium has been found ineffective in the treatment of pulseless electrical activity. Calcium is not recommended for the routine management of cardiopulmonaray arrest in children but is indicated for documented hypocalcemia, hyperkalemia, hypermagnesemia, and calcium channel blocker overdose. Calcium chloride provides greater bioavailability than calcium gluconate. The recommended dose is 20 mg/kg of a 10% solution.

Glucose

Infants and young children have high glucose requirements but minimal glycogen stores and easily become hypoglycemic during periods of stress. Therefore, blood glucose is carefully monitored during resuscitation. In hypoglycemic patients, the dose of glucose is 0.5 to 1.0 mg/kg, which can be provided by 2 to 4 mL/kg of a 25% solution.

Lidocaine

Lidocaine is used to suppress ventricular ectopy and raise the threshold for ventricular fibrillation. It is indicated in ventricular tachycardia associated with a pulse. It is also indicated for the treatment of pulseless ventricular tachycardia and ventricular fibrillation. In each of these situations, defibrillation takes precedence over the administration of lidocaine. Primary ventricular tachycardia and ventricular fibrillation are very rare in the pediatric age group.

If indicated, the dose of lidocaine is 1 mg/kg. It can be administered as a continuous infusion at a rate of 20 to 50 μg/kg/min. Excessive plasma concentrations of lidocaine can cause disorientation, muscle twitching, and seizures.

Bretylium

There are no published data supporting the use of bretylium in the pediatric age group. In some adults, it has been useful in refractory ventricular fibrillation. If both defibrillation and lidocaine are ineffective, it can be administered in a dose of 5 mg/kg. If ventricular fibrillation persists, a bolus of 10 mg/kg can be given.

Transcutaneous Pacing

Noninvasive transcutaneous pacing is used in children with profound symptomatic bradycardia refractory to basic and advanced life support. It requires an external pacing unit and two adhesive-backed electrodes. The negative electrode is placed over the heart on the anterior chest and the positive electrode behind the heart on the back. Alternatively, the negative electrode is placed near the apex of the heart and the positive elecrode on the right side of the anterior chest under the clavicle. If the child weighs less than 15 kg, small or medium electrodes are recommended. Both output and sensitivity will need adjustment. The pacemaker must function so that every paced impulse results in ventricular depolarization, or capture.

Defibrillation

Defibrillation is the unsynchronized depolarization of the myocardium. It is the primary treatment of ventricular fibrillation and pulseless ventricular tachycardia. Its usefulness in the pediatric age group is limited by the fact that both of these entities are very uncommon. Defibrillation is not useful for asystole, which is common in pediatric arrests.

In children weighing less than 10 kg, pediatric paddles are used. Adult paddles are used for all other children. The paddle-chest interface can be an electrode cream or paste, saline-soaked gauze, or self-adhesive defibrillation pads. Alcohol pads can result in severe burns and are not used. Bare paddles are ineffective. One paddle is placed over the right side of the upper chest and the other over the apex of the heart. The initial defibrillation is at 2 J/kg. If that is unsuccessful, the patient is defibrillated twice more in rapid succession at 4 J/kg. If a perfusing rhythm is not restored, epinephrine is administered and defibrillation again attempted at 4 J/kg. If that does not succeed, lidocaine is administrered, and the patient is once more defibrillated at 4 J/kg (Fig. 4-3).

Management of Pulseless Electrical Activity

Cardiopulmonary collapse with organized electrical activity but no palpable pulse is termed *pulseless electrical activity* (PEA). It is managed in the same manner as is asystole (Fig. 4-3). Treatable causes of PEA to consider are tension pneumothorax, pericardial tamponade, severe hypovolemia, hypoxemia, and hypothermia.

Management of Supraventricular Tachycardia

Supraventricular tachycardia (SVT) is the most common tachydysrhythmia that causes cardiovascular instability during infancy. Usually due to a reentrant mechanism, SVT produces heart rates in infants from 220 to 300 beats per minute with no beat-to-beat variability. In older children with SVT, heart rates are lower. In general, the electrocardiogram reveals a narrow QRS complex without discernible P waves. Occasionally it is difficult to distinguish SVT from sinus tachycardia, and when the electrical impulse is aberrantly conducted, the QRS complex can be wide and SVT difficult to distinguish from ventricular tachycardia (Table 4-2).

The child in shock or severe congestive heart failure from SVT requires immediate synchronized cardioversion. The initial dose is 0.5 to 1 J/kg. If SVT persists, the dose is increased to 2 J/kg. Adenosine may be used to treat the infant in cardiogenic shock due to SVT before going to cardioversion if vascular access is

TABLE 4-2 Differentiating Types of Tachycardia

	Sinus tachycardia	Supraventricular tachycardia	Ventricular tachycardia
Rate	Usually < 220	Usually > 220	120–400
QRS complex	Narrow	Usually narrow	Wide
Beat-beat variability	Yes	No	No
P waves	Yes (although they may be difficult to see)	No	No

readily available. However, cardioversion should not be delayed while IV access is attempted.

Adenosine is an endogenous nucleoside that interrupts the reentrant pathway. It has a half-life of 10 s. It is administered in a dose of 0.05 to 0.1 mg/kg. If the initial dose is unsuccessful, the second dose is doubled. The maximum dose is 12 mg.

Patients with stable SVT may respond to vagal maneuvers such as carotid massage or induction of the diving reflex by placing an ice bag over the face. Ocular massage is not used in children. If vagal maneuvers are unsuccessful, adenosine is the drug of choice. The use of verapamil is discouraged in children because it has been associated with profound hypotension and death.

Cerebral Resuscitation

Since survivors of pediatric cardiorespiratory arrest often have significant neurological impairment, a major goal is resuscitation of the brain as well as the heart. Some brain cells are damaged during the primary insult, but a cascade of processes follow arrest that can lead to further loss of brain cells over the hours following the arrest. Experimental treatment modalities aimed at preventing or ameliorating secondary injury have been proposed. Hyperventilation is the quickest way to decrease intracranial pressure. Levels of P_{CO_2} should be maintained between 25 and 28 torr. Excessive hyperventilation can result in drastic reduction of cerebral blood flow, with resultant brain ischemia. Other promising modalities are induction of mild hypothermia and use of pharmacologic agents such as thiopental, calcium channel blockers, and free radical scavengers.

For a more detailed discussion, see Primm PA, Lynn RR: Cardiopulmonary resuscitation, chap. 4, p. 17, in *Pediatric Emergency Medicine: A Comprehensive Study* Guide.

5 Neonatal Resuscitation

Collin Goto / Brian A. Bates

Since it is inevitable that the emergency department physician will be confronted with precipitous deliveries, expertise in resuscitation of the newborn is an important part of emergency department practice (Fig. 5-1).

NEWBORN PHYSIOLOGY

Multiple complex changes occur in the cardiovascular and respiratory systems at the moment of birth. The stimuli responsible for the first fetal breath include decreased P_{O_2} and PH and increased P_{CO_2} due to interpretation of the placental blood flow. Decreased body temperature and tactile stimulation also contribute. Pulmonary artery pressure decreases and systemic blood pressure increases. Blood that had bypassed the fetal lungs through the ductus arteriosus is distributed to the pulmonary circulation, and the ductus begins to close.

HISTORY

Pertinent information regarding the mother includes the date of her last menstrual period and the number of previous pregnancies and living children. Any history of diabetes or hypertension is elicited. A history of drug abuse alerts the physician to the possibility of narcotic-induced respiratory depression in the newborn or the potential development of a withdrawal syndrome.

Prolonged rupture of membranes, foul-smelling amniotic fluid, and maternal fever indicate a potentially septic newborn. Meconium-stained amniotic fluid increases the risk of meconium aspiration syndrome. Vaginal bleeding is associated with placenta previa or abruption of the placenta. Lack of prenatal care always implies a high-risk delivery.

ASSESSING THE NEWBORN

Appropriate supplies and equipment are listed in Table 5-1. The Apgar score is used to assess the overall status of the newborn (Table 5-2). The most important aspects of the score are heart rate, respiratory effort, and color.

The heart rate is evaluated by auscultating the chest or counting the pulse when palpating the umbilical cord. Bradycardia is virtually always due to hypoxia. Virtually all babies have peripheral cyanosis, which can be distinguished from central cyanosis by assessing the tongue, which should be pink. The quality of muscle tone is an indication of the degree of intrauterine ischemia. An extremely hypotonic newborn has usually suffered prolonged hypoxia.

Resuscitative efforts are guided by the 1-min Apgar score. Newborns with 1-min Apgar score of 7 or greater require only gentle

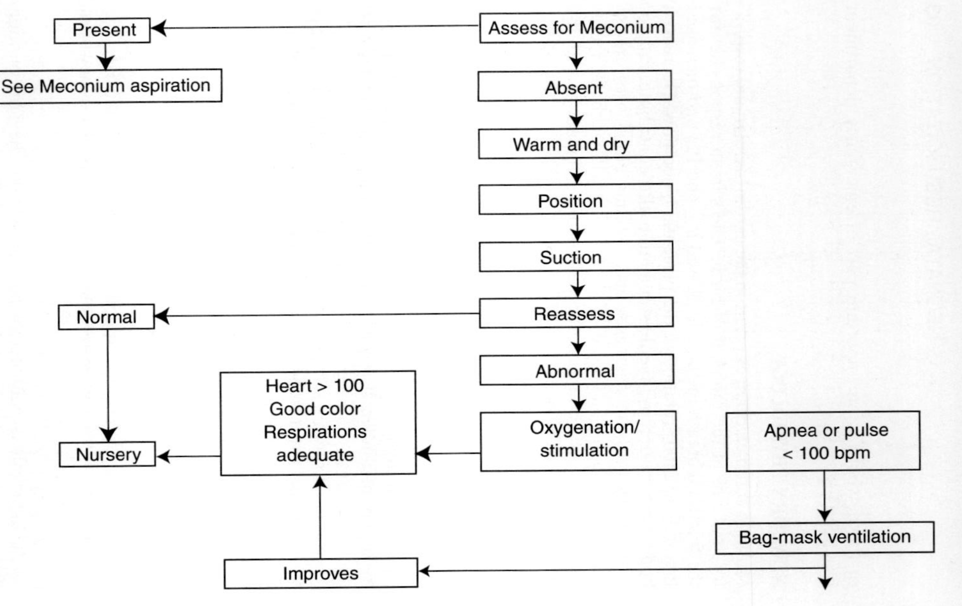
Assess for Meconium
Present
See Meconium aspiration
Absent
Warm and dry
Position
Suction
Reassess
Normal
Abnormal
Oxygenation/ stimulation
Heart > 100
Good color
Respirations adequate
Nursery
Apnea or pulse < 100 bpm
Bag-mask ventilation
Improves

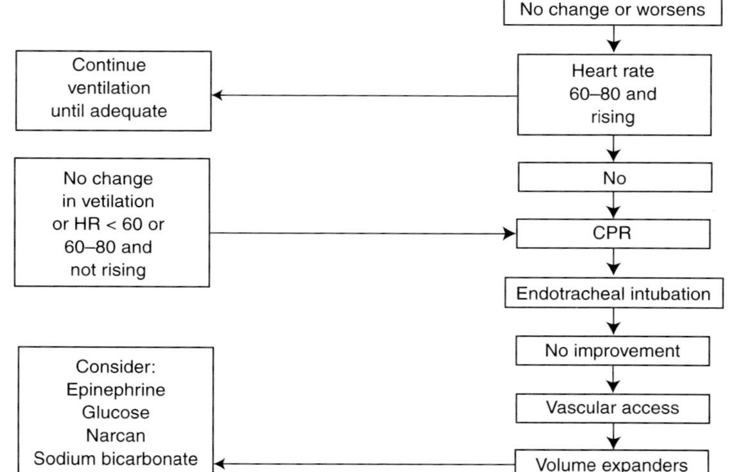

FIG. 5-1 Summary of neonatal resuscitation.

TABLE 5-1 Supplies for Neonatal Resuscitation

Resuscitation tray (sterile)	Resuscitation equipment
Bulb syringe	Radiant warmer
DeLee suction trap	Wall suction with manometer
Meconium aspirator	Oxygen source
Endotracheal tubes (2.0, 2.5, 3.0, and 3.5 mm)	Resuscitation bag (250 to 500 mL) with manometer
Suction catheters (5F, 8F)	Face masks (newborn and premature sizes)
Endotracheal tube stylet	Laryngoscope
Umbilical catheter (5F)	Laryngoscope blades (Miller 0 and 1)
Syringes (5, 10, and 20 mL) Three-way stopcock	Charts with proper drug doses and equipment sizes for various-sized neonates
Feeding tubes (5F, 8F)	
Towels	
Umbilical cord clamps	
Scissors	

stimulation, drying, and suctioning of the mouth and nose. If the newborn has a 1-min Apgar score of 4 to 6, mild to moderate asphyxia has occurred. Vigorous stimulation, supplemental oxygen, and other resuscitative efforts will be necessary. If the Apgar score is 3 or less, the neonate has been subjected to moderate to severe asphyxia, and aggressive resuscitation is initiated. All infants should be watched closely for deterioration.

RESUSCITATION

Positioning the Newborn

The newborn is placed on its back in a radiant warmer. The newborn has a relatively large tongue, which can result in significant obstruction of the airway. Placing the head in the sniffing position, with a towel under the shoulders, can open the airway. Care is taken to avoid hyperextension of the neck.

Suctioning

After the head is positioned, the newborn's mouth and nose are suctioned to remove amniotic fluid and mucus. A bulb syringe or

TABLE 5-2 The Apgar Score

Parameter	0	1	2
Color	Blue, pale	Body pink, extremities blue	Totally pink
Muscle tone	None, limp	Slight flexion	Active, good flexion
Heart rate	0	<100	>100
Respirations	Absent	Slow, irregular	Strong, regular
Reflex irritability (response to nasal catheter)	None	Some grimace	Good grimace, crying

DeLee trap is usually adequate for this purpose. If wall suction is used, pressure should not exceed 100 mm Hg (136 cmH_2O). Deep suctioning can cause a relax bradycardia; therefore the heart rate is monitored during the procedure, and suctioning is continued for only 5-s intervals and is discontinued if severe bradycardia develops.

Tactile Stimulation

Most infants with mild to moderate cardiorespiratory depression will respond to tactile stimulation with increased heart rate and the development of adequate respiratory efforts. Vigorous drying is often sufficient. More aggressive methods of stimulation include rubbing the infant's back and slapping the soles of its feet.

Thermoregulation

The newborn is at great risk for hypothermia as amniotic fluid evaporates. Hypothermia results is increased oxygen consumption, hypoglycemia, and, if severe, respiratory and metabolic acidosis. Premature and asphyxiated newborns are especially vulnerable to the deleterious effects of hypothermia.

Heat loss is prevented by placing the infant under a radiant warmer and quickly drying off the amniotic fluid. The baby's body is then wrapped in warm blankets, and the head is covered with a cap.

Oxygen

In any infant with even mild cardiorespiratory depression at delivery, oxygen is the first drug administered. In infants with mild bradycardia and respiratory depression, oxygen can be administered by holding the tubing close to the baby's face, with a flow rate of 5 L/min. Oxygen can also be delivered via a mask connected to an anesthesia bag placed over the nose and mouth. Some self-inflating bags may not deliver sufficient oxygen unless squeezed. There is no contraindication to short-term oxygen administration for any newborn.

Bag-Valve-Mask Ventilation

Indications for initiating assisted ventilation with a bag-valve-mask device are apnea or gasping respirations and bradycardia (heart rate less than 100 beats/min) that do not respond to tactile stimulation and supplemental oxygen. Central cyanosis unresponsive to supplemental oxygen is also an indication for assisted ventilation.

Ventilations are performed with a tight-fitting mask with a cushioned seal. If a self-inflating bag is used, the pop-off valve is bypassed, since the initial pressures required to inflate the lungs can be as high as 70 cmH_2O. Subsequent breaths usually require less pressure. A pressure manometer is useful to gauge the minimum inspiratory pressure required to produce adequate chest expansion.

The initial rate of assisted ventilation is 40 to 60 breaths per minute. After 15 to 30 s of assisted breaths, the baby is reassessed. If resuscitation has been successful, improvement will be noted in muscle tone and, most importantly, heart rate, and the infant will begin to establish spontaneous respirations. Color will generally improve, although peripheral cyanosis can persist. If improvement is not apparent and the heart rate is less than 60 beats/min or persists at 60 to 80 beats/min despite continued assisted ventilation, chest compressions are begun and the infant is intubated.

Endotracheal Intubation

If there is an inadequate response to assisted ventilation, endotracheal intubation is indicated. Other indications for intubation are a requirement for endotracheal suctioning, a need for prolonged positive pressure ventilation, and extreme prematurity.

The size of the endotracheal tube depends on the patient's weight (3.5 mm for a 3 to 4-kg neonate, 3.0 mm for a 2-kg neonate, and 2.5 mm for a 1-kg premie). Intubation is performed with a 0 or 1 straight blade. Proper tube positioning is assured by adequate chest expansion, equal bilateral breath sounds on auscultation, and improvement in heart rate, muscle tone, and color. In neonates, it is common to accidently intubate either of the mainstem bronchi, in which case breath sounds are heard preferentially over one hemithorax. Complications of positive pressure ventilation include gastric distention and pneumothorax.

Chest Compressions

Infants are dependent on heart rate to sustain adequate cardiac output. Indications for chest compressions in neonates are a heart rate less than 60 beats/min and a heart rate that persists between 60 and 80 beats/min despite adequate ventilation with 100% oxygen.

There are two techniques for providing chest compressions in neonates and infants. In the two-finger technique, the ring and middle fingers are placed on the sternum just below the nipple line and the chest is compressed to a depth of 1/2 to 3/4 in. In the preferred technique, the hands are wrapped around the chest, and both thumbs are placed over the middle one-third of the sternum, again just below the nipple line. The chest is compressed to the same depth as in the two-finger technique. Compression of the lower sternum or xiphoid is avoided because of the potential for injury to abdominal organs. The ratio of chest compressions to ventilations is 3 to 1, with 90 compressions and 30 ventilations per minute. Ventilation with 100% oxygen is continued during chest compressions.

Vascular Access

The preferred site of access is the umbilical vein, which is easily located and cannulated. The vein is distinguished from the umbilical arteries by the fact that it is single, with a thin, distensible wall.

To insert an umbilical vein catheter, the umbilical cord is trimmed with a scalpel blade to 1 cm above the skin. The umbilical stump is encircled with a tie that is secured tightly enough to prevent excessive bleeding. A 3.5 or 5 French umbilical catheter is inserted just below the skin. Effective combination is assured by the free flow of blood or aspiration. Deep insertion of the catheter is avoided, as this result can result in the infusion of hypertonic fluids into the liver. The catheter is sutured in place to avoid inadvertent dislodgment and hemorrhage.

Pharmacologic Agents

Epinephrine

Epinephrine is the most important drug used in neonatal resuscitation. Indications for its use are asystole and a heart rate that remains at 80 beats/min or less despite effective ventilation with 100% oxygen and chest compressions. The dose of epinephrine is 0.01 to 0.03 mg/kg of the 1 : 10,000 solution intravenously. Epinephrine can also be given intratracheally. In newborns, the same dose is recommended for intravenous and intratracheal administration. Epinephrine is given every 3 to 5 min. An intratracheal dose can be diluted to 1 to 2 mL with normal saline.

Sodium Bicarbonate

Sodium bicarbonate buffers hydrogen ion and reverses metabolic acidosis. There is currently no evidence that it has a role in the resuscitation of the newborn.

Naloxone Hydrochloride

Naloxone is a direct narcotic antagonist without respiratory depressant activity. It is indicated to reverse respiratory depression in the newborn that results from administration of narcotics to the mother, usually within 4 h of delivery. Since the duration of action of naloxone is exceeded by that of narcotics, infants with narcotic-induced respiratory depression are observed closely for several hours after delivery. In infants of narcotic-addicted mothers, naloxone can induce a severe drug withdrawal syndrome.

The dose of naloxone is 0.1 mg/kg given intravenously, intratracheally, intramuscularly, or sublingually. The standard form of 0.4 mg/mL is utilized.

Glucose

Hypoglycemia commonly occurs in infants born to diabetic mothers and in premature infants. Signs of hypoglycemia include jitteriness, hypotonia, hypertonia, seizures, and coma.

Neonatal hypoglycemia is defined as a blood glucose less than 40 to 50 mg/dL. If the newborn is symptomatic due to hypoglycemia, intravenous glucose administration is recommended. A 2- to 3-mL/kg bolus of a 10% glucose solution is used to correct hypoglycemia. Higher concentrations may lead to untoward hyperosmolar effects such as intraventricular hemorrhage, particularly in premature infants. Intravenous glucose is continued as an infusion at a dose of 6 to 8 mg/kg per min. Once the infant is stable and can tolerate oral feeding without risk, a 10% solution can be initiated orally, with close blood glucose monitoring.

Volume Expanders

Volume expansion is indicated to restore circulating blood volume. Conditions that can produce acute blood loss in the newborn are placenta previa, abruption of the placenta, and twin-twin transfusion. Significant blood loss can also occur if the umbilical cord is clamped prematurely, interrupting placental transmission.

The detection of acute anemia in the newborns can be extremely difficult. Profound vasoconstriction may cause the infant to appear pale despite adequate oxygenation, and peripheral pulses may be diminished. In the face of placental disruption, the initial hemoglobin may be normal.

Volume resuscitation is initiated with 10-mL/kg aliquots of normal saline, Ringer's lactate, or 5% albumin administered over 10 min. Whole blood is rarely required, but packed red blood cells, crossmatched with maternal or neonatal blood, may be indicated.

Special Situations

Meconium

The aspiration of meconium can cause airway obstruction, severe pneumonitis, and, in severe cases, persistence of the fetal circulation. Meconium aspiration syndrome is more likely if the material is thick and particulate as opposed to thin and nonviscous.

If thick meconium is present in the amniotic fluid, the newborn's oropharynx is suctioned as the head is delivered, prior to clamping of the cord. After delivery, the trachea is suctioned prior to the onset of respirations, since a significant number of patients will have meconium in the trachea. Under largyngoscopic visualization, the trachea is intubated with an endotracheal tube connected to a meconium aspirator and wall suction. Suction is applied as the tube is slowly withdrawn. The process is repeated until the trachea is free of meconium. In the event that the infant becomes bradycardic, clinical judgment is used to determine when suctioning is discontinued and positive pressure ventilation is instituted. The management of newborns with thin meconium in the amniotic fluid remains controversial.

Prematurity

A newborn is considered premature if born before 37 weeks of gestation. Birth asphyxia is more likely in preterm labor. The immature lungs are deficient in surfactant, which leads to decreased lung compliance, atelectasis, and the respiratory distress syndrome of prematurity. The premature infant is extremely vulnerable to hypothermia after delivery.

The determination of viability has become very complex as new technology has developed. Unfortunately, the emergency physician is not usually in a position to consider long-term viability or quality of life prior to acting. Whenever a baby is born with a pulse and spontaneous respiration, initial resuscitation efforts should be started. The decision to discontinue support should be made on the basis of the infant's response to resuscitation and after consultation with a neonatologist.

Diaphragmatic Hernia

The combination of a scaphoid abdomen, cyanosis, and respiratory distress suggests a diaphragmatic hernia. Diaphragmatic hernias occur most commonly on the left side (Bochdalek type). The presence of abdominal contents in the left hemithorax results in varying degrees of hypoplasia of the left lung. Breath sounds are diminished or absent on the left, and heart sounds can be heard in the right chest.

In the presence of a diaphragmatic hernia, bag-valve-mask ventilation is contraindicated, since this can fill the stomach and bowel with gas and further compromise respiratory status. The infant is intubated, and the lungs are expanded and ventilated. A nasogastric tube is placed to deflate the stomach. Early transport to a tertiary care facility is imperative, since many of these infants will require extracorporeal membrane oxygenation.

Infant of a Diabetic Mother

Diabetes remains a significant cause of perinatal morbidity and mortality. High maternal blood glucose results in high fetal insulin levels, which can lead to fetal macrosomia, functional immaturity, and a host of other problems. Metabolic complications include hypocalcemia and severe hypoglycemia.

Gastroschisis and Omphalocele

These congenital malformations occur when there is herniation of the abdominal contents through the umbilical ring. Herniation usually involves only the intestines, but in severe cases it can involve other abdominal organs. An omphalocele is covered by a thin layer of peritoneum, while a gastroschisis is not.

The protrudring organs are not forced back into the abdominal cavity. They are covered with a sterile, saline-soaked dressing and a sterile plastic bag to prevent evaporation and desiccation. Volume resuscitation may be indicated. After the baby is stabilized, a nasogastric tube is placed. Urgent pediatric surgical consultation is indicated.

For a more detailed discussion, see Goto C, Bates BA: Neonatal resuscitation, chap. 5, p. 26, in *Pediatric Emergency Medicine: A Comprehensive Study Guide.*

6 Sudden Infant Death Syndrome and Acute Life-Threatening Event

Thomas T. Mydler / Collin Goto

Sudden infant death syndrome (SIDS) is the unexpected death of a previously well infant whose death remains unexplained after review of the clinical history, performance of an autopsy, and examination of the death scene. In the United States, the overall incidence of SIDS is about 2 per 1000 live births. It is the leading cause of postperinatal mortality during the first year of life. Victims range in age from 1 month to 1 year, with a peak between 2 and 4 months of age. About 95 percent of cases occur before 1 year of age. The incidence of SIDS is higher during the winter months.

There is considerable ethnic variation in the incidence of SIDS in the United States. The rates per 1000 live births are 5.9 among American Indians, 2.9 among blacks, 1.7 among Hispanics, 1.3 among whites, and 0.5 among Asians.

Mutliple epidemiologic risk factors have been associated with SIDS (Table 6-1). It is important to note that these are associations and do not necessarily imply a cause-and-effect relationship. Certain infants are recognized to be at significantly greater risk, including survivors of an apparent life-threatening events (ALTE). Other known risk factors are a history of a sibling with SIDS, maternal drug dependency, and a history of prematurity, especially when complicated by bronchopulmonary dysplasia. Recent studies of SIDS victims have identified tissue markers of chronic hypoxia. These findings support the possibility of central apnea as one cause of SIDS. The incidence of dysplastic, dysmorphic, and anomalous features is significantly higher in SIDS than in non-SIDS deaths (Table 6-2).

The classic victim is found by the parents in his or her bed after having been put down for the night—hence the term *crib death*. During the resuscitation, the parents should be continuously informed regarding the medical situation. Information solicited from the parents includes past medical history, present illnesses, current medications, and any history of trauma, however trivial. The child is carefully examined for any congenital abnormalities or signs of abuse.

In an unsuccessful resuscitation, the baby's body is referred to the coroner or medical examiner for an autopsy. The parents should be allowed to see and hold the baby, and the details of the resuscitation and the nature of SIDS should be explained. Any

TABLE 6-1 Epidemiologic Factors Associated with SIDS

Infant factors	Maternal factors
Preterm birth	Age less than 20 years
Low birth weight	Short interpregnancy interval
Low Apgar scores	Unmarried
Treatment in an intensive care unit	Low socioeconomic status
Congenital defects	Low educational level
Neonatal respiratory abnormalities	Illness during pregnancy
Recent viral illness	Smoking during pregnancy
Prone sleeping position	Use of addictive drugs
Previous ALTE	
Sibling who died of SIDS	

suggestion that the parents were at fault is inappropriate unless the physical evidence unequivocally reveals otherwise. It is important to stress the importance of the autopsy. All parents should be referred to a SIDS support group.

APPARENT LIFE-THREATENING EVENT

An apparent life-threatening event is an episode characterized by a combination of apnea, color changes, choking, gagging, and

TABLE 6-2 Morphologic Variations in SIDS Victims

Dysplastic Lesions
- Nevi
- Hemangiomas
- Nodular renal blastoma
- Neuroblastoma

Dysmorphic Lesions
- Hernias
- Club foot
- Pectus excavatum

Minor Anomalies
- Meckel's diverticulum
- Polydactyly
- Ectopic adrenal or pancreatic tissue
- Atrial septal defect
- Small membranous ventricular septal defect

alteration in muscle tone. The infant recovers either spontaneously or with some degree of resuscitation. The exact relationship between ALTE and SIDS is not known.

The majority of infants who suffer an ALTE appear well, and the challenge is to differentiate between a true ALTE and a non-life-threatening problem. Parents are questioned closely about the details of the incident, especially about the baby's respiratory effort, color, and mental status. True apnea must be distinguished from the normal periodicity of breathing that occurs during infancy. Apnea or respiratory difficulty associated with cyanosis or mottling is significant. Periodic breathing is not associated with cyanosis or mottling. A history of apnea that required physical stimulation or cardiopulmonary resuscitation (CPR) is extremely ominous. An infant who remains awake and alert during an event is unlikely to have suffered prolonged hypoxia or an acute neurological event. Hypotonia associated with apnea or color change can imply primary hypoxia or decreased perfusion, while hypertonicity is characteristic of seizures.

Information is also gathered concerning any acute illness. Vomiting and diarrhea can lead to serious electrolyte abnormalities. Fever implies sepsis. Significant regurgitation with feedings is compatible with gastroesophageal reflux and aspiration.

Laboratory Studies

The laboratory studies obtained reflect the broad differential diagnosis. A complete blood count can provide evidence for a blood-borne infection or profound anemia. Serum electrolytes, blood urea nitrogen, and serum creatinine, calcium, magnesium, and phosphorus are obtained. A serum glucose is essential. A baseline electrocardiogram can exclude the presence of an acute dysrhythmia or prolonged QT syndrome. Cultures of blood, spinal fluid, and urine are obtained. Consideration is given to obtaining a drug screen, computed tomography of the head, and a skeletal survey. A serum ammonia is useful for detecting certain inherited metabolic disorders.

Any infant in whom the history supports the ALTE is admitted to the hospital and, at a minimum, placed on a cardiopulmonary monitor. Any infant who requires resuscitation is observed in a pediatric intensive care unit. Infants in whom sepsis is suspected receive age-appropriate antibiotics.

Further workup may include a pneumogram to evaluate the potential for central or obstructive apnea, an electroencephalogram to exclude seizures, and barium studies and esophageal pH-probe monitoring to exclude gastroesophageal reflux.

Upon discharge, the patient may be sent home on a portable cardiopulmonary monitor. This is often a controversial decision and is left to the patient's personal physician.

For a more detailed discussion, see Mydler TT, Goto C: Sudden infant death syndrome and apparent life-threatening event, chap. 6, p. 33, in *Pediatric Emergency Medicine: A Comprehensive Study Guide.*

---

7 Discontinuation of Life Support

Brian A. Bates

To withhold or withdraw life from a child is a very difficult decision for both parents and physicians. It is especially difficult in an emergency department. Even in patients with obvious terminal disease, there is often no do-not-resuscitate (DNR) order, and the patient's personal physician may be unavailable.

In the emergency department, the decision to terminate resuscitation is usually based on the patient's response to advanced life support. Death is defined by the failure to generate a spontaneous perfusing rhythm despite standard resuscitative measures. However, once cardiopulmonary resuscitation is initiated, there are no absolute guidelines that determine how long the effort is continued until death is declared. In children, the failure to respond to two standard doses of epinephrine is highly correlated with death, but this is not an "official" standard. Prolonged resuscitative efforts may ultimately succeed in generating a perfusing rhythm in a patient with severe neurologic impairment, who then languishes in a vegetative state.

There are certain medical situations that appear to justify prolonged resuscitations. Cold-water drowning is perhaps the most common clinical situation in which very long resuscitations have occasionally produced viable survivors. In any situation in which the patient is hypothermic, resucitation is generally continued until the patient is adequately warmed. Resuscitation is not indicated in patients with rigor mortis, dependent lividity, or decapitation.

Terminally ill children may have advance directives in the form of DNR orders. Such directives require a written statement from the patient's attending physician and are revocable at any time. When a patient arrives in the emergency department with a DNR order, it is reviewed by the attending physician with the parents or legal guardian. There are often time limits on DNR orders.

In the event that patients who undergo resuscitation in the emergency department develop a perfusing rhythm, they are transferred to an intensive care unit, where a definitive assessment of the neurologic status of the patient is carried out. The ability of technology to sustain cardiopulmonary function despite cessation of neurologic activity has led to the development of criteria for brain death. Brain death is generally considered as the irreversible cessation of all neurologic activity and justifies the withdrawal of medical support. In some situations, such as severe head trauma, it may be obvious that a terminal neurologic insult has occurred, and it may be appropriate to advise the parents or guardians of this. Patients who suffer brain death but who are candidates for organ donation may be identified in the emergency department, and it may be justifiable to approach family members to discuss the possibility of organ donation.

For a more detailed discussion, see Bates BA: Discontinuation of life support, chap. 7, p. 36, in *Pediatric Emergency Medicine: A Comprehensive Study Guide.*

SECTION II
TRAUMA CARE

8 Evaluation and Management of the Multiple Trauma Patient

Michael J. Gerardi

Trauma is the leading cause of death in children above 1 year of age in the United States. In developed countries, traumatic injuries are the leading cause of morbidity and mortality in children between the ages of 1 and 14 years. The costs in terms of dollars and lives are impressive: 22,000 lives lost; 600,000 hospitalized, and 16 million seen in emergency departments each year.

The health care cost is approximately $160 billion per year nationally. There are additional costs to the emotional and financial status of the patients and their families, attributable to the devastating nature of many traumatic injuries. Therefore, the physical, emotional, and psychological needs of the child and family must be considered.

NATURE OF INJURIES AND UNIQUE PEDIATRIC ASPECTS

Motor vehicle occupant injuries are the leading cause of death from injury among children aged 0 to 19 years.

Blunt injuries account for 87 percent of all childhood trauma. Penetrating trauma accounts for 10 percent, with the remaining 3 percent due to drownings. Motor vehicle–related incidents account for 40 percent of blunt trauma and are the leading cause of severe injury in children; falls are the second most common etiology.

Children have psychological and physiologic responses to trauma that are different from those seen with adults. An understanding of these anatomic and physiologic differences is fundamental in providing appropriate, expert care for children.

Because of a child's smaller mass, kinetic energy is distributed over a smaller area, and therefore it affects a greater proportion of the total body volume. Musculoskeletal compliance is greater in children, and children have less protective muscle and subcutaneous tissue. Internal injury must always be considered even in the absence of external signs of trauma.

A child's head represents a larger percentage of total body mass

TABLE 8-1 Comparison of Infant and Adult Airways

	Infant	Adult
Head	Large, prominent occiput, assumes sniffing position when supine	Flat occiput
Tongue	Relatively larger	Relatively smaller
Larynx	Cephalad position, opposite C2-C3	Opposite C4-C6
Epiglottis	"Ω" or "U" shaped, soft	Flat, flexible
Vocal cords	Short, concave	Horizontal
Smallest diameter	Cricoid ring, below cords	Vocal cords
Cartilage	Soft	Firm
Lower airways	Smaller, less developed	Larger, more cartilage

Source: Used with permission from the American Academy of Pediatrics, American College of Emergency Physicians. *APLS: The Pediatric Emergency Medicine Course*, 2d ed. Elk Grove Village, IL: American Academy of Pediatrics, 1993.

than that of an adult. Head injuries in children are common and account for a large percentage of serious morbidity and mortality. The occiput is more prominent in young children, decreasing in prominence from birth until approximately age 10. This should be taken into account when positioning the head for intubation and airway management. The child's brain, having a higher percentage of white matter than gray matter, may have greater resilience in withstanding blunt trauma. However, it is more susceptible to axonal shearing forces and cerebral edema.

A child's neck is shorter than an adult's and a younger child's short, fat neck makes the evaluation of neck veins and tracheal position difficult.

The most dramatic and critical differences between children and adults are in the airway (Table 8-1). A child's larynx is located in a more cephalad and anterior position. The glottis is the narrowest portion of the upper airway in the adult, and the cricoid cartilage is the narrowest portion of the airway in the child. This limits the size of the endotracheal tube in the child and is why uncuffed tubes should be used in patients below 8 years of age.

The pediatric thorax is more pliable because the ribs and cartilage are more flexible. A greater amount of blunt force is transmitted to underlying tissues.

The diaphragm inserts at a nearly horizontal angle from birth until about 12 years of age, contrasting with the oblique insertion in the adult. This causes abdominal organs to be more exposed and less protected by ribs and muscle. Therefore, insignificant forces can cause serious internal injury.

The spleen and the liver are in a more caudal and anterior position in the child. They are more subject to injury because of increased motion at impact.

Long bones in children are different because of the presence of growth plates or epiphyses and increased compliance. The Salter-Harris classification system was created to assist in the diagnosis and management of growth plate injuries. The physical examination is often more sensitive than radiographs for growth plate injury. Blood supply to bones can also be easily disrupted, resulting in limb length disparity.

PREHOSPITAL CARE ISSUES

Considerations in the field care of the traumatized child include endotracheal intubation, IV access, immobilization, and rapid transport. Which procedures should be attempted in the field is controversial. The prehospital success rate for endotracheal intubation varies from 48 to 89 percent. Rural systems require more aggressive initial treatment in the field because transport times are three to four times greater than those in urban areas.

Vascular access is a difficult procedure under the best of circumstances and is often a reason for delay in transport of a critically ill child. It is reasonable for traumatized children to be transported immediately without vascular access if a short transport time is expected. Intraosseous (IO) infusion should be used as a quick access for crystalloid infusion if attempts at intravenous cannulation are unsuccessful after 90 s. Some 80 percent of the time, IO lines can be placed successfully in the field.

INITIAL ASSESSMENT AND MANAGEMENT GUIDELINES FOR THE INJURED CHILD

The highest priority in caring for an injured child is determining whether there are life-threatening disturbances and providing immediate treatment. The next priority is identifying injuries requiring operative intervention and initiating that process. Finally, the child is examined for non-life-threatening injuries and specific therapy is initiated (Table 8-2).

The *primary survey* and initial *resuscitation* focus on diagnosing and treating life-threatening disorders. The *secondary survey* continues the assessment, with more thorough physical examination

TABLE 8-2 Initial Approach to the Pediatric Trauma Patient

1. BEFORE ARRIVAL
   - Prepare all equipment
   - Mobilize trauma team
   - Call for assistance (respiratory, radiology)
   - Request O-negative blood on standby
2. FIRST 5 MIN—PRIMARY SURVEY AND RESUSCITATION
   - Airway maintenance, cervical spine control
     Assess respiration
     Maintain cervical spine immobilization
   - Breathing
     Ventilate if necessary
     Assess oxygenation (pulse oximetry)
     Needle thoracostomy for tension pneumothorax
     Occlusive dressing for sucking chest wounds
     Endotracheal intubation (or needle cricothyrotomy)
     Consider end-tidal CO_2 monitoring
   - Circulation
     Attach cardiac monitor
     Direct pressure for external hemorrhage
3. SECOND 5 MIN—PRIMARY SURVEY AND RESUSCITATION
   - Reassess airway, ventilation, and oxygenation
   - Circulation
     Assess perfusion status
     Volume resuscitation: 20 mL/kg of crystalloids
       Repeat as needed
       Consider O-negative blood
     Pericardiocentesis if indicated
     Thoracotomy and aortic clamping if indicated
     Collect and send specimens for laboratory testing:
       Type and crossmatch, CBC, amylase, liver transaminases, BUN, creatinine, glucose, electrolytes, arterial blood gases, urinalysis
     Nasogastric catheter
     Foley catheter
   - Disability
     Assess neurologic status
   - Exposure
     Remove all covering
     Assess temperature and maintain normothermia
4. NEXT 10 MIN—SECONDARY SURVEY AND DEFINITIVE CARE
   - Reassess ABCDE
   - Head-to-toe physical examination
   - Tube thoracostomy if indicated
   - Reduce dislocations compromising the circulation
   - Initial x-rays: lateral cervical spine, chest, pelvis
   - ECG
   - Administer analgesics, antibiotics, tetanus toxoid
   - Initiate admission, transfer, or movement to OR

TABLE 8-2 *Continued*

5. NEXT 10 MIN—SECONDARY SURVEY AND DEFINITIVE CARE
   - Reassess ABCDE
   - Complete documentation
   - Talk to family
   - Splint fractures
   - Dress wounds
   - Additional diagnostic tests: IVP, CT, and diagnostic peritoneal lavage as indicated
   - Consider central and arterial lines

and diagnostic testing. Children with serious injuries require continual reassessment. Repeat vital signs should be performed every 5 min during the primary survey and every 15 min while the patient is in the ED awaiting transfer or operative intervention.

Primary Survey

The primary survey includes the following:

- Airway and cervical spine stabilization
- Breathing and ventilation
- Circulation and hemorrhage control
- Disability (neurologic screening examination)
- Exposure and thorough examination

A guide to pediatric vital signs is provided in Table 8-3.

Airway

The airway is secured while concomitantly stabilizing the neck. The jaw-thrust maneuver is used to open the airway, and the oropharynx is cleared of debris and secretions.

Although injuries of the bony cervical spine are less common in children, children are at high risk for cervical cord injuries. Cervical spine injury should be assumed until an adequate cervical spine series and normal examination are obtained.

Ventilation with a bag-valve-mask device is initiated to treat inadequate ventilation. Cricoid pressure must be applied when ventilating a patient with a bag and mask to prevent gastric insufflation.

Indications for endotracheal intubation in the trauma patient are:

TABLE 8-3 Pediatric Vital Signs

Age	Weight,[a] kg	Respiratory rate	Heart rate	Systolic BP[b]
Preterm	2	55–65	120–180	40–60
Term newborn	3	40–60	90–170	52–92
1 month	4	30–50	110–180	60–104
6 months–1 year	8–10	25–35	120–140	65–125
2–4 years	12–16	20–30	100–110	80–95
5–8 years	18–26	14–20	90–100	90–100
8–12 years	26–50	12–20	60–110	100–110
>12 years	>40	12–16	60–105	100–120

[a] Weight estimate: 8 + [2 × age (years)] = weight (kg).
[b] Blood pressure minimum: 70 + [2 × age(years)] = systolic blood pressure; ⅔ × systolic pressure = diastolic pressure.

Source: From Fitzmaurice LS: *Pediatric Emergency Medicine, Concepts and Clinical Practice*. St. Louis, MO: Mosby-Yearbook Inc. Modified with permission.

- Inability to ventilate the child by bag-valve-mask methods
- The need for prolonged control of the airway
- Prevention of aspiration in a comatose child
- The need for controlled hyperventilation in patients with serious head injuries
- Flail chest with pulmonary contusion
- Shock unresponsive to fluid administration

An uncuffed tube should be used in children under 8 years of age. Appropriate tube size is approximated by the diameter of the nostril. General guidelines based on age are given in Table 8-4. Emergency intubation should always be accomplished via the oral approach in traumatized children. Nasotracheal intubation, besides being extremely difficult in an acutely injured child, is contraindicated because of the acute angle of the posterior pharynx. Other disadvantages are a high complication rate and high failure rate.

Rapid Sequence Induction

Intubation may be difficult owing to poor airway visualization, seizures, or the child's combativeness. Prolonged intubation procedures can lead to elevation of intracranial pressure (ICP), pain, bradycardia, regurgitation, and hypoxemia. Rapid sequence induc-

Table 8-4 Equipment Sizes for Pediatric Trauma

Age	Mask	Oral airway	Nasal airway	Laryngoscope blade	Endotracheal tube, mm	Foley catheter	Orogastric tube	Suction catheter	Chest tube	Vascular catheter	Intraosseous needle
Newborn	Infant	0	—	0	3–3.5	5–8	5 or 8	8	12–18	20–22	—
6 months	Infant/ child	1	12	1	3.5	8	8	8	14–20	20–22	17
1 year	Child, small	1–2	12	1	4.0	8	10	8	14–24	20–22	17
3 years	Child, small	2	16	2	4.5	10	10	10	16–28	18–22	15
5 years	Child, medium	3	16	2	5.0	10	10–12	10	20–32	18–20	15
6 years	Child, medium	3	16	2–3	5.5	10–12	12	10	20–32	18–20	—
8 years	Small to medium	4	20	2–3	6.0	12	14	12	24–32	16–20	—
12 years	Medium to large	4–5	24–28	3	6.5	12–16	14	12	28–36	16–20	
16 years	Medium to large	5	28–30	3–4	7.0–8.0	14–18	16–18	12–14	28–40	14–18	—

Source: Reprinted with permission from Shafermeyer RW: Advances in trauma: Pediatric trauma. *Emerg Med Clin North Am* 11:187, 1993.

tion (RSI) can greatly facilitate intubation and reduce adverse effects significantly.

Rapid sequence intubation is defined as the simultaneous administration of a neuromuscular blocking agent and a potent sedative for the purpose of facilitating endotracheal intubation and reducing adverse effects of the procedure. Following below is a series of steps required for use of RSI.

1. *Brief assessment.* The history in a trauma patient needs to be concise yet provide key information. The mnemonic "AMPLE" provides an adequate framework for a history prior to intubation:
   - *A*llergies
   - *M*edications
   - *P*ast medical history
   - *L*ast meal
   - *E*vents leading to the injury

   Head, neck, cervical spine, face, nose, throat, and teeth should all be checked.
2. *Preparation of equipment (Table 8-5) and medications (Table 8-6).* Prepare needed equipment as soon as possible. The mnemonic "SOAP ME" is useful for remembering the critical equipment:
   - *S*uction
   - *O*xygen
   - *A*irway (laryngoscope, endotrachael tube, stylet, bag-valve-mask)
   - *P*harmacology (mix, drawup, and label all anticipated drugs)
   - *M*onitoring *E*quipment (cardiorespiratory monitor, pulse oximeter)
3. *Preoxygenation.* Preoxygenation with 100% oxygen as discussed in Chap. 2.
4. *Premedication with adjunctive agents.*
   - *Atropine* decreases secretions and vagal tone. Bradycardia can be profound in infants and children during airway management. It may be caused by hypoxia, succinylcholine (SCH), or vagal stimulation. Indications for atropine include all children younger than 1 year of age, children receiving SCH, adolescents and adults receiving a second dose of SCH, and any patient with bradycardia at the time of intubation. The dose is 0.02 mg/kg (1 mg maximum, 0.15 mg minimum).
   - *Lidocaine* blunts the ICP response to intubation. Give 1.5 mg/kg intravenously 2 min before paralytic agents are given, since maximum mucous membrane anesthesia is reached in 3 to 5 min.

TABLE 8-5 Equipment for Intubation and Rapid Sequence Induction

Equipment	Specifications
Laryngoscope handles/blades	Straight, 0, 1, 2, 3, 4 Curved, 2, 3, 4
Endotracheal tubes	Uncuffed, 3.0 through 6.0 mm Cuffed, 5.0 through 8.5 mm
Stylets	3–16F
Magill forceps	
Suction catheters	Rigid and flexible 6–18F
Suction source	
Ventilation self-inflating bag with oxygen reservoir tail and positive end-expiratory pressure valve attachment	Oxygen reservoir PEEP valve attachment 750 and 1000 mL
Clear plastic masks	Infant, child, adult—small, medium, large
Orogastric tubes	8–18F
Nasogastric tubes	8–18F
Pulse oximeter	
Cardiac monitor	
Automatic sphygmomanometer	
Oral airways	0–5
End-tidal CO_2 monitor	
Tracheostomy tubes	
Tracheostomy surgical set	
Transtracheal jet ventilation	Preassembled set
Cricothyrotomy catheter/needle	Large-bore

- *Fentanyl* blunts the heart rate and the mean arterial blood pressure effects of intubation, is well tolerated hemodynamically, and may be a good choice for blunting the intracranial pressure response to intubation. The dose is 3 to 5 μg/kg about 1 to 3 min before laryngoscopy and intubation. Larger doses may cause hypoventilation and hypercarbia.

5. *Priming or defasciculating muscle relaxant step (optional).* Nondepolarizing agents may be used as a pretreatment to abolish

TABLE 8-6 Medications Used in Rapid Sequence Induction

Premedication	
Medication	**Dosage**
Atropine	0.02 mg/kg; 0.15 mg minimum
Lidocaine[a]	1.5 mg/kg IV; 2 min preparalysis
Fentanyl[a]	1–5 μg/kg; 1–3 min preintubation

Medication	Dose, IV	Onset	Duration
Sedation			
Thiopental[a,b]	3–5 mg/kg	10–30 s	10–30 min
Fentanyl[a]	6–10 μg/kg	1 min	30–60 min
Ketamine[a,d]	1–2 mg/kg	1–2 min	15–30 min
Diazepam[b]	0.25–4 mg/kg	2–4 min	30–90 min
Midazolam[b]	0.1–0.2 mg/kg	1–2 min	30–60 min
Propofol	1.5–2.5 mg/kg	30–60 s	10–15 min
Etomidate[c,e]	0.2–0.4 mg/kg	1 min	30–60 min
Muscle Relaxation			
Succinylcholine	>10 kg: 1.0–1.5 mg/kg <10 kg: 1.5–2.0 mg/kg	30–60s	4–10 min
Vecuronium	RSI: 0.15–0.3 mg/kg Standard: 0.1 mg/kg Defasciculation: 0.01 mg/kg	60–90 s 2–3 min	90–120 min 25–40 min
Pancuronium	0.1 mg/kg Defasciculation: 0.01 mg/kg	2–5 min	45–90 min
Atracurium	0.4 mg/kg	2–4 min	25–40 min
Rocuronium	0.6–1.0 mg/kg	30–60 s	25–60 min

[a] Good choice in the presence of head trauma.
[b] Use with caution in the presence of hypotension.
[c] Good choice in the presence of hypotension.
[d] Good choice in the presence of bronchospasm.
[e] Good choice in the presence of head trauma *and* hypotension.

Source: Used with permission from the American Academy of Pediatrics, American College of Emergency Physicians. *APLS: The Pediatric Emergency Medicine Course*, 2d ed. Elk Grove Village, IL: American Academy of Pediatrics, 1993.

fasciculations due to subsequent administration of SCH. A dose that is 10 percent of the usual dose for paralysis is used:

- *Pancuronium* 10% of 0.1 mg/kg = 0.01 mg/kg
- *d-Tubocurarine* 10% of 0.5 mg/kg = 0.05 mg/kg
- *Vecuronium* 10% of 0.1 mg/kg = 0.01 mg/kg

6. *Prepare for ventilation.* Provide a seal over the nose and mouth with a bag-valve-mask device. Provide cricoid pressure and assisted ventilation if patient has inadequate respiratory rate.
7. *Administer* ***sedative*** *to induce unconsciousness.* An ideal sedative will rapidly induce unconsciousness and have short duration. No sedative is free of cardiovascular depression, especially in the hypovolemic or hypotensive patient. Such patients should receive reduced doses or no sedative at all. Options for sedation are as follows:
   - ***Thiopental*** is a short-acting barbiturate which has a rapid onset of action (10 to 20 s) and reduces ICP and cerebral oxygen demands. Disadvantages include hypotension due to vasodilation and myocardial depression. It should be used in lower doses or avoided altogether in hypotensive or hypovolemic patients. It is a poor analgesic and may cause dose-dependent respiratory depression, coughing, laryngospasm, and bronchospasm. It is contraindicated in asthma.
   - ***Ketamine*** is a dissociative anesthetic which produces rapid sedation, amnesia, and analgesia. Its unique characteristics make it useful in hypovolemic, non-head-injured patients because it increases systemic blood pressure through catecholamine release. It is useful in patients with hypotension, hypovolemia, or status asthmaticus. It may cause cardiovascular depression in hypotensive patients because of its sedative effects. Adverse effects include ICP elevation, intraocular pressure elevation, hallucinations, excessive airway secretions, and laryngospasm. The patient should be premedicated with atropine to decrease excessive secretions. Ketamine should not be used in patients with hypertension, head injury, psychiatric problems, glaucoma, or open globe injury.
   - ***Fentanyl*** is a potent synthetic short-acting narcotic analgesic, reversible with naloxone. It rapidly produces analgesia and unconsciousness with duration of 30 min or longer. It blocks sympathomimetic responses. Adverse effects include chest wall rigidity, which can occur with rapid injection but is reversible with muscle relaxants or naloxone. It causes dose-dependent respiratory depression and seizurelike activity. Fentanyl is unreliable as an anesthetic induction agent when used as the sole sedative and should not be used with monoamine oxidase inhibitors.

- ***Diazepam*** has a slower onset than other sedatives but is capable of induction anesthesia at higher doses. It causes less cardiovascular and respiratory depression than barbiturates but may cause antegrade amnesia. It has a highly variable effective dose (0.2 to 1.0 mg/kg), and titration is required.
- ***Midazolam*** has a faster onset, shorter duration, and narrower dosing range than diazepam. It may cause a moderate decrease in cerebrospinal fluid pressure. It has a broader dosing range (0.1 to 0.3 mg/kg), requiring titration. The need for titration of benzodiazepines severely limits their usefulness in RSI.
- ***Propofol*** is a relatively new anesthetic induction agent which is very short-acting. Although it is being used for deep sedation and induction for anesthesia, it causes significant decreases in mean arterial blood pressure.
- ***Etomidate*** causes much less cardiovascular depression than the barbiturates or propofol. It is a good agent for the management of patients with elevated intracranial pressure. It can suppress the synthesis of cortisol after as little as one dose. Nevertheless, in a volume-depleted or hemodynamically unstable patient, it is becoming a more popular choice. The dose is 0.2 to 0.4 mg/kg.

The selection of the best agent depends on the specific clinical situation. Table 8-6 provides a useful comparison of agents for use in commonly encountered situations. The following recommendations are also provided:

- No hypotension/hypovolemia (excluding status asthmaticus): thiopental 3 to 5 mg/kg
- Mild hypotension/hypovolemia with suspected head injury: thiopental 2 to 4 mg/kg; etomidate 0.2 to 0.4 mg/kg
- Mild hypotension/hypovolemia without head injury: ketamine 1 to 2 mg/kg; etomidate 0.2 to 0.4 mg/kg
- Severe hypotension/hypovolemia: no sedative; ketamine 0.35 to 0.7 mg/kg; etomidate 0.2 mg/kg
- Status asthmaticus: ketamine 1 to 2 mg/kg

8. *Muscle relaxation.* The ideal muscle relaxant should have rapid onset and short duration of action or be reversible. Prior sedation is critical, since paralysis should never be induced in patient who is conscious.
   - ***Succinylcholine*** is rapid-acting and has a short duration. Bradycardia and excessive bronchial secretions can be prevented by premedicating with atropine. Other side effects are negative inotropic and chronotropic effects, which are exacerbated by repeat dosing. Succinylcholine is also associated with malignant hyperthermia, hypertension, and dysrhythmias. Reliable reversal agents are not approved for

use in the United States, but reversal is rarely needed because of the short duration of action. Succinylcholine is contraindicated in crush injuries, glaucoma, penetrating eye injuries, significant neuromuscular disease, history or family history of malignant hyperthermia, or pseudocholinesterase deficiency. It can result in severe hyperkalemia when used in patients with established paralysis or after the acute phase of a major burn.

- ***Vecuronium* and *atracurium*** are the nondepolarizing are the nondepolarizing muscle relaxants with the fastest onset and shortest duration of action. Atracurium may cause histamine release, resulting in hypotension. Vecuronium has minimal cardiovascular effects and is not associated with histamine release, making it the drug of choice as an alternative to SCH. The onset of action is as fast as 90 s, with a duration of 25 to 60 min.
- ***Pancuronium*** causes tachycardia via muscarinic blockade. Its duration of action is at least 60 min, and it is longer-acting than either atracurium or vecuronium.
- ***Rocuronium*** is a new nondepolarizing neuromuscular blocker which has a more rapid osnet of paralysis than other nondepolarizing agents. It has a slightly shorter duration of action than vecuronium. The dose is 0.6 to 1.0 mg/kg.

Selection of a Muscle Relaxant (Table 8-6)

Succinylcholine has the fastest onset time, but vecuronium has the desirable properties of the nondepolarizing agents, and the time to intubation with vecuronium is only slightly longer than that for SCH alone. Vecuronium avoids the risks of SCH and avoids the histamine release and longer duration of action of the other nondepolarizing agents. Use of vecuronium without priming may be the quickest and easiest technique by which to paralyze for RSI. However, vecuronium has a longer duration than SCH, which could lead to problems if an airway is not secured. In addition, SCH has been used more extensively than vecuronium.

The following sequence of events then occurs:

1. Sellick maneuver. The Sellick maneuver helps prevent regurgitation and aspiration. Release only after endotracheal tube placement is confirmed.
2. Intubate when full relaxation is achieved.
3. Secure endotracheal tube, begin appropriate mechanical ventilation, order chest radiograph.
4. Consider gastric decompression.

5. If reversal of vecuronium is desired, use
   - Atropine 0.02 mg/kg (1 mg maximum, 0.15 mg minimum)
   - Edrophonium 0.5 to 1.0 mg/kg
6. If unable to perform orotracheal or nasotracheal intubation, an airway must be secured by one of the following techniques:
   - *Cricothyrotomy* has a role in patients with extensive facial or upper airway injury. However, it is difficult and hazardous in children. It is not recommended under the age of 10, and complication rates are as high as 10 to 40 percent.
   - *Tracheostomy* is time-consuming, is hazardous in the ED, and requires significant surgical skill.
   - *Needle cricothyrotomy and transtracheal jet ventilation (TTJV)* currently is the preferred method for securing an emergency airway in children when endotracheal intubation is not possible. The technique allows adequate ventilation for at least 45 to 60 min. Complications include subcutaneous emphysema, bleeding, and catheter dislodgment. The issue of CO_2 retention is overstated and of relative unimportance when airway access and oxygenation are critical. The TTJV technique should be adequate for 45 min to 2 h until endotracheal intubation is possible. To perform the procedure, a 14-gauge angiocath is connected to a 5-mL syringe containing 3 mL of saline. The trachea is stabilized with the nondominant hand, and after the region is prepped, the cricothyroid membrane is punctured at a 30 to 45° angle caudally. Placement is verified with aspiration of air. Special care is required to avoid puncturing the posterior wall of the trachea. The catheter is slid off the needle, and placement is reconfirmed with the syringe. The cathether must be constantly held or secured in place, and the jet ventilation tubing is attached to the O_2 source. This O_2 source *must be a high-pressure source* directly from the wall and not from a regulator valve. The pounds per square inch (PSI) of oxygen pressure can then be adjusted on the pressure gauge. There are no well-studied guidelines for PSI settings for TTJV in children. Table 8-7 provides generally accepted guidelines. A low PSI must be used initially in children, and the provider should look for adequate chest excursion. The PSI can be adjusted upward until adequate chest rise is observed. The inspiration : expiration ventilation ratio is 1 : 3 or 1 : 4.

BREATHING

Acceptable ventilation occurs if there is adequate spontaneous air exchange with normal O_2 saturation and carbon dioxide levels.

TABLE 8-7 Parameters for Transtracheal Jet Ventilation

Age	Initial PSI	Estimated tidal volume, mL
Adult	30–50	700–1000
8 years–adolescents	10–25	340–625
5–8 years	5–10	240–340
<5 years	5	100

Pulse oximetry is mandatory, and end-tidal CO_2 monitoring is an increasingly available technology which should be considered.

Reasons for compromised ventilatory function include depressed sensorium, airway occlusion, restriction of lung expansion, and direct pulmonary injury. Restriction of lung expansion by gastric distension is more likely to occur in children because of the increased importance of the diaphragmatic excursion to ventilation in children. This problem is addressed by early placement of a nasogastric or orogastric tube.

In an obtunded or comatose child, ventilation using bag-valve-mask device, endotracheal tube, or transtracheal-jet-ventilation needle should be via a high-flow oxygen source capable of producing chest rise and adequate O_2 saturation. Immediate recognition and treatment of tension pneumothorax or hemopneumothorax is required. Children are especially sensitive to mediastinal shift with tension hemopneumothoraxes. Needle decompression should be performed immediately if any of the following are present: decreased breath sounds, refractory hypotension, hypoxia, or radiographically confirmed hemopneumothoraxes.

CIRCULATION

During the primary survey, the major goals of circulatory assessment and treatment are to diagnose and control external and internal hemorrhage and assess pulses and perfusion. Vascular access for fluid infusions and phlebotomy are additional goals. Volume status, blood pressure, and perfusion are estimated by assessment of pulse, skin color, and capillary refill time. A palpable peripheral pulse correlates with a blood pressure above 80 mmHg, and a palpable central pulse indicates a pressure above 50 to 60 mmHg. A normovolemic euthermic patient's capillary refilling time, assessed after blanching, will be 2 to 3 s. If the extremities are cool distally and warm proximally, changes in volume status and perfusion can be followed during therapy by the change in temperature as perfusion of the distal extremities improves or worsens.

External hemorrhage is controlled by direct pressure. Application of extremity tourniquets or hemostats to bleeding vessels should be avoided. Application and inflation of a pneumatic antishock garment is controversial but may be useful to help control bleeding in the pelvis or lower extremities. As in adults, Trendelenburg position may be of benefit in low-perfusion states to help maintain central circulation.

Vascular access is discussed below under "Resuscitation."

DISABILITY (NEUROLOGIC FUNCTION)

Neurologic function is assessed by performing a rapid neurologic examination to determine level of consciousness and pupillary size and reaction. The Glasgow Coma Scale (Table 8-8) is a more quantitative measure of level of consciousness. It is an extremely useful tool for detecting improvement or deterioration.

Early in a trauma resuscitation, the AVPU system is quicker and can be quite helpful in grossly following mental status changes (Table 8-9).

EXPOSURE

The patient is completely undressed in order to perform a thorough assessment. Children have a larger ratio of body surface area to weight, so maintaining the patient's body heat is a constant concern when he or she is exposed.

RESUSCITATION

Resuscitation occurs simultaneously with the primary survey, but it is separated in presentation for clarity.

Adequate oxygenation and ventilation must be ensured. Vascular access is essential for administration of drugs and fluid. Establishing an intravenous line can be difficult. A protocol for establishment of vascular access should be adhered to so that an excessive amount of time is not used in attempting to gain access by one technique. The first approach to attempt to start a peripheral intravenous line using an over-the-needle catheter, preferably in the hand, forearm, or antecubital fossa. Lower extremity lines may be used, but pooling of blood in the inferior vena cava during resuscitation can lead to poor distribution of drugs given through lower extremity lines. If this approach is not successful in the first 90 s, attention should be directed toward establishing central venous access, access via a saphenous vein cutdown, or access via intraosseous cannulation.

TABLE 8-8 Pediatric Glasgow Coma Scale

Eye Opening		
Score	0–1 year	>1 year
4	Spontaneously	Spontaneously
3	To shout	To verbal command
2	To pain	To pain
1	No response	No response

Best Motor Response		
Score	0–1 year	>1 Year
6		Obeys command
5	Localizes pain	Localizes pain
4	Flexion withdrawal	Flexion withdrawal
3	Decorticate	Decorticate
2	Decerebrate	Decerebrate
1	No response	No response

Best Verbal Response			
Score	0–2 years	2–5 years	>5 years
5	Appropriate cry Smiles, coos	Appropriate words and phrases	Oriented, converses
4	Cries	Inappropriate words	Disoriented, converses
3	Inappropriate cry	Cries/screams	Inappropriate words
2	Grunts	Grunts	Incomprehensible sound
1	No response	No response	No response

Note: A score is given in each category. The individual scores are then added to give a total of 3–15. A score of <8 indicates severe neurologic injury.

TABLE 8-9 AVPU Method for Assessing Level of Consciousness

A	Alert
V	Vocal stimuli: responds
P	Painful stimuli: responds
U	Unresponsive

During cardiopulmonary resuscitation, the femoral approach to central venous access is the most practical because it can be attempted without interruption of CPR. In the nonarrest situation, the internal jugular, subclavian, and external jugular approaches can be used. In experienced hands, all of these techniques are safe and efficacious. Choice is based largely on the experience and preference of the physician performing the procedure. Saphenous vein cutdown at the ankle is an alternative approach, especially in children over the age of 3 years, in whom intraosseous infusion is less applicable.

Intraosseous cannulation is an excellent alternative for vascular access in the child below the age of 3 years. With short-term use, complications of intraosseous infusion are extremely rare. Epinephrine, lidocaine, atropine, sodium bicarbonate, calcium, pressors, antibiotics, digitalis, heparin, anticonvulsants, and whole blood all can be infused via the intraosseous route.

Intraosseous cannulation is achieved with an intraosseous (IO) needle with a stylette. The preferred site is 1 to 3 cm distal to the tibial tuberosity on the medial or anterior surface of the tibia. The needle is directed perpendicularly or slightly caudally to prevent injury to the epiphyseal plate.

By using this stepwise protocol for establishment of vascular access, access should be achieved in less than 5 min in the majority of cases.

Blood is then sent for typing and crossmatching, complete blood count, electrolytes, liver transaminases, and amylase. Liver transaminase elevation in the acute trauma setting serves as a marker of liver injury that might not be clinically apparent. A blood gas is indicated in any patient with significant volume loss, respiratory compromise, or concomitant toxic exposure, such as carbon monoxide poisoning in a burn patient.

An assessment for shock is performed, adequacy of organ perfusion is determined. Shock after trauma is usually hypovolemic. Determination of the extent of volume depletion is difficult in children, and multiple parameters must be used (Table 8-10). Hematocrit, which can be normal in the face of acute blood loss, and blood pressure are insensitive indicators of shock.

Cardiogenic shock after a major childhood injury is rare but could occur as a result of cardiac tamponade or cardiac contusion. It should be suspected if there are dilated neck veins in a patient who has sustained a decelerating injury, penetrating chest trauma, or sternal contusion. Neurogenic shock presents with hypotension without tachycardia or vasoconstriction. Isolated head injury does not produce shock unless there is significant intracerebral hemorrhage in an infant. Distributive or septic shock should not be a consideration immediately after trauma, even if there is contamination of the abdominal cavity.

Guidelines for fluid resuscitation in shock are given in Table 8-11. The initial resuscitative fluid should be crystalloid isotonic solution such as Ringer's lactate or normal saline. An initial infusion of 20 mL/kg is given as rapidly as possible. This is best accomplished by using a three-way stopcock and pushing boluses rather than infusing via a pump or gravity, especially if the cannulation device is smaller than 18 gauge. After a rapid 20-mL/kg bolus, the child should be reassessed. The fluid bolus should be repeated up to four times if necessary. If the child continues to be unstable, 10 to 20 mL/kg of packed red blood cells or whole blood is infused. The 3:1 rule is commonly used in replacing lost blood with crystalloid: 300 mL of crystalloid for each 100 mL of blood loss. If the initial hemoglobin value is 7 or less, blood should be given immediately, since compensatory mechanisms are ineffective below this level and cellular hypoxia develops.

Volume and perfusion status are clinically assumed during resuscitation. Vital signs are checked before and after bolus therapy. If a child is not responding appropriately, continued bleeding, tension pneumothorax, or hypoxemia are looked for. A Foley catheter is inserted and urinary output is monitored. Adequate output is 1 mL/kg/h for children >1 year of age and 2 mL/kg/h for children under 1 year of age. The appropriate size of the Foley catheter can be estimated by doubling the size of the endotracheal tube. Guidelines are provided in Table 8-4.

While restoring or immediately after attaining adequate perfusion, urinary and gastric catheters should be placed. Blood at the urethral meatus or in the scrotum or abnormal position of the prostate on rectal examination prohibit catheterization until retrograde urethrogram (RUG) has proved that the urethra is intact. The RUG is done by instilling gastrografin via a partially inserted Foley catheter.

Nasogastric tube insertion should be avoided or performed with

TABLE 8-10 Therapeutic Classification of Hemorrhagic Shock in the Pediatric Patient

Blood Loss, % volume[a]	Up to 15%	15–30%	30–40%	>40%
Pulse rate	Normal	Mild increase	Moderate increase	Severe increase
Blood pressure	Normal or increased	Decreased	Decreased	Decreased
Capillary refill	Normal	+	+	+
Respiratory rate	Normal	Mild increase	Moderate increase	Severe increase
Urinary output, mL/kg/h	1–2	0.5–1	0.25–0.5	Negligible
Mental status	Slightly anxious	Mildly anxious	Anxious, confused	Confused, lethargic
Fluid replacement (3 : 1 rule)	Crystalloid	Crystalloid	Crystalloid, blood	Crystalloid, blood

[a] Assume blood volume to be 8–9% of body weight (80–90 mL/kg).

TABLE 8-11 Guidelines for Fluid Resuscitation in Shock

	Initial volume	Total volume	Maintenance
Mild shock (15–25% loss)	20 mL/kg LR or NS; repeat if no improvement	After response, 5 mL/kg for several hours	<10 kg: 100 mL/kg/24 h 10–20 kg: 1000 mL + 50 mL/kg/24 h
Moderate shock (25–40% loss)	20 mL/kg LR or NS; repeat if no improvement 40 mL/kg LR or NS if not improved 10–20 mL/kg PRBC if not improved or HCT <7.0 Consider operative intervention	After response, 5 mL/kg for several hours Adjust toward maintenance Consider transfusion	As above
Severe shock (>40% loss)	Push LR or NS until colloid available Push PRBC or whole blood surgery	Replace with type-specific blood	As above

the utmost care when a patient has blood coming from the ears, nose, or mouth. A cribriform plate fracture may allow passage of the catheter into the brain.

The patient's body temperature is measured and monitored. Hypothermia must be avoided or corrected. Radiant warmers, warmed IV fluids, and covering of exposed body parts will prevent or correct hypothermia.

Radiographs should be obtained during the primary survey, but they should be limited to cervical spine, chest, and pelvic films. More extensive radiographs should be delayed until the patient is stabilized.

A trauma surgeon, an intensivist, an orthopedist, and an anesthesiologist should be consulted as needed. Initiation of a transfer protocol, if warranted, should be activated as soon as the need for a higher level of care is realized. Table 8-12 outlines the reasons for transfer of pediatric trauma patients.

SECONDARY SURVEY AND DEFINITIVE CARE

Once life-threatening conditions identified in the primary survey are stabilized, a directed evaluation of each body area is performed, proceeding from head to toe. Vital signs and abnormal conditions identified in the primary survey are reassessed at least every 15 min. The components of the secondary survey are complete examination, history, laboratory studies, radiographic studies, and problem identification.

History

An AMPLE history is used to determine the mechanism of injury, time, status at scene, changes in status, and complaints that the child may have.

Diagnostic Studies

Complete laboratory and radiologic studies not obtained during the resuscitation phase are ordered.

Physical Examination

Head

Pupillary size and reactivity are reevaluated. A conjunctival and fundal examination for hemorrhage or penetrating injury is performed. Visual acuity is assessed. A thorough palpation of the skull and mandible should be done, looking for fractures or dislocations. As long as the airway is not obstructed by maxillofacial trauma, its management is a lower priority.

TABLE 8-12 Reasons for Transfer of Pediatric Trauma Patients for Tertiary Care

I. Mechanism of trauma
  A. Falls
    1. Greater than 10 ft involving patients <14 years old
    2. Falls from second floor or higher
  B. Motor vehicle craches
    1. Evidence of high-impact incident
      a. Shattered windshield
      b. Intrusion into passenger compartment
      c. Bent steering wheel
    2. Rollover incident with unrestrained victim
    3. Ejection from the vehicle
    4. Death of an occupant
    5. Extraction time >20 min
  C. Auto versus pedestrian incident at >20 mph and victim <15 years old
  D. Major burns
  E. Blast injuries
II. Physiology
  A. Total trauma score of 12 or less
  B. Pediatric Trauma Score of 8 or less
  C. Unstable vital sign (age-appropriate)
  D. Compromise of airway, breathing, or circulation or need for protracted ventilation
  E. Severely compromised neurologic function, with Glasgow Coma Scale score of 8 or less
III. Injuries
  A. Penetrating injuries of the head, neck, chest, abdomen, or groin
  B. Two or more proximal long bone fractures
  C. Traumatic amputation proximal to either the wrist or the ankle
  D. Evidence of neurologic deficit due to spinal cord injury
  E. Flail chest, major chest wall injury, or pulmonary contusion
  F. Open head injury/CSF leak
  G. Suspicion of vascular or cardiac injury
  H. Severe maxillofacial injuries
  I. Depressed skull fracture

Cervical Spine

Injuries of the cervical spine are not common in children, but the presence of any of the following conditions increases the risk:

- Injuries above the clavicles
- Falls from a height of one or more floors
- Motor vehicle–pedestrian crashes that occur at >30 mph

- Unrestrained or poorly restrained occupant of a motor vehicle crash
- Sports injuries

The sensitivity of the lateral cervical spine radiograph is reported to be between 82 and 98 percent. A normal lateral x-ray does not clear the cervical spine but does allow the physician to proceed with essential evaluation and management and complete the series during the secondary survey and definitive care phases of the workup. Cervical spince films must show all seven cervical vertebrae. The series should contain at least three views: anteroposterior (AP), odontoid, and lateral views. Children tend to have injuries of the upper cervical spine and cord.

The incomplete development of the bony spine, the relatively large size of the head, and the weakness of the soft tissues of the neck given the larger head size predispose to spinal cord injury without radiographic abnormality (SCIWORA). Patients with altered sensorium cannot be cleared despite negative films, and the collar should remain in place.

Special considerations are required in four situations. First, the child who requires immediate intubation should not have airway management delayed while waiting for a lateral cervical spine film. Second, if a child who is intubated is at high risk for cervical spine injury, a CT scan of the upper cervical vertebrae should be done along with a head CT scan. Third, if an injured patient arrives with a helmet in place and does not require immediate airway intervention, the lateral cervical spine film can be done prior to removing the helmet. Cervical spine immobilization is maintained while the helmet is removed. Finally, penetrating injuries to the neck requiring operative intervention should have entry and exit sites denoted with opaque markers on AP and lateral films of the cervical spine.

Chest

The chest is inspected for wounds. Sucking chest wounds require a sterile occlusive dressing. A flail segment may be splinted, but the patient will usually require intubation. The patient is rolled while maintaining in-line spine immobilization and inspected for posterior thoracic wounds. The lungs are auscultated. Tension pneumothorax is suggested by contralateral tracheal shift, distended neck veins, and diminished breath sounds. However, auscultation is an insensitive tool for detecting pneumothorax. Neck vein distension is also difficult to appreciate. Therefore, any hemodynamically unstable child should undergo needle decompression if there has been blunt or penetrating injury to the thorax. After thoracentesis, tube thoracostomy should be done. An appropriate size for a chest tube can be approximated by multiplying the internal diameter of the endotracheal tube by 4 or by referring to Table 8-4. Impaled objects protruding from the chest should be left in place until the child undergoes surgery. If the chest x-ray reveals a widened mediastinum or apical cap and there is a history of significant deceleration injury, aortography is indicated. First or second rib fractures also increase the likelihood of a vascular injury. Any penetrating injury to the abdomen or lower chest carries a risk of diaphragmatic injury.

Abdomen

During the secondary survey, determining the exact etiology of an abdominal injury is secondary to determining whether or not an injury actually exists. Signs suggesting abdominal injury include abdominal wall contusion, distension, abdominal or shoulder pain, signs of peritoneal irritation, and shock. Penetrating wounds to the abdomen usually require immediate operative intervention.

The role of abdominal CT scanning and diagnostic peritoneal lavage (DPL) in the evaluation of abdominal trauma is controversial. Computed tomography with IV, oral, and colonic contrast may be the most sensitive and useful diagonstic modality. However, DPL provides rapid, objective evaluation of possible intraperitoneal injury. It is considered more sensitive than a CT in diagnosing hollow viscus injuries, especially early in the evaluation of a child who is a victim of a deceleration injury while wearing a seatbelt. It is much less sensitive than CT in diagnosing injuries to the pancreas, duodenum, genitourinary tract, aorta, vena cava and diaphragm. The indications, advantages and disadvantages of DPL are discussed in Chap. 12.

Diagnostic peritoneal lavage is most valuable in deciding whether or not a patient needs immediate laparotomy. It should be considered in the patient requiring urgent anesthesia and nonabdominal surgery, such as evacuation of an epidural hematoma or treatment of a penetrating upper chest injury.

After the bladder is emptied with a Foley catheter, DPL is performed using a midline approach above or below the umbilicus. If the initial aspirate is not grossly bloody, 10 mL/kg of Ringer's lactate is instilled. An aspirate is considered positive if it shows more than 100,000 red blood cells/μL, more than 500 white blood cells/μL, or a spun hematocrit greater than 2 percent, or if bile, bacteria, or fecal material is found. False-positive tests most commonly occur in the face of a pelvic fracture. Lacerations of the liver or spleen are not necessarily an indication for surgery. More than 80 percent of these patients will stop bleeding without operative intervention. A CT scan is more valuable for evaluating and assessing damage and determining a treatment plan in the stable patient.

Pelvis

The bony prominences of the pelvis should be palpated for tenderness or instability. The perineum is examined for laceration, hematoma, or active bleeding.

Rectum

A rectal examination, is performed to determine sphincter tone, rectal integrity, prostatic position, evidence of a pelvic fracture, or the presence of blood in the stool.

Extremities

All extremities are examined for deformity, contusions, abrasions, sensation, penetrating injuries, pulses, and perfusion. The presence of a pulse does not exclude a proximal vascular injury or a compartment syndrome. The long bones are palpated circumferentially, assessing for tenderness, crepitation, or abnormal movement. Severe angulations of the extremities are straightened and immobilized. Open fractures and wounds should be covered with sterile dressings. Soft tissue injuries are inspected for foreign bodies and irrigated to minimize contamination, and devitalized tissues are debrided.

Back

The back is examined for hematomas, penetrating wounds, or spine tenderness. The patient should be rolled for the examination while maintaining spinal immobilization.

Skin

The skin is examined for evidence of contusions, penetration sites, burns, petechiae, and signs of abuse. A traumatized child may have concomitant burn or inhalation injuries (Chap. 113). The depth, location, and types of burns and the extent of body surface area involved need to be documented. The burns should be covered with sterile dressings and intravenous fluid resuscitation initiated appropriate for the extent of the burns.

Neurologic

A repeat Glasgow Coma Score is obtained and an in-depth evaluation of motor, sensory, and cranial nerves is performed. The fundi are checked and rhinorrhea is looked for. Level of consciousness, pupillary examination, and sensorimotor examination, as quantified in the Glasgow Coma Scale, are invaluable in identifying a change in mental status. The presence of paresis or paralysis suggests a major neurologic injury. Conversely, lack of neurologic findings does not eliminate the possibility of a cervical cord injury, especially when the patient has a distracting injury.

Throughout the primary and secondary surveys, the injured child is at risk for exposure to cold. Because of the child's relatively larger body surface area, hypothermia can develop in the prehospital setting or in the emergency department. Hypothermia may impair circulatory dynamics and coagulation, worsen metabolic acidosis by increasing metabolic demand, and increase peripheral vascular resistance. The likelihood and risks of hypothermia can be minimized with the use of overhead warmers, warmed intravenous fluids, and warm blankets.

Tetanus Prophylaxis

Upon completion of the secondary survey, tetanus prophylaxis, if indicated, should be given.

Psychosocial Considerations

Parents should be allowed to be at the child's bedside as soon as the child is stabilized.

IMAGING

A child with major blunt trauma needs three basic radiographs immediately:

- Lateral cervical spine
- Chest
- Pelvis

In smaller children, chest films are much more sensitive than clinical examination in detecting hemopneumothoraxes. Widening of the mediastinum and fractured ribs should be checked for. Pelvic fractures are important clinical indicators, since 80 percent of children with multiple fractures of the pelvis have concomitant abdominal or genitourinary injuries.

During the secondary survey, thoracolumbar and extremity films can be completed as indicated. Computed tomography and ultrasonography are also considered during the secondary survey.

A CT scan of the head is indicated when there is significant head trauma. Indications are outlined in Chap. 9.

A CT scan of the abdomen is indicated for a hemodynamically stable victim of blunt trauma with clinical signs of intraabdominal injury, hematuria greater than 20 RBCs per high-powered field (or minimal hematuria with a history of deceleration injury), and a worrisome mechanism of trauma in the presence of neurologic compromise. The likelihood of positive findings on abdominal CT is significantly increased if three or more of the following are present:

- Gross hematuria
- Lap-belt injury
- Assault or abuse as a mechanism of trauma
- Abdominal tenderness
- Trauma score less than or equal to 12

Other indicators alone increase the positive predictive value of abdominal CT: positive abdominal findings, worrisome mechanism of trauma, and significant neurologic compromise (GCS score <10).

In trauma patients, double-contrast CT should be performed. Dilute gastrografin is instilled via a nasogastric tube 20 min prior to CT scan, and intravenous contrast is administered after the initial survey. During the CT, the Foley catheter should be pulled into the esophagus to avoid artifact. Doses for contrast media are given in Table 8-13.

Ultrasonography may be an alternative to CT in selected cases or when CT is not available. Ultrasound can diagnose most injuries to the liver, spleen, and kidneys and can document intraperitoneal fluid. An experienced ultrasonographer is essential for proper performance and interpretation of the scan.

TABLE 8-13 Dose of Contrast Media for Radiographic Studies

Age, years	Dose
Intravenous: 60% Hypaque	
0 to 9	1 mL/0.45 kg bolus
10 or more	50 mL, followed by infusion of 50 to 100 mL during scan
Oral: 1.5% hypaque (20 mL to 1 L of fluid given PO or NG)	
0–2	100 mL
3–5	150–200 mL
6–9	200–250 mL
>9	300–1000 mL
Adult	1000 mL
Oral: gastrografin, 20 mL/kg via NG tube 20 min prior to scan	

If intraperitoneal fluid is found by CT or ultrasound but there is no apparent injury to the spleen or liver, a DPL should be performed. A limitation of CT scanning is its lack of sensitivity in diagnosing injuries to hollow organs. Therefore, other diagnostic modalities should be considered for victims of motor vehicle accidents who have transverse ecchymoses of the abdominal wall with or without abdominal pain or tenderness (which may be seen with lap-belt injuries) or symptoms or signs of lumbar spine injury with or without spinal cord injury. The CT scans will also miss lumbar spine injuries in 77 percent of cases. Therefore, if a patient is hemodynamically stable, evaluation should include thoracolumbar spine films, especially a lateral, in the resuscitation area; a decubitus abdominal film looking for free air; a cystogram; and a DPL. If injury to bowel or bladder is confirmed, laparotomy is indicated. If plain films are negative but there is evidence of retroperitoneal injury, double-contrast CT is indicated.

When a patient has gross blood at the meatus or the integrity of the urethra is in doubt due to possible pelvic fracture, a retrograde urethrogram should be performed. There is high correlation between blood at the meatus and pelvic fractures. A Foley catheter is inserted in the distal urethra, and the balloon is partially inflated (0.5 to 1.0 mL). Contrast is then instilled. The catheter can be advanced to perform a cystogram if the urethra is not found to be damaged.

A "one-shot" intravenous pyleogram is a very useful and reasonable test to perform in the ED for evaluation of renovascular status if the patient is too unstable for CT. To do this, 2 to 4 mL/kg of 50% diatrizoate sodium (Hypaque) is injected, and a film of the abdomen is taken 5 min later. This will demonstrate blood supply to the kidneys and may also show the function of the upper ureters. Knowledge of the status of the blood supply is very important because an intimal tear with occlusion or vascular disruption must be identified immediately. The warm ischemic time in which to diagnose, repair, and avoid irreparable damage to a devascularized kidney is only 6 h.

MEASURES OF INJURY SEVERITY

The Trauma Scores

The Revised Score (Table 8-14) was developed for rapid assessment, triage, measuring progression of injury, predicting outcome, and assisting in quality assessment. It is useful in the overall management of patients with multiple-system trauma but it is a less sensitive indicator of severe injury to a single organ system. It is straightforward to calculate, and it allows for standardization of

TABLE 8-14 Revised Trauma Score

Revised trauma score	Glasgow coma scale score	Systolic blood pressure	Respiratory rate
4	13–15	>89	10–20
3	9–12	76–89	>29
2	6–8	50–75	6–9
1	4–5	1–49	1–5
0	3	0	0

Note: A score of 0–4 is given for each variable then added to give a range of 0–12. A score of 11 or less indicates potentially significant trauma.

triage protocols and for scientific comparisons between groups of patients and institutions. The Pediatric Trauma Score was developed to reflect the unique injury pattern in children and incorporates age into the score (Table 8-15).

In a study by Nayduch and Noylan, the Revised Trauma Score (Table 8-14) had a better predictive value for overall outcome, whereas the Pediatric Trauma Score (Table 8-15) was a better predictor for appropriate ED disposition. Unfortunately, no trauma score is totally reliable in predicting extent of injuries or outcomes. Therefore, the Revised Trauma Score or Pediatric Trauma Score can be used to triage patients and predict outcome,

TABLE 8-15 Pediatric Trauma Score

Variables	+2	+1	−1
Airway	Normal	Maintainable	Unmaintainable
CNS	Awake	Obtunded or transient LOC	Coma
Body weight	>20 kg	10–20 kg	<10 kg
Systolic BP	>90 mmHg	90–50 mmHg	<50 mmHg
Open wound	None	Minor	Major
Skeletal injury	None	Closed fracture	Open/multiple fractures

Note: A score of +2, +1, or −1 is given to each variable, then added to give a range of −6 to +12. A score of 8 or less indicates potentially significant trauma. A score of >8 is associated with 100% survival, while a score of <0 is associated with 100% mortality.

but caution should be exercised in using it to predict functional outcome.

DISPOSITION/TRANSFER

Facilities that receive trauma victims should have the appropriate personnel and patient care resources committed to the care of trauma at all times. The majority of seriously injured children are not, however, brought to comprehensive trauma centers. If the receiving hospital does not have pediatric anesthesia or pediatric surgical consultants, early transfer to a pediatric trauma center, adult trauma center, or pediatric intensive care unit should be considered. Plans for transfer and referral agreements between institutions should be established prospectively. Guidelines for stabilization and reasons to transfer to a pediatric trauma center are available (Table 8-12).

When dealing with a traumatized child, the physician must communicate openly and clearly with the family. Psychological support is needed through the entire hospital course. Parents should be allowed to see the child as soon as is practical and to accompany the child whenever possible during transports.

Children who have clinical brain death should be considered for continued resucitation, since they may be candidates for organ procurement. If heart, heart-lung, kidney, pancreas, or liver transplantation is considered, premortem management is key to the viability of the organs. Sensitive parental consultation and support are paramount. Organ donation may provide traumatized families some consolation and strength in the face of their tremendous grief.

For a more detailed discussion, see Gerardi MJ: Evaluation and Management of the Multiple Trauma Patient, Chap. 8, p. 37, in *Pediatric Emergency Medicine: A Comprehensive Study Guide.*

---

9 Head Trauma

Kimberly S. Quayle

Each year approximately 22,000 children aged 1 to 19 years die from trauma in the United States, and 600,000 sustain injuries necessitating hospital admission. Of children who die from multiple trauma, 80 percent have significant head injury, compared to 50 percent of adult trauma victims. Pediatric brain injury leads to major morbidity from physical disability, seizures, and mental retardation.

PATHOPHYSIOLOGY

Primary brain injury occurs as a result of direct mechanical damage inflicted during the traumatic event. Secondary injuries occur from metabolic events such as hypoxia, ischemia, or increased intracranial pressure.

ANATOMY

Cerebrospinal fluid surrounds the brain within the subarachnoid space. Approximately 72 percent of the adult intracranial volume of 1200 to 1500 mL is attained by age 2, 90 percent by age 8, and 96 percent by adolescence.

The outer structures protect the brain during everyday movements and minor trauma. Movement of the brain within the vault along the uneven base of the skull may injure brain tissue. The unyielding, mature skull can contribute to brain injury when brain edema or an expanding hematoma develops. Subsequently, herniation across compartments can cause compression of vital structures, ischemia for vascular occlusion, and infarction.

In infants, the open sutures and thin calvarium produce a more flexible skull capable of absorbing greater impact. This flexibility permits more severe distortion between the skull and dura and the cerebral vessels and brain, increasing susceptibility to hemorrhage.

SPECIFIC INJURIES

Scalp injuries may bleed profusely, which can lead to hemodynamically significant blood loss from relatively small lacerations. Open scalp wounds should be carefully explored for skull integrity, depressions, or foreign bodies.

Linear nondepressed skull fractures occur at the point of impact. The presence of a skull fracture indicates a significant blow to the head but does not necessarily imply brain injury. The absence of a skull fracture does not exclude the presence of intracranial injury. Skull fractures usually prompt a computed tomography (CT) scan of the head. "Growing fractures" are unique to infants and young children. They occur after a skull fracture in children under 2 years of age and are associated with a dural tear. Rapid brain growth during the postinjury period may be associated with the development of a leptomeningeal cyst, which is an extrusion of cerebrospinal fluid or brain tissue through the dural defect. Thus, children less than 2 years old with a skull fracture require follow-up to detect a growing fracture.

Basilar skull fractures typically occur at the petrous portion of the temporal bone, although they may occur anywhere along the base of the skull. Clinical signs suggesting a basilar skull fracture include hemotympanum, cerebrospinal fluid otorrhea, cerebrospinal fluid rhinorrhea, periorbital ecchymosis ("raccoon's eyes"), or postauricular ecchymosis (Battle sign). Radiologic diagnosis often requires detailed CT imaging of the temporal bone, as plain skull radiographs or routine head CTs may not be diagnostic.

Epidural hematomas occur as commonly in children as in adults, although they are more likely to be clinically occult in children. Eighty percent occur in combination with a skull fracture and meningeal artery bleeding; the remainder are venous in origin. Signs and symptoms include headache, vomiting, and altered mental status, which may progress to signs and symptoms of uncal herniation with pupillary changes and hemiparesis.

Acute subdural hematomas occur four times more commonly in adults than in children. Acute interhemispheric subdural hematomas occur more commonly in infants and young children; they are often caused by shaking/impact injuries of abuse. Subdural hematomas usually result from tearing of the bridging veins and typically occur over the cerebral convexities. The mechanism of injury is usually acceleration-deceleration; therefore, subdural hematomas are often associated with more diffuse brain injury. Subdural hematomas progress more slowly than epidural bleeds, with common symptoms including irritability, vomiting, and lethargy.

Parenchymal contusions are bruises or tears of brain tissue. Bony irregularities of the skull cause these cerebral contusions as the brain moves within the skull. Intraparenchymal hemorrhages may also occur from shearing injury or penetrating wounds. Signs and symptoms may include decreased level of consciousness, focal neurologic findings, and seizures.

Penetrating injuries occur as a result of sharp object penetration or gunshot wounds. Extensive brain injury is common, and severity depends on the path of the object, associated hemorrhage, and brain injury.

A concussion is defined as a transient loss of awareness and responsiveness following head trauma. Transient symptoms may include loss of consciousness, vomiting, headache, and dizziness.

Diffuse brain swelling occurs three times more often in children than in adults. The swelling usually occurs as the result of a shearing acceleration-deceleration injury. Prolonged coma or death may occur, as the increased intracranial pressure may compromise cerebral blood flow.

INTRACRANIAL PRESSURE AND HERNIATION SYNDROMES

The total volume of the intracranial contents is constant. Approximately 70 percent of this volume is brain, 20 percent is cerebrospinal and interstitial fluid, and 10 percent is blood. If one of these three components increases in volume, then the other two compartments must decrease or intracranial pressure rises. The main component of compensation is a displacement of cerebrospinal fluid into the spinal canal. Any additional increases in volume cause elevation of intracranial pressure to abnormal levels (greater than 15 to 20 mmHg). Cerebral perfusion becomes impaired, and irreversible ischemic damage to the brain ensues.

An intracranial mass or hematoma will occupy the fixed intracranial space and compress the normal brain tissue and reduce blood flow. Cytotoxic cerebral edema occurs with fluid accumulation within damaged brain and glial cells. Interstitial cerebral edema results from decreased absorption of fluid following brain trauma. Vasogenic cerebral edema occurs as the endothelial cell barrier is compromised and leakage of fluid into the perivascular brain tissue occurs.

The volume of cerebrospinal fluid may also increase despite the compensatory redistribution of the fluid into the spinal canal. As brain and blood volumes increase, the ventricular spaces become compressed until redistribution is not possible.

Cerebral blood volume in head-injured children may be increased as a result of brain injury. The autoregulation of cerebral blood flow is complex. Hypoxia and hypercapnea for hypoventilation of the injured patient also increase cerebral blood flow. Cerebral hyperemia occurs more commonly in children than in adults and may account for the presentation of brain swelling in children in the first 24 h postinjury.

Diffusely or focally increased intracranial pressure may produce herniation. Cingulate herniation occurs as one cerebral hemisphere is displaced underneath the falx cerebri to the opposite side. A transtentorial or uncal herniation is of major clinical significance (Fig. 9-1). A mass lesion or hematoma forces the ipsilateral uncus of the temporal lobe through the space between the cerebral peduncle and the tentorium. This causes ipsilateral compression of the oculomotor nerve and an ipsilateral dilated, nonreactive pupil. The cerebral peduncle is compressed, causing a contralateral hemiparesis. As the intracranial pressure increases and the brainstem is compressed, consciousness wanes. If hereniation continues, on-

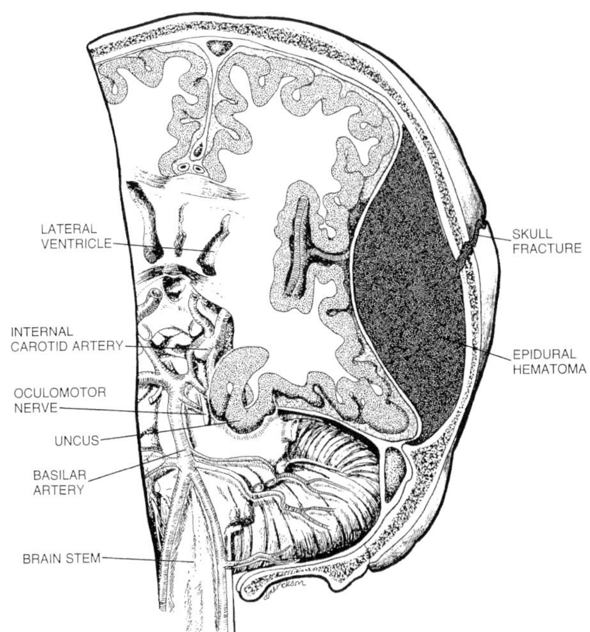

FIG. 9-1 Anterior view of transtentorial uncal herniation caused by a large epidural hematoma. (From American College of Emergency Physicians: *Emergency Medicine: A Comprehensive Study Guide*, 3d ed. New York: McGraw-Hill, 1992. Reproduced with permission of McGraw-Hill.)

going brainstem deterioration occurs, progressing to apnea and death. Uncal herniation may be bilateral if there are bilateral lesions or diffuse edema. Herniation of the cerebellar tonsils downward through the foramen magnum occurs infrequently in children. Medullary compression from this herniation causes bradycardia, respiratory arrest, and death.

ASSESSMENT

Assessment begins with a detailed history the traumatic event. As many details about the mechanism of injury of a possible should be obtained. The time and location of injury are also important.

Symptoms and signs occurring since the injury should be noted, including loss of consciousness, seizures, vomiting, headache, visual changes, altered mental status, weakness, and amnesia. Past medical history should include prior history of seizures, neurologic abnormalities, bleeding disorders, and immunization status.

Physical evaluation begins with the primary assessment. Airway obstruction by the tongue commonly occurs in unconscious children with serious head injury. Blood, vomitus, teeth, foreign bodies, or other debris may be present as well. An airway is established by positioning, suctioning, placing an oral airway, or intubation. Cervical spine control must be maintained in a child with significant head injury until cervical spine injury is excluded. The cervical spine should be manually stabilized during laryngoscopy.

Once the airway is established, ventilation is assessed. Chest expansion is observed, breath sounds are auscultated, and the patient is assessed for cyanosis or respiratory distress. Hypoventilation is treated with 100% oxygen, bag-valve-mask ventilation, and subsequent intubation of the trachea with consideration of rapid sequence technique. Rapid sequence induction (RSI) is used to protect the brain from increased intracranial pressure during the intubation procedure.

The general procedure for RSI is discussed in Chap. 8. There are a few points of special note regarding the use of RSI in head trauma patients.

Ketamine is contraindicated in head-injured patients because it increases intracranial pressure. Succinylcholine may also lead to increased intracranial pressure as a consequence of its depolarizing effect. Vecuronium is a better choice for head trauma victims. Rapid sequence induction for intubation is contraindicated in patients with major facial or laryngeal trauma and with distorted facial and airway anatomy. These conditions may lead to a situation in which intubation or mask ventilation is unsuccessful.

Circulation should be assessed by evaluating the heart rate, peripheral pulses, and perfusion. Life-threatening hemorrhage must be controlled and blood pressure maintained, so that adequate cerebral perfusion occurs. Hypovolemic shock is rare after an isolated head injury, although it is possible in infants and young children. Other sources for hypovolemia must be sought.

After the rapid ABC (airway, breathing, circulation) assessment, a primary survey of neurologic disability follows. Level of consciousness should be ascertained and categorized as alert, responsive to verbal stimulus, responsive to painful stimulus, or unresponsive (AVPU). Pupillary response is then evaluated. The remainder of the primary survey is completed prior to returning to a more detailed secondary neurologic examination. Decorticate posturing signifies damage to the cerebral cortex, white matter, or basal ganglia. Decerebrate posturing suggests damage lower in the midbrain.

In adults and older children, the Glasgow Coma Score is commonly used to assess and follow the level of consciousness in head-injured patients. The Glasgow Coma Scale evaluates for eye opening, best motor response, and best verbal response (see Table 8-8). Use of the Glasgow Coma Scale in infants and young children is limited by the verbal skills of this age group. Many specialized coma scores for use in children have been developed; however, none have been validated. Evaluation of young children and infants following head injury may be difficult, particularly the assessment of mental status and the neurologic examination.

The neurologic status of a head-injured child must be regularly reassessed, particularly with regard to level of consciousness and vital signs. The frequency of reassessment is dictated by the condition of the child. In 1984, a study described 42 children who developed neurologic deterioration after "minor head injury" following a lucid or symptom-free period. Only one of these patients had an intracranial hematoma. Brain edema was hypothesized as a causative factor in the other patients. In 1990, a study described four children with head trauma who each talked postinjury and then suffered a rapid neurologic decline leading to death. No space-occupying intracranial hematomas were present. Postmortem examination of two of the children revealed multiple cerebral contusions, diffuse brain edema with herniation, and hypoxic-ischemic injury.

DIAGNOSTIC STUDIES

Computed tomography of the head has become the diagnostic method of choice for the identification of intracranial pathology in acute victoms of head trauma. The role of skull radiographs in evaluation of children with head injury remains controversial. Opinion on the value of skull radiographs in head-injured children is divided.

Many authors have investigated predictive clinical criteria for intracranial injury in adults, but fewer have focused on children, and all pediatric studies have been retrospective. In 1987, a multidisciplinary panel provided recommendations for the management of head trauma patients, and then prospectively gathered information on over 7,000 patients (Table 9-1). Children below 2 years of age were assigned to the moderate-risk group unless the injury was trivial. No clarification of trivial injury was given.

In the absence of definitive information, skull radiographs may

TABLE 9-1 Management Strategy for Radiographic Imaging in Patients with Head Trauma[a]

Low-risk group	Moderate-risk group	High-risk group
Possible findings	Possible findings	Possible findings
Asymptomatic	History of change of consciousness at the time of injury or subsequently	Depressed level of consciousness not clearly due to alcohol, drugs, or other cause (e.g., metabolic and seizure disorders)
Headache	History of progressive headache	Focal neurologic signs
Dizziness	Alcohol or drug intoxication	Decreasing level of consciousness
Scalp hematoma	Unreliable or inadequate history of injury	Penetrating skull injury or palpable depressed fracture
Scalp laceration	Age less than 2 years (unless injury very trivial)	
Scalp contusion or abrasion	Posttraumatic seizure	
Absence of moderate-risk or high-risk criteria	Vomiting	
	Posttraumatic amnesia	
	Multiple trauma	
	Serious facial injury	
	Signs of basilar fracture[b]	
	Possible skull penetration or depressed fracture[c]	
	Suspected physical child abuse	

Recommendations	Recommendations	Recommendations
Observation alone: discharge patients with head-injury information sheet (listing subdural precautions) and a second person to observe them.	Extended close observation (watch for signs of high-risk group). Consider CT examination and neurosurgical consultation. Skull series may (rarely) be helpful, if positive, but do not exclude intracranial injury if normal.	Patient is a candidate for neurosurgical consultation or emergency CT examination or both.

[a] Physician assessment of the severity of injury may warrant reassignment to a higher-risk group. Any single criterion from a higher-risk group warrants assignment of the patient to the highest risk group applicable.

[b] Signs of basilar fracture include drainage from ear, drainage of cerebrospinal fluid from nose, hematotympanum. Battle sign, and "raccoon eyes."

[c] Factors associated with open and depressed fracture include gunshot, missile, or shrapnel wounds; scalp injury from firm, pointed object (including animal teeth); penetrating injury or eyelid or globe; object stuck in the head; assault (definite or suspected) with any object; leakage of cerebrospinal fluid; and sign of basilar fracture.

Source: From Masters SJ, McClean PM, Arcarese JS, et al: Skull x-ray examinations after head trauma: Recommendations by a multidisciplinary panel and validation study. Reprinted by permission of the *New England Journal of Medicine* 316:84, 1987.

be useful in possible child abuse and in infants with large scalp hematomas. Head CT scans should be obtained, as this is the most important study in children with severe headaches, recurrent vomiting, bulging fontanelles, seizures, focal neurologic signs, altered mental status, pentrating injuries, or palpable depressed skull fractures.

TREATMENT

The goal of management of head injury in children is to prevent secondary injury to the brain. Prevention of hypoxia, ischemia, and increased intracranial pressure is essential. Prompt neurosurgical intervention is necessary in most of the seriously head-injured or multisystem-injured children.

As discussed earlier, endotracheal intubation is almost always required for serious head injury. Hypoxemia and hypercarbia will increase cerebral blood flow and intracranial pressure, and must be avoided. By following arterial blood gases and adjusting ventilator settings accordingly, it is possible to keep arterial P_{O_2} and P_{CO_2} near normal levels unless the child has underlying pulmonary disease or injury. If the intracranial pressure continues to rise, more vigorous hyperventilation to decrease the P_{CO_2} to no lower than 25 torr may reduce the intracranial pressure to more acceptable levels.

Brain perfusion must be preserved by maintaining a normal intracranial pressure and a normal mean arterial pressure. Cerebral perfusion pressure is equal to mean arterial pressure minus intracranial pressure. An arterial catheter should be inserted for close monitoring of arterial pressure. More invasive cardiovascular monitoring is infrequently necessary. Urine output is also a useful indirect measure of cardiac output and is best measured with an indwelling bladder catheter.

A state of relative dehydration will decrease intracellular water and reduce intravascular pressure and fluid leakage from blood vessels in the brain. This can be accomplished by fluid restriction and diuretics to maintain serum osmolarity at 300 to 310 mOsm with normal cardiac output. Syndromes of inappropriate antidiuretic hormone secretion or diabetes insipidus may occur in children with serious head injury. Therefore, fluid balance and electrolyte status must be followed closely.

Seizures may occur following brain injury. Most children with serious injuries are treated with phenytoin either to control active seizures or for prophylaxis. Studies in adults have concluded that phenytoin is effective in preventing early posttraumatic seizures; however, studies in children are still in progress. Phenytoin is given as a dose of 15 mg/kg, infused at a rate of 1 mg/kg per min.

Seriously brain-injured children must be monitored in an intensive care setting. Cardiopulmonary monitors, noninvasive blood pressure monitors or indweling arterial catheters, and urinary catheters are commonly used. Direct intracranial pressure monitors are often utilized. The patient should be positioned with a 30° elevation of the head. Coordination of care for these children should involve neurosurgical, pediatric, and critical care physicians, most often in a tertiary care pediatric center.

The care for children with less serious injuries varies. Many children are admitted for observation with serial neurologic examinations. The majority of children who have only minor head injuries can be observed safely at home by an adult caretaker, with careful, detailed instructions to return if there is a change in condition. If a responsible caretaker cannot be identified, hospital admission to observe the child for the first 24 h is warranted.

PROGNOSIS

Although children have a greater likelihood of surviving a severe head injury and are more likely to recover from focal brain injury than adults, they may be more vulnerable than adults to long-term cognitive and behavioral dysfunction after diffuse brain injury. Early identification of neurobehavioral deficits is an important part of follow-up in children in significant head injury.

For a more detailed discussion, see Quayle KS: Head Trauma, Chap. 9, p. 58, in *Pediatric Emergency Medicine: A Comprehensive Study Guide.*

---

10 Evaluation for Cervical Spine Injuries

David M. Jaffe

There are approximately 200,000 persons with spinal cord injury in the United States. The annual direct medical costs of these injuries exceed $4 billion, and the estimated annual lost earnings are $3.4 billion. The emergency physician must maintain a high level of suspicion for possible cervical spine injury to avoid inadvertently causing or worsening cord damage by permitting unnecessary neck motion when a spine injury is present.

EPIDEMIOLOGY

There are approximately 1100 newly spine-injured children annually. The incidence of spinal cord injury in children has been estimated at 18 per million, as compared to 28 to 50 per million for Americans of all ages.

Motor vehicle–related injuries and falls are the leading situational causes of spinal cord injuries. Most sports-related injuries occur among adolescents and young adults.

The case fatality rate was reported as 59 percent in a carefully done epidemiologic study in California. All children in this study who sustained their cord injuries in auto-bicycle or auto-motorcycle crashes died, as did 76 percent of pedestrians struck by an automobile.

Brain injury is associated with 80 percent of traumatic deaths in children. A rough estimate of the incidence of brain injury in children is 1850 per million, approximately 100 times that of spine injury. Since head injury is so common among seriously injured children, the emergency physician will often need to evaluate for spine injury in the presence of head injury. Cervical spine injury should also be suspected in the multiply injured child with absent vital signs.

ANATOMY AND PHYSIOLOGY

The major anatomic components of the cervical spine consists of the base of the skull, and the first eight vertebrae, C1–C7 and T1 (Fig. 10-1). C1 and C2 have unique characteristics (Figs. 10-2 and 10-3). C1 is a ringlike structure, and the occiput articulates with articular facets on the lateral arches of C1. The odontoid process of C2 is articulated with the inner surface of the anterior arch of C1 and serves as a pivot point for rotation of C1 on C2. The atlantoaxial joint is stabilized by a transverse ligament. Other ligaments that connect the vertebrae are depicted in Fig. 10-4.

Because the vertebral column undergoes significant developmental changes in childhood, the patterns of injury also differ between children and adults. The biomechanical and anatomical features of the spine approach adult patterns between the ages of 8 and 10 years; however, the adult patterns of injury are not fully manifest until age 15 years. The pediatric spine is characterized

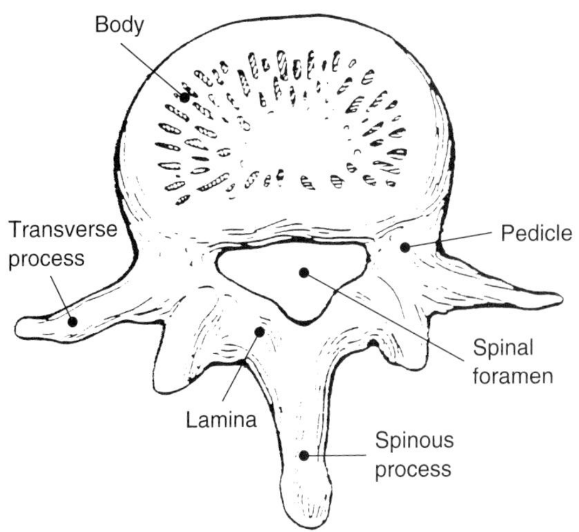

FIG. 10-1 Anatomy of a typical cervical vertebra. (From Bonadio WA: Cervical spine trauma in children: Part I. General concepts, normal anatomy, radiographic evaluation. *Am J Emerg Med* 11:158–165, 1993. Reproduced by permission of W. B. Saunders Company, copyright © 1993.)

by greater elasticity of ligaments, joint capsules, and cartilaginous structures; a relatively more horizontal orientation of facet joints and uncinate processes; and wedged anterior surfaces of vertebral bodies (Figs. 10-5 and 10-6). There is a greater vulnerability of the vertebral arteries to ischemia, thought to be due to relative instability of the atlantooccipital joint. The major differences in injury patterns between children and adults that result from these anatomic and biomechanical features are a predisposition for upper cervical spine injuries and for spinal cord injury without radiographic abnormality (SCIWORA). Fractures below the level of C3 account for only about 30 percent of spinal lesions among children less than 8 years old, whereas they account for 85 percent of those in adults. The reported prevalence of SCIWORA ranges from 1 to 67 percent, but most studies report SCIWORA in 25 to 50 percent of pediatric spinal cord injuries. Autopsy studies have revealed muscular and ligamentous disruptions, growth plate avulsions, epiphyseal separations, spinal instability, and subdural

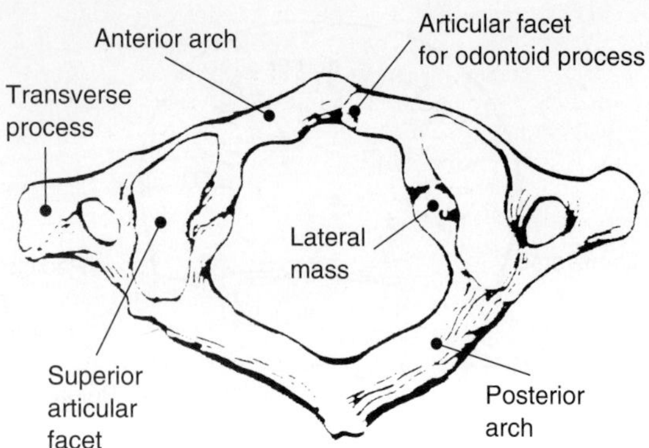

FIG. 10-2 Anatomy of C1 (atlas). (From Bonadio WA: Cervical spine trauma in children: Part I. General concepts, normal anatomy, radiographic evaluation. *Am J Emerg Med* 11:158–165, 1993. Reproduced by permission of W. B. Saunders Company, copyright © 1993.)

or epidural spinal hematomas. Some of these injuries can be unstable despite the absence of bony injury. Magnetic resonance imaging (MRI) may show some but not all of these abnormalities.

EVALUATION AND MANAGEMENT

Spinal cord injury should be suspected whenever there has been severe multiple trauma; significant trauma to the head, neck, or back; or any trauma associated with high-speed vehicular crashes or falls from heights. One useful mnemonic is to evaluate the "6 P's": pain, position, paralysis, paresthesia, ptosis, and priapism. Conscious children who are old enough to talk may complain of pain localized to the vertebrae involved. Head injury with diminished level of consciousness, intoxication, or significant injury of another part of the body may make the localization of pain unreliable. The patient's position may indicate a spine injury. A head tilt may be associated with a rotary subluxation of C1 on C2 or a high cervical injury. The prayer position (arms folded across the chest) may signify a fracture in the C4 to C6 area. Parasthesia, "pins and needles" sensation, or numbness or burning may sometimes seem inconsequential, but they should always be taken as potential indicators of spine injury. Some patients complain of an electric shock passing down the vertebral column, especially when attempting to flex the head. Horner syndrome (ptosis and a miotic pupil) suggests a cervical cord injury. Priapism is present only in about 3 to 5 percent of spine-injured patients but indicates that the sympathetic nervous system is involved. Absence of the bulbocavernosus reflex in the presence of flaccid paralysis carries a grave prognosis for recovery. To elicit the bulbocavernosus reflex, a finger is inserted into the rectum. Then the glans of the penis or the head of the clitoris is squeezed. A normal response is a reflex contraction of the anal sphincter.

There are also characteristic cord syndromes: spinal shock, Brown-Séquard, central cord, and anterior cord (Table 10-1). The anterior cord syndrome is associated with severe flexion injuries, especially teardrop fractures, in which a fragment of the fractured vertebral body is driven posteriorly into the anterior portion of the spinal cord (Fig. 10-7).

Upper extremity position and function may provide clues not only to the presence of a cervical cord injury but also to the level of injury. Patients with injuries at C5 can flex at the elbows but are unable to extend; with injuries at C6-C7, they can flex and

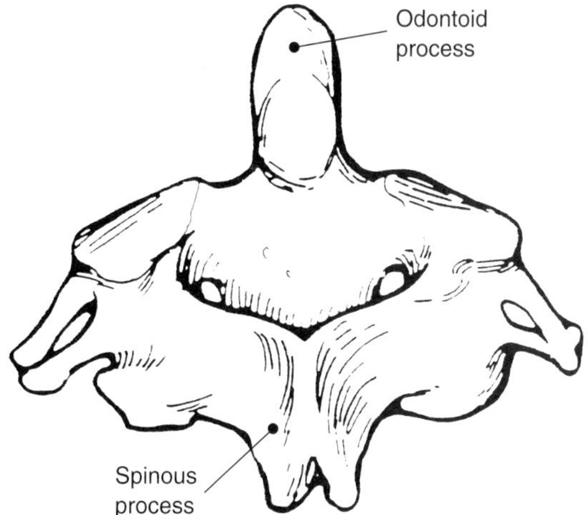

FIG. 10-3 Anatomy of C2 (axis). (From Bonadio WA: Cervical spine trauma in children: Part I. General concepts, normal anatomy, radiographic evaluation. *Am J Emerg Med* 11:158–165, 1993. Reproduced by permission of W. B. Saunders Company, copyright © 1993.)

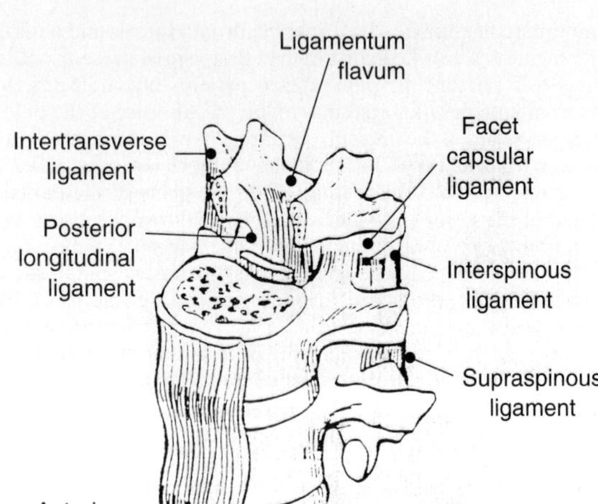

FIG. 10-4 Multilayered section of cervical spine anatomy with anterior and posterior compartments delimited by posterior longitudinal ligament. (From Bonadio WA: Cervical spine trauma in children: Part I. General concepts, normal anatomy, radiographic evaluation. *Am J Emerg Med* 11:158–165, 1993. Reproduced by permission of W. B. Saunders Company, copyright © 1993.)

extend at the elbows; and with injuries at T1, they have preserved finger and wrist flexion.

ANALYSIS OF RADIOGRAPHS

The standard screening series for adults consists of three views: the cross-table lateral view (CTLV), the anterioposterior (AP) view, and the open-mouth (OM) view to visualize C1, C2, and the atlantoaxial and atlantooccipital articulations. Because it is difficult to obtain in younger children, the value of requiring the OM view in cervical spine screening has been questioned. The Waters view can be substituted to allow visualization of the odontoid projected through the foramen magnum. The steps in evaluating the CTLV are presented in Table 10-2. On the AP view, symmetry of longitudinal alignment of vertebral bodies, facets, pillars, and spinous processes is assessed. On the OM view, the alignment of the atlantooccipital and atlanto-axial joints, the margins of the lateral arches of C1 with C2, and the position of the odontoid between the lateral arches of C1 are evaluated.

The sensitivity and specificity of the CTLV as compared to a "gold standard" of thin-layer computerized tomography in adults have been reported as 82 percent and 70 percent, respectively. Adding the AP and OM views increased sensitivity to 93 percent and specificity to 71 percent. The predictive value of negative tests was 97 percent for CTLV alone and 99 percent for three views. In a retrospective study of 59 spine-injured children, the AP and CTLV views were sufficient to identify all the children who had spine injuries, although other views were necessary to delineate the extent of injury fully.

Other imaging modalities are available when the standard views fail to delineate the cervical anatomy adequately or when clinical suspicion of a cervical spine injury is high despite a negative screening series. These include the swimmer's view, flexion and extension views, supine oblique views, thin-section tomography, computed tomography, and MRI. Some of these techniques, especially flexion

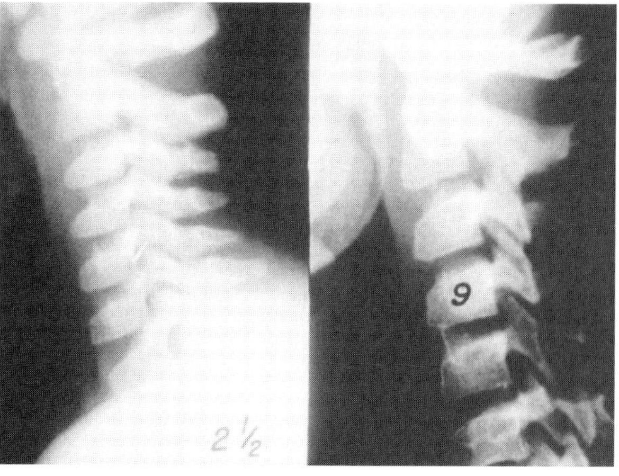

A *B*

FIG. 10-5 CTLV radiographs of 2-year-old (*A*) and 9-year-old (*B*) children, for comparison.

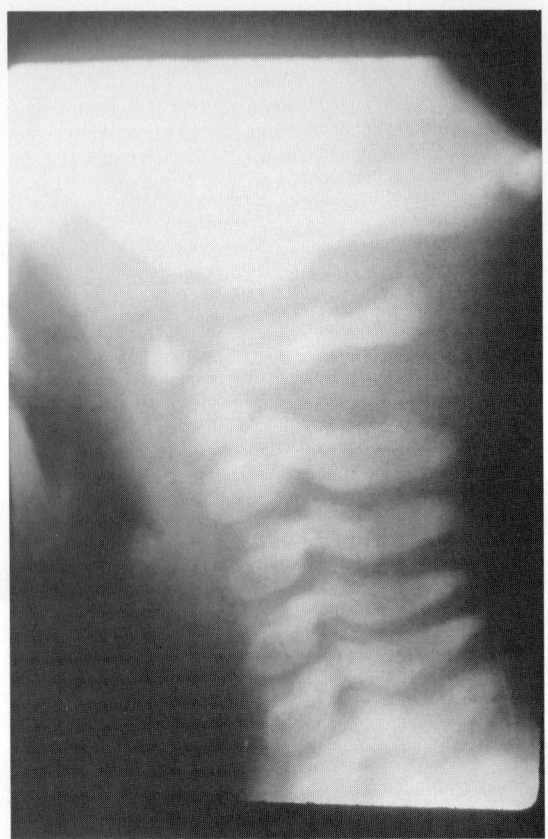

FIG. 10-6 CTLV radiograph of neonate.

and extension (stress) views, require positioning the head and neck out of neutral position and must be performed under careful medical supervision. It is unwise to perform stress imaging of the cervical spine in patients who have altered mental status or who are otherwise incapable of clear communication about the effect of such manipulation.

MANAGEMENT

A widely held view regarding the pathogenesis of spinal cord injury is that there are two phases of injury: direct damage that is largely irreversible and a second phase consisting of ischemia, hypoxemia, and tissue toxicity. Therefore, good trauma management is also good management for spinal cord injuries. The ABC (airway, breathing, circulation) mnemonic establishes priorities of care. Careful attention to oxygenation and ventilation is critical. Airway obstruction is common in trauma victims. The mandibular block of tissue often obstructs the airway of the supine, unconscious child. Also, the child may be unable to cough or expectorate to clear mucus, vomitus, blood, or other debris. Lifting the mandible with a jaw-thrust maneuver often improves the airway. At the same time, the emergency practitioner must be cognizant of the possibility of a cervical spine injury, which could be worsened by excessive motion of the spine. It is often possible to provide a jaw-thrust maneuver and stabilize the cervical spine at the same time (Fig. 10-8).

Most injured children arrive at the emergency department with good immobilization of the cervical spine. Stiff collars are now made for children as young as 1 year of age. However, the cervical collar alone does not provide adequate immobilization. Cloth tape or straps across the forehead and external orthoses, including a rigid backboard, are usually employed to complete the immobiliza-

TABLE 10-1 Cord Syndromes

Spinal shock	Brown-sequard

· Flaccid below level of lesion
· Absent reflexes
· Decreased sympathetic tone
· Autonomic dysfunction (including hypotension)
· Sensation may be preserved; if absent = total cord transection (poor prognosis)
	· Hemi section
	· Ipsilateral loss of
	  · motor function
	  · proprioception
	· Contralateral loss of sensation:
	  · pain
	  · temperature

Central cord	**Anterior cord**
· Diminished or absent upper extremity function · Preservation of lower extremity function · Associated with extension injuries	· Complete motor paralysis · Loss of pain and temperature sensation · Preservation of position and vibration · Associated with severe flexion injuries

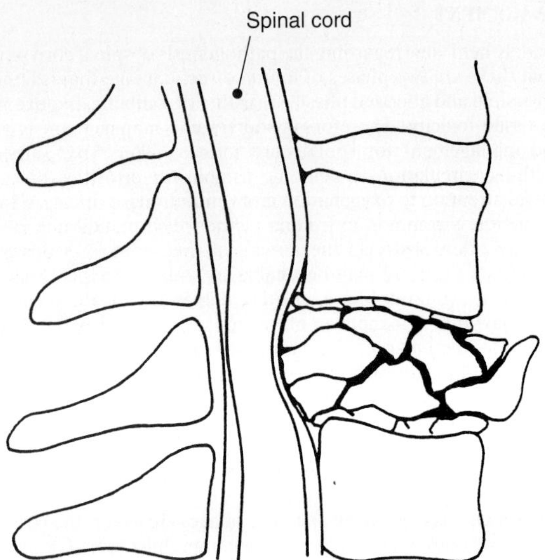

FIG. 10-7 Burst fracture with anterior cord compression.

tion (Fig. 10-9). Concern has been raised regarding the immobilization of younger children, who have disproportionately large heads. Use of a flat board may force the head forward, causing the neck to flex. The ideal backboard would be modified with a recess for the young child's occiput. Alternatively, the chest may be raised by an extra mattress pad or even a support made of sheets or towels (Fig. 10-10). Schafermeyer recently demonstrated that full supine immobilization reduced the forced vital capacity of healthy children between ages 6 and 15 years to 80 percent of unrestricted values (Fig. 10-11). Therefore, it is important for prehospital and emergency care providers to evaluate the effect of immobilization on ventilation, especially when a significant injury or embarrassment of the respiratory system is likely.

The spine-injured patient may have hypoventilation because of diminished diaphragmatic activity or because of intercostal muscle paralysis. Concomitant head or chest injuries and aspiration of gastric contents may further compromise ventilation. Therefore, supplemental humidified oxygen should routinely be provided.

Ventilation should be assisted whenever hypoventilation is suspected. If prolonged assisted ventilation is likely, the trachea should be intubated to facilitate ventilation, to protect the airway, and to reduce the hazards associated with gastric air accumulation.

Although the bag-mask technique will permit ventilation, its prolonged use increases the likelihood of aspiration of gastric contents. The emergency practitioner, therefore, often faces the need to intubate the trachea prior to completing full evaluation of the cervical spine. There have been a number of studies on cadavers and adult volunteers that suggest that some cervical mobility occurs with laryngoscopy. These studies also suggest that manual in-line stabilization is the best method for minimizing this mobility during laryngoscopy. In children, blind nasotracheal intubation is unreliable because it can be exceedingly difficult technically. Emergency cricothyrotomy is relatively contraindicated in young children because of the small size of the cricothyroid membrane and the likelihood of causing permanent tracheal damage. When intubation of the trachea is needed, both pediatric surgeons and emergency physicians have adopted the strategy of oral intubation with in-line manual stabilization, which can be

TABLE 10-2 Criteria for Clearing the Cervical Spine; Cross-Table Lateral View

1. All seven vertebral bodies must be clearly seen, including the C7 to T1 junction.
2. Evaluate proper alignment of the posterior cervical line and the four lordotic curves: anterior longitudinal ligament line, the posterior longitudinal ligament line, the spinolaminal line, and the tips of the spinous processes.
3. Evaluate the predental space (3 mm in adults, 4–5 mm in children).
4. Evaluate each vertebra for fracture and increased or decreased density (e.g., suggestive of a compression fracture, metatistic lesion, osteoporosis).
5. Evaluate the intervertebral and interspinous spaces. (Abrupt angulation of more than 11° at a single interspace is abnormal).
6. Evaluate if there is fanning of the spinous processes, suggestive of posterior ligament disruption.
7. Evaluate prevertebral soft-tissue distance. (Less than 7 mm at C2 and less than 5 mm at C3–C4 is considered normal.) Note: in children less than 2 years old, the prevertebral space may appear widened if it is not an inspiratory film.
8. Evaluate the atlantooccipital region for possible dislocation.

Source: From Van Hare RS, Yaron M: The ring of C2 and evaluation of the cross-table lateral view of the cervical spine. *Ann Emerg Med* 21:734, 1992. Reproduced by permission.

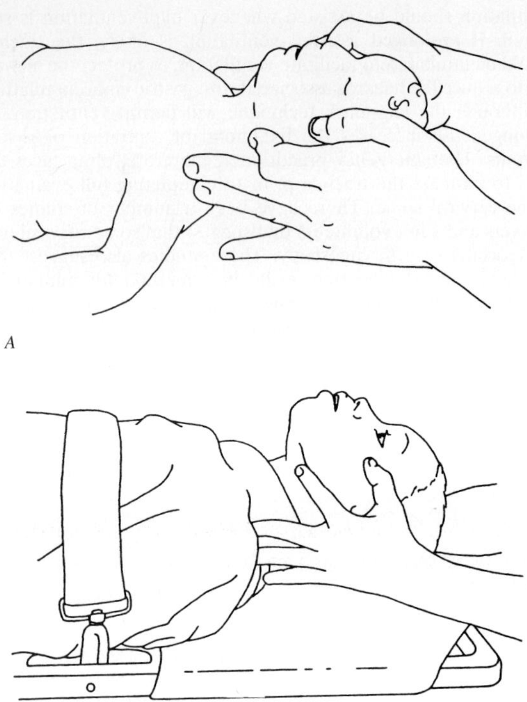

FIG. 10-8 Manual jaw thrust and cervical spine stabilization in infant (*A*) and child (*B*).

provided from either below or above the patient (Fig. 10-12). The rapid sequence induction technique is often indicated, especially when significant brain injury is suspected (see Chap. 9). The emergency physician should never fail to provide an adequate airway for an injured child in order to wait for the cervical spine to be cleared.

Hypotension may be secondary to either hypovolemic or spinal shock. A clue to differentiating these is the pulse. Often the pulse is slow in spinal shock, whereas it is rapid in hypovolemic shock. Adequate fluid (crystalloid, colloid, and blood) is administered to

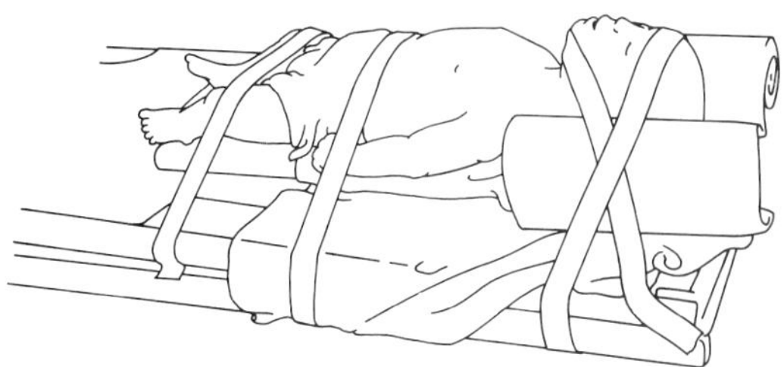

FIG. 10-9 A method for immobilization of an infant.

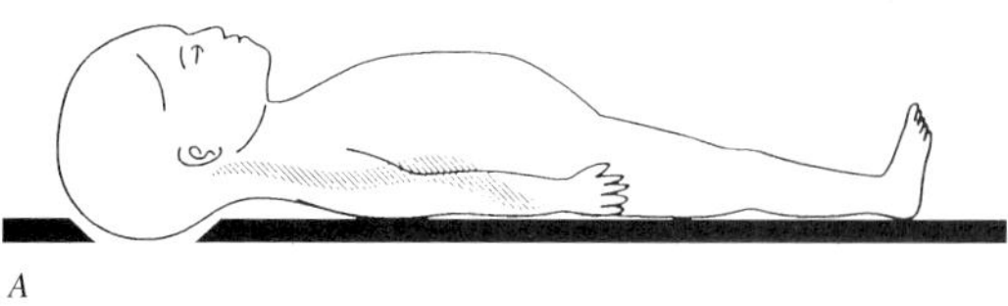

A

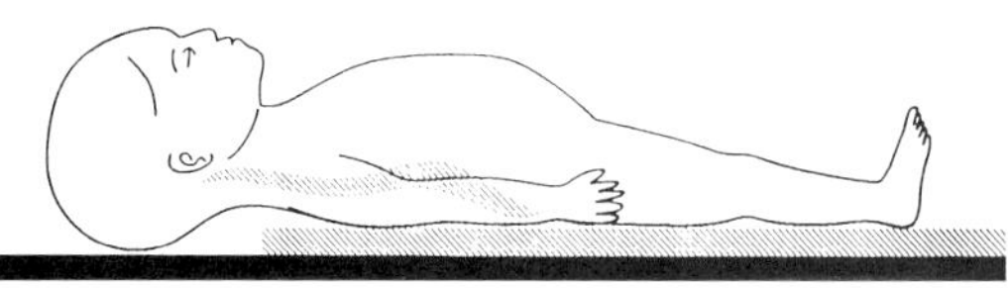

B

FIG. 10-10 Emergency transport and positioning of young children: backboard modifications for infants. *A*. Young child on a modified backboard that has a cutout to recess the occiput, obtaining a safe supine cervical positioning. *B*. Young child on a modified backboard that has a double-mattress pad to raise the chest, obtaining a safe supine cervical positioning. (From Herzenberg JE, Hensinger RN, Dedrick DK, et al: Emergency transport and positioning of young children who have an injury to the cervical spine: The standard backboard may be hazardous. *J Bone Joint Surg* 17:15, 1989. Reproduced by permission.)

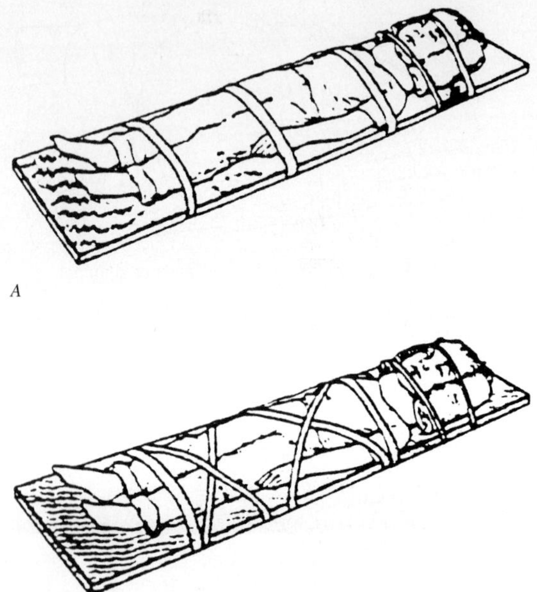

A

B

FIG. 10-11 Illustrations of (*A*) lateral- and (*B*) cross-strap techniques. (From Schafermeyer RW, Ribbeck BM, Gaskins J, et al: Respiratory effects of spinal immobilization in children. *Ann Emerg Med* 20:1018, 1991. Reproduced by permission.)

combat hypovolemia. In the case of spinal shock, atropine and vasopressors such as dopamine may be needed.

The patient with spinal shock may be more sensitive to temperature variations than other patients and may require warming or cooling if subjected to extreme environmental temperatures either at the scene or in transport. Care should be taken to protect areas of the body that may have lost sensation from hard, protruding objects, as these may cause skin necrosis, especially on long transports.

The results of the second National Acute Spinal Cord Injury Study were reported in May 1990. The investigators reported that high-dose methylprednisolone (30 mg/kg) followed by 5.4 mg/

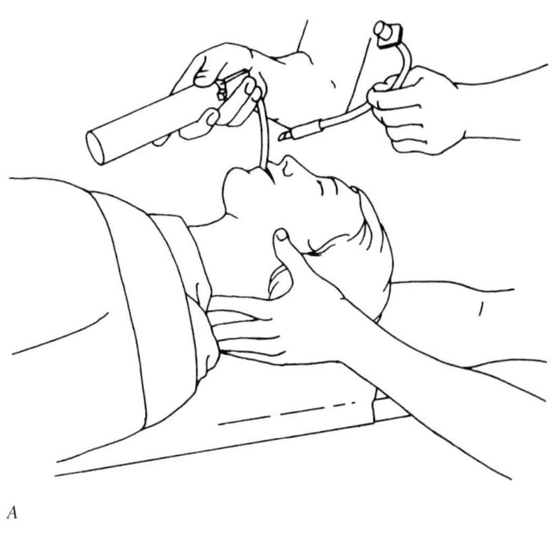

A

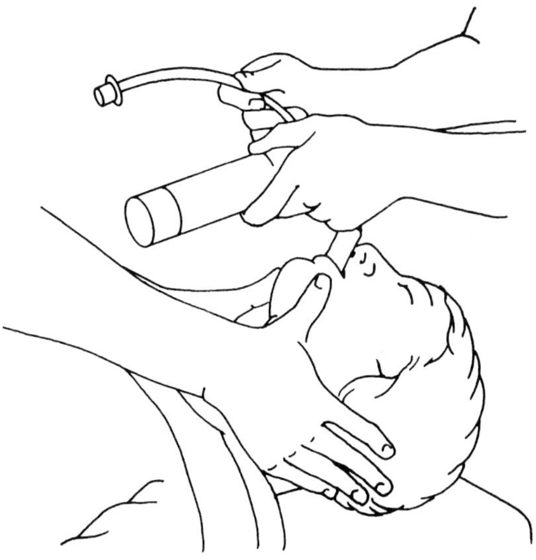

B

FIG. 10-12 In-line stabilization for endotracheal intubation: above (*A*) and below (*B*).

kg/h for 23 h, if given within 8 h of acute spinal cord injury, improved the neurologic recovery as compared to placebo or naloxone. Children under the age of 13 years were excluded from the study. The putative mechanism of action is the ability of the steroid at these doses to inhibit oxygen free radical–induced lipid peroxidation. New drugs with similar protective properties but with potentially fewer side effects are currently under investigation.

For a more detailed discussion, see Jaffe D: Evaluation for Cervical Spine Injuries, Chap. 10, p. 66, in *Pediatric Emergency Medicine: A Comprehensive Study Guide.*

---

11 Thoracic Trauma

Wendy Ann Lucid / Todd Brian Taylor

Serious thoracic injuries are relatively less common among children, and only 15 percent require more than simple chest tube placement. Nevertheless, children surviving to reach an emergency department require rapid evaluation and management.

The decision to discharge, admit, or transfer to a higher level of care must take into account the mechanism of injury as well as the clinical status of the child. Facility expertise and regional protocols will often dictate these decisions.

MECHANISM OF INJURY

Blunt Thoracic Trauma

Blunt trauma accounts for the vast majority of serious chest injuries in children. The National Pediatric Trauma Registry statistics reveal 83 percent blunt versus 15 percent penetrating trauma. Of the blunt injuries, more than three-fourths are caused by motor vehicle accidents and the remainder by falls and bicycle accidents. The mechanism of injury is important because of the recognizable patterns of trauma associated with particular types of injury.

Multisystem trauma mortality is 10 times higher when associated with chest injury and therefore serves as a marker of injury severity.

Penetrating Thoracic Trauma

Penetrating trauma accounts for only about 15 percent of thoracic trauma in childhood. Hemorrhagic shock from massive hemothorax accounts for the vast majority of deaths with gunshot wounds, whereas stab wounds more often lead to death from tension pneumothorax. Cardiac injury with associated tamponade and major vascular injuries are more often associated with death and account for the remainder of deaths associated with penetrating thoracic injuries.

Thoracic and concomitant abdominal injury should be suspected with penetrating trauma at or below the level of the sixth rib; when stomach contents, chyme, or saliva are recovered from the chest tube; or when the upper abdomen has been penetrated.

PATHOPHYSIOLOGY

Children are somewhat anatomically protected against blunt thoracic trauma, although it remains the second most common cause of traumatic death (15 percent), after head injury. This is due in part to the compliance of the cartilaginous ribs, which dissipates the force of impact. The same anatomic characteristics, however, can complicate pediatric thoracic trauma. Compliant ribs allow significant injury to occur to intrathoracic structures (heart, lungs, airways, and vessels) with little apparent sign of external trauma. The mobility of the mediastinal structures can lead to rapid ventilatory and circulatory collapse should tension pneumothorax develop.

Several factors lead to a decreased respiratory compensation in children sustaining thoracic trauma:

- Risk of hypoxia is increased by a proportionally larger oxygen consumption and smaller functional residual capacity of the lungs.
- Tachypnea is the chief physiologic response to hypoxia due to limited pulmonary compliance and greater chest wall compliance.
- Younger children are diaphragmatic breathers due to horizontally aligned ribs and immature intercoastal muscles. Multisystem trauma in which air swallowing results in gastric distension limits diaphragm excursion.

Pulmonary injuries are the most common result of thoracic trauma in children. Blunt trauma tends to cause pulmonary contusion, while penetrating trauma tends to cause lacerations, and either can cause hematoma. Pulmonary lacerations have a cavitary appearance on chest radiograph, but require surgical repair only when associated with ongoing bleeding or air leak.

MANAGEMENT OF THORACIC INJURY

A variety of conditions can cause airway compromise, all of which can be immediately life-threatening. The obvious causes include airway obstruction from foreign body, unconsciousness, and neck trauma. This section assumes that the "ABCs" of trauma resuscitation have already been initiated.

Diagnostic studies and treatment will vary depending on the clinical situation. With thoracic injury and as part of a multisystem trauma evaluation, an arterial blood gas, hemoglobin/hematocrit, supine chest radiograph, pulse oximetry, cardiac monitoring, supplemental oxygen, and two large-bore intravenous lines are a minimum. Upright posteroanterior chest radiograph is the mainstay in the evaluation of chest trauma and is most likely to facilitate the diagnosis of small apical pneumothorax or small hemothorax. The clinical situation may dictate immediate treatment without a radiograph or reliance on the more easily obtained supine portable chest radiograph initially.

SPECIFIC INJURIES AND MANAGEMENT

Pneumothorax

Traumatic pneumothorax is often associated with significant pulmonary injury that may not resolve as readily as a spontaneous pneumothorax and is more prone to expansion. There may be an associated hemothorax, and even a small pneumothorax can quickly develop into a more serious tension pneumothorax.

Conservative treatment includes placing a large-caliber, lateral, posteriorly directed chest tube for even a small traumatic pneumothorax. A small-caliber, lateral or anteriorly placed tube can be used to evacuate a pneumothorax if an underlying hemothorax is not suspected. Even with a very small pneumothorax, a chest tube is mandatory if the patient is to undergo mechanical ventilation (for surgery or respiratory failure) or emergency transport, particularly by air ambulance, as the changes in atmospheric pressure will tend to increase the pneumothorax. Less invasive treatment for isolated small traumatic pneumothorax includes observation for 6 h with a repeat chest radiograph. If there is no increase, the patient is discharged to return in 24 h for another chest radiograph. This approach may be reasonable in selected cases.

Hemothorax

The mechanism of injury for a hemothorax is similar to that for a pneumothorax. Injury to the intercostal or internal mammary vessels or lung parenchyma may result in significant bleeding. A chest tube is invariably necessary to evacuate the hematoma and observe for ongoing bleeding. Removal of the hematoma also prevents delayed complications due to fibrosis.

Massive Hemothorax

Massive hemothorax requires rapid evaluation and treatment. Clinical findings include decreased breath sounds and dullness to percussion on the affected side with or without obvious respiratory distress. Pneumothorax may coexist, presenting features of tension pneumothorax and hemothorax. Hypovolemic shock may be an early or late presenting feature. A hemothorax requires a minimum of 10 mL of blood per kilogram of body weight to be visualized on chest radiograph. Any abnormal fluid collection in the traumatic setting is assumed to be blood.

Fluid resuscitation should begin with crystalloid administered in the field. Preparation for transfusion should begin immediately, and blood is given as the clinical situation warrants. Critical patients may require type-specific or O-negative blood, while more stable patients may be able to wait for crossmatched blood or may not need a transfusion at all. Both vital signs and the amount of output from the chest tube should be taken into account in the decision on the need for immediate transfusion. Hemoglobin and hematocrit may not be useful initially, as rapid blood loss does not allow for equilibration and they may not accurately reflect current blood volume.

Thoracostomy tubes should be placed as soon as the diagnosis of massive hemothorax is suspected. A large-caliber (about as wide as the intercostal space) tube placed laterally and directed posteriorly to allow for drainage of blood should be used. Consideration should be given to using an autotransfusion chest tube collection system, as this may be the most rapidly available source for blood transfusion. A chest radiograph should be taken soon after chest tube placement to confirm the position of the tube and to ensure reexpansion of the lung.

The decision to proceed with a thoracotomy will generally be made by the consulting surgeon. Guidelines include an initial evacuated volume exceeding 10 to 15 mL of blood per kilogram of body weight, continued blood loss exceeding 2 to 4 mL/kg per hour or continued air leak. Aggressive blood resuscitation and continued chest tube suction is a reasonable alternative until a physician with expertise in emergency thoracotomy is available.

Open Pneumothorax

Open pneumothorax (sucking chest wound) is created when the chest wall is sufficiently injured to create bidirectional flow of air between the pleural cavity and the environment. The normal expansion of the lung is impossible due to the equalization of pressures between the chest cavity and the atmosphere.

Management of an open pneumothorax depends on the size of the defect in the chest wall and respiratory status. Breathing patients with small injuries such as knife or gunshot wounds can be treated by covering the chest wall defect with a sterile petroleum dressing and placing a thoracostomy tube through a fresh incision. Small chest wall defects will seal and heal spontaneously and generally do not require surgical repair.

Prehospital treatment may consist of placing a petroleum dressing with only three sides taped to create a flutter valve to decompress the chest and eliminate the sucking chest wound. This should be converted to a sealed dressing and thoracostomy tube as soon as possible. Chest wall defects too large to seal adequately (such as in a blast injury) or in patients who are not spontaneously breathing will require intubation and ventilatory support. Large wounds will often require urgent thoracotomy to repair the chest wall defect and underlying injuries.

Tension Pneumothorax

Tension pneumothorax occurs when the lung or airway develops a leak, allowing air to enter the pleural cavity without a means of escape. As the amount of air increases, the pressure against the mediastinal structures shifts the mediastinum toward the opposite side and causes vascular compromise of the heart and great vessels. The result is cardiac decompensation from mechanical impingement of blood flow and hypoxia from respiratory compromise. Immediate action must be taken to relieve the tension to avoid the patient's imminent demise.

Many patients with tension pneumothorax present with severe respiratory distress, decreased breath sounds and hyperresonance on the ipsilateral side. As the tension progresses, mediastinal shift leads to contralateral tracheal deviation and distended neck veins due to compromised venous return. Subcutaneous emphysema may dissect superiorly into the neck or inferiorly into the abdomen and scrotal area. Circulatory collapse with hypotension and narrow pulse pressure will result if the tension is not decompressed quickly.

Diagnosis of tension pneumothorax in children is complicated by false transmission of breath sounds. This can confuse the clinical diagnosis; however, uncertainty as to the side of the tension pneumothorax should not prohibit initiation of empirical treatment if the patient is deteriorating. Decompression of the other side should be done if immediate improvement is not seen with the initial needle or tube thoracostomy.

Definitive treatment is accomplished using a large-caliber (appropriate for age) thoracostomy tube placed laterally and directed posteriorly to allow drainage of the hemothorax that often accompanies tension pneumothorax in trauma patients.

Pulmonary Contusion

Pulmonary contusion may be caused by blunt trauma to the chest wall or by high-speed penetrating trauma, such as a gunshot or shotgun wound to the chest.

Initial symptoms range from minimal to severe respiratory distress, and the mechanism of injury may be the only early clinical indicator of pulmonary contusion. The initial chest x-ray may not show the classic patchy infiltrate, and physical examination may not reveal signs of pulmonary consolidation because of the contracted state of circulation often present in a multisystem injury.

Treatment is aimed at preventing hypoxia and respiratory failure. Search for concomitant injuries is prudent, as a force capable of causing a pulmonary contusion often causes other injuries as well. In the isolated case, however, supplemental oxygen and close monitoring are often all that is required. Those meeting the usual blood gas criteria for intubation require ventilation with positive end-expiratory pressure (PEEP) of 5 to 10 cmH_2O.

Spontaneous resolution of pulmonary contusion is the usual course unless acute respiratory distress syndrome (ARDS) supervenes. Excessive administration of crystalloid and aspiration of gastric contents are two factors that predispose to ARDS, and these should be avoided.

Traumatic Asphyxia

Traumatic asphyxia is not as ominous as its name would suggest. It is thought to arise from a severe blow to the chest that results in transmission of pressure through the superior vena cava into the capillaries of the head and neck. This results in a deep violet color of the skin in the head and neck and is associated with bilateral subconjunctival hemorrhages and facial edema. The patient's appearance can be quite dramatic, but the condition itself is benign. The significance is as a marker for associated thoracic trauma. About one-third of these patients will experience a loss of consciousness, but intracranial hemorrhages are rare. Transient and permanent visual disturbances can occur due to retinal hemorrhages and edema.

Traumatic Tracheal and Bronchial Disruption

Traumatic bronchial disruption is rare in children but is highly lethal. Half of these patients die within the first hour after injury.

It is caused by a shearing force associated with a crush injury to the chest or, more commonly, from severe compression of the chest against a closed glottis. The disruption nearly always occurs adjacent to the carina.

Ipsilateral tension pneumothorax is common, and a persistent large air leak or failure of reexpansion of the lung after chest tube placement may be seen. Hemoptysis may also be present. Bronchoscopy is diagnostic and should be considered in any patient with these findings.

Establishment of an airway can be complicated by disruption of the trachea or by a peritracheal hematoma distorting the airway anatomy. A surgical airway may be necessary and should be placed below the level of the disruption via tracheostomy or cricothyrotomy. Inability to ventilate once an airway has been established requires emergency thoracotomy.

TRAUMATIC ESOPHAGEAL RUPTURE

Traumatic esophageal rupture is virtually unknown in children. It occurs with severe blunt upper abdominal trauma in which stomach contents are forcefully injected into the esophagus against a closed cricopharyngeus muscle, causing a rupture of the esophageal wall into the mediastinum. Clinically similar to Boerhaave syndrome, it progresses rapidly to mediastinitis, sepsis, and death if unrecognized.

Clinical signs include pain and shock out of proportion to the apparent severity of injury. Traumatic esophageal rupture may be associated with a pneumothorax that drains stomach contents or bubbles equally and continuously throughout the respiratory cycle. Subcutaneous emphysema may dissect into the neck and be palpable. Although rarely heard in children, the Hamman sign (mediastinal crunch) may be appreciated, with a crunching sound accompanying heartbeats.

Urgent surgical repair with mediastinal drainage is required. Delayed definitive repair may be necessary with extensive esophageal damage, and temporary esophageal diversion may be required.

Traumatic Diaphragmatic Hernia

Traumatic diaphragmatic herniation in children is part of the "lap-belt" complex and occurs predominately on the left in the acute setting. Symptoms result not from the hernia itself but from herniation of abdominal contents into the chest. Right-sided herniation is often delayed, and symptoms appear after the abdominal contents have been drawn into the chest. The diagnosis may be obscured

TABLE 11-1 Chest Radiographic Findings in Traumatic Diaphragmatic Hernia

Acute herniation of abdominal contents
Bowel and/or stomach presenting within the chest cavity
Presence of the nasogastric tube in the chest
Diaphragmatic tear, but delayed herniation of abdominal contents
Unexplained elevation of the hemidiaphragm
Unrelieved acute gastric dilatation
Loculated subpulmonic hemopneumothorax
Presence of the nasogastric tube in the chest

until this event occurs, resulting in as many as 90 percent of these injuries being overlooked on the initial evaluation.

Signs may include contusions and abrasions of the upper abdomen and lower chest wall, but herniation can occur without external signs of trauma. Breath sounds may be decreased or bowel sounds heard on the affected side. Chest radiographic findings depend on the status of the abdominal contents and are outlined in Table 11-1.

Acute traumatic diaphragmatic herniation requires surgical repair. However, initial management should concentrate on assuring respiratory status and stabilizing other injuries. A nasogastric tube should be placed to decompress the stomach and intubation with positive-pressure ventilation performed if respiratory status deteriorates.

Rib Fractures

Rib fractures are uncommon in children. They can occur, however, with severe direct blows to the chest. Without a good trauma history and particularly if there are multiple fractures in various stages of healing, child abuse should be suspected. The posterolateral aspect of the ribs is the most susceptible to fracture for all causes.

No specific treatment is indicated. Simple rib fractures are well tolerated in children. Pain medication may be necessary, depending on the clinical setting.

Flail Chest

Severe blunt trauma to the chest wall can cause two or more fractures to the same rib. When this occurs in two or more adjacent ribs, the structural integrity of the chest wall is compromised, causing a "flail chest." Concomitant pulmonary contusion is common, and children tolerate this condition poorly.

Symptoms and signs include varying degrees of respiratory distress and hypoxia along with the classic "paradoxical" chest wall motion. Tenderness, bruising, and crepitus overlying the flail segments may also be present. Muscle spasm and respiratory splinting may obscure the clinical diagnosis by "stabilizing" and concealing the flail segments on physical examination.

Chest radiograph confirms the diagnosis and often reveals associated pulmonary contusion. Treatment is aimed at preventing hypoxia and respiratory failure and is dependent on the extent of injury and the child's ability to compensate. Supplemental oxygen and close monitoring may be all that is required. The addition of intercostal or epidural nerve block for pain control is preferable to narcotic analgesia because of the potential for respiratory depression. Those meeting the usual blood gas criteria for intubation require ventilation with PEEP of 5 to 10 cmH_2O. External stabilization with Hudson traction and towel clips has proved to be less effective than the above methods and should no longer be used.

Cardiac and Vascular Injuries

Cardiac and great vessel injuries are uncommon in children. The most common injury from blunt trauma is myocardial contusion and from penetrating trauma, pericardial tamponade. Traumatic aortic rupture is the most common great vessel injury and is probably underreported, as more than 50 percent of patients with this injury die before reaching the hospital. Injuries to other vessels are rare except in cases of penetrating trauma involving projectiles.

Cardiac Tamponade

Cardiac tamponade is a life-threatening condition that occurs when fluid (blood or serous fluid) fills the pericardial space to such an extent that venous return is compromised. The laceration of the pericardium can be quite small, and since the coronary arteries and cardiac chambers are at or near arterial pressure, the pericardial sack fills quickly with blood, causing normovolemic shock and death.

Clinical findings include the presence of a precordial wound, tachycardia, muffled or distant heart sounds, narrow pulse pressure, pulses paradoxus, and jugular venous distension (which may be absent in the presence of hypovolemia). Hypotension progressing to pulseless electrical activity (PEA) results unless prompt treatment is initiated.

The chest radiograph typically shows the classic "water bottle" cardiac silhouette. The electrocardiogram may show evidence of acute myocardial infarction if a coronary artery has been lacerated or may simply show tachycardia with extremely low voltage.

Bedside echocardiography is diagnostic and is usually available in trauma centers. However, treatment should not be delayed while waiting for an echocardiogram. Definitive treatment requires thoracotomy, pericardiotomy, and repair of the underlying injury. In certain circumstances, pericardiocentesis is both diagnostic and therapeutic. There is a high incidence of false negatives, however, so a negative pericardiocentesis does not necessarily rule out a hemopericardium. Repeated aspirations may be necessary, so the needle or plastic angiocath is generally left in place until a thoracotomy can be done.

In certain circumstances, an emergency thoracotomy may be necessary to open the pericardium, control the bleeding, and buy time until definitive treatment can be performed. Bleeding may be controlled by directly clamping the injured area. However, the coronary arteries are easily damaged even under the best of circumstances. Therefore, this should be performed only by those trained in these procedures.

Myocardial Contusion

The most common cause of myocardial contusion in adults is striking the steering wheel at moderate to high speed. This probably explains why this problem is rare and does not often cause significant morbidity in children.

Clinical diagnosis is often necessary, and the mechanism of injury is the most significant clue. Typically there is significant tenderness in the anterior chest or poorly localized chest pain. Electrocardiographic findings are less common in children, and tachycardia is the most common finding. Echocardiograms, while often diagnostic in adults, rarely show abnormalities in children. Myocardial enzymes may be diagnostic, but, as in adults, there usefulness and significance are difficult to ascertain. Radionuclide angiography may be useful in selected cases.

If the diagnosis of myocardial contusion is suspected, cardiac monitoring should be utilized and significant dysrhythmias treated appropriately. Children injured with a mechanism significant enough to potentially cause a cardiac contusion will usually be observed for other reasons, and cardiac monitoring should be instituted in these cases.

Traumatic Rupture of the Great Vessels

Rupture of great vessels is extremely rare in children, in part because of the higher elastin content in the connective tissue. However, children and adults with Marfan syndrome are more susceptible because of the intrinsic weakness of their un-cross-

TABLE 11-2 Chest Radiographic Findings in Aortic Injury

Widened mediastinum with obliteration of the aortic knob
Dilatation of the ascending aorta
Deviation of the trachea (as evidenced by the endotracheal tube) to the right
Deviation of the esophagus (as evidenced by the nasogastric tube) to the right
Evidence of first and/or second rib fracture
Apical pleural cap (blood at the apex of the lung, more commonly on the left)

linked collagen. Aortic disruption at the level of the ligamentum arteriosum is the most common injury in children and may be associated with aortic dissection. As in adults, morbidity and mortality are high with injuries to the great vessels.

Blunt Trauma

Aortic injury is most commonly caused by rapid deceleration, as seen in high-speed automobile accidents and falls from extreme heights. Greater than 50 percent of patients with such an injury die at the scene. Clinical signs include chest pain that may be localized to the anterior chest, back, or upper abdomen and a murmur radiating to the back (rarely appreciated). Chest radiographic findings (Table 11-2), although sometimes subtle, can increase suspicion for aortic injury.

Penetrating Trauma

The vena cava and pulmonary vessels are more commonly injured by penetrating trauma. The aorta is equally susceptible to these types of injuries, although it is injured more commonly with blunt trauma. A vascular injury should be considered when obvious wounds to the chest are associated with hypotension. Associated hemopneumothorax is invariably present.

With isolated venous or pulmonary vessel injuries, death is usually not immediate and patients often survive to surgery even with severe injuries. Hypovolemic shock is often present initially and may respond to fluid resuscitation, only to recur as the slow venous bleeding progresses.

Making the diagnosis can be difficult, especially in children, who are not prone to aortic injury. A widened mediastinum is the most common finding but, alone, does not confirm the diagnosis or necessarily warrant an angiogram. Computed tomography of the chest may confirm the diagnosis and is less invasive, but can miss small tears. In the appropriate clinical setting, early surgical consultation plus angiography is the diagnostic modality of choice for suspected aortic rupture or dissection.

Definitive treatment requires immediate surgical repair. Initial treatment should be directed toward the ABCs of trauma care and aggressive fluid resuscitation while the surgical team prepares for surgery. Hemopneumothorax should be treated with a thoracostomy tube unless an emergency department thoracotomy is indicated.

PROCEDURES

These procedures should be performed only by physicians trained in the techniques and for the appropriate indication.

Thoracostomy Tube Placement for Traumatic Pneumothorax or Hemothorax

The technique is identical for all ages except for the size of the tube and depth of insertion. Obviously a postinsertion chest radiograph should be obtained to confirm proper placement of the tube and reexpansion of the lung.

Pericardiocentesis

The technique for pericardiocentesis is the same for adults and children. The only essential equipment is a simple 20-mL syringe attached to an 18-gauge, 3 1/2-in. spinal needle. Special kits are available that include sterile drapes, large-bore angiocath needle, syringes, three-way stopcock, and an alligator clip with a wire for cardiac monitor guidance. Using cardiac monitor guidance, one will see atypical ventricular depolarizations as the needle is advanced toward the myocardium. For the subxyphoid approach, the needle is inserted just left of the xyphoid process, aiming for the sternal notch at a 30 to 45° angle. Variations of the technique abound, and experience is very helpful.

Emergency Department Thoracotomy

When cardiac arrest occurs after penetrating trauma, immediate thoracotomy may be lifesaving. Thoracotomy should be used only for cases where vital signs have initially been documented and arrest has supervened. Cardiac tamponade is another indication. Outcome with use in blunt trauma victims has been dismal. External chest compressions, along with attempts to control bleeding and restore blood volume, are a better alternative in the victim of blunt trauma. Cross-clamping of the distal thoracic aorta has been all but abandoned even in adults. Direct finger compression of the proximal abdominal aorta via laparotomy is as effective, with less potential for collateral injury.

LAW ENFORCEMENT

Most states require reporting of stab wounds, gunshot wounds, and assaults. Child abuse statutes also require reporting of suspected abuse. As we consider pediatric trauma, we should also consider our duty to report these injuries to the local authorities and to child protective services.

For a more detailed discussion, see Lucid WA, Taylor TB: Thoracic Trauma, Chap. 11, p. 75, in *Pediatric Emergency Medicine: A Comprehensive Study Guide.*

---

12 Abdominal Trauma

Wendy Ann Lucid / Todd Brian Taylor

Serious abdominal injuries are relatively common in childhood. Only 15 percent of these injuries require surgery. Abdominal trauma is the third leading cause of traumatic death behind head and thoracic injuries.

Penetrating abdominal trauma accounts for only about 15 percent of the total cases, and of these patients, 6 percent will die primarily from the penetrating wound. Blunt trauma accounts for 85 percent of pediatric abdominal trauma, with 9 percent of these dying primarily of other associated injuries.

Children are susceptible to different types of injuries than are adults. Blunt trauma due to automobile accidents causes more than half of the abdominal injuries in children and is also the most lethal. Penetrating injuries in the pediatric population are increasing. Gunshot and stab wounds are particularly common in young adolescents.

Management of pediatric abdominal trauma requires a coordinated effort between the emergency physician, trauma surgeon, and pediatric referral center.

PATTERNS OF INJURY

Motor Vehicle Crashes

Multisystem trauma, along with abdominal injury, is common when children are struck by an automobile. In countries where people drive on the right side of the road, left-sided injuries are most common, often resulting in splenic injuries. Presumably liver injuries would be more common in countries in which people drive on the opposite side of the road.

The "lap-belt complex" (bursting injury of solid or hollow viscera and, rarely, disruption of the diaphragm or lumbar spine) is characterized by ecchymosis across the abdomen and flanks (the Grey-Turner sign) and occurs in up to 10 percent of restrained children.

Bicycle Crashes, Sports Injury, and Falls

Handlebar injuries to the abdomen are particularly obscure, as most children show no serious sign of injury for hours to days after the impact. The mean elapsed time to onset of symptoms is almost 24 h, and as many as one-third of these patients are discharged home initially. The seriousness of these injuries is illustrated by a mean length of stay for those children requiring admission for a handlebar injury that exceeds three weeks.

Sports-related trauma typically produces isolated organ injury due to a direct blow to the abdominal area. It has been reported that falls from heights up to five stories have predominantly caused injury to other body systems.

Child Abuse

Significant abdominal injury occurs in only about 5 percent of child abuse cases, but it represents the second most common cause of death after head injury. The diagnosis can be obscured by the inherent delay in seeking treatment, the surreptitious nature of the visit, and the lack of external signs of trauma in up to one-half of these patients.

PATHOPHYSIOLOGY

Certain anatomic features predispose children to multiple rather than single injuries. Proportionally larger solid organs; a poorly muscled, protuberant abdomen; and flexible, thin ribs contribute to the increased incidence of significant abdominal injury and potential for hemorrhage. External signs of injury, abdominal tenderness, and absence of bowel sounds seldom give clues as to the need for surgery. Abdominal distension may be due to hemoperitoneum, peritonitis, or, most commonly, gastric distension, which can confound examination by masking or mimicking serious abdominal injury or bleeding. Gastric dilatation results from crying and air-swallowing. Severe dilatation can result in respiratory compromise due to interference with diaphragm motion, gastric aspiration, or vagal dampening of the normal tachycardic response. In children, the primary response to decreased cardiac output is increased heart rate; therefore vagal dampening can lead to precipitous circulatory collapse in the presence of hypovolemia.

MANAGEMENT

General Principles

In the evaluation and treatment of abdominal injuries, a team approach that includes the emergency physician, trauma surgeon, anesthesiologist, and surgical subspecialists is ideal. In reality, many times the emergency physician is the *only* physician initially and must approach the injured child in a systematic way, utilizing consultants appropriately and expeditiously. Abdominal injuries resulting from blunt trauma rarely require surgical intervention. Penetrating trauma frequently requires surgery. All unstable patients need immediate surgical consultation.

The basic principles of trauma evaluation and resuscitation are followed in all cases of abdominal trauma. Evaluation of the abdomen is included in both the primary and secondary surveys. The following are particularly important interventions:

- Insertion of a nasogastric tube to decompress the stomach and to check for blood or bile
- Insertion of a Foley catheter to check for blood and urinary retention
- A rectal examination to check for blood, prostate position in males, and rectal tone
- Keep the child NPO considering possible surgery or the development of paralytic ileus

Blood should be obtained for typing and crossmatching, CBC, serum amylase, and liver transaminases.

The mechanism of injury is important and will guide the secondary survey and ordering of specific tests and procedures. With penetrating injury, it is important to log-roll the patient to inspect the posterior torso for additional wounds. External injuries such as abrasions, lacerations, bruising, and characteristic markings such as tire tracks and seat-belt marks should be noted.

Penetrating Abdominal Trauma

The diagnosis and treatment of penetrating abdominal injuries in children does not differ greatly from that in adults, and the initial management is not dependent on identifying any specific injury.

Penetrating wounds between the nipples and the groin potentially involve the peritoneal cavity and should be considered contaminated, with potential for infection. Surgical evaluation, debridement, and possibly exploration, along with broad-spectrum intravenous antibiotics, are necessary except in the most minor wounds. At a minimum, with any *significant* penetrating abdominal trauma, a nasogastric tube and Foley catheter should be placed, and an upright posteroanterior chest radiograph with a lateral view obtained, if possible; supine, upright, and cross-table abdomen radiographs should also be obtained. A "one-shot" intravenous pyelogram is required if there is significantly deep penetration with a stab wound and in all gunshot wounds.

Gunshot wounds to the abdomen require immediate exploration. Vascular injuries are the greatest threat with stab wounds. Commonly injured vessels include the aorta, inferior vena cava, portal vein, and hepatic veins. However, stab wounds enter the peritoneal cavity only one-third of the time, and only one-third of these require a visceral repair. Local exploration may therefore be possible to rule out peritoneal penetration in minor stab wounds. This conservative management can be entertained if the patient meets the following criteria:

- No sign of shock or peritonitis with observation for 12 to 24 h
- No blood in the stomach, rectum, or urine
- No evidence of free abdominal or retroperitoneal air on x-ray
- No history or evidence of bowel evisceration
- Close observation with surgical consultation

Blunt Abdominal Trauma

Both isolated abdominal and multisystem trauma present a challenge in the pediatric patient, where information is inherently difficult to obtain. For the emergency physician, the key to management is suspecting the diagnosis and obtaining appropriate studies and consultation. Minor mechanisms (such as falling 2 ft to the ground from a hammock) can result in significant splenic injury with minimal symptoms. Therefore, emergency department observation, repeated abdominal examinations, and vital signs are warranted even with minimal evidence of injury.

A supine (or preferably upright) posteroanterior with lateral chest radiograph and a supine abdomen/pelvis radiograph can give

TABLE 12-1 Abdominal Radiograph Clues in Abdominal Trauma

A ground-glass appearance of the abdominal cavity may suggest intraperitoneal blood or urine.
Medial displacement of the lateral border of the stomach as evidenced by the nasogastric tube suggests splenic laceration or hematoma as the enlarged spleen pushes the stomach aside.
Obliteration of the psoas shadow or renal outline and fracture of the lower ribs suggest renal trauma.
Bleeding from the short gastric vessels gives the fundic mucosa a "sawtooth" appearance.
With a nasogastric tube in place, the relative lack of gas in the distal small intestine may suggest a duodenal or proximal jejunal hematoma.
Air injected via the nasogastric tube may increase the chance of detecting a pneumoperitoneum indicative of perforated viscus.

important clues to the diagnosis of abdominal injury (Table 12-1). Hemoglobin and hematocrit determinations are seldom useful early in the evaluation and treatment and are better used for comparison after serial determinations. However, if the initial hematocrit is less than 30 percent with other signs of impending shock, this suggests significant hemorrhage. An initial hematocrit of less than 24 percent is associated with a high mortality, and transfusion should be initiated.

Computed Tomography

Computed tomography (CT) has eliminated much of the difficulty surrounding the diagnosis of abdominal injuries (Table 12-2). It is useful for evaluation of liver, kidney, spleen, retroperitoneum, and (to a lesser extent) gastrointestinal injuries. Use of oral and intravenous contrast media increases the sensitivity of the study, but oral contrast has obvious problems with suspected abdominal injuries, and it takes up to 20 to 30 min to become adequately distributed. As with all suspected intestinal perforations, a water-soluble oral contrast medium should be used.

To avoid unnecessary delay in definitive treatment, specialized studies should be ordered in consultation with the trauma surgeon in the stable trauma patient.

Diagnostic Peritoneal Lavage

Close observation, serial physical examinations, and particularly abdominal CT are utilized to the virtual exclusion of diagnostic peritoneal lavage (DPL) in pediatric patients. However, DPL may still be useful if these other modalities are unavailable or if the child must undergo immediate general anesthesia for other injuries. Under these circumstances, DPL can often be performed in the operating suite. The usefulness of DPL remains questionable. It is neither organ- nor injury-specific, it cannot reliably assess retroperitoneal injury, and, in children, the decision to operate for liver or splenic injuries is not based on the amount of intraperitoneal blood. In addition, the introduction of air and fluid into the abdomen and the resulting peritoneal irritation make subsequent radiographic and physical examinations more difficult.

The technique for DPL in children is similar to that for adults, although a small supraumbilical incision to avoid the bladder is preferred over the usual infraumbilical approach.

Abdominal Ultrasound

Abdominal ultrasound is useful when CT is not available and is most sensitive for the evaluation of pancreatic injuries and for detecting intraperitoneal hemorrhage. Bedside ultrasound is becoming more readily available in trauma centers and may further reduce the need for DPL.

Nuclear Scans

Nuclear scans are not typically used for the acute abdominal injury but can be useful as a follow-up for liver or splenic injuries previously diagnosed by CT.

SPECIFIC INJURIES AND MANAGEMENT

Solid Organs

Spleen

The spleen ranks first among solid abdominal organs for major hemorrhage and significant injury in blunt pediatric trauma and second only to the liver in lethal injury. A right-sided blow or fall can cause a contrecoup splenic injury. Mononucleosis, common in children, can result in splenic enlargement and predispose to splenic rupture. Patients with this condition should be warned about contact sports or any activity that could cause a blow to the abdomen until the spleen has returned to normal size—at a minimum, 4 to 6 weeks.

Although diffuse abdominal pain may be the presenting complaint, typical findings with splenic injury are left upper quadrant abdominal pain radiating to the left shoulder associated with palpa-

TABLE 12-2 Comparison of Techniques for Evaluation of Abdominal Trauma

	Abdominal CT	Diagnostic peritoneal lavage	Abdominal ultrasound
Indication	Relatively stable patient Multiple trauma or major thoracic or orthopedic (pelvic) injury Physical findings or a mechanism suggesting possible abdominal injury Unexplained hypotension Hematuria CNS injury, spinal injury, or mental status alteration precluding serial abdominal examination Declining hematocrit or unaccountable fluid and blood requirements	Relatively unstable patient otherwise the same as for CT	Evaluation of pancreatic injury and intraabdominal fluid (presumably blood) May also reveal other intraabdominal injuries when CT is not readily available.

Advantage	Relatively noninvasive High sensitivity and specificity Evaluates multiple organ systems simultaneously	May be performed on a patient who is relatively unstable or who needs to undergo urgent general anesthesia for other reasons Easily and rapidly performed	More readily available than CT in some locales Can be used at the bedside for a "quick look" to evaluate peritoneal fluid/blood
Disadvantage	Generally requires oral and intravenous contrast Time delay	Unless grossly positive, lab results may delay definitive treatment Neither organ- nor injury-specific Cannot assess retroperitoneal injury Decision to operate is not generally based on the amount of peritoneal blood Introduction of air and fluid into the abdomen may alter future diagnostic tests Local peritoneal irritation may alter serial abdominal exams	Not as sensitive as CT

ble tenderness on examination. Significant tenderness in the left upper abdomen and/or splenic enlargement should prompt surgical consultation and consideration of a CT scan. Frank splenic rupture may lead to shock and posttraumatic cardiac arrest. Persistent unexplained leucocytosis or hyperamylasemia also suggests splenic injury. Abdominal CT is the study of choice to identify splenic injury.

Once a splenic injury has been identified in the stable patient, management is focused on salvaging the spleen. The thick, elastic splenic capsule in children and the usual transverse orientation of lacerations parallel to the vessels commonly results in spontaneous cessation of bleeding and allows nonoperative management in most cases.

Conservative management includes initial hospitalization for 7 to 10 days of bed rest followed by a regimen of limited activity. Although spontaneous healing of splenic lacerations and subcapsular hematomas occurs in the overwhelming majority of cases, delayed spontaneous rupture can occur at any time, most commonly on the third to fifth day. The commitment to conservative management includes close observation and frequent examination.

Children who develop hypotension not responsive to volume resuscitation obviously require surgery to control bleeding. When surgery is required for persistent bleeding, all efforts are made to salvage as much spleen as possible. The results of splenorrhaphy or partial splenectomy have been as good as the results of nonoperative management. There is a marked increase in infection and a 65-fold increase in lethal sepsis in children with splenectomy, particularly with encapsulated organisms (*Streptococcus pneumoniae, Haemophilus influenza, Neisseria meningitides, Staphylococcus aureus,* and *Escherichia coli*). The pneumococcal and *H. influenza* (HIB) vaccines should be given in any patient undergoing partial or complete splenectomy even though the antibody response may be inconsistent and impermanent.

Liver

The liver ranks second among solid abdominal organs for major hemorrhage and significant injury, but it is the most common source of *lethal* hemorrhage. Mortality from serious liver injuries may be as high as 10 to 20 percent. Computed tomography has revolutionized the diagnosis of liver injury and accounts for the increased recognition of this problem.

The mechanisms of injury are those common to splenic trauma. Symptoms depend largely on the extent of injury and range from nonspecific, diffuse abdominal pain to posttraumatic cardiac arrest. Significant tenderness in the right upper abdomen and/or liver enlargement should prompt surgical consultation and consideration of a CT scan.

Children with liver injuries who are not in shock or who respond to volume resuscitation rarely require surgery to control bleeding. Nonoperative management is not without complication, however. Those requiring late laparotomy have transfusion requirements greater than 50 percent of total blood volume (TBV) during the first 24 h after injury, and bleeding into the biliary tract (hematobilia) is not uncommon. Conservative management includes careful monitoring of vital signs, serial abdominal examinations, and serial hematocrit measurement.

Large stellate liver lacerations and subcapsular hematomas that have eroded through Glisson's capsule rarely stop bleeding without surgery. In preparation for surgery, circulating blood volume should be restored, since rapid hemorrhage can occur during surgery as blood clots are evacuated during repair.

Pancreas

The pancreas is in a fixed position anterior to the vertebral column and is vulnerable to a direct blow to the upper central abdomen, as seen with bicycle handlebar injury.

Traumatic pancreatitis without major pancreatic injury is most common, followed by pancreatic hematomas and (rarely) transection of the body or duct. Pancreatic transections often lead to pancreatic pseudocyst formation within 3 to 5 days and result in chronic intermittent attacks of abdominal pain, nausea, vomiting, and weight loss.

Computed tomography may help identify severe pancreatic injury and reveal evidence of pancreatic edema as an early indication of trauma.

Simple traumatic pancreatitis is treated similarly to other types of pancreatitis, with bowel rest, nasogastric suction, intravenous fluids, and pain medication. Severe pancreatic injury will typically require surgical drainage with repair or partial resection of the pancreas. Pancreatic pseudocyst treatment involves 6 to 8 weeks of total parenteral nutrition followed by a surgical drainage procedure.

Hollow Organs

Hollow visceral organs are injured in only 1 to 5 percent of children with blunt abdominal trauma. Of those requiring laparotomy, up to 16 percent may have such injuries. Perforations of the duodenum and proximal jejunum are the most common and are usually associated with a "lap-belt" or bicycle handlebar injury. Penetrating trauma is more obvious and more likely to show early signs of injury, such as free air.

Without obvious evidence of free air on a radiograph, the diagnosis of a perforated viscus in blunt trauma can be difficult. Tenderness may initially be localized and may slowly worsen over 6 to 12 h, accounting for the time necessary for peritonitis or obstruction to occur. Abdominal CT is not particularly sensitive for these injuries, and repeated physical examinations remain the most reliable indicator of enteric disruption. Surgical consultation for observation or treatment should be obtained early in the management of these patients. Once the suspected diagnosis of perforated abdominal viscus has been made, treatment is straightforward, with laparotomy to repair the injury. Most injuries can be repaired primarily; however, colonic perforations often require a diverting colostomy.

Intramural hematomas of the duodenum or jejunum can cause symptoms of intestinal obstruction, with pain, bilious vomiting, and gastric distension. The diagnosis can be made with ultrasound or an upper GI series, which reveals the "coiled spring sign." This problem rarely requires surgery. It may cause traumatic pancreatitis with involvement of the ampulla of Vater. Treatment is conservative and supportive, including nasogastric suction and parenteral nutrition for up to 3 weeks.

For a more detailed discussion, see Lucid WA, Taylor TB: Abdominal Trauma, chap. 12, p. 84, in *Pediatric Emergency Medicine: A Comprehensive Study Guide.*

---

13 Genitourinary and Pelvic Trauma

Wendy Ann Lucid / Todd Brian Taylor

The incidence of urinary tract injury in children with multiple trauma is second only to injury of the central nervous system. Most serious genitourinary (GU) injuries result from motor vehicle and pedestrian crashes, but penetrating injuries continue to increase with the overall increase in violence. Sports-related injuries and child abuse are less frequently recognized mechanisms.

Hematuria heralds the possibility of injury to the kidneys, ureter, bladder, or urethra. As in all major trauma, management of GU injuries begins with the basics of trauma assessment and life support. Care must be taken to revisit the GU system after more critical systems have been addressed.

GENERAL MANAGEMENT PRINCIPLES

Blunt Genitourinary Trauma

After stabilization of the patient's vital functions, specific organ systems are evaluated. The definitive diagnosis of blunt GU injuries may be difficult and demands a systematic approach regardless of whether the patient presents with multiple trauma or isolated injuries to the abdomen, pelvis, or flank. Complications of GU trauma include hemorrhage, urinary extravasation, renal parenchymal damage, infection, delayed hypertension, and renal dysfunction. Many other organ systems take precedence over the GU system initially, but these potential injuries must be considered in the overall evaluation.

During the physical examination, attention to the abdomen, flank, pelvis, and genitalia will provide clues to possible GU injuries. As in all trauma patients, the genital and rectal examination (looking for blood at the meatus and a high-riding prostate indicative of urethral injuries) should precede the insertion of a Foley catheter.

The usual trauma blood panel, chest radiograph, anteroposterior pelvic film, and abdominal flat plate utilized in the evaluation of the multiply injured patient may give clues to possible GU injuries. The abdominal radiograph may show loss of the psoas shadow, indicating retroperitoneal blood; scoliosis with concavity to the side of injury; or lower rib or transverse process fractures, all of which are associated with renal trauma. The location of the injury is also a clue to the potential site of injury. Urethral injury may present with blood at the meatus or a high-riding prostate; a pelvic fracture may herald a bladder injury. A retrograde urethrogram to evaluate the urethra and, if it is disrupted, a suprapubic catheter may be needed.

A urinalysis should be performed on all major trauma patients as well as those suspected of having an isolated renal injury. If a urine dipstick is positive for blood, a microscopic urinalysis should be performed. Although hematuria heralds the possibility of GU trauma, it may also be present without significant injury if there is an underlying renal malformation. Hematuria may also be *absent* with renal pedicle injury. Therefore, there is no direct correlation between the degree of hematuria and the severity of renal injury. Indications for further GU evaluation include gross or microscopic

TABLE 13-1 Indications for Diagnostic Evaluation of the Genitourinary Tract in Pediatric Trauma

Blunt Trauma
Multiple trauma
Gross or microscopic hematuria (>20 RBCs/high-power field) or shock
Palpable flank mass, hematoma, ecchymosis, or tenderness
Lower rib, thoracic, or lumbar spine fractures
Deceleration injuries (motor vehicle crash or fall from a height) with crush injuries to the abdomen or pelvis with or without other signs
Pelvic fracture
Penetrating Trauma
Any injury that can reasonably be expected to injure the GU tract
Anticipated surgery for lower chest, abdomen, or pelvis for gunshot or deep stab wound

hematuria [>20 RBC/high-power field (hpf) in children versus >50 RBC/hpf in adults]; abdominal or flank pain, hematoma, mass, flank ecchymosis (Grey Turner sign), or periumbilical ecchymosis (Cullen sign); and penetrating trauma that could reasonably be expected to injure the GU system (Table 13-1). Urine output should be monitored to assure renal perfusion and to exclude bilateral renal artery occlusion or other obstructing process.

Finally, sexual and physical abuse should be considered when evaluating perineal injuries. These injuries may result from the caretaker's ignorance of proper toilet training or from overt abuse. In particular, burns to the perineum, inconsistent mechanism of injury, evidence of previous injury, or the child's own history should prompt further investigation and report to child protective services and local authorities.

Penetrating Genitourinary Trauma

Penetrating trauma between the nipples and perineum requires at least a preliminary "one-shot" intravenous pyelogram (IVP) prior to surgery to rule out GU injuries (Table 13-1).

DIAGNOSTIC STUDIES

Computed Tomography

A computed tomography (CT) scan of the abdomen with intravenous contrast is an excellent study for evaluation of the kidneys, with an accuracy of 98 percent. Nonionic contrast media should be considered in patients less than 1 year of age, those with a history of previous reaction to contrast, unstable patients, and those with underlying renal disease, diabetes, sickle cell anemia, heart or lung disease, dehydration, or other significant medical conditions. Use of nonionic media may, however, lead to overestimation of the amount of urinary extravasation, and results of such studies should not be used as absolute criteria for surgery. In addition to identifying specific renal injuries, CT provides information about function and may be more valuable than arteriography when vascular injuries are suspected. A simple IVP may be more appropriate for isolated renal injuries without shock or significant physical findings (Fig. 13-1, Tables 13-1 and 13-2).

Intravenous Pyelography

An intravenous pyelogram (IVP) of the kidneys, ureter, and bladder ("scout KUB") followed by injection of dye (1 to 2 mL/kg, depending on the agent used) and films at 1, 5, and 10 min makes up the typical routine emergency IVP. A "one-shot IVP" at 5 min can be substituted in unstable patients in order to document two functioning kidneys. These limited IVPs often do not correlate well with the findings at operation, and a more formal IVP is more appropriate in patients who do not require close observation.

Other Procedures

If CT is unavailable or does not clearly define the injury, other procedures may be useful. Renal ultrasound is less accurate than CT but may be useful for following perirenal hematomas or to limit radiation exposure in pregnancy. Retrograde pyelography is useful for delineating ureteropelvic disruption if the IVP is indeterminate. Renal angiography has been virtually replaced by CT and digital subtraction angiography, which are less invasive. Radioisotope renal scanning can be used as an alternative for the evaluation of renovascular injuries in patients who are allergic to ionic contrast media.

SPECIFIC INJURIES AND MANAGEMENT

Kidney

Pathophysiology

The kidneys are the second most commonly injured solid organ in blunt pediatric trauma. The substantial force required to cause significant renal injury frequently results in associated abdominal injuries, which may cause hypovolemic shock. Shock due to isolated renal fracture is uncommon.

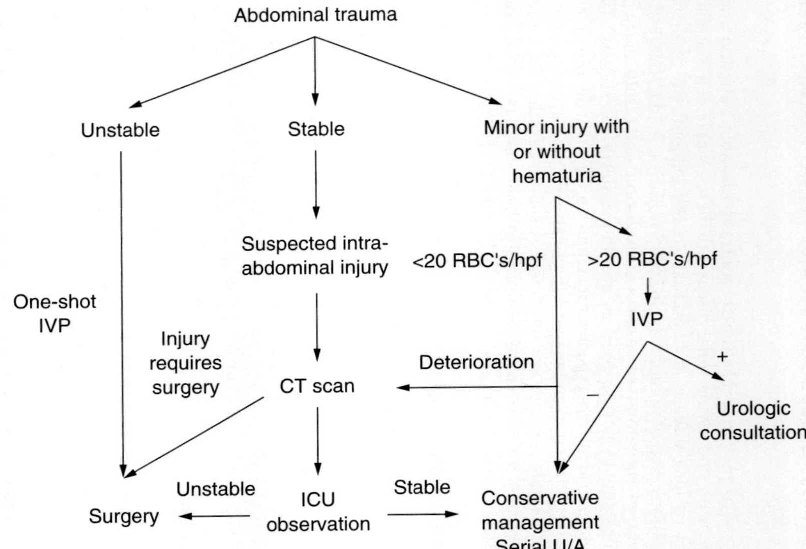

FIG. 13-1 Renal evaluation after trauma.

TABLE 13-2 Abdominal Computed Tomography versus Intravenous Pyelography

Patients Meeting Criteria for GU Evaluation	
Abdominal CT	IVP
Stable patient	Unstable patient
Multiple trauma	Isolated GU trauma
IVP equivocal or severe injury requiring better definition	Penetrating wounds Suspected ureteral injury

Management

Blunt trauma patients without significant concomitant injuries who present with microscopic hematuria (less than 20 RBC/hpf in children or 50 RBC/hpf in adults) in the absence of shock require only a follow-up urinalysis within 48 h to ensure resolution of the hematuria. If bleeding persists, a formal evaluation should be performed. More significant bleeding, and certainly gross hematuria, requires urgent investigation. Significant renal injuries or suspicious mechanisms of injury require hospital observation to detect potential progression or associated injuries (Table 13-3 and Fig. 13-1).

Serious renal bleeding occurs in less than 3 percent of cases and requires immediate surgery. Serious bleeding may be due to direct communication between the renal arterioles and calyx, injury to the renal pedicle, expanding retroperitoneal hematoma, severe kidney laceration causing extensive extravasation, and frank transection of a portion of the main collecting system. Less serious injuries, which may require delayed surgical intervention, include retroperitoneal extravasation secondary to communication between the renal calyx and the perinephric space and persistent or infected "urinoma" resulting from a small urinary leak. There is considerable controversy regarding management of grade IV and V injuries (Table 13-3). Ironically, efforts to save the injured kidney with early surgical intervention usually result in nephrectomy. Therefore, many urologists recommend conservative management unless there is a definite surgical indication. Associated injuries may require laparotomy in up to 89 percent of the cases. Management of moderate and severe renal injuries must be individualized, and early consultation with the appropriate surgeon is important to determine the best course of action.

Trauma to anomalous kidneys (hydronephrosis, tumor, horseshoe kidney, polycystic kidney disease) can present with hematuria

TABLE 13-3 Classification of Renal Injury

Grade	Minor renal injury	Observation, 85% of renal injuries
I	Contusion	Parenchymal injury without fracture of the parenchyma or capsule as evidenced by delayed or underfilling of the renal calyces on IVP
II	Shallow cortical laceration	Intact capsule with superficial parenchymal laceration without extension into the collecting system; no urinary extravasation on IVP
III	Deep cortical lacerations	Lacerated capsule with superficial parenchymal laceration without extension into the collecting system; no urinary extravasation on IVP
IV	Forniceal laceration	Disruption of the collecting system and parenchymal junction without injury to the parenchyma and capsule
	Major renal injury	**Consider surgery, 15% of renal injuries**
IV	Deep parenchymal laceration	Extension of the laceration into the collecting system with intact or disrupted capsules
V	Shattered kidney	Parenchyma ruptured in multiple fragments with distortion of the intrarenal collecting structures, with intact or disrupted capsule
VI	Renal pedicle injury	Laceration or thrombus at the pedicle involving the renal artery or vein as evidenced by lack of contrast in the affected kidney on IVP

of varying degrees, and these kidneys are more easily injured with minor trauma. In children, the incidence of anomalous kidneys with renal trauma has been reported to be as high as 15 percent. Because of this high incidence, evaluation by IVP for lower levels of microscopic hematuria than adults (20 versus 50 RBCs/hpf) has been recommended.

Delayed Findings

Renal trauma can lead to acute tubular necrosis with renal failure, delayed bleeding, infection secondary to urinary extravasation and abscess, and renin-mediated hypertension within weeks to months after the injury. Arteriovenous fistula, chronic pyelonephritis, hydronephrosis, chronic calculi, pseudocyst, and hypertension can also occur. Therefore, repeat IVP or CT should be done 3 to 6 months after significant renal injuries to reevaluate the kidneys.

Ureter

Ureteral injuries are uncommon in children, occurring in less than 5 percent of those suffering GU trauma. Avulsion occurs most commonly at the right ureteropelvic junction or in the proximal 4 cm of the ureter. It occurs more commonly in children and is invariably due to blunt trauma. The diagnosis is difficult to make and often delayed, since hematuria can be absent or transient. Intravenous pyelography will usually show extravasation of contrast at the level of the kidney without filling of the ureter, but retrograde pyelography may be necessary to differentiate avulsion from a forniceal tear and to identify the level of the avulsion. Abdominal CT may raise the suspicion for ureteral avulsion, but an IVP or retrograde pyelogram is usually necessary to make the definitive diagnosis. Delayed symptoms include fever, ileus, hematuria, and flank or abdominal pain.

Ureteral transection, irrespective of the cause, is treated with prompt ureteropyelostomy with or without proximal drainage. The kidney salvage rate is greater than 95 percent. When diagnosis is delayed, nephrectomy is frequently necessary. Other complications, such as fistulas, ureteral strictures, and abscesses, may also result when diagnosis is delayed.

Bladder

Pathophysiology

Bladder injury represents about one-fourth of all urologic injuries and is often associated with multisystem trauma. There is a high mortality due to associated injuries. Bladder trauma is associated with pelvic fractures about three-fourths of the time, and about one-fourth of pelvic fractures will result in bladder injury. The bladder has a more abdominal position in childhood; it is more vulnerable to rupture, especially when full.

Bladder rupture is associated with a high mortality rate (11 to 44 percent), which increases with delayed diagnosis. Persistent hematuria, sepsis, and renal failure following trauma suggest delayed diagnosis. Bladder rupture is divided into extraperitoneal, intraperitoneal, and combined. With all types, abdominal pain may be absent initially or related to pain associated with other abdominal injury or pelvic fracture. Delayed diagnosis results in

TABLE 13-4 Indications for Cystogram in Pediatric Trauma Patients

Penetrating injury to lower abdomen and pelvis
Blunt lower abdominal or perineal trauma with significant microscopic hematuria (>20 RBC/hpf), gross hematuria,[a] or blood at the meatus[a]
Significant pelvic fracture[a]
Unable to void[a] or little urine with Foley catheterization

[a] A retrograde urethrogram should be considered before attempting urethral catheterization in these instances.

peritonitis due to infection and associated azotemia and acidosis. Intraperitoneal absorption of urine leads to elevated or rising levels of blood urea nitrogen (BUN), which can be used as a sensitive indicator for this injury.

Management

In general, one should consider bladder rupture in children with abdominal trauma if there is gross hematuria, blood at the urethral meatus, inability to void, or little urine upon urinary catheter placement (Table 13-4). Microscopic hematuria suggests potential bladder contusion, but hematuria may be absent even with bladder rupture.

A cystogram is the radiographic study of choice for suspected bladder rupture and has an accuracy of greater than 96 percent (Table 13-5). However, an IVP or abdominal/pelvic CT should

TABLE 13-5 Cystogram Findings with Bladder Injury

	Radiographic finding
Bladder contusion	Teardrop shape or elevation of the bladder due to a perivesical hematoma without extravasation of contrast. Lateral deviation and obliteration of the soft tissue planes by pelvic hematoma may also be present.
Extraperitoneal bladder rupture	Postvoid films with significant rupture reveal a typical "sunburst" pattern as the contrast extravasates outside the peritoneal cavity. However, there may only be small streaks of contrast with minor bladder ruptures.
Intraperitoneal bladder rupture	Extravasation into the peritoneal cavity around the bowel and intraabdominal organs and/or in the pericolic gutters giving a typical "hourglass" appearance.

be performed before the cystogram to avoid obscuration of the IVP findings by extravasation of dye from the bladder. An abdominal/pelvic CT is useful in multiple trauma, but may not be sensitive enough for bladder injury unless the bladder is fully distended with contrast. A retrograde urethrogram should also precede attempts to pass a Foley catheter in males because of the high incidence of urethral injuries associated with bladder trauma. Cystography should include maximally full, postdrainage, and oblique films to provide the best chance for diagnosis, because false-negative cystograms may occur, especially with penetrating bladder injuries.

Intraperitoneal bladder rupture requires surgical exploration, repair, debridement, and bladder drainage. In male infants, a suprapubic catheter is preferred for management in order to avoid complications associated with long-term transurethral catheter drainage.

Urethra

Pathophysiology

Urethral injuries predominantly occur from blunt trauma and, due to a more flexible pelvis, are less common in children. Causes include pelvic fractures, straddle injuries, and urethral manipulation, which can result in strictures, incontinence, impotence, diverticulae, fistulas, and chordee.

Proximal urethral injuries in males occur when the bladder is pulled upward, resulting in shearing forces against the relatively fixed portions of the urethra at the urogenital diaphragm, the symphysis pubis, and the bladder neck. Partial or complete vesicourethral avulsion may occur. Female urethral injuries are extremely rare but can occur at the bladder neck and vesicourethrovaginal septum, resulting in urethrovaginal fistula or vaginal stricture. Some 90 percent of posterior urethral injuries are associated with pelvic fractures.

Less commonly, distal urethral injuries result from direct blows, such as straddle injuries, where the bulbous urethra is forced against the symphysis pubis. With significant straddle injury, examination under sedation or anesthesia is essential to assess the extent of urethral injury and possible vaginal involvement in females.

Symptoms of proximal urethral injury include difficulty voiding; blood at the urethral meatus (90 percent); abdominal pain; instability of the pelvis, indicating pelvic fracture; and, in males, a high-riding, floating, or boggy prostate. Symptoms of distal urethral injury include difficulty voiding and discoloration and edema due

TABLE 13-6 Indications for Retrograde Urethrogram in Pediatric Trauma Patients

Penetrating injury to lower abdomen and pelvis suspected of involving the lower genitourinary tract
Blunt lower abdominal or perineal trauma with significant microscopic hematuria (>20 RBC/hpf), gross hematuria, or blood at the meatus
Significant pelvic fracture
Unable to void
High-riding, floating, or boggy prostate in males
Discoloration or edema due to extravasation of blood or urine into the scrotum, perineum, or abdominal wall, or along the shaft of the penis
Laceration of the vagina secondary to significant trauma

to extravasation of blood or urine into the scrotum, perineum, or abdominal wall, or along the shaft of the penis.

Management

Early urologic consultation is recommended. It is most important for the emergency physician to recognize the potential for urethral injury and to avoid iatrogenic complications. Indications for retrograde urethrogram prior to catheter placement are listed in Table 13-6. Care should be taken to avoid converting partial tears of the urethra into transections by injudicious attempts to pass urethral catheters.

Male Perineal Trauma

Scrotal and Testicular Injuries

Pathophysiology Injuries to the external male genitalia result from the testis being forced against the ramus of the pubic bone. Common mechanisms of injury include straddle injury and the impact of bicycle handlebars [particularly from bicycle motocross (BMX) racing], seats, or center bars. Salvage of the testis and/or fertility is dependent on rapid differentiation between testicular torsion, rupture, and dislocation from other nonsurgical injuries. Examination of the testis is often complicated by the presence of a hematoma or hematocele. In addition edema, ecchymosis, and tenderness of the testis may be present with any of the common etiologies.

Management Significant straddle injuries should be screened with an x-ray of the pelvis to rule out fracture of the ramus. Testicular tissue is fragile and vulnerable to rapid necrosis. Failure to diagnose testicular torsion or rupture can lead to atrophy, loss of spermatogenesis and hormonal function, and psychological consequences. Obvious cases of testicular torsion, rupture, and dislocation require immediate urologic consultation and surgical exploration. Epididymitis, hematocele, hematoma, hydrocele, and testicular appendage torsions may be treated conservatively, but may require surgical exploration to differentiate them from a more serious problem. Diagnostic tests, only if immediately available, should be used for those cases where the possibility of serious injury or torsion is less likely. A delay of 4 to 6 h in obtaining diagnostic tests may result in the loss of the testis. Therefore, urologic consultation should be obtained prior to ordering diagnostic tests to determine the feasibility and logistics of the evaluation.

A radionucleotide scan with technetium 99m is the preferred test for differentiation of torsion from epididymitis. It may also reveal evidence of testicular rupture, although it is not often diagnostic until 24 h after injury. Surgical exploration, however, remains the most rapid and definitive method for evaluation of significant scrotal trauma, and these other modalities should be reserved for less obvious cases.

Testicular or epididymis rupture results from direct trauma as the testis is forced against the pubic ramus, resulting in tearing of the inelastic tunica albuginea with extrusion of the seminiferous tissue. Although somewhat rare in children, it is probably underdiagnosed and is often confused with hematocele and treated nonoperatively. Early surgical exploration should be performed when rupture is suspected. The recurrence of pain and delayed onset of scrotal swelling, from several hours to 3 days after the injury, suggests rupture. Complications include epididymoorchitis, which is characterized by localized redness, warmth, swelling, and fever. Delayed exploration and orchiectomy are frequently required.

Testicular dislocation occurs when the testis is forcibly displaced from the scrotum into the inguinal, acetabular, crural, perineal, penile, or abdominal region or extruded from the scrotum through a laceration. The mechanisms for this injury are similar to those for other scrotal injuries, and, while rare, dislocation should be considered when an empty hemiscrotum is present after trauma. Frequent symptoms include scrotal pain, nausea, and vomiting. Closed relocation of the testis may be possible, and a urologic consultation should be obtained along with diagnostic tests to evaluate the integrity of the testis.

Penile Injuries

Pathophysiology Penile injuries occur from a variety of mechanisms; causes include direct blows (from toilet seats, falls, and sports injuries), zipper entrapment of the foreskin, and tourniquet injuries. The vast majority of these injuries are minor and can be treated conservatively. Major trauma to the perineum may require fluid resuscitation, surgical intervention, and consideration of associated genitourinary trauma. Urinalysis should be performed with any significant penile injury.

Management *Superficial lacerations* of the penis can be repaired similarly to any other laceration, but injury to deeper structures should be considered if there is marked swelling, ecchymosis, or blood at the meatus.

Fracture of the penis occurs with rupture of the corpora cavernosa from a tear in the tunica albuginea, resulting in a large subcutaneous hematoma. It most often occurs when the erect penis is forced against a solid object, such as the pubis, during sexual intercourse. The patient hears a "cracking" sound followed by pain, swelling, and deformity of the penis. Urologic consultation is important to determine the best management in individual cases.

Zipper injuries to the foreskin occur when a zipper entraps the skin of an uncircumcised male and retraction of the zipper is either impossible or too painful. Boys 3 to 6 years of age are most susceptible as they quickly zip up their pants after urinating. Treatment involves using bone cutters to break the small bridge of the sliding piece of the zipper, allowing it to fall apart and release the trapped foreskin. Local anesthesia and sedation are usually not required.

Tourniquet injuries are often heralded by balanitis, paraphimosis, or cellulitis of the penis in an infant. They result when a band of hair surrounds the coronal groove and cuts into the shaft of the penis. The injury is usually localized, but may extend into the urethra and corpora. Removal of the band and treatment of infection is usually all that is required. Follow-up with urology is necessary if deeper injury is suspected.

Female Perineal Trauma

Vulvar and Vaginal Injuries

Pathophysiology Perineal trauma in girls is not uncommon and often results from blunt trauma, such as straddle injuries. Stretching of the perineum from sudden abduction of the legs (doing the splits) can cause tears, and various penetrating injuries can also occur. Child abuse should be considered in cases where the reported mechanism or history does not match the injuries. Typical injuries include vulvar hematomas; vaginal tears or lacerations; and urethral, rectal, or bladder injuries. Complications of perineal trauma include urinary retention, secondary infection, and urinary tract infection.

Management *Vulvar injuries* are usually minor and can be treated with rest and cold packs. Significant straddle injuries should be screened with a pelvic radiograph to rule out fracture of the ramus. Large or expanding vulvar hematomas may require surgical drainage and are susceptible to secondary infection. Vulvar hematoma and edema can also result in urinary retention; a urethrogram or cystoscopy may be required to rule out urethral injury, or a suprapubic catheter may be necessary. Minor linear abrasions of the vulva or vagina may result from masturbation and can become secondarily infected, requiring antibiotics.

Vaginal injuries usually result from penetration through the hymenal opening, although severe blunt injury to the pelvis may also cause damage, as noted earlier in this chapter. Most vaginal injuries are minor, but complete examination of the vagina is warranted to exclude significant injury. Large lacerations can occur, causing significant bleeding and shock. Injury to adjacent organs is also possible and can result in bladder, urethral, ureter, peritoneal, or rectal injuries and retroperitoneal hematoma. The principles mentioned earlier in this chapter should be followed for evaluation of these severe vaginal injuries.

Sexual abuse is estimated to occur in one out of five girls during childhood. Abuse should be considered with all perineal injuries and the possibility of sexually transmitted disease recognized. The injuries seen with sexual abuse are usually minimal; the forensic aspect of these injuries is usually more important.

Rectal Trauma

Pathophysiology

Rectal injuries are very uncommon in childhood and are primarily caused by impalement. The injuries are often significant and lead to frequent surgical intervention for either diagnostic evaluation or repair of the injury. Lacerations can occur anywhere from the anal sphincter to well within the rectum. Lesions as far as 10 cm from the anal margin have been reported and may show minimal signs of external trauma. Concomitant vaginal injury may be present in females.

Management

Complete evaluation of rectal impalement is necessary, and few children will cooperate with anoscopy without sedation or general anesthesia. Therefore, with a history of impalement with or without significant signs of external trauma, a surgical consultation is warranted. In younger children, the history of impalement may be absent as they present with an acute abdomen or ileus. The rectal perforation may be discovered only on laparoscopy.

For a more detailed discussion, see Lucid WA, Taylor TB: Genitourinary and Pelvic Trauma, chap. 13, p. 91, in *Pediatric Emergency Medicine: A Comprehensive Study Guide.*

---

14 Maxillofacial Trauma

Stephen A. Colucciello

Accurate bony alignment is important in the growing child, and missed fractures or inappropriate treatment may result in permanent facial deformity. A child with severe maxillofacial injury requires a team approach involving emergency physicians, pediatricians, general surgeons, maxillofacial specialists, and radiologists. Emergency specialists must recognize and prioritize injuries, manage the airway, stabilize the patient, read initial radiographs, and make appropriate consultations.

INCIDENCE

Children have a lower incidence of facial fractures than adults. Great structural differences exist between birth and 10 years of age, with marked changes in bone composition and anatomy.

Fracture site distribution tends to shift from the upper aspect of the face in younger children to the lower face in older children. Development of paranasal sinuses weakens the anterior facial skeleton. In one study, no LeForte fracture or unclassified maxillary sinus fracture occurred in children under 5 years of age, prior to pneumatization of paranasal sinuses. For this reason, in children under 5, orbital and frontal skull fractures predominate, whereas in older children, maxillary and mandibular fractures become more prominent. The highest incidence of facial fractures in children occurs between ages 8 and 10, and the most frequently fractured bones include the nose (45 percent), mandible (32 percent), orbit (17 percent), and zygoma/maxilla (5 percent). By the early teen years, the frequency and pattern of maxillofacial injury begin to mirror those found in adults.

ASSOCIATED INJURIES

Up to 55 percent of seriously injured children with facial trauma may also have intracranial injury, a much higher percentage than in adults. This is due to the high energy necessary to disrupt the pediatric facial skeleton. Periorbital fractures lead to intraocular injury in up to 10 percent of patients, mandating a careful ophthalmologic exam in these situations.

EMERGENCY MANAGEMENT

The most urgent complication of facial trauma is airway compromise, which is most often associated with middle and lower face injury. Simple maneuvers, such as chin lift–jaw thrust and oropharyngeal suctioning, provide immediate benefit.

Infants under the age of 3 months are obligate nose breathers and nasal or midface trauma can lead to complete airway obstruction. Mandibular fractures can result in loss of support of the tongue and occlusion of the upper airway. These fractures may also produce hematomas of the floor of the mouth, which can displace the tongue and obstruct the airway. In this situation, the physician should open the mouth and pull the tongue forward, either manually or with a large suture or towel clip. If cervical spine injury is not a consideration or has been ruled out, the child should be allowed to sit up and lean forward.

If simple airway maneuvers do not suffice, orotracheal intubation with in-line immobilization is necessary. Nasotracheal intubation should be avoided with midface trauma to prevent passage of the tube into the cranial vault. If severe oropharyngeal bleeding persists, the pharynx must be packed with absorbent gauze to prevent aspiration when uncuffed endotracheal tubes are utilized.

If the child cannot be intubated, the physician must open the airway surgically. Emergency cricothyroidotomy should be avoided in children under 12. In children below this age, there are numerous complications, including subglottic stenosis and tracheolaryngeal injury. Emergency tracheostomy results in fewer long-term complications but is time-consuming and requires great expertise. Percutaneous transtracheal jet ventilation is an excellent temporizing measure in these situations. A needle is inserted into the cricothyroid membrane, and oxygen at 50 PSI is used (directly from the wall without a Christmas tree adaptor) with a 1-to-3 inspiration to expiration ratio.

Severe nasal hemorrhage may lead to aspiration and should initially be controlled by applying pressure to the external nares. If bleeding continues, nasopharyngeal packing should be considered. A Foley catheter is an effective emergency intervention. The catheter is inserted along the floor of the nose, and the balloon is inflated in the nasopharynx and pulled anteriorly; an anterior pack is then placed. A calming interaction, touching and reassuring the child, will assist in the management of a conscious, fearful patient.

HISTORY

A history regarding the circumstances of injury is obtained from parents and prehospital care providers as well as from the child. The mechanism and time of injury are determined and an assessment for loss of consciousness is made. The child is questioned about any visual problems, facial anesthesia, or pain with jaw movement.

PHYSICAL EXAMINATION

Inspection of the face may reveal areas of swelling, ecchymosis, or deformity. In addition to face-to-face inspection, a view from the child's head looking down or from the chin looking up may reveal otherwise unappreciated asymmetries. Posttraumaic Bell's palsy provides evidence of a temporal bone fracture. The entire face is carefully palpated, starting with the skull. Areas of bony deformity and crepitus will guide x-ray studies.

The eyes must be evaluated for the presence of the pupillary light reflex. Hyphema, subconjunctival hemorrhage, and extraocular motion must be assessed. The presence of proptosis or enophthalmos should be noted. Unequal pupil height may indicate orbital floor fracture. Lids must be retracted for adequate visualization of the globe, and visual acuity must be documented. Complete ocular examination is important in periorbital trauma because of the high incidence of globe injury (Chap. 15).

The *entire* orbital rim must be carefully palpated for tenderness or deformity. Many physicians neglect careful palpation of the superior orbital rim, concentrating instead on the inferior rim. Anesthesia above or below the eye may be secondary to supraorbital or infraorbital nerve injury and often occurs in conjunction with fractures.

Telecanthus, an increased width between the medial canthi of the eyelids with flattening of the medial canthus, is associated with nasal ethmoidal injury. In this situation, the medial canthal ligaments are torn or underlying bone is avulsed from the nasal orbital complex.

Subcutaneous emphysema about the eyes and maxillary area indicates a communication with a sinus or nasal antrum and may erupt when the child blows his or her nose.

The pinnae are examined for presence of subperichondral hematoma. The ear canal must be examined for lacerations and CSF leak. The Battle sign—ecchymosis over the mastoid area—appears several hours after injury resulting in basilar skull fracture. The presence of hemotympanum should also raise suspicion for this injury.

Nose

The examining physician must carefully palpate the nose for crepitus and deformity, as edema often obscures bony anatomy. The inside of the nose is examined for septal hematoma, which may be recognized by a bluish, bulging mass on the septum or by the subjective impression of an abnormally wide septum. Pressure with a cotton swab will detect the presence of a soft, doughy swelling.

With any significant facial trauma, it is important to assess for CSF rhinorrhea. A drop of bloody nasal secretions on a sheet, towel, or tissue paper will form a double ring in the presence of CSF leak. This ring or halo sign, however, is not specific for cerebrospinal fluid and may occur in the presence of normal nasal secretions.

Intraoral and Mandibular Examination

The emergency physician must observe movement of the patient's jaw through a full range of motion. Deviation to one side usually indicates ipsilateral subcondylar fracture, since dislocation of the jaw occurs infrequently in children. Difficulty in jaw movement may be secondary to mandibular fractures, injury to the temporomandibular joint, or a depressed zygoma impinging upon the mandible or muscles of mastication. Trismus and malocclusion also occur.

Children, unlike adults, may suffer traumatic diastasis of the hard palate along the midline; to detect this injury, the physician must apply a distracting pressure upon the dental arches. Each tooth is grasped and manipulated to assess for laxity, and teeth that are in danger of falling into the airway are removed. Permanent teeth may be saved in saline-moistened gauze.

Facial Lacerations

Key to evaluating facial lacerations is an understanding of the relationship between the skin and underlying vital structures. Injuries to the medial third of the upper or lower eyelids may result in disruption of the lacrimal apparatus. Laceration of the parotid duct should be suspected if saliva enters the wound or if blood is expressed at Stinson's duct. These signs may be elicited by massage of the parotid gland. Parotid duct injury is possible if a deep wound crosses a line drawn from the tragus to the midportion of the upper lip. The buccal branch of the facial nerve also parallels this line. Facial nerve injuries must be surgically repaired if they occur posterior to a vertical line drawn from the lateral canthus. Injuries anterior to such a line are usually not repaired.

RADIOGRAPHY

The choice of radiographic studies depends on the degree of injury and the clinical stability of the child. Management of associated intracranial, thoracic, and abdominal injuries always takes precedence over imaging of the face. In the severely injured child, radiographs of the face, including computed tomography (CT), may be deferred for several days, until life-threatening injuries have been addressed and the child's condition is stabilized. Multiple diagnostic modalities may be required.

Utilizing three radiographic views of the face—the Waters, posteroanterior, and lateral films—the vast majority of facial bone fractures can be detected. These plain films provide an excellent screening tool for maxillofacial trauma.

The submental vertex view (jug-handle or zygomatic arch view) demonstrates the zygomatic arches and the base of skull, while the Towne view images the ramus of the mandible and condyles.

X-rays of the nose are of relative usefulness only. Nasal radiographs may be inaccurate, with many false positives and false negatives. Surgical decisions are based more upon cosmetic appearance and ability to breathe through the nose than upon radiographic findings.

Computed Tomography

The CT scan has become the definitive diagnostic test for precise delineation of maxillofacial fractures. Computed tomography further defines injuries seen on plain film, or it may be the initial imaging study of choice for patients with clinically obvious complex fractures. Specialized CT techniques, such as coronal views, thin-slice scans (1.5 to 3 mm), and three-dimensional reconstruction, assist in surgical planning for these complex injuries. Computed tomography is particularly helpful in the presence of orbital fractures and evaluates the status of orbital contents.

To obtain a high-quality scan, children may require sedation and, in some cases, paralysis and intubation. Agents useful in sedation include narcotics, such as fentanyl; benzodiazepines, such as midazolam; barbiturates; sedative hypnotics, such as chloral hydrate; and combination agents. Short-acting, intravenously administered, reversible agents are the safest choice. Avoid ketamine in patients with head trauma, as it may raise intracranial pressure.

SPECIFIC INJURIES

Nasal Fractures

Nasal fractures are the most commonly encountered pediatric facial fracture. Initial control of hemorrhage is obtained with external digital pressure. If nasal packing is used, care must be taken to assure that the packing is not placed intracranially. A particularly severe type of nasal fracture that occurs mostly in children is the "open book" type fracture, where nasal bones separate in the midline along the suture.

Initially, nasal fractures may go undiagnosed secondary to edema and the difficulty in interpreting radiographs. If radiographs are deferred, the child should be rechecked in 3 to 4 days after swelling has subsided to reassess for deformity or septal deviation. This reexamination may be performed by the emergency specialist or the consultant. For optimal repair of displaced nasal fractures, consultation should take place within 5 to 6 days postinjury, past which time fractures begin to unite and manipulation becomes increasingly difficult.

It is critical that emergency physicians recognize and treat septal hematomas. An untreated septal hematoma results in collapse of the septum and a "saddle" deformity of the nose. Upon diagnosing a septal hematoma, the physician should use a #11 blade to make an L-shaped incision through the mucoperiosteum along the floor of the nose and extend the incision vertically. The hematoma will then be evacuated through the flap. Subsequent packing of the nasal antrum prevents reaccumulation, and the child must be referred to the appropriate specialist. Timely referral of nasal fractures is of significant medical and legal concern, as these injuries may have a profound effect on subsequent nasal and maxillofacial development.

Nasal-Ethmoidal-Orbital Fractures

Nasal-ethmoidal-orbital (NEO) fractures occur when the bony structures of the nose are driven backward into the intraorbital space. Fortunately, these injuries are rare in children. Telecanthus presents secondary to avulsion of one or both medial canthal ligaments. In this situation, the bimanual test for mobility is performed. Associated injuries include orbital and optic nerve problems as well as lacrimal system disruption. Computed tomography scans are useful in evaluating these injuries.

Orbital Fractures

The most common orbital fracture is the blowout, which occurs when a blunt object, often a ball or fist, strikes the globe. The intraorbital pressure increases suddenly, and the contents decompress through the thinnest portion of the orbit, which is the floor. This may lead to entrapment of the inferior ocular muscles, with subsequent diplopia on upward gaze. Evaluation for associated ocular injury such as hyphema, retinal contusion, lens dislocation, and corneal lacerations must be performed and visual acuity documented (see Chap. 15).

Patients with NEO or orbital fractures should be instructed not to blow their nose. Because patients with subcutaneous emphysema have a fracture into a sinus or the nasal antrum, many practitioners use antibiotics to cover common sinus pathogens. Such prophylaxis, however, has not been conclusively proven to reduce complications. First-generation cephalosporins, trimethoprim/sulfamethoxazole, amoxicillin, or erythromycin are frequently utilized in outpatients. Urgent consultation is required in the presence of exophthalmus or extraocular muscle entrapment. In these situations, the orbital contents must be surgically released and the area of blowout covered with implants or bone grafts. Many cases of posttraumatic diplopia associated with blowout fractures may be due to muscle or nerve injury and not true mechanical entrapment. Evaluation with CT and the forced duction test help distinguish these conditions.

Frontal Sinus and Supraorbital Fractures

Supraorbital fractures involve the superior orbital rim or orbital roof. The superior orbital fissure syndrome results in paralysis of extraocular muscles, ptosis, and anesthesia in the ophthalmic division of the trigeminal nerve. The orbital apex syndrome is a combination of the superior orbital fissure syndrome and optic nerve damage and results in blindness.

Linear, undisplaced fractures of the anterior wall of the frontal sinus may be treated by observation and antibiotics in either an inpatient or an outpatient setting. If the posterior wall is involved, a CT scan will evaluate the possibility of depression and underlying brain injury. Posterior wall fractures should prompt neurological as well as maxillofacial consultation.

Maxillary Fractures

Maxillary fractures are very uncommon in young children. Because of the high degree of energy required to fracture the pediatric face, associated injuries, particularly intracranial, must be suspected.

Malar Fractures

The malar complex is often broke in a tripod fashion, with a fracture at the infraorbital rim, across the zygomatic frontal suture, and along the zygomatic temporal junction. Inward displacement of this fragment may result in impingement upon the mandible, giving rise to impaired mouth opening and trismus.

LeFort Fractures

Fractures to the midface are classified according to the LeFort system, based upon the horizontal level of the fracture. LeFort I is a transversed fracture which separates the hard palate from the lower portion of the pterygoid plate and nasal septum. Traction on the upper incisors produces movement of only the hard palate and dental arch. LeFort II or pyramidal fracture separates the central maxilla and palate from the rest of the craniofacial skeleton. Mobilization of the upper incisors will move the central pyramid of the face, including the nose. LeFort III, also known as craniofacial disjunction, separates the facial skeleton from the rest of the cranium. The entire face, including inferior and lateral portions of the orbital rim, moves with mobilization maneuvers. "Pure" LeFort fractures are found more often in textbooks than in clinical practice. Fractures often do not fit the LeFort classification and demonstrate a mixed pattern—perhaps a LeFort II on one side and a LeFort III on the other. LeFort fractures may result in lengthening of the midface and occlusal abnormalities, and may be associated with basilar skull fractures; CT scans are useful in their evaluation.

Children with LeFort fractures must be admitted and carefully assessed for associated injury. A maxillofacial specialist should be involved in their care.

Mandible Fractures

Mandible fractures are the second most common facial fracture, following nasal bone injury. Blows or falls to the chin result in symphyseal or perisymphyseal injury, whereas lateral blows are more likely to produce body or angle fractures on the injured or contralateral side. Younger children suffer isolated condylar fractures and may present with deviation of the jaw to the affected side and trismus. Unlike the situation with adults, dislocation of the temporomandibular joint (TMJ) is very unusual in this age group. Physical examination is key in diagnosing these injuries, as radiographs may be nondiagnostic. Greenstick fractures, especially in the area of the condyles, are not well visualized on plain films. Because the panorex view does not visualize the symphyseal area well, an occlusal view of the mandible is helpful in suspected symphyseal injury. The Towne and lateral oblique views delineate the body and ramus.

The mandible is the facial bone most frequently involved in posttraumatic developmental deformities. Crush injuries to the condyle prior to the age of 5 have the greatest potential for developmental arrest. Arrested development results in severe facial deformity, micrognathia, and ankylosis of the TMJ. The possibility of subsequent growth disturbances should be raised with the parents—the younger the child, the more likely the complications.

Treatment of mandibular fractures is based upon age, state of dentition, fracture location, bony integrity, and the presence of associated injuries.

CONCLUSION

Maxillofacial trauma in children more often results in soft tissue injury than in facial fractures. When fractures do occur, associated injuries, particularly intracranial, may be present. Fractures heal rapidly over 2 to 3 weeks, and repair must be undertaken before bony union occurs. Conservative management is often the rule.

Late reduction of a fracture may result in unsatisfactory cosmesis secondary to arrested growth and distorted dentition. Aggressive airway management, assiduous search for associated injuries, and early consultation are the keys to successful emergency management of pediatric facial trauma.

DENTAL INJURIES

Injuries to the teeth are common in childhood and cause anxiety for both patients and parents. As with all forms of trauma, attention to the ABCs must be given first priority. Ensure airway patency and ventilation, circulation, and hemostasis. Assess the skull, facial bones, oropharynx, and neck for associated injuries. Although many dental injuries are seen by a physician initially, most require dental follow-up for definitive care. Delay in dental follow-up may adversely affect outcome. The most common dental emergencies include soft tissue lacerations, dental fractures, and avulsions, tooth displacement, alveolar fractures, and maxillary or mandibular fractures.

Displacement is the most common injury to the primary dentition, with peak periods of incidence between ages 2 and 5 years. The maxillary incisors are the most commonly displaced followed by the mandibular incisors. Displacement can cause disruption of the neurovascular supply, resulting in pulp necrosis and apical abscess formation. Damage to unerupted permanent teeth can also occur. Concussion is a mild blunt injury with no tooth motion and pain to percussion. Subluxation causes pain with tooth movement and requires splinting and dental follow-up. In an intrusion injury, the tooth is pushed into the alveolar socket, requiring radiographic and early dental evaluation. In an extrusion injury, a tooth may be torn from its apical neurovascular bundle, and requires urgent dental evaluation and splinting.

Primary simple dental fractures involving enamel only (Ellis Class I) have no apparent symptoms and can be referred to a dentist to have the rough edges smoothed. If the child complains of cold sensitivity, the fracture extends at least into the dentin (Ellis Class II). If the surface is dull with reddish marking, there is extension into the pulp (Ellis Class III), which requires dental evaluation for application of a temporary zinc oxide or calcium hydroxide cap. A root fracture extends into the gingival groove and alveolar socket, and requires prompt dental evaluation and removal of fragments to prevent pulp necrosis.

Avulsion of the primary teeth occurs more frequently as root resorption occurs, and these teeth should not be replaced. Use direct pressure or a 4–0 chromic gut suture to control bleeding. Identify the whole teeth or all of its fragments. This occasionally requires dental radiographs to identify intruded pieces or fragments in the lacerated lip or gingival spaces, or a chest-abdomen scout film to identify an aspirated or ingested tooth.

Permanent teeth are most commonly injured in boys aged 8 to 12 years, and most commonly involve the maxillary incisors. Displacement of permanent teeth is common, and is controlled with adequate hemostasis, digital reduction, and dental wax as a temporary splint until the child can be seen by the dentist. A majority of patients will require root canal therapy and periodic evaluation for pulp necrosis. All intruded teeth will require root canal therapy to prevent ankylosis and inflammatory root resorption. Fractures of the permanent teeth are classified and managed in much the same way as primary teeth. Enamel fractures of the permanent teeth do, however, require radiographic assessment to rule out an occult root fracture, and periodic evaluation for pulp vitality by a dentist is recommended. Avulsion injuries of permanent teeth are true emergencies, and the success of reimplantation is inversely proportional to the time the tooth is out of its socket. If the tooth is dirty, rinse it gently to remove debris, while paying attention not to injure the periodontal membrane remnants. If there is a clot in the socket, irrigate gently with normal saline to remove it. Relocate the tooth with a dental wax splint until the dentist arrives, or if unable to do so, place the tooth in the child's or parent's buccal pouch. Other alternatives include placing the tooth in a glass of milk or normal saline while awaiting dental care. If the tooth is reimplanted within 30 minutes, there is a good long-term prognosis.

Always assess occlusion and check for temporomandibular joint tenderness or pain to palpation and movement of the jaw. This may help to identify subtle mandibular fractures or mild tooth displacement.

For a more detailed discussion, see Coluccciello SA: Maxillofacial Trauma, chap. 14, p. 100, in *Pediatric Emergency Medicine: A Comprehensive Study Guide.*

---

15 Eye Trauma

Stephen A. Colucciello

Ocular trauma is the leading cause of monocular blindness in children, and if unilateral visual impairment occurs before the age of 7, deprivational amblyopia may result. In preschool children, most injuries are due to falls, motor vehicle crashes, and accidental blows to the eye. In the older child, sports-related injuries become important, especially baseball, tennis, soccer, archery, and fishing injuries. The notorious BB gun remains a significant cause of pediatric eye injury.

HISTORY

A full history should be obtained and any preexisting eye abnormality noted, along with whether or not the child normally wears glasses. A history of exposure to power tools or metal striking metal should raise a suspicion of an intraocular foreign body.

PHYSICAL EXAMINATION

Visual Acuity

Visual acuity should be assessed and documented in every child with an ocular injury. This should be done *before* intervention except in the case of major trauma or caustic exposure. If the child wears glasses, acuity is measured with glasses on; if they have been lost or damaged, refractive error may be corrected by having the child look through a pinhole in a piece of paper. An older child may look through an ophthalmoscope and, by experimenting with different magnifications, correct for refractive problems. Preliterate children are evaluated with an Allen or "E" chart, and a toy is moved to test the young child's ability to track with each eye. If the child is unable to read an eye chart, he or she is asked to finger count at 3 ft or, if that fails due to visual loss, light perception is assessed. Older children cooperate with visual field examination in the usual confrontation method, while younger children will glance toward a toy brought into the field of view.

Pupillary Exam

The pupils are examined for any asymmetry or irregularity. Congenital anisocoria may be detected by obtaining a history from the parents, or by examining a picture of the child taken prior to the traumatic event. Pupillary dilatation may occur with direct blows to the eye (posttraumatic mydriasis) and various atropine-like medications. Pilocarpine will constrict a pupil that is dilated secondary to a third nerve lesion but will have no effect on pharmacologic mydriasis.

The swinging flashlight test is exquisitely sensitive for optic nerve injury. The flashlight is swung from eye to eye. A pupil that initially dilates when illuminated by light has a sensory (afferent) defect (Marcus Gunn pupil).

Adenexae

The lids are examined for swelling or penetrating injury and inspected for ecchymosis. Swollen lids can be retracted with a finger in most cases, but lid retractors or bent paper clips serve in the case of massive lid edema. Periorbital soft tissue air indicates fracture into a sinus or nasal antrum and is most commonly seen with a blowout fracture. The eye is examined for normal lacrimal drainage. Epiphora—tears spilling over the lid margins—may be secondary to injury of the canicular system.

Globe

The sclera is examined for injection and the presence of capillary blush around the iris (perilimbal injection), which indicates a significant insult to the eye. The presence and location of any subconjunctival hemorrhage is observed, and the anterior chamber is examined for abnormal shallowness or depth.

The lens should be transparent, and the margins should not be visible. A careful fundoscopic exam should reveal a clear vitreous and good visualization of the retina. Intraocular pressure should not be measured if globe rupture or penetrating injury is apparent, as this may herniate ocular contents.

EQUIPMENT

The basic equipment for a standard pediatric eye exam includes the following:

- Visual acuity charts (Snellen and Allen "E")
- Penlight
- Ophthalmoscope
- Wood's lamp
- Slit lamp
- Lid retractors
- Ocular spud
- Ophthalmic burr
- Fluorescein strips
- Shitz tonometer
- Morgan lens
- Metal eye shields

MEDICATIONS

Topical anesthetics such as 0.5% tetracaine or proparacaine are useful in the patient with blepharospasm and allow an adequate exam. Topical anesthetics should never be prescribed for home use, as they delay corneal epithelialization. Cycloplegics (mydriatics) such as homatropine (2 to 5%) and cyclopentolate hydrochloride (1 to 2%) dilate the eye and decrease pain by overcoming ciliary spasm. The use of such medications should always be documented. The use of atropine drops should be avoided because of their extremely long duration of action (over a week in some cases). Steroids are useful in some inflammatory conditions but may lead to glaucoma, cataract formation, and acceleration of fungal and herpetic infections, resulting in ultimate visual loss or blindness. Ocular steroids must never be used without first consulting an ophthalmologist. The need for tetanus prophylaxis should be evaluated in all patients with ocular injuries.

SPECIFIC INJURIES

Lid Lacerations

Minor lid lacerations may mask serious intraocular injury and underlying globe disruption. If fat appears in a wound located in the palpebral fornices, underlying globe injury is to be anticipated.

Lacerations involving the medial third of the upper or lower lids must be approached cautiously, as they may involve the lacrimal system. Injuries to the canthal structures or lid margins result in deformity of the lids and abnormal lid movement. If the levator muscle is injured and not repaired, posttraumatic ptosis will result. Specialty consultation must be obtained for any laceration involving the lacrimal system, tarsal plate, lid margins, or canthi. Minor lacerations superficial to the tarsal plate may be repaired by the emergency physician.

Subconjunctival Hematoma

In the presence of significant blunt trauma, a subconjunctival hemorrhage may hide a scleral rupture. Occasionally a bloody chemosis occurs that prevents complete closure of the lids. In this situation. antibiotic ointment is applied to prevent drying. Parents should be reassured that the subconjunctival hemorrhages are benign and warned of the dramatic color changes that will occur with resolution over the following 2 weeks.

Corneal Abrasion

Children with corneal abrasions complain of a foreign-body sensation, pain, and photophobia and present with marked blepharospasm and a red eye. Tetracaine or proparacaine is used prior to examination to decrease blepharospasm.

A few drops of fluorescein placed in the conjunctival sac, followed by examination under a Wood's lamp or the cobalt blue light of a slit lamp, will result in marked fluorescence of corneal abrasions. Multiple vertical striations (ice-rink sign) usually indicate a retained foreign body under the upper lid. Careful examination with double lid eversion should reveal the offending agent.

Corneal abrasions in the absence of known trauma may, in fact, represent herpetic dendrites, and patients may have concurrent oral or genital herpes. The involved cornea will be anesthetic to light touch when brushed with a wisp of cotton as compared to the opposite cornea (decreased corneal reflex).

Ophthalmic antibiotics are used as prophylaxis against infection. Several drops of a mydriatic agent such as cyclopentolate 1 to 2% or homatropine 2 to 5% will decrease ciliary spasm and provide comfort.

Eye patching was the traditional standard of care, but some recent studies question the necessity of patching. If the eye is not patched, mydriatic agents and topical antibiotics for home use are prescribed. Abrasions are rechecked in 24 to 48 h to assess healing. If the corneal basement membrane has been damaged, epithelial cells may not adhere, and recurrent erosions can develop.

Blunt Trauma

Patients with posttraumatic iritis present 1 to 2 days after a blow to the eye complaining of photophobia, pain, and tearing and often have marked blepharospasm and perilimbal injection. One can test for pain on accommodation by having patients first look across the room at a distant object and then quickly focus upon the examiner's finger held several inches away. If near gaze causes pain, there is a high probability of iritis. Posttraumatic miosis develops secondary to spasm of the pupillary sphincter muscle, while posttraumatic mydriasis results when sphincter fibers are ruptured. High-magnification slit-lamp examination reveals cells or a flare reaction in the anterior chamber.

Topical mydriatic agents and oral anti-inflammatory medication may safely be prescribed by the emergency physician to treat the pain of iritis, and dark sunglasses can be used for photophobia.

Although ocular steroids decrease inflammation, they should be prescribed only after consultation with the ophthalmologist who will see the patient in flow-up.

Hyphema

A hyphema is defined by blood in the anterior chamber. Hyphemas are almost always secondary to blunt trauma. The blood may layer out or may present initially as a diffuse red haze that takes hours to settle. A 100 percent hyphema, known as an "eight ball," may cause complete loss of light perception. Hyphemas are easily overlooked in cases of massive lid edema, and in those cases lid retraction is necessary. Although hyphemas may cause marked somnolence, decreased mental status must prompt the consideration of intracranial injury. Other injuries associated with hyphema include lens dislocation, vitreous hemorrhage, and retinal damage. A large untreated hyphema may result in permanent corneal staining, with resultant loss of visual acuity and deprivational amblyopia. Often it is not the initial hyphema that causes serious morbidity but the rebleed that occurs several days later upon clot lysis. Rebleeding occurs in up to 16 to 25 percent of patients and clogs the aqueous outflow system, with a subsequent rise in intraocular pressure. Hemoglobinopathies, particularly sickle cell disease, sickle cell trait, and sickle thalassemia, predispose to rebleeding and other complications. It is critical to determine through history or laboratory testing whether any of these conditions exists.

The patient with a hyphema is placed at bed rest in the head-up position and the involved eye is shielded, with care being taken not to touch or apply pressure to the eye. An ophthalmology consultation must be obtained on all patients with hyphemas. Traditionally, patients with hyphemas have been admitted and placed at strict bed rest with head elevation. Some specialists utilize antifibrinolytics such as aminocaproic acid. The use of mydriatics, ocular steroids, osmotic agents, or acetazolamide should be left to the ophthalmologist. Acetazolamide and osmotic agents are contraindicated in patients with sickle cell disease because of the increase risk of bleeding. Aspirin and other platelet-active medications are also avoided, as these also increase the risk of rebleeding.

Lens Injury

Blunt ocular trauma may result in subluxation and subsequent monocular diplopia, secondary glaucoma, or cataracts. The lens may sublux either posteriorly or anteriorly, resulting in a deep or shallow anterior chamber and a visible lens margin. Iridodonesis is a shimmering/shaking of the iris provoked by rapidly changing gaze and is associated with lens dislocation.

Retinal Injury

Retinal injury often occurs in conjunction with other eye injuries, and older children with retinal injury complain of light flashes or a "curtain" over the visual field. Central visual acuity will be spared if the macula is unaffected. Fundoscopy may reveal a variety of hemorrhage patterns. Preretinal hemorrhages are boat-shaped with a horizontal "deck," while superficial flame-shaped hemorrhages are distinguishable from deeper round, purple-gray lesions. The shaken-baby syndrome causes linear retinal hemorrhages and associated exudates.

Retrobulbar Hemorrhage

Bleeding behind the globe may result in compromise of extraocular motions and lead to proptosis or bulging of the eye. Subsequent compromise of the optic nerve produces a Marcus Gunn pupil. In cases of severe proptosis and optic nerve injury, surgical decompression may be necessary, and, in rare instances, a lid release procedure may be required in the emergency department. The presence of a bruit accompanying proptosis indicates a traumatic arteriovenous fistula.

Foreign Bodies

A careful history is taken to evaluate patients with ocular foreign bodies. Exposure to power tools or metal striking metal (such as a hammer upon a nail) predisposes to an occult *intraocular* foreign body. A foreign-body sensation persists even after removal because of an underlying corneal abrasion. The lids are doubly everted and the cornea anesthetized for a thorough examination. More tenacious foreign bodies are removed with a cotton applicator soaked in tetracaine. In older cooperative children, foreign bodies may be removed under slit-lamp guidance using an eye spud or 25-gauge needle on a tuberculin syringe. Iron-containing foreign bodies may leave rust rings that result in photophobia and decreased visual acuity. Experienced emergency physicians may remove these rust rings in the emergency department, or alternatively patients may be referred to specialists.

After a foreign body is removed, additional foreign bodies and abrasions are checked for. A mydriatic agent and a topical antibiotic are instilled, the eye is patched, and the child is rechecked in 24 h. Appropriate analgesia is prescribed, including narcotic agents if appropriate. If a foreign body penetrates the corneal stroma, an ophthalmologist must be consulted.

Intraocular Foreign Body

Intraocular foreign bodies are vision-threatening injuries that may be easily overlooked. Certain foreign bodies place the patient at greater risk than others. Iron (siderosis) and copper (chalcosis) are particularly toxic to the eye, whereas glass and plastic are less inflammatory. Organic foreign bodies pose a high risk for intraocular infection. Occasionally a condition known as sympathetic ophthalmia develops several weeks after a penetrating injury. This autoimmune response occurs in the uninjured eye, leading to photophobia, inflammatory changes, and visual loss.

Children with intraocular foreign bodies may have decreased visual acuity, pupillary distortion, and relatively little pain. A teardrop pupil will "point" to the perforation site. Iridodialysis, a tear in the iris, produces a "second pupil."

A number of imaging modalities can detect intraocular foreign bodies. While larger metallic objects may be seen on a radiograph, computed tomography (CT) of the orbit provides greater resolution if the foreign body is small. Ocular ultrasound is highly sensitive for both metallic and nonmetallic penetrations. Magnetic resonance imaging (MRI) accurately detects organic, plastic, and glass particles but may cause further injury if mistakenly used in the case of metal objects, as the MRI magnet may move the foreign body.

The involved eye is covered with a metal eye shield, and the child is kept at rest. Broad-spectrum intravenous antibiotics are administered, usually a first-generation cephalosporin and an aminoglycoside. Foreign bodies that protrude from the eye must be left in place and removed in the operating room. Topical antibiotics are not indicated; in particular, antibiotic ointments should be avoided, as they produce intraocular granulomas.

Should a child with penetrating globe injury require emergency intubation, a nondepolarizing blocker such as vecuronium or pancuronium should be used instead of a depolarizing blocker such as succinylcholine. Succinylcholine and ketamine increase intraocular pressure and could theoretically cause extrusion of the intraocular contents.

Conjunctival and Scleral Lacerations

A slit-lamp examination is performed on all children with conjunctival lacerations to assess for scleral violation. To perform the Seidel test for scleral laceration, fluorescein is placed on the cornea and the suspicious area is observed under the cobalt blue light of the slit lamp. A swirling dilution of fluorescein secondary to leaking aqueous humor denotes scleral disruption. If a globe laceration is seen, tonometry is contraindicated, as additional pressure against the eye may cause extrusion of the iris. A combination of decreased visual acuity, media opacity, and an abnormal anterior chamber, or low intraocular pressure (less than 6) is accurate in the clinical diagnosis for scleral rupture. Blunt scleral rupture often occurs at the insertions of the intraocular muscles or at the limbus.

Small conjunctival lacerations are treated with topical antibiotic drops alone; sutures are not usually necessary. If the patient has deeper injury, an eye shield is placed on the child, intravenous antibiotics are administered, and adequate sedation is provided.

Chemical Injuries to the Eye

A caustic injury to the eye is one of the few situations in which treatment must precede examination and visual acuity testing. Copious irrigation with normal saline takes precedence over all but lifesaving interventions. The extent of caustic injury relates to the quantity of exposure, the pH, and the duration of the exposure (i.e., time to irrigation). Alkali injuries result in the most serious damage to the eye. Acids produce a coagulation necrosis that results in a protein barrier that blocks further penetration. Alkalis cause liquefaction necrosis with saponification of ocular tissues and deep penetration. Complications of caustic injuries include blindness, corneal neovascularization, secondary glaucoma, cataract formation, and retinal damage.

Irrigation is begun in the prehospital setting immediately after injury. Upon arrival in the emergency department, the child may require sedation with a rapid-acting intramuscular or intravenous agent to allow irrigation of the eye, but topical anesthesia alone may be adequate. The eyes are irrigated with normal saline using a Morgan lens. Alternatively, a nasal oxygen cannula placed upon the bridge of the nose allows bilateral irrigation of the eyes through the nasal prongs. One must never attempt to neutralize acids with alkalis or vice versa, as the resultant release of heat will further damage the eye. The eyes are lavaged for at least 20 min in the case of acid exposure and irrigated continuously in the case of severe alkali injury. Irrigation may be beneficial for up to 24 h after alkali exposure. Double lid eversion is performed to expose the fornices, and any caustic particulate matter is irrigated or swabbed out. Litmus paper is used to check the pH in the conjunctival sac after 20 min of irrigation, and irrigation is continued until the pH is between 7.0 and 7.5. If irrigation is stopped, the pH must be rechecked 10 min later to ensure a stable level.

Hydrofluoric acid exposure is a unique situation and may require irrigation with a magnesium oxide solution. A poison center should be consulted for the latest recommendations.

Ultraviolet Keratitis

Ultraviolet (UV) keratitis occurs when children stare at an eclipse or are exposed to the prolonged glare of snow. Older children who watch a welder's torch or use tanning booths without special glasses may also suffer this injury. They complain of photophobia and eye pain, usually 8 to 12 h after exposure; for this reason, patients with UV keratitis generally present at night. They exhibit both scleral and perilimbal injection accompanied by tearing and blepharospasm. A slit-lamp exam using fluorescein shows thousands of punctate, shallow lesions on the cornea (keratitis). Treatment is with cycloplegia, oral analgesia, and eye patching. Ultraviolet keratitis is usually bilateral and generally heals in 24 to 48 h.

Thermal Burns

Because of reflex blinking, lids are more often damaged from thermal injury than is the globe. Eyelashes and eyebrows are often burned. Corneal injury is diagnosed with the slit lamp with and without fluorescein staining, and topical antibiotics are applied to burned lids. Third-degree burns to the eye and periorbital tissues require admission to the hospital.

CONCLUSION

The emergency physician plays a central role in the management of pediatric eye injuries. He or she must perform a careful history and physical exam, document visual acuity, and use the slit lamp where appropriate. Early and liberal specialty consultation will prevent both medical and legal mishaps. In addition to early recognition and management of ocular trauma, the emergency physician must be active in patient education and community prevention programs. The most consistent means of decreasing pediatric eye morbidity is prevention of injury, and the use of safety goggles during sports must be encouraged.

For a more detailed discussion, see Colucciello SA: Eye Trauma, chap. 15, p. 107, in *Pediatric Emergency Medicine: A Comprehensive Study Guide.*

---

16 Orthopedic Injuries

Russell H. Greenfield

THE PEDIATRIC SKELETON

Growing bone is less dense and more malleable than mature bone. When a fracture does occur, propagation of the fracture line is diminished, making comminution less likely. These properties account for injuries that are unique to children, such as incomplete (greenstick) and torus fractures, as well as plastic deformation or bowing injuries, in which bending of the bone occurs without fracture.

New bone is laid down at fracture sites according to local stresses. This remodeling corrects some longitudinal malalignment and permits the acceptance of greater degrees of angulation with metaphyseal fractures. Remodeling will occur if a fracture is adjacent to a hinged joint, if angulation is less than 30° in the plane of motion, and if the child has at least 2 more years of bone growth remaining. However, the potential for bony remodeling does not obviate the need for precise anatomic fracture reduction in the presence of the following: rotational deformities, excessive degrees of angulation, or displaced intraarticular fractures.

The periosteum enveloping growing bones is stronger and thicker than mature periosteum and contributes to the lower incidence of open fractures in children.

The presence of physes (growth plates) and epiphyses accounts for the location of some childhood fractures, as well as for specific complications associated with pediatric orthopedic injuries. The growth plate is the weakest structure in the pediatric skeleton and also the place where anatomic alignment of fracture fragments is most critical in order to avoid growth imbalance and deformity.

Physeal injuries occur more often than ligamentous tears in children because the developing ligaments are more resistant to stress than the adjacent bony structures. Situations in which a sprained ligament would be diagnosed in an adult should prompt the diagnosis of a growth plate injury in a child. Forces capable of producing joint subluxations or dislocations in adults result in epiphyseal separations in children.

TERMINOLOGY

The precise anatomic location and morphology of a given fracture should be described using specific terminology. Table 16-1 outlines terms commonly used to describe fractures. Figure 16-1 is a diagram demonstrating anatomic terms related to the immature bone.

A break in the skin overlying a fracture converts the injury to an open fracture. The major treatment principles concerning open fractures in adults apply to children as well. Operative wound debridement, fracture reduction, and antibiotic administration are mandated in order to promote healing and prevent infectious complications.

PHYSEAL INJURIES

Physeal injuries are more common than is generally appreciated, accounting for up to 18 percent of all pediatric fractures. In the early 1960s, Salter and Harris developed the most widely used classification system for fractures involving the growth plate. Modifications were introduced by Ogden years later. Both systems are based upon the radiographic appearance of the fracture and describe the degree of involvement of the growth plate, epiphysis, and joint. These classifications have both prognostic and therapeutic implications (Table 16-2, Fig. 16-2).

Any fracture that involves the growth plate may result in growth disturbance, limb length inequality, and deformity. Parents should be made aware of this fact at the time a physeal injury is diagnosed.

Most fractures classified as Salter-Harris type I or II can be treated with closed reduction. Growth disturbances often complicate fracture types III to V, and these injuries often require operative intervention. Due to severe injury to the growth plate in type V fractures, growth disturbances can occur regardless of the method of treatment.

BIRTH TRAUMA

Fractures of the clavicle, humerus, hip, and femur occur frequently during difficult deliveries. The initial diagnosis is often infection or pseudoparalysis until a radiograph confirms the presence of a fracture.

CHILD ABUSE

A high index of suspicion for nonaccidental trauma must always be maintained when an injured child is evaluated. Most child abuse occurs between birth and 2 years of age. Up to 50 percent of fractures in children less than 1 year of age are the result of nonaccidental trauma.

Historical aspects of the injury, physical and radiographic findings, and an evaluation of the social interactions between family members must all be pooled in making the diagnosis of nonaccidental trauma. Certain radiographic findings are suggestive of nonaccidental trauma but not confirmative in and of themselves (Table 16-3). The presence of long bone fractures in a young child should raise the possibility of child abuse. Femur fractures in the nonambulatory child and nonsupracondylar fractures of the humerus are both very suggestive of abuse.

Fractures of the metaphyseal-epiphyseal junction are virtually pathognomonic for child abuse. These long bone "corner" frac-

TABLE 16-1 Fracture Terminology

Anatomic location

Epiphyseal—present at the end of each long bone; completely cartilaginous at birth except at distal femur; secondary ossification centers develop which replace cartilage over time

Apophyseal—traction epiphysis; nonarticular site of ligament and tendon attachment (example: distal humeral condyles); not directly involved in longitudinal growth but contribute to bony contour

Physeal (growth plate)—cartilaginous structure between epiphysis and metaphysis responsible for longitudinal bone growth; injury may result in growth disturbance or arrest

Metaphyseal—flared end of diaphysis adjacent to physes representing new bone; structurally weak area

Diaphyseal—central shaft of long bone

Articular—involves portion of epiphysis comprising joint surface

Epicondylar—distal humeral site of muscle attachments

Supracondylar—part of metaphysis located cephalad to condyles and epicondyles

Transcondylar—across the condyles of humerus or distal femur

Intercondylar—intraepiphyseal; fracture disrupts articular surface and separates condyles from one another

Subcapital—metaphyseal area of proximal femur and radius

Fracture pattern

Avulsion—bone fragment pulled off by action of tendon or ligament

Longitudinal—fracture line follows long axis of bone

Transverse—fracture line at right angle to long axis of bone

- Oblique—fracture line angled at 30 to 60° from long axis of bone
- Spiral—encircling oblique fracture (has torsional component)
- Impacted—fracture ends compressed together
- Comminuted—any fracture with more than two fracture fragments
- Bowing—(plastic deformation) significant bend in bone without fracture; commonly seen in ulna and fibula in association with fracture of respective paired bone
- Torus—"buckle fracture"; metaphyseal compaction of trabecular bone and buckling of cortical bone
- Greenstick—incomplete fracture of cortex on convex (tension, elastic phase) side of bone with only a bend in cortex of concave side (compression, plastic phase); most common fracture pattern in children
- Pathologic—fracture through abnormal, weakened bone (examples: tumors, osteomyelitis, cysts, inherited metabolic disorders)

Fracture fragment positions

- Alignment—refers to longitudinal relationship of one fragment to another
- Displacement—deviation of fracture fragments from anatomic position (displacement of distal fragment described in relation to proximal one; varus displacement—toward midline of body; valgus displacement—away from midline of body)
- Angulation—direction of apex of angle formed by fracture fragments (will be opposite to direction of displacement of distal fragment)
- Distraction—degree to which fracture surfaces are separated
- Bayonet deformity—overlapping fracture surfaces with resultant shortening
- Butterfly fragment—wedge-shaped fragment arising at apex of force applied to shaft of long bone

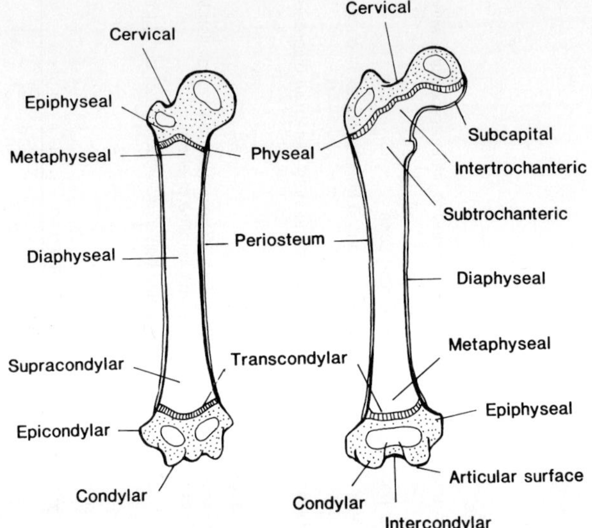

FIG. 16-1 Illustration of a pediatric humerus and femur depicting specific anatomic sites and descriptive terminology.

tures are frequently bilateral and result from periosteal avulsion of bone and cartilage secondary to violent twisting forces or a downward pull on an extremity. The injury may not be visible on initial radiographs but will be identifiable 7 to 10 days later as new subperiosteal bone formation (Fig. 16-3).

A skeletal survey should be performed on any child under 2 years of age when abuse is suspected. The survey should include anteroposterior (AP) views of the chest and pelvis; AP views of all extremities, including the hands and feet; and AP and lateral views of the skull.

CLINICAL EVALUATION

Resuscitative efforts and attention to potentially life-threatening injuries take precedence. Once the patient has been stabilized, a complete history and physical examination can be performed.

Pain and fear complicate the evaluation of the injured child.

TABLE 16-2 Classification of Epiphyseal Injuries

The Salter-Harris Classification System	
Type I:	Complete separation of the epiphysis and most of the physis from the metaphysis. Prognosis for normal growth is good. Commonly results from shearing force in newborns and young infants. May be seen in victims of abuse. Diagnosis may be difficult; if radiographic studies are normal but patient is tender over the growth plate, immobilization and orthopedic referral are recommended.
Type II:	Fracture line propagates along the physis and extends into the metaphysis; result is displaced metaphyseal fragment, often with epiphyseal displacement. Most common epiphyseal injury; associated with low risk of growth disturbance. Usually occurs in children over 10 years of age.
Type III:	Fracture line extends from the physis through the epiphysis to the articular surface to the joint. Anatomic reduction necessary to restore normal joint mechanics and prevent growth disturbance, bony bridging, and posttraumatic arthritis.
Type IV:	Fracture line begins at articular surface, crosses the epiphysis and growth plate, and extends into the metaphysis, splitting off a metaphyseal fragment (example: humeral lateral condyle fractures). Open reduction and internal fixation usually required to ensure anatomic reduction and avoid angular deformity and loss of joint function. Significant incidence of growth disturbance.
Type V:	Results from longitudinal compression of the growth plate. Rare injury associated with apparently normal x-rays. Diagnosis usually made in retrospect when premature closure of the physis and growth abnormalities develop.
Additional fracture types from the Ogden Classification System	
Type VI:	Peripheral shear injury to borders of growth plate. Angular deformity may develop due to formation of osseous bridge between metaphysis and epiphysis.
Type VII:	Intraarticular intraepiphyseal injury where ligament pulls off distal portion of epiphysis rather than tearing.
Type VIII:	Fracture through region of metaphysis with temporary disruption of circulation.
Type IX:	Fracture involving significant damage to or loss of periosteum.

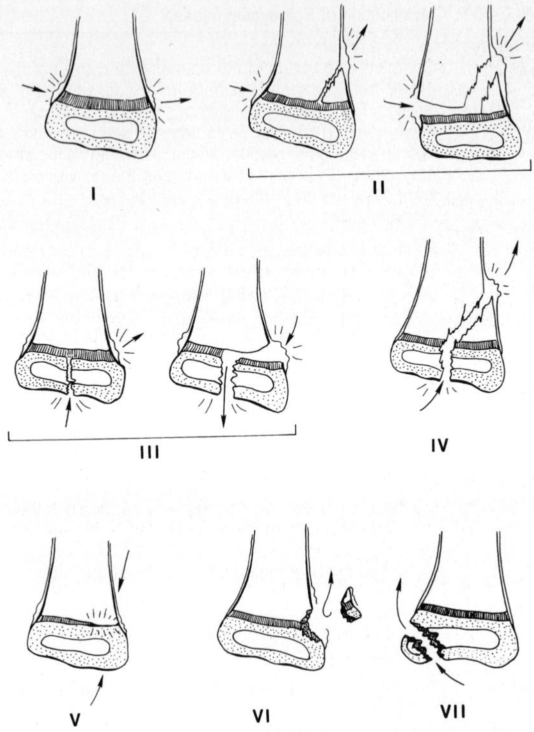

FIG. 16-2 Classification of growth plate injuries described by Salter and Harris (I to V) and Ogden (VI and VII).

History should be obtained both from the patient, if age-appropriate, and from any witnesses to the injury. Histories that are vague or inconsistent with the injury suggest the possibility of nonaccidental trauma. Past medical history and developmental milestones should also be addressed.

The injured limb should be observed and palpated, thereby checking for deformity, swelling, pain, and abnormal motion. Examination of both the joint above and the joint below the site of injury must be included in the evaluation. Careful inspection of the surrounding soft tissues may reveal a break in integrity that signals open communication with the fracture site. A thorough assessment of the neurovascular status of the extremity should be performed prior to and after any attempts at manipulative reduction. Serial assessments during the patient's course will ensure that a developing compartment syndrome is discovered early.

Liberal use of radiographs is advisable because of the difficulty in performing an adequate history and physical examination on young children and because of the relative paucity of physical findings associated with certain childhood fractures. At least two views perpendicular to each other should be obtained, usually an AP and lateral view. The films should include the joints above and below the injury site, since dislocations can occur with diaphyseal fractures (e.g., Monteggia fractures). To prevent further injury, the injured extremity should be splinted *before* the patient goes to the radiographic suite. Comparison views of the noninjured extremity may be helpful but are not routinely recommended.

THERAPEUTIC CONSIDERATIONS

Pain medication should be provided as needed and local or regional blocks considered after a thorough neurovascular assessment has been performed. Immobilization of the injured extremity, including the joints above and below the fracture, will prevent further injury and may make the patient more comfortable. Open fractures, fractures that are significantly displaced or angulated, frac-

TABLE 16-3 Radiographic Findings Suggestive of Child Abuse

High Risk for Abuse
Metaphyseal lesions
Posterior rib fractures
Scapular fractures
Spinous process fractures
Sternal fractures
Moderate Risk for Abuse
Multiple fractures, especially bilateral
Fractures of different ages
Epiphyseal separation
Vertebral body fractures and subluxations
Digit fractures
Complex skull fractures
Low Risk for Abuse
Clavicular fractures
Fractures of long bone shaft
Linear skull fractures

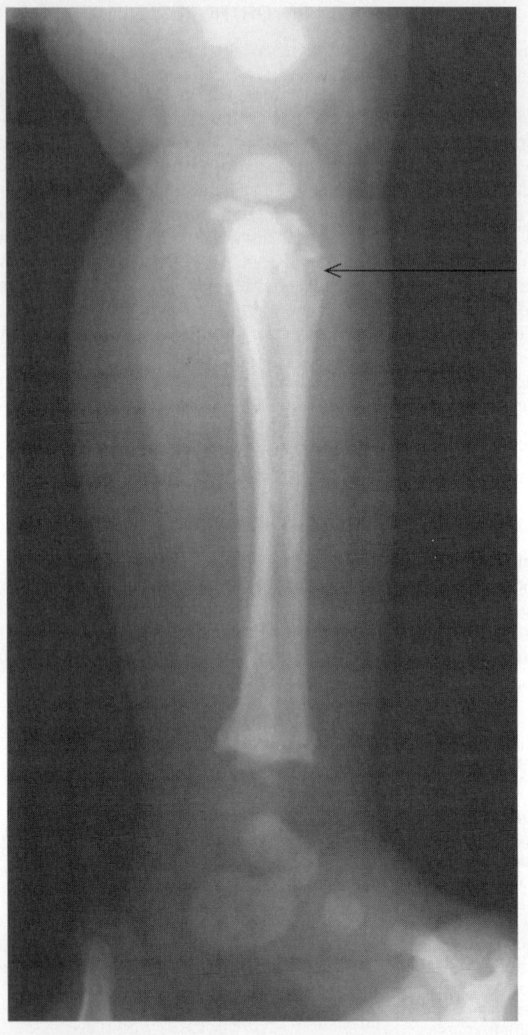

FIG. 16-3 Periosteal reaction with metaphyseal irregularity in a 3-month-old (*arrow*). This metaphyseal corner fracture is very suggestive of nonaccidental trauma.

tures associated with neurovascular compromise, and fractures involving a growth plate require immediate orthopedic consultation. Most nondisplaced fractures can be splinted by the primary care physician and referred for definitive care within 3 days.

A sling and swathe provide sufficient immobilization for most injuries between the sternoclavicular joint and the elbow, whereas posterior arm splints are useful with elbow, forearm, and wrist injuries. In both cases the elbow should be flexed to 90° and the forearm placed in neutral position. An ulnar gutter splint immobilizes fractures of the fourth and fifth fingers, while a thumb spica splint stabilizes injuries involving the scaphoid bone and thumb. Long posterior leg splints immobilize the knee and stabilize the distal femur as well as the proximal and middle tibia and fibula. Short posterior leg splints provide stable immobilization for ankle and foot injuries.

Prior to discharge, the proper use of ice and elevation should be described and instructions given to return immediately for repeat evaluation should severe pain, swelling, or change in color develop. Children's fractures heal much more quickly than similar injuries in adults, so fracture reduction and orthopedic follow-up must take place as soon as possible after the injury.

For a more detailed discussion, see Greenfield RH: Orthopedic Injuries, chap. 16, p. 113, in *Pediatric Emergency Medicine: A Comprehensive Study Guide.*

17 Injuries of the Upper Extremities

Russell H. Greenfield

THE CLAVICLE AND ACROMIOCLAVICULAR JOINT

The most common pediatric orthopedic injury is the clavicle fracture, usually resulting from a fall onto a shoulder or outstretched hand. The vast majority of injuries involve the area between the middle and distal thirds of the clavicle (>90 percent). Young children sustain incomplete injuries (greenstick or torus fractures), whereas older children and adolescents present more often with displaced fractures.

A careful search for associated vascular injury is mandatory in the presence of a clavicular fracture. Pulse changes and significant swelling may signal laceration or compression of the subclavian vessels, especially with posterior displacement of the fracture fragments, prompting emergent consultation with a vascular surgeon.

Most clavicular fractures heal well without complication, and reduction is rarely necessary unless significant overriding is present. Injuries due to birth trauma require only careful handling of the infant. Young children are placed in either a sling or a shoulder strap, while older patients can be managed with a sling and swathe. Operative intervention is indicated in the presence of an open fracture or vascular complication.

Direct trauma to the distal clavicle produces metaphyseal fractures in young children rather than true acromioclavicular joint separations, as seen in adolescents and adults. Avulsion of bone and periosteum occurs rather than ligamentous tearing. Weighted radiographic views are not routinely recommended. The fracture heals well with the use of a sling and swathe, and surgery is only rarely indicated.

SHOULDER DISLOCATIONS

The same trauma that results in shoulder dislocation in adults usually causes physeal fractures of the proximal humerus in young children.

Inspection of the anteriorly dislocated shoulder reveals loss of the normally rounded contour and a squared-off appearance. The arm is held in slight abduction and external rotation, and the humeral head may be palpated anterior to the glenoid fossa. Radiographs should include an anteroposterior (AP) view of the shoulder and either a true scapular lateral or transaxillary view. In general, adequate analgesia and relaxation should be provided before attempting reduction with either traction-countertraction, scapular manipulation, or external rotation techniques. Posterior shoulder dislocations can occur following seizures or electrical injuries. The arm is held in adduction and internal rotation. The anterior shoulder appears abnormally flat, and the displaced humeral head may be palpable posteriorly. Orthopedic consultation is recommended in all cases of posterior shoulder dislocation.

Axillary nerve damage may accompany shoulder dislocation. Sensation over the deltoid muscle should be assessed before and after any joint manipulation. Other complications include greater tuberosity fractures, damage to the glenoid labrum, the Hill-Sachs deformity (a compression fracture of the posterolateral humeral head), and recurrent dislocation.

HUMERAL FRACTURES

Nearly 80 percent of the longitudinal growth of the humerus takes place at the proximal humeral epiphysis. Accordingly, fractures involving the growth plate of the proximal humerus may result in growth disturbances. Fortunately, Salter-Harris fracture types III, IV, and V are rare in this region.

Salter-Harris type I and II fractures of the proximal humerus are encountered frequently. Type I fractures and proximal metaphyseal injuries, including greenstick and torus fractures, occur in youngsters aged 5 to 11 years. Children between the ages of 11 and 15 suffer the majority of proximal humerus fractures, usually type II injuries. The majority of proximal humerus fractures are nondisplaced due to the presence of a strong periosteal sleeve.

Routine radiographic evaluation should include at least two views of the humerus at right angles to one another. Films should include the distal clavicle and acromion to rule out associated injury.

Most fractures of the proximal humerus heal well with only a sling and swathe. If the proximal humeral epiphysis is displaced more than 1 cm, angulation is greater than 40°, or significant malrotation is present, internal fixation may be required.

Proximal and distal humeral fractures are much more common than diaphyseal injuries. Most fractures of the humeral shaft are the result of a direct blow to the area.

Because of bony remodeling and longitudinal overgrowth that occurs in response to the fracture, midshaft fractures heal well even with angulation of up to 15 to 20° and as much as 2 cm of overriding. A sling and swathe should be applied to young children, and a sugar-tong splint can be used for adolescents.

Fractures involving the junction of the middle and distal thirds of the humerus are associated with injury to the radial nerve. Motor and sensory functions should be assessed initially and following any manipulation.

THE ELBOW

With injury in the area of the elbow, radiographic interpretation is complicated by the presence of numerous epiphyses and ossification centers that appear and fuse at different but characteristic ages. Matters are further complicated by the need for precise anatomic reduction of fracture fragments in order to avoid both early and late complications.

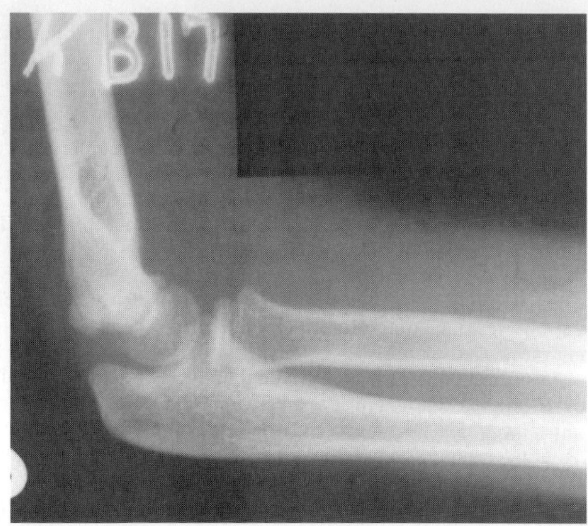

FIG. 17-1 Fracture through the medial epicondyle extending into the olecranon fossa. Note the posterior fat pad sign, signifying the presence of blood within the joint space.

An adequate radiographic evaluation of the elbow consists of an AP view with the joint in extension and a true lateral view with the elbow flexed at a right angle. The anterior fat pad is located within the coronoid fossa and normally appears as a small lucency just anterior to the fossa on a true lateral radiograph of the elbow. The posterior fat pad sits deep down in the olecranon fossa and is not visible under normal circumstances. The presence of a posterior fat pad on a true lateral view of the elbow is always abnormal and suggests blood within the joint capsule. Joint space fluid collections may also cause the anterior fat pad to be pushed away from the joint and appear as a windblown sail—the "sail sign." These abnormal fat pad signs are radiographic evidence of occult fracture of either the distal humerus or the proximal ulna or radius (Fig. 17-1) and can be detected only with the elbow in a full 90° of flexion.

The paths of two lines on plain elbow radiographs may provide additional evidence of an occult elbow fracture. The anterior humeral line, drawn along the anterior cortex of the distal humerus on a true lateral view of the elbow, should normally intersect the posterior two-thirds of the capitellum distally. Variation in this linear relationship points to the presence of a nondisplaced supracondylar fracture, an injury in which the fracture line is often not evident on a radiograph. Most supracondylar fractures occur in extension and are associated with some degree of posterior displacement of the distal humeral fragment. In the presence of minimal displacement, the fracture can be detected by noting that the anterior humeral line transects only the anterior third of the capitellum or misses it altogether. The radiocapitellar line is drawn through the middle of the proximal radius and should bisect the capitellum on any radiographic view of the elbow. Failure to do so suggests the presence of an occult radial neck fracture or radial head dislocation.

SUPRACONDYLAR HUMERAL FRACTURES

A fall onto an outstretched hand causing violent hyperextension of the elbow is the usual mechanism of injury with supracondylar fractures of the distal humeral metaphysis (Fig. 17-2). Supracondylar fractures account for 50 to 60 percent of all elbow injuries in children aged 3 to 10 years.

Supracondylar humeral fractures are associated with a high incidence of early neurovascular complications. Signs of significant distal ischemia include severe pain in the forearm or hand, paresthesias, pallor and cyanosis of the fingers, forearm pain exacerbated by passive finger extension, and absence of the radial pulse. Prompt reduction of the fracture fragments may be corrective, but if the vascular status is not improved following reduction, surgical exploration is indicated. If attention to vascular compromise is delayed, compartment syndrome and Volkmann's ischemic contracture, a permanent disability, may develop. Nerve damage occurs in 10 to 20 percent of children with supracondylar fractures, yet the prognosis for return of function is good. Radial, median, and ulnar nerve injuries, in descending order of frequency, have all been reported. A late complication of supracondylar humeral fractures is a change in the carrying angle of the elbow (cubitus varus).

The potential for significant complications with supracondylar humeral fractures mandates accurate diagnosis and urgent orthopedic consultation. Rotational and angular deformities must be meticulously reduced in order to preserve normal elbow function and prevent vascular compromise. Most children are admitted for 24 to 48 h of observation so that the neurovascular status of the extremity can be reassessed frequently. Open reduction and internal fixation may be necessary.

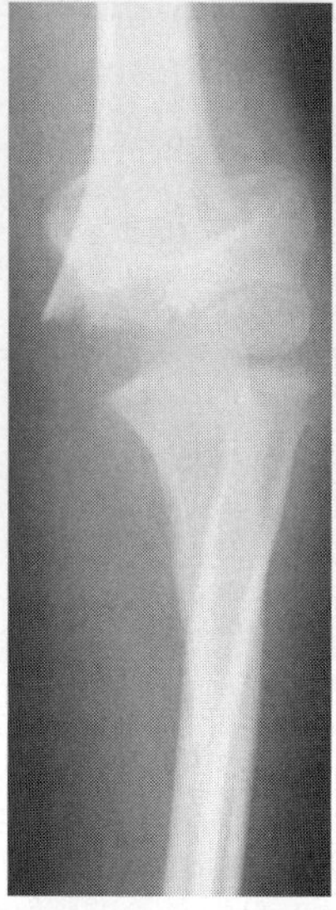

A

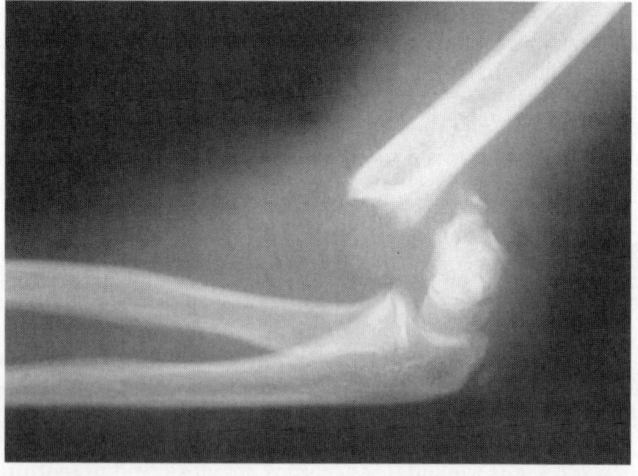

B

FIG. 17-2 *A* and *B*. Comminuted supracondylar fracture with large joint effusion. The patient required fasciotomy and skin grafting because of neurovascular compromise.

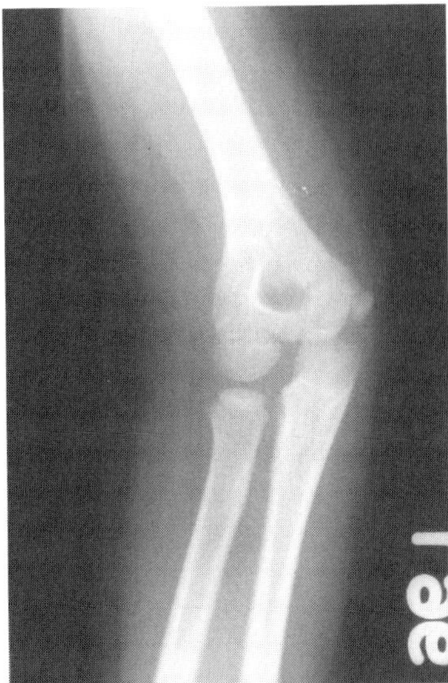

FIG. 17-3 Nondisplaced fracture of the medial condyle in a 5-year-old.

THE MEDIAL AND LATERAL CONDYLES

Fractures involving the articular surface of the lateral condyle (capitellum) represent 15 percent of all pediatric elbow fractures and peak in incidence at 6 years of age. Salter-Harris type IV fractures are common. These unstable intraarticular injuries require aggressive intervention to prevent complications such as nonunion, loss of mobility, and growth arrest of the lateral condylar physis, resulting in cubitus valgus. Management is usually operative.

Fractures of the articular surface of the medial condyle, or trochlea, occur only rarely, but when present require precise anatomic reduction because of the intraarticular nature of the injury (Fig. 17-3). The most frequent complications associated with medial condylar fractures are nonunion and ulnar nerve neuropraxia.

THE EPICONDYLES

The epicondyles are located just proximal to the articulating surface of the distal humerus and are the origins of the flexor and

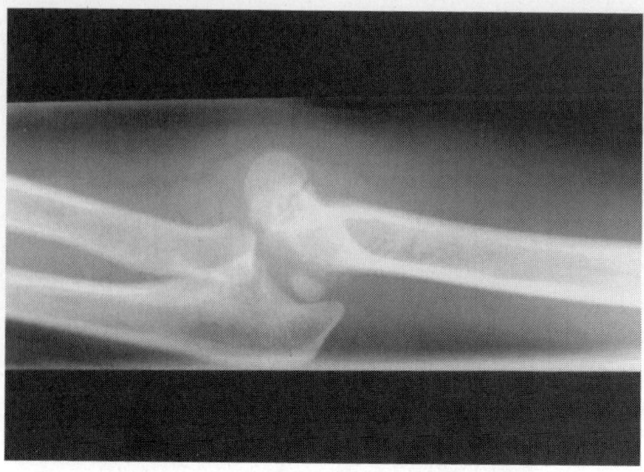

FIG. 17-4 Posterior elbow dislocation with avulsion of the medial epicondyle.

extensor muscles of the forearm. Fractures of the medial epicondyle are rarely encountered in patients under 4 years of age and occur most commonly in children aged 7 to 15 years. The vast majority of medial epicondylar fractures occur in association with elbow dislocations (Fig. 17-4), and intraarticular fracture fragments may block relocation. Avulsion injuries result from forceful contraction of the wrist flexors or secondary to the pull of the ulnar collateral ligament following a repetitive valgus stress (Little Leaguer's elbow). Ulnar nerve neuropraxia commonly accompanies this apophyseal fracture, and concomitant radial neck and olecranon fractures can be seen. Operative intervention is required only when the attached musculature exerts traction on the fragment, resulting in significant displacement (>0.5 to 1.0 cm). Injury to the lateral epicondyle is relatively rare.

ELBOW DISLOCATIONS

Pediatric elbow dislocations occur infrequently, since most forces that result in dislocations in adults usually cause fractures in children. When elbow dislocations do occur, they are usually the result of an adolescent's fall onto a slightly flexed, outstretched arm. Most dislocations are posterior, as with adults.

Associated fractures are the rule and most commonly involve the medial epicondyle, coronoid process, radial head, or olecranon (Fig. 17-4). Significant damage to the surrounding soft tissues also occurs, with damage to the neighboring nerves more common than brachial artery injury. Recovery of function of the ulnar nerve can be expected, but the prognosis is less optimistic with median nerve damage. Vascular compromise complicates up to 7 percent of pediatric elbow dislocations.

Most dislocations can be reduced after adequate analgesia and muscle relaxation are provided. The elbow should be flexed to 60 to 70° and the forearm placed in supination. The proximal humerus is then stabilized by an assistant while longitudinal traction is applied at the wrist. Upon successful relocation, the elbow should be gently flexed and immobilized and the neurovascular status of the arm reappraised. A postreduction radiograph should be obtained.

RADIAL HEAD SUBLUXATION

This most common pediatric elbow injury is also called *nursemaid's elbow* or *pulled elbow*. It occurs when abrupt axial traction is applied to the wrist or hand of the extended, pronated forearm of a child under 5 years of age, causing the annular ligament to slip free of the radial head and become entrapped between the radial head and capitellum.

On presentation, the child appears comfortable yet refuses to reach for objects with the affected arm. On examination, the forearm is held in pronation with the elbow in slight flexion. There is a remarkable lack of swelling and only mild tenderness over the radial head. The child resists all attempts at passive supination. Radiographic evaluation is not necessary unless an alternative diagnosis is being strongly considered.

Whether by supination or pronation, successful reduction of the subluxed radial head usually occurs after one or two attempts. A time-honored method is to place one finger over the radial head while the forearm is supinated and then flexed at the elbow. A palpable or audible "pop" usually signals successful relocation. Typically the patient again reaches for objects with the affected arm within 5 to 10 min of relocation. No further treatment is necessary. If radiographs have been obtained, the child often returns with normal arm movement after active positioning by the technologist.

Several attempts at reduction may be necessary before the patient regains normal use of the arm. If the subluxation occurred several hours prior to relocation, it may take a longer period of time for normal arm function to return. If relocation is still unsuccessful, alternative diagnoses should be considered. Recurrence rates have been reported to be as high as 30 percent.

FRACTURES OF THE RADIUS AND ULNA

Three-quarters of all injuries involve the distal third of the forearm. While an isolated fracture of one of the bones can occur, a high index of suspicion must be maintained for concomitant injury to the paired bone. The force precipitating a readily apparent injury may be transmitted to the paired bone, resulting in bowing, a greenstick fracture, or dislocation, often at a location distant from the obvious fracture site. For this reason forearm radiographs should always include the wrist and elbow. Most fractures of the radius and ulna heal without significant complications.

The appearance of an abnormal fat pad sign or abnormal radiocapitellar line on a radiograph points to the presence of an occult radial head or radial neck fracture, respectively. Minimally displaced or nondisplaced fractures can be treated in a posterior splint, with the elbow flexed at 90°. Complications include restriction of pronation and supination as well as myositis ossificans.

Olecranon fractures occur commonly in combination with other elbow injuries, such as radial head dislocations, radial neck fractures, and fractures of the medial epicondyle. Isolated olecranon epiphyseal fractures are rare; they are usually due to a direct blow to the posterior elbow. Nondisplaced injuries may be treated in a posterior splint. Healing usually takes place without complications, although nonunion and ulnar nerve neuropraxia do occur infrequently.

Most forearm diaphyseal fractures are either greenstick or bowing injuries. One or both bones may suffer greenstick or bowing injuries, or one bone may have a greenstick fracture while the paired bone is bowed (Fig. 17-5). The potential for remodeling of a bowing injury—or plastic deformation—is minimal in children over 4 years of age. Bowing may restrict pronation and supination as well as result in permanent deformity of the extremity.

Overriding of fracture fragments in the presence of an isolated fracture of one of the forearm bones suggests either a Monteggia or Galeazzi fracture. An isolated fracture of the proximal ulna may be associated with concomitant dislocation of the radial head (*Monteggia fracture*). This combined injury can be overlooked initially because attention is focused on the displaced ulnar fracture. An aberrant radiocapitellar line on plain radiograph is evidence of the accompanying radial head dislocation (Fig. 17-6). Closed reduction is usually successful. A fracture at the junction of the middle and distal thirds of the radius in association with distal radioulnar joint dislocation is called a *Galeazzi fracture* and is rare in children (Fig. 17-7).

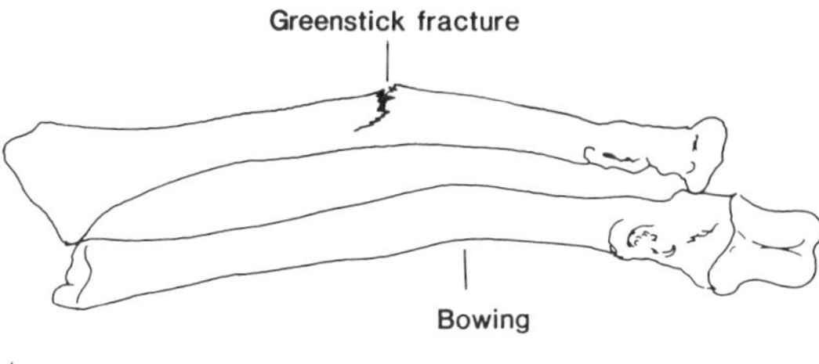

A

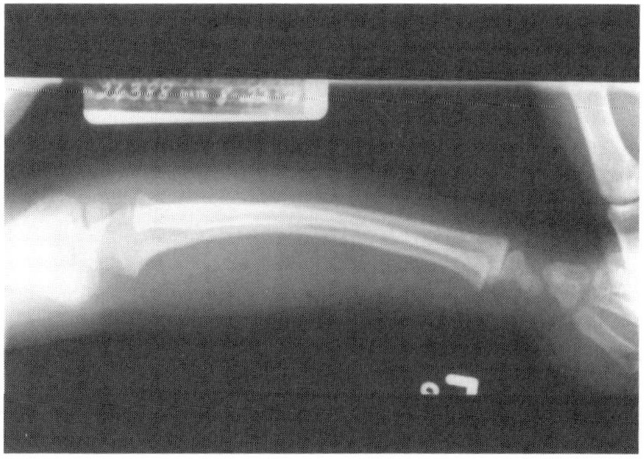

B

FIG. 17-5 *A.* Illustration depicting a greenstick fracture of the radius with associated plastic deformity of the ulna. *B.* Radiographic appearance of midshaft bowing injury of both the radius and ulna.

Torus fractures of the distal radius and ulna are frequently encountered and can be treated in a long arm splint (Fig. 17-8). The distal radial physis accounts for almost 80 percent of the longitudinal growth of the radius, but significant growth disturbance secondary to injury rarely occurs. Tenderness over the growth plate of the distal radius with a normal radiograph should prompt the diagnosis of a Salter-Harris type I injury.

The capacity for remodeling in the forearm is significant, but rotational abnormalities must be corrected. The strong periosteal sleeve of the bones makes nonunion rare. Complications are un-

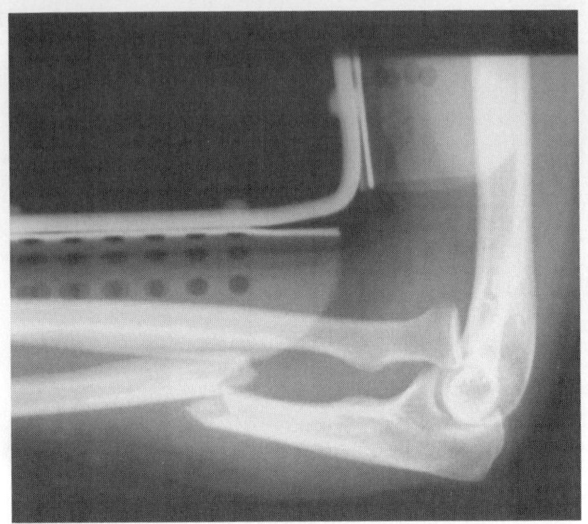

FIG. 17-6 Fracture of the proximal ulna with radial head dislocation (Monteggia fracture). A line bisecting the proximal radius completely misses the capitellum.

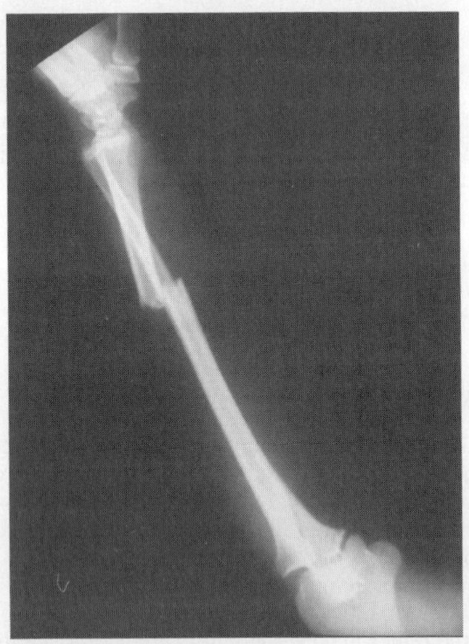

FIG. 17-7 Galeazzi fracture in a 16-year-old.

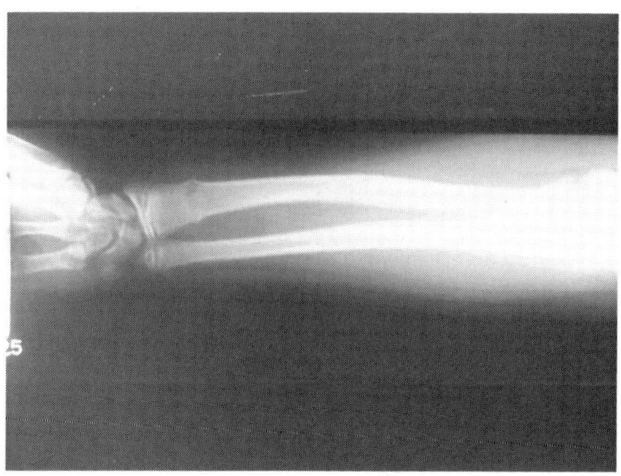

FIG. 17-8 Torus fracture of the distal radius.

common, but vascular compromise can develop with any forearm fracture.

For a more detailed discussion, see Greenfield RH: Injuries of the Upper Extremities, chap. 17, p. 119, in *Pediatric Emergency Medicine: A Comprehensive Study Guide.*

18 Injuries of the Hand and Wrist

Russell H. Greenfield

Most information about a young child's hand is garnered through observation and palpation. Tendon injuries, rotational defects, and bony deformities can be detected with a thorough inspection of the injured part. The position in which the digits are held can provide a wealth of information. Increasing degrees of flexion are normally present at rest as one travels from the index finger to the little finger. A tendon injury should be suspected if this digital cascade is interrupted. Rotational defects are often clinically evident yet difficult to detect radiographically. Malrotation becomes more obvious during flexion, when all fingertips should normally point toward the scaphoid tubercle. Thus, radiographs should be obtained liberally and should include anteroposterior, lateral, and oblique views.

Proper evaluation of the motor function of the hand requires testing of each individual tendon separately. Testing should be performed against force, because partial tendon injuries can be discovered by detecting weakness in flexion or extension.

The flexor digitorum profundus (FDP) tendon flexes the distal interphalangeal (DIP) joint. The middle phalanx and proximal interphalangeal (PIP) joint of the digit being tested must be stabilized and the metacarpophalangeal (MCP) joint held in extension in order to properly assess the function of the FDP. The flexor digitorum superficialis (FDS) tendon flexes the PIP joint. Function is evaluated by holding all digits in full extension except for the finger being tested, thus blocking the common action of the FDP to the finger being examined. Flexor pollicis longus function is assessed by testing flexion of the interphalangeal joint while stabilizing the proximal phalanx of the thumb. About 40 percent of the population has only one flexor tendon of the little finger.

Extensor tendon function is evaluated with the joint in flexion. The examiner stabilizes the digit just proximal to the joint being tested, and the patient is then asked to extend the finger. The index and little fingers have double extensor tendons, so injury to one often will not result in an observable extension deficit.

The evaluation of nerve function of the hand can prove to be extremely difficult in the young child. Motor and sensory functions of the radial, medial, and ulnar nerves must each be assessed individually.

The radial nerve permits extension of the wrist and the MCP joints. Motor function is assessed by either testing wrist extension while pushing down on the dorsum of the hand or testing finger extension with the wrist extended. The radial nerve provides sensory innervation to the dorsum of the hand radial to the third metacarpal, including the dorsal surfaces of the thumb, index, and middle fingers at least as far as the DIP joints. Measuring two-point discrimination in the proximal dorsal thumb web space provides the best assessment of radial nerve sensory function.

The motor function of the median nerve can be evaluated by testing thumb abduction away from the palm, during which the muscles of the thenar eminence should normally contract. The median nerve also supplies the FDS, which can be tested as described earlier. Sensory innervation essentially mirrors that of the radial nerve, but on the volar surface of the hand as well as to both the dorsal and volar tips of the thumb and first two fingers. The most reliable method of assessing median nerve sensory function is testing two-point discrimination on the volar pad of the index finger.

The ulnar nerve controls the dorsal and palmar interosseous muscles and supplies sensation to the entire ulnar aspect of the hand. Motor function is evaluated by having the patient abduct and adduct the fingers against resistance, thereby testing the dorsal and volar interossei, respectively. Sensory function is best assessed by measuring two-point discrimination on the volar pad of the little finger.

Harrison's tactile adherence test addresses local sweat gland activity and can be useful in evaluating nerve function in fearful, uncooperative patients. Innervated skin will adhere slightly to a smooth object, such as a pen, being drawn across the surface, causing some drag. Denervated skin is dry, slick, and smooth, with loss of the characteristic tactile adherence. Intact innervation can also be assumed in the presence of skin wrinkling after the injured part is submerged in water.

A finger laceration that is pumping blood implies concomitant digital nerve injury, because the nerve courses superficial to the digital artery. The artery should not be clamped for fear of causing further injury to the adjacent nerve. The integrity of the vascular supply of the hand can be assessed by palpating the radial and ulnar arteries, noting the color and warmth of the digits, performing Allen's test, and testing capillary refill.

Amputated digits should be wrapped in saline-soaked gauze and enclosed in a plastic bag. The bag should then be placed in an iced liquid bath until definitive treatment can be performed. If the amputated finger is immersed directly in iced fluid, cold injury and maceration of the cut edges of the digit can occur, lessening the chances for successful replantation. Indications for replantation in children include proximal phalanx amputations, thumb amputations, index finger amputations, and amputation of multiple digits. Most amputations secondary to crush injuries are not suitable for replantation because of accompanying soft tissue damage.

TENDON INJURIES

The general principles of tendon injury management in adults also apply to children. All flexor tendon injuries should be evaluated by an orthopedic specialist.

The mallet finger deformity results from injury to the conjoined extensor tendon at the DIP. Salter-Harris type I fractures predomi-

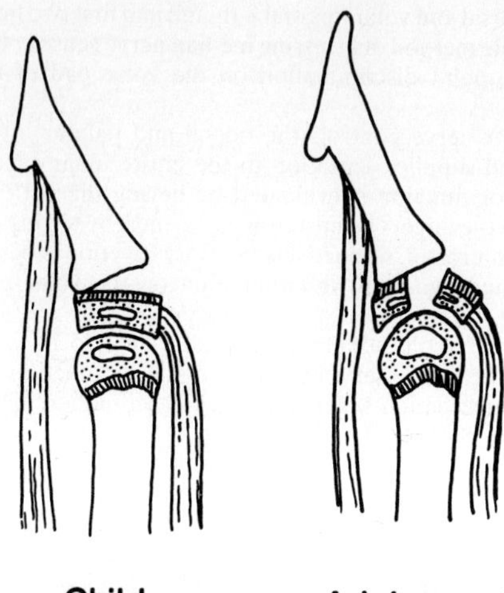

FIG. 18-1 A finger demonstrating loss of active extension at the DIP joint and a flexion deformity is called a *mallet finger.* In adults, the injury is due to avulsion of the extensor tendon from its insertion at the base of the distal phalanx. In children and adolescents, respectively, Salter-Harris type I and type III fractures predominate.

nate in the very young, while type III fractures are more common in adolescents (Fig. 18-1). The DIP joint assumes a flexion deformity and exhibits loss of active extension. Treatment involves 6 weeks of immobilization with the DIP in mild hyperextension. If the fracture involves more than 25 percent of the joint surface or if significant subluxation is present, internal fixation may be necessary.

Disruption of the central portion of the extensor mechanism overlying the PIP joint in association with volar subluxation of the lateral bands causes the "boutonniere," or "buttonhole," deformity, usually as a result of a direct blow to the finger. Findings include loss of active extension at the PIP joint, a flexion deformity of the PIP joint, and hyperextension of the DIP joint. The digit should be splinted in extension and follow-up with an orthopedist arranged in anticipation of surgical repair.

FRACTURES AND JOINT INJURIES

Unlike other childhood fractures, only minimal deformity will be tolerated in the hand. Most hand fractures in children can be managed with closed reduction. Open reduction is indicated when an articular surface or epiphysis is damaged. Adequate immobilization of a child's injured hand is difficult to guarantee, so the entire upper extremity is usually casted or splinted to prevent further injury.

Fractures of the proximal and middle phalangeal shafts are the most common childhood hand injuries. Salter-Harris type II fractures of the proximal and middle phalanges are commonly encountered (Fig. 18-2). Distal tuft fractures secondary to local crush injury require no special treatment other than management of associated soft tissue damage and splinting.

In splinting or casting proximal phalangeal fractures, care should be taken to maintain flexion of the collateral ligaments so as to preserve normal hand function. The wrist should be placed in 30° of extension, the MCP joint flexed 60 to 90°, and the interphalangeal joints placed in 15° of flexion.

Metacarpal shaft fractures are frequently unstable, but management with closed reduction is usually successful. Rotational deformities, if present, may necessitate open reduction and internal fixation. Fracture of the metaphysis of the distal fifth metacarpal is analogous to a boxer's fracture in adults and should be reduced if angulation is greater than 40°. Reduction is accomplished by flexing both the MCP and PIP joints to 90° and pushing on the head of the proximal phalanx. When metacarpal fractures are splinted or casted, flexion should be maintained at the MCP joint to prevent the development of stiffness. Fourth and fifth metacarpal fractures that are well aligned can be placed in an ulnar gutter splint until seen by an orthopedist.

Falls onto an outstretched hand after age 7 often result in fracture of the scaphoid bone (carpal navicular). The initial radiographs may be normal, but if "snuffbox" tenderness is present on examination, a thumb spica splint should be placed and the patient referred to an orthopedist.

Complete disruption of the ulnar collateral ligament (UCL) of the thumb, or Salter-Harris type I or III fractures at the base of the thumb proximal phalanx, results in "gamekeeper's thumb." Swelling and tenderness over the thumb MCP joint are present. A lateral stress applied to the joint will exacerbate discomfort and may reveal gross instability. Cast immobilization is adequate treatment for type I fractures, but operative repair is necessary to restore proper joint function with type III fractures. Surgical

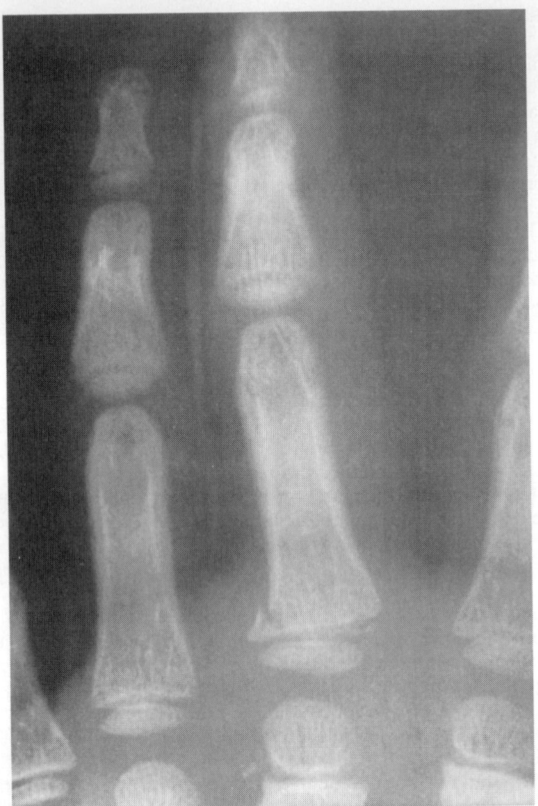

FIG. 18-2 Salter-Harris type III fracture of the proximal.

intervention is frequently required in older adolescents and adults because the ligament, which has been avulsed from its distal insertion, often gets caught over the edge of the extensor aponeurosis when the joint spontaneously reduces.

Bennett's fracture is an intraarticular fracture-dislocation of the trapeziometacarpal joint of the thumb. Pediatric Bennett's fractures are Salter-Harris type III injuries and result in bony bridging and joint incongruity if not treated carefully. This injury is unstable and requires open reduction.

Interphalangeal joint dislocations can usually be reduced by hyperextending the joint and then repositioning the distal bone in a dorsal-to-palmar direction. The digit should be splinted in extension for 2 weeks.

Most MCP joint dislocations can be reduced by applying longitudinal traction to the digit followed by flexion of the joint. Operative reduction is required for index finger MCP joint dislocations when there is dorsal dislocation of the proximal phalanx on the metacarpal head. Attempts at closed reduction fail because the metacarpal head gets trapped volarly between the flexor tendons and the transverse metacarpal ligament, while the volar plate gets caught dorsally between the metacarpal head and the base of the proximal phalanx.

For a more detailed discussion, see Greenfield RH: Injuries of the hand and wrist, chap. 18, p. 126, in *Pediatric Emergency Medicine: A Comprehensive Study Guide.*

19 Fractures of the Pelvis and Femur

Russell H. Greenfield

Properties unique to the immature pelvis account for the different types of pelvic fractures found in children.

The three primary ossification sites of the pelvis—located within the ilium, ischium, and pubis—meet at the acetabulum and form the triradiate cartilage. Lateral compression fractures of the pelvis or acetabular fractures may damage the triradiate cartilage, resulting in growth arrest and a shallow, dysplastic acetabulum. Injury to the triradiate cartilage is easily missed on a radiograph (Fig. 19-1), prompting the recommendation that children with pelvic fractures be reevaluated frequently for at least 12 months.

Examination of the pelvis must be performed within the context of care of the multiple trauma victim. The degree of force required to cause pelvic fractures is sufficiently great that concomitant injury to vital organs is common. Resuscitative efforts and attention to possible intraabdominal, bladder, urethral, and vascular injuries

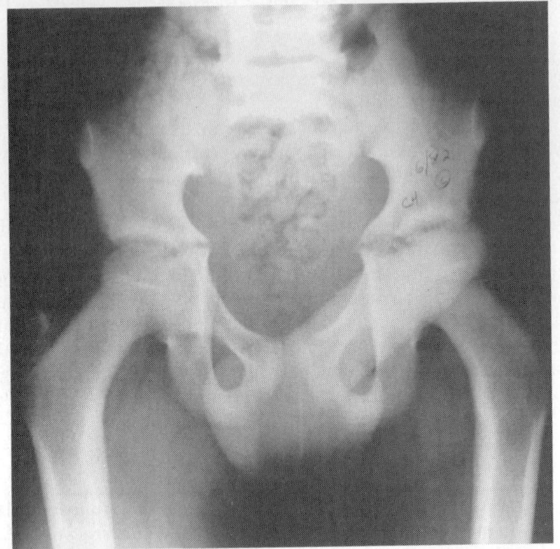

A

B

FIG. 19-1 An unusual case of fracture through the triradiate cartilage of the left acetabulum (*A*) followed by a similar fracture involving the right acetabulum (*B*) almost one year later. Growth arrest is a common complication of this type of injury.

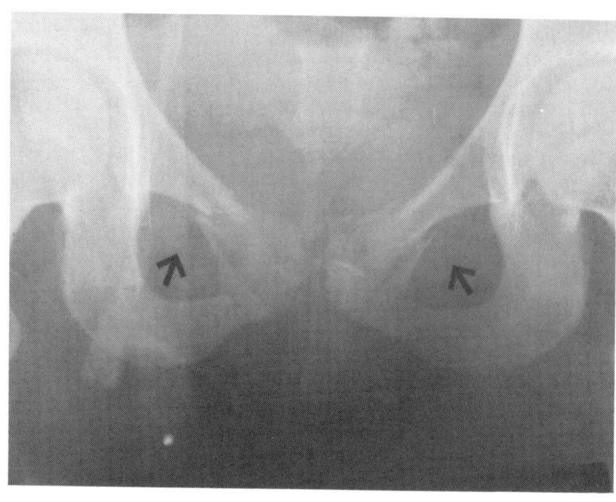

FIG. 19-2 Bilateral fractures of the superior pubic rami. Associated injury to the bladder and urethra should be suspected.

take precedence. The circulatory status of the patient must be carefully monitored, since hemorrhagic shock from associated vascular injury is common.

Gentle posterior pressure on or lateral compression of the iliac crests will cause pain at the site of a pelvic fracture. Direct pressure on the symphysis pubis may elicit pain, crepitus, and movement if a free section of pelvic ring is present. In the presence of a pelvic fracture, careful rectal and vaginal examinations should be performed to detect open injuries.

Isolated unilateral superior and inferior fractures of the pubic rami and diastasis pubis are stable injuries that are adequately treated with bed rest and pain management. Severe anteroposterior compressive forces result in bilateral fractures of the pubic rami and a free-floating segment of bone (Fig. 19-2). A fracture-dislocation or double vertical break of the pelvic ring is termed a *Malgaigne fracture* and typically involves either diastasis pubis or pubic rami fractures with concomitant sacroiliac joint disruption or sacral fracture. This unstable anterior and posterior pelvic injury is more common in adults and is associated with increased morbidity and mortality.

Avulsion fractures are the most common pediatric pelvic injuries and are frequently seen in adolescent athletes. Strong contractions of the sartorius and hamstring muscles cause traction damage to the anterior superior iliac spine, anterior inferior iliac spine, or ischial tuberosity. Physical examination is remarkable for localized swelling and tenderness as well as painful range of motion. The diagnosis is confirmed by plain radiographic findings, and treatment is conservative.

THE HIP

Pediatric hip dislocations are rare but occur more often than hip fractures. Greater force is required to produce hip dislocation after age 6. As with adults, posterior dislocation is more common than anterior dislocation. The incidence of avascular necrosis is related to the severity of injury and to delays in reduction. Closed reduction is most successful within 8 to 12 h of injury. Other complications of hip dislocation include sciatic nerve injury, degenerative arthritis, and myositis ossificans.

Pediatric hip fractures have been classified into four categories. A type I injury is a transepiphyseal separation with or without dislocation of the femoral head from the acetabulum and is uncommon. A type II injury is a transcervical fracture and is the most common hip fracture occurring during childhood. Most type II fractures are displaced, and the degree of displacement correlates well with the subsequent development of avascular necrosis. Because of the unstable nature of this injury, internal fixation is usually required. Type III fractures are cervicotrochanteric fractures, analogous to fractures at the base of the femoral neck in adults, and are frequently complicated by avascular necrosis. Type IV injuries (intertrochanteric fractures) are associated with rapid union and few complications.

SLIPPED CAPITAL FEMORAL EPIPHYSIS

Slipped capital femoral epiphysis (SCFE) and type I proximal femur transepiphyseal fracture-separations are variations on the same injury pattern. Type I fractures usually occur in younger children secondary to major trauma, whereas SCFE occurs primarily in obese black males aged 12 to 16 years. Small amounts of slippage can occur over a period of months, and an acute slip may be superimposed on chronic slippage after relatively minor trauma. Bilateral SCFE is common. Patients usually present with hip, knee, or groin pain, especially with movement, and may not report any precipitating event. The correct diagnosis is reached by main-

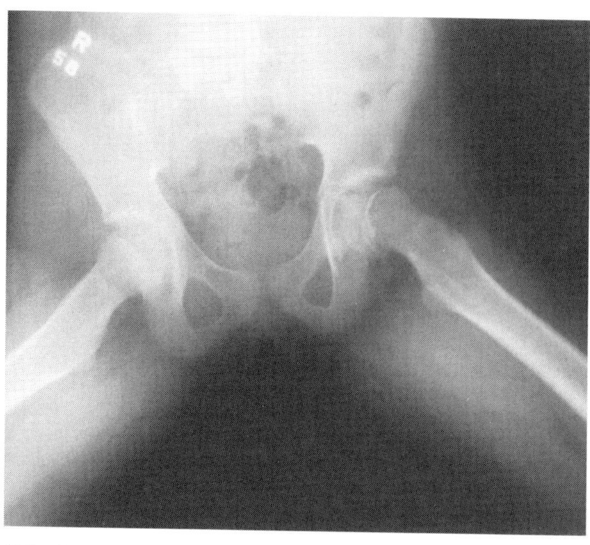

FIG. 19-3 Frog-leg view of the pelvis revealing a slipped left capital femoral epiphysis.

taining a high index of suspicion for the injury and recognizing associated radiographic findings.

Both anteroposterior (AP) and frog-leg views of the pelvis should be obtained. Irregular widening of the epiphyseal line may be discernible and suggest the diagnosis. The single best radiographic method for diagnosing an SCFE is to draw a line from the lateral edge of the femoral neck cephalad toward the joint on the frog-leg view. In a normal hip, the line will transect at least the lateral 25 percent of the epiphysis, whereas with an SCFE the line will not intersect the epiphysis (Fig. 19-3). Slips are defined as mild, moderate, or severe based on the degree of displacement of the femoral head.

The most dreaded complication of SCFE is avascular necrosis, the development of which is related to the severity of the slip and the amount of manipulation performed. Gradual reduction over a few days can be attempted, with traction and internal rotation, but operative pinning and immobilization is still necessary in most cases. Prophylactic pinning of the uninvolved side is not routinely

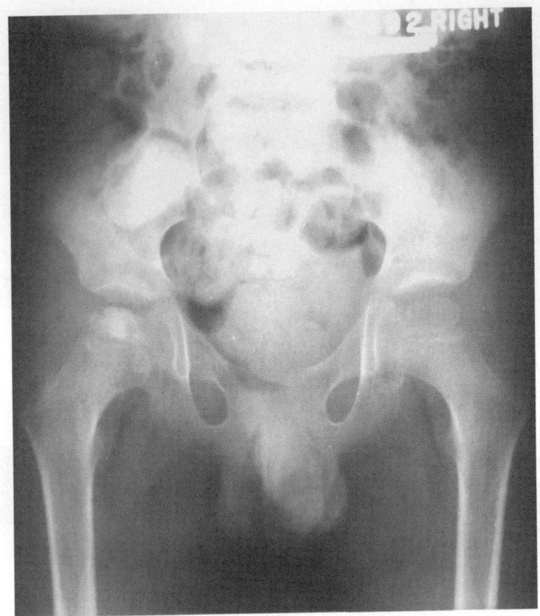

FIG. 19-4 Legg-Calvé-Perthes disease of the right femoral head.

recommended. Other complications include premature closure of the epiphysis and the development of degenerative arthritis.

LEGG-CALVÉ-PERTHES DISEASE

Avascular necrosis of the femoral head without known precipitating event in children aged 5 to 9 years is called Legg-Calvé-Perthes Disease. Boys are affected more commonly than girls. Patients may present with a limp or knee pain that is exacerbated by strenuous activity. Radiographs may be normal in the early stages of the disease, but later findings include demineralization and ultimately collapse of the femoral head (Fig. 19-4). Bilateral involvement occurs in 15 percent of cases.

FRACTURES OF THE FEMUR

Pediatric fractures of the femur are common and peak in incidence at age 3. Fractures of the femur in infants are due to birth trauma, underlying pathology, or nonaccidental trauma. Abuse should be strongly considered in the nonambulatory child.

Performance of a femoral nerve block may provide significant pain relief for patients with midshaft femoral fractures. Splinting prevents further injury and usually helps make the patient more comfortable. The management of femoral fractures may include skeletal traction followed by casting for children, while adolescents usually undergo intramedullary fixation.

Distal femoral epiphyseal fractures are not as common as epiphyseal fractures in other parts of the body, but the incidence of growth disturbance after injury is very high. Premature closure of the epiphysis can have serious consequences for the patient, since almost 65 percent of the longitudinal growth of the lower extremity can be traced to this area. Salter-Harris type II fractures of the distal femoral epiphysis occur most often, usually in older children, and characteristically heal well. Type III and type IV injuries are uncommon, but when present they require exact anatomic reduction. Type V fractures are usually diagnosed retrospectively when growth disturbances are detected.

For a more detailed discussion, see Greenfield RH: Fractures of the Pelvis and Femur, chap. 19, p. 130, in *Pediatric Emergency Medicine: A Comprehensive Study Guide.*

---

20 Injuries of the Lower Extremities

Russell H. Greenfield

THE KNEE

Children's ligaments are more resistant to stress than the bones to which they are attached. Pediatric ligamentous injuries do occur, however, often in conjunction with fractures of the adjacent bone. Avulsion of the intercondylar eminence of the tibia (tibial spine) is analogous to anterior cruciate ligament disruption in adults, and injury to the medial or lateral collateral ligament is frequently associated with fracture of the distal femoral epiphysis.

THE TIBIA AND FIBULA

The most common pediatric injuries of the lower extremities are fractures of the tibia and fibula. Rotational and angular deformities do occur, however, and must be carefully reduced to preserve normal function of the knee and ankle joints. An uncommon but potentially devastating complication associated with lower extremity fractures is the development of a compartment syndrome. Pressure within this enclosed space can rise in response to closed injuries, especially fractures of the tibia. Pain on passive dorsiflexion of the ankle is an early sign of impending anterior compartment syndrome that, when present, signals the need for emergent measurement of compartmental pressures by an orthopedist.

Patients with nondisplaced tibial fractures can be placed in a posterior splint, given crutches, and instructed not to bear weight on the affected leg. Isolated fractures of the fibula can be managed in a short leg walking cast. Healing of pediatric tibial and fibular fractures is usually complete after 6 weeks. Surgical intervention is indicated for open fractures, inadequate closed reduction, and some injuries involving the epiphysis.

Avulsion of the tibial tuberosity may be more common in active children who intermittently cause microscopic injury to the tibial tubercle, also known as Osgood-Schlatter disease or traumatic tibial apophysitis. Children with Osgood-Schlatter disease are usually 11 to 15 years of age and experience recurrent localized pain and swelling after running. The disease is self-limited, and treatment is symptomatic.

Proximal tibial metaphyseal fractures are associated with significant complications, including damage to the posterior tibial artery and subsequent valgus growth deformity (Fig. 20-1). This common posttraumatic limb deformity may occur even after precise anatomic reduction of the fracture fragments is accomplished.

Midshaft tibial fractures can be treated with closed reduction and casting. Healing usually takes place without complication even in the presence of an associated fibular fracture. Overnight admission or a period of observation is recommended, so that serial neurovascular examinations can be performed to detect a developing compartment syndrome.

A Salter-Harris type I fracture should be diagnosed in any child who has posttraumatic swelling and tenderness over the growth plate of the distal tibia or fibula without a visible fracture on a radiograph. The extremity should be splinted and orthopedic referral arranged. Radiographic evaluation of the ankle should include at least anteroposterior (AP), lateral, and mortise views.

The growth plate of the medial malleolus is the weakest compo-

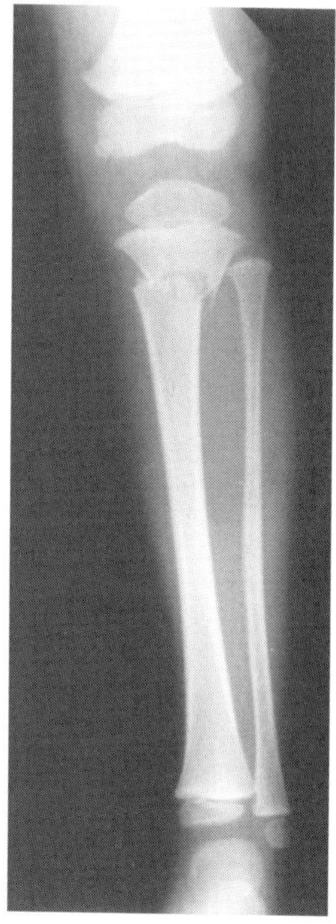

FIG. 20-1 This patient suffered a fracture of the proximal tibial metaphysis after being struck by a car. Complications associated with this injury include damage to the posterior tibial artery and the development of a valgus deformity.

nent of the pediatric ankle. Isolated Salter-Harris type I fractures of the distal tibia are rare, but type II fractures occur commonly (Fig. 20-2), often with an associated greenstick fracture of the fibula. Type II fractures may be accompanied by occult type V injury; however, discrepancies in leg length develop more frequently with type IV fractures (30 percent). Type I and II injuries are managed with closed reduction and casting. Most Salter-Harris type III and IV fractures require operative intervention. Most fractures in this area occur in conjunction with distal tibial injuries.

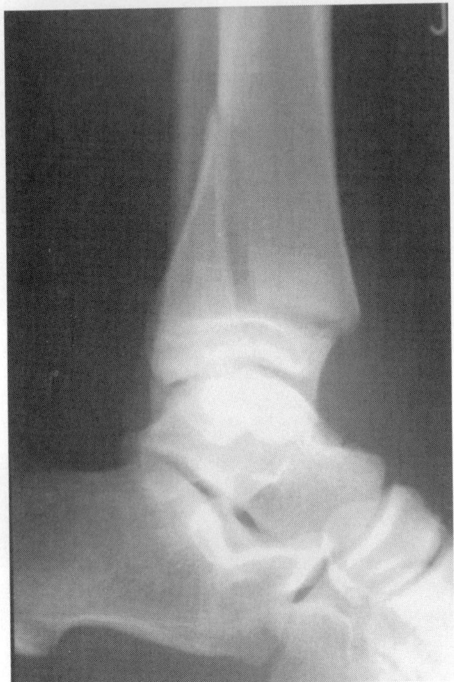

FIG. 20-2 Salter-Harris type II fracture of the distal tibia. An associated greenstick fracture of the fibula commonly occurs with this injury.

Salter-Harris type I distal fibular fractures are common. Type I and II fractures usually heal without complication when placed in a short leg cast for 3 to 6 weeks. Type III and IV fractures of the distal fibula are rarely seen. As the physis begins to fuse, avulsion fractures of the distal fibula occur more frequently.

FOOT FRACTURES

Most childhood fractures of the foot involve the forefoot and occur secondary to falls, crush injuries, or lawnmower accidents. Radiographic evaluation of the injured foot should include AP, lateral, and oblique views.

The most common pediatric hindfoot fractures involve the calcaneus. Diagnosis can be difficult, since over 30 percent of calcaneal fractures are not readily apparent on plain radiographs. A flattened Bohler angle is indicative of occult fracture of the calcaneus in adolescents and adults but is an unreliable sign in young children, who normally have a small angle. Ski-jump views of the ankle or computed tomography may be needed to make the diagnosis. Treatment is avoidance of weight bearing for 4 to 6 weeks.

Fractures of the neck of the talus occur secondary to forced dorsiflexion of the foot. If the blood supply to the body of the talus is disrupted, avascular necrosis can ensue. Minimally displaced talar neck fractures usually result in only minor vascular damage and can be treated with closed reduction and avoidance of weight bearing. Displaced talar neck fractures and osteochondral fractures of the dome of the talus require operative intervention.

Forefoot fractures occur commonly in children but usually heal without complication. Most metatarsal injuries can be treated with a hard-soled postoperative shoe or short leg walking cast, crutches, and elevation. Significant displacement of proximal metatarsal fractures is rare due to the presence of strong interosseous ligaments. The second metatarsal anchors the foot, and a fracture at its base is indicative of occult damage to the tarsometatarsal joint. An associated torus fracture of the cuboid and marked soft tissue damage may also be present. The presence of multiple metatarsal fractures or significant crush injury to the foot warrants overnight observation, so that serial neurovascular assessments can be performed to detect signs of a developing compartment syndrome.

The apophysis of the proximal fifth metatarsal becomes visible after 8 years of age and fuses by age 15. The long axis of the apophysis is parallel to the axis of the shaft of the bone and is frequently mistaken for a fracture. Transverse avulsion fractures commonly occur at the base of the fifth metatarsal due to the actions of the plantar aponeurosis and the abductor digiti minimi. A transverse fracture just distal to the tuberosity of the fifth metatarsal is called a Jones fracture and is not an avulsion injury.

Fractures and dislocations of the foot phalanges can be reduced with longitudinal traction. Once rotational deformities have been corrected, splinting can be accomplished by placing interdigital padding and then buddy-taping the injured digit to an adjacent toe.

For a more detailed discussion, see Greenfield RH: Injuries of the Lower Extremities, chap. 20, p. 134, in *Pediatric Emergency Medicine: A Comprehensive Study Guide.*

21 Soft Tissue Injury and Wound Repair

Jordan D. Lipton

HISTORY AND PHYSICAL EXAMINATION

In assessing a child with a minor wound, one must first exclude more serious, sometimes occult, injuries that will take precedence in management. The history of the injury should include whether the inciting force was blunt or sharp, the time and mechanism of the injury, whether there are other injured areas, and whether there are any possible contaminants or foreign bodies in the wound. Other important information to ascertain is the child's tetanus immunization status, whether the child has any medical problems or allergies, any medications that the child takes, and what wound care was received prior to arrival in the emergency department (ED). Child abuse must always be considered, especially when the history and the injury are inconsistent.

Physical examination of the wound must include assessment of the length and depth of the injury, circulatory status, motor and sensory function, the presence of foreign bodies and contaminants, and the involvement of underlying structures (nerves, tendons, muscles, ligaments, vessels, bones, joints, and ducts). Although the sensorimotor examination must precede the administration of anesthesia, the remainder of the examination should rarely be performed without adequate anesthesia.

Sensation is tested by measurement of two-point discrimination distal to an injury. For children younger than 3 years of age, the use of a noxious stimulus, such as a pinprick, may be necessary to provide a sensory and partial motor assessment. Since normal autonomic tone produces a degree of normal sweating, denervated fingers do not sweat, which provides a clue to injury. The ophthalmoscope can assist in spotting sweat beads on the fingers. Circulation is evaluated by palpation of peripheral pulses and skin temperature, observation of skin color, and rapidity of capillary refill. Tendons, muscles, and ligaments are tested distal to an injury, with special attention to hand and forearm injuries. With cooperative older children, it is possible to test these structures' functions individually; however, with younger, less cooperative children, one must rely on observation of posture, symmetry, and function and on exploration of the wound. A toy or penlight that requires manipulation by the child can be used to help in evaluating motor function.

MANAGEMENT

Instruments, Sutures, Staples, Tape, and Adhesives

Most wound repairs can be accomplished with a few basic instruments and supplies. The essentials include a needle holder, forceps, a number 15 scalpel (number 11 for puncture wounds), scissors, sutures (see Table 21-1), sterile drapes, anesthetic agents, topical antiseptic, normal saline, irrigation equipment (large syringe with 18- to 20-gauge needle or plastic cathether), and sterile gauze.

Staples have become a frequently used alternative for suturing selected wounds. Sharp lacerations of the scalp, trunk, and extremities are rapidly and effectively closed using staples, which induce a minimal inflammatory reaction and produce similar cosmetic results to suturing. Staples should not be used for repair of hand or face lacerations, and they should be avoided in areas of the body that will undergo computed tomography (CT) or magnetic resonance imaging (MRI). They should also not be placed in areas of the scalp that will be subject to prolonged pressure, as they will be uncomfortable for the patient.

Tape (Steri-Strip) is an effective alternative for the closure of small linear lacerations that are under minimal tension. Taped wounds are more resistant to infection than sutured wounds, and tape often does not require injection of local anesthetic for application, and does not require return to an ED for removal. If applied with an adhesive such as tincture of benzoin, tape should remain in place for several days. Benzoin must be kept out of the wound, however. Tape can also be used for skin closure of partial-thickness wounds and of wounds that are closed in a layered fashion with well-approximated wound edges. Tape closure is a preferred technique for the repair of multiple tangential skin flaps such as those produced when a child's face hits the windshield in a motor vehicle accident.

Tissue adhesives such as fibrin glue and cyanoacrylate are not currently available in the United States, but are used frequently in Europe and Canada. A recent prospective randomized study of 81 children undergoing repair of facial lacerations with butyl cyanoacrylate as compared with sutures noted similar cosmetic results, faster repair, and less pain to the child. However, caution must be used in repairing lacerations near the eyes.

Analgesia, Local Anesthesia, Nerve Blocks, and Sedation

Most wounds are adequately anesthetized using local infiltration of lidocaine 1% to 2%, with or without epinephrine, and this is still the standard approach. Lidocaine has a rapid onset of action

TABLE 21-1 Suture Materials

Type	Material	Properties
Nonabsorbable	Silk	Easy to handle; lies flat when tied; forms secure knot due to presence of braid; induces more tissue reaction and has higher infection potential than other nonabsorbables
	Cotton	Similar to the properties of silk sutures
	Nylon	Synthetic; less tissue reactivity and infection potential; does not tend to lie flat; more difficult to handle than silk/cotton; decreased knot security due to lack of braid requires more throws per knot
	Polypropylene	Similar to the properties of nylon sutures, although slightly easier to handle
	Polyester	Infection potential greater than nylon and polypropylene, but less than silk and cotton; easier to handle and better know security than nylon and propylene
	Metal	Low tissue reactivity and infection potential; difficult to handle; uncomfortable for patient during healing
	Polybutester	Equivalent to nylon and polypropylene in tensile strength and low infection potential; streches easily, thus advantageous for wounds that tend to swell

Absorbable	Plain gut	Phagocytosed by macrophages; maintains tensile strength for ~7 days; high tissue reactivity and infection potential
	Chromic gut	Similar to the properties of plain gut sutures, but maintains tensile strength for 2–3 weeks
	Fast-absorbing gut	Similar to the properties of plain gut sutures, but breaks down within 5–7 days, thus does not require removal with scrissors
	Polyglycolic acid and polyglactin	Synthetic; causes less tissue reactivity and has lower infection potential than gut sutures; absorbed by enzymatic hydrolysis; braided, thus holds knots well, but has lots of drag through tissues if not coated with materials that reduce friction; gradually loses tensile strength over ~4 weeks
	Polydioxanone, polyglyconate, and glycolide trimethylene carbonate	Synthetic monofilament (passes more smoothly through tissues); causes less tissue reactivity than gut sutures; absorbed by enzymatic hydrolysis; retains ~60 percent of tensile strength at 28 days

and a duration of action of approximately ½ to 2 h. Duration of action is prolonged by using epinephrine, but epinephrine may increase the risk of infection and should not be used in regions that are supplied by end arteries (fingers, nose, lip, ears, genitalia, toes). In order to spare a patient repeated injections, the use of a longer-acting agent such as bupivacaine should be considered if wound repair may be interrupted. Bupivacaine's onset of action is moderate, and its duration of action is approximately 2 to 6 h. Regardless of the local anesthetic agent used, care must be taken not to use more than the recommended dose per kilogram. For plain lidocaine and lidocaine with epinephrine, 4.5 mg/kg and 7 mg/kg, respectively, are the recommended maximum doses.

Infiltration is achieved by means of a 25- to 27-gauge needle, injecting slowly into the wound margins. Buffering 9 to 10 mL of 1% lidocaine with 1 mL of 8.4% sodium bicarbonate reduces the pain of injection significantly. When possible, infiltration is performed prior to irrigation; however, for grossly contaminated wounds, it is occasionally necessary to irrigate prior to infiltration.

Topical tetracaine, adrenaline, and cocaine (TAC) as well as adrenaline-cocaine and adrenaline-lidocaine mixtures can provide effective anesthesia for pediatric facial and scalp lacerations. Care should be taken to avoid contact of these mixtures with mucous membranes, and they should not be used in regions supplied by end arteries because of the vasoconstrictive effect of the adrenaline. The mixture is applied to the wound by using saturated sponges, gauze pads, or cotton swabs held in place by a parent or caregiver wearing gloves. Transient anesthesia can also be obtained by applying a solution of 4% lidocaine to a wound prior to infiltration or to an abrasion that requires mechanical scrubbing.

Regional nerve blocks that anesthetize the nerve or nerves that supply a specific anatomic area are used for large lacerations and lacerations in areas whose anatomy will be distorted if local infiltration is performed. Blocks are especially useful for anesthetizing digits.

Conscious sedation is usually not required for the management of wounds in most children. However, for the child who is too uncooperative to permit adequate wound management, chemical sedation with agents such as midazolam, fentanyl, nitrous oxide, or ketamine may be used. Both cardiac and respiratory monitoring is essential during sedation. Airway management equipment and reversal agents (naloxone, flumazenil) should be available at the bedside, and patients should be discharged only when the agents have worn off and the child has returned to his or her presedation level of consciousness.

Some form of physical restraint during wound assessment and

management is used for children under the age of 2 years; it is sometimes necessary for children up to 5 or 6 years of age. One method used to immobilize a child involves the use of a folded sheet, although commercially available papoose boards may be more convenient. Neither method provides adequate immobilization of the head.

Wound Cleaning and Preparation

Controversy exists as to the proper physician attire during wound care. Some advocate routine donning of goggles, mask, gloves, cap, and gown. Certainly, gloves, mask, and eye protection should always be worn, in keeping with universal precautions.

Hemostasis

Hemostasis is necessary during all stages of wound management and is usually achieved by applying direct pressure with sterile gauze for 10 to 20 min. Other methods utilized for the control of more brisk bleeding include elevation of the wound, application of dilute epinephrine solution (1 : 100,000) to the wound, infiltration of lidocaine with epinephrine, and packing with absorbable gelatine powder or sponge. Persistent arterial bleeding in an extremity wound is controlled with proximal placement of a blood pressure cuff and inflation to slightly higher than the patient's systolic blood pressure. Alternatively, a tourniquet formed from a Penrose drain, an elastic band, or a cut sterile glove can be used for proximal control of bleeding from an injured digit or small extremity. Close attention must be paid to time limits when using these methods, however (generally no longer than 30 to 45 min). Electrocauterization of small oozing vessels can also be used for successful hemostasis.

Vessels must not be sutured or clamped blindly because of the risk of injuring adjacent structures. Persistently bleeding small arteries do, however, require ligation. Arteries in the wrists or hands should not be clamped and ligated; these require consultation with a hand or vascular surgeon.

Foreign-Body Evaluation

After anesthesia, wound exploration is performed on all injuries to determine the extent of damage and to remove foreign material. Inert foreign bodies such as glass or metal should be removed if possible. Radiographs are occasionally required for precise localization of a foreign body, which can be aided by taping a radioopaque marker such as a paper clip to the skin overlying the suspected location. Other studies that can aid in the localization of foreign bodies include xeroradiography, ultrasonography, CT, and MRI. If an inert foreign body is small and cannot be removed easily, it may be left in place and the patient or parent informed of its presence. Organic foreign bodies such as wood unequivocally require removal to prevent inflammatory reactions and infection.

Hair Removal

Since infection rates are significantly greater in wounds that are shaved, hair should be removed by clipping if it interferes with the procedure. For most wounds, even those to the scalp, removal of hair is not necessary. Moistening the hair in the area of the laceration with lubricating jelly usually keeps it out of the way. The eyebrows should never be shaved or clipped. They serve as valuable landmarks for alignment during wound repair, and can take 6 to 12 months to grow back.

Irrigation

Irrigation with between 5 and 8 psi of normal saline is the method of choice for removing bacteria and debris from most wounds. Low-pressure irrigation with a bulb syringe does not adequately remove bacteria and debris from a wound. The pressure delivered by a simple assembly consisting of an 18- to 20-gauge plastic catheter or needle attached to a 30-mL syringe is 6 to 8 psi. Commercial systems to facilitate irrigation are available, including spring-loaded syringes with one-way valves connected to a standard intravenous (normal saline) setup. Regardless of the system used, the tip of the needle should be maintained somewhere between the wound surface and 5 cm above the intact skin; 200 to 300 mL of fluid is used for an average-sized low-risk wound. For increasing size or contamination, more fluid is used.

A consequence of and disincentive to irrigation is splatter, which can be minimized using one of many techniques. Irrigating through the first web space of the irrigator's hand while cupping the hand above the wound will avoid splatter but will also diminish visualization of the wound during irrigation. Attaching a 4 × 4 in gauze to the irrigation catheter or needle will also provide protection. Commercially available plastic shields (Zerowet) that attach directly to the irrigation syringe provide good protection against splatter while permitting visualization of the wound. An inexpensive version of these plastic shields is formed by puncturing the base of a sterile plastic medication cup with the irrigation needle.

Antisepsis and Scrubbing

The skin surrounding the wound is cleansed prior to wound irrigation and repair. Various antiseptic skin cleansers can be used, including povidone-iodine (Betadine scrub) and chlorhexidine gluconate (Hibiclens). Nonionic surfactants, such as Shur-Clens and Pharma Clens, mechanically lift bacteria from the skin but possess no bactericidal activity. A gauze sponge folded and placed into the wound will prevent the entry of detergents into the wound itself.

Large debris is removed from the wound with forceps, and devitalized tissue and foreign matter are debrided if needed. Mechanical scrubbing of the wound should be avoided unless there is gross contamination. Although scrubbing can remove debris from the wound, it increases wound inflammation. If it is decided to perform scrubbing, a fine-pore sponge (i.e., Optipore) is used to minimize tissue abrasion, along with a nonionic surfactant to minimize tissue toxicity and inflammation.

Debridement

Debridement is often necessary in the management of contaminated wounds or wounds with nonviable tissue. Through removal of contaminants and devitalized tissue, debridement increases a wound's ability to resist infection, shortens the period of inflammation, and creates a sharp, trimmed wound edge that is easier to repair and more cosmetically acceptable. If the devitalized edge of an irregular wound is debrided, the wound can be undermined to avoid a wide scar.

Primary Closure

Primary closure using sutures, staples, or tape is performed on lacerations that have been recently sustained (less than 24 h on the face and 12 h on other areas of the body), are relatively clean, and have minimal tissue devitalization.

Prior to beginning closure, all the injured layers, such as fascia, subcutaneous tissue, muscle, tendon, and skin, should be identified. During repair, each layer edge is always matched to its counterpart, making sure that when the sutures are placed, they enter and exit the appropriate layer at the same level, so that there is no overlapping of layers.

The size of suture used for wound closure depends on the tensile strength of the tissue in the wound. A 3-0 suture is used for tissues with strong tension, such as fascia in an extremity, and a 5-0 suture for tissues with light tension, such as the subcutaneous tissue of the face.

Buried Stitch

Deep (buried) sutures serve four key functions and are required for repair of many facial lacerations to ensure the best cosmetic result. First, they provide 2 to 3 weeks of additional support to

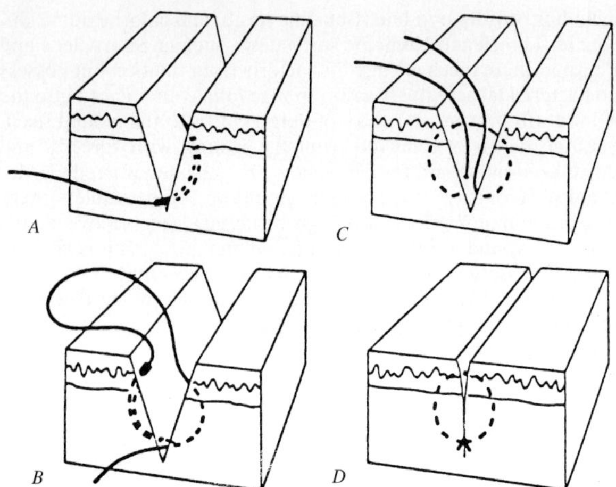

FIG. 21-1 The buried-knot suture. The loop is constructed so that the knot lies at the bottom, leaving the upper surface that the skin will rest on smooth and flat. The needle enters the deep portion of the tissue to be repaired first and exits at a more superficial plane. Next the needle enters the opposite side of the wound at the same superficial place and exits at the deep plane, and the knot is tied beneath the dermis. (From Simon RR, Brenner BE: *Procedures and Techniques in Emergency Medicine,* 2d ed. Baltimore, MD: Williams & Wilkins, 1987, p 308. By permission.)

the wound after the skin sutures are taken out or the tape is removed. This prevents widening of the scar. Second, they help to preserve the normal functioning of the underlying or involved muscles if the muscular fascia is sutured. Third, they reduce the likelihood of the development of a hematoma or abscess by minimizing the dead space. Fourth, they avoid the development of pitting in the injured region caused by inadequate healing of the deep tissues. Unfortunately, deep sutures can result in damage to nerves, arteries, and tendons; in the extremities, they can increase the risk of infection. Since suture material is a foreign body, only a few deep sutures should be used even in clean or minimally contaminated wounds. The most common deep suture for laceration repair is the buried-knot stitch, where one begins and ends at the base of the wound so as to bury the knot (Fig. 21-1).

The subcuticular stitch is a running buried suture at the dermal-epidermal junction that is actually used for skin closure (Fig. 21-2).

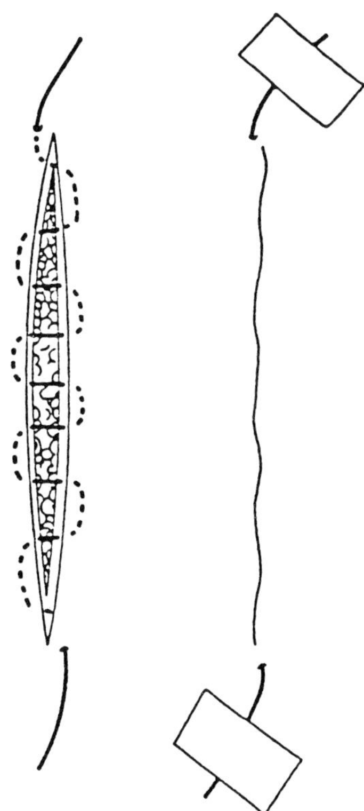

FIG. 21-2 The subcuticular suture. The skin is entered 3 to 4 mm from one end of the laceration; then the needle burrows through the deep tissue to emerge in the subcuticular plane at the apex of the wound. Next, the suture is made to pass through the subcuticular tissue on alternate sides of the wound. The point of entry of each stitch should be directly across from or slightly behind the exit point of the previous stitch. When the repair is completed, the needle again burrows through the dermis and is made to exit the skin. Prior to securing the suture ends in place, the tension along the wound should be carefully adjusted to ensure that there is no puckering of the skin. The free suture at both ends of the laceration can then be taped into place. (From Simon RR, Brenner BE: *Procedures and Techniques in Emergency Medicine*. Baltimore, MD: Williams & Wilkins, 1987, p 307. By permission.)

It is important to ensure that there is no skin puckering. The free suture is then taped in place at both ends of the laceration. This stitch can be left in place permanently if absorbable suture is used, or it can be removed in 2 to 3 weeks if nonabsorbable suture is used. Use of the subcuticular stitch avoids skin suture marks but takes more time than simple interrupted or running sutures.

Skin Closure

The epidermis and superficial layer of the dermis are repaired with nonabsorbable synthetic sutures. Sutures are placed such that the same depth and width is entered on both sides of the incision. A key to cosmetically acceptable closure is edge eversion, which is obtained by entering the skin at a 90° angle and, in some cases, by using a skin hook. For wounds whose edges tend to invert despite proper technique, vertical mattress stitches can be used (see below). The number of sutures used to repair a laceration will vary with each case. For facial lacerations, sutures are generally placed 2 to 4 mm apart and 2 to 3 mm from the wound edge.

The simple interrupted stitch is used most frequently for skin closure. It involves placing separate loops of suture using proper eversion technique (i.e., entering skin at 90°, including sufficient subcutaneous tissue), followed by tying and cutting each stitch. Although this is time-consuming, if one stitch in the closure fails, the remaining stitches will hold the wound together. This stitch is useful for stellate lacerations, wounds with multiple components, and lacerations that change direction. It is also helpful for approximation of landmarks on the skin.

Running Stitch The running or continuous stitch is well suited for pediatric laceration repair for numerous reasons (Fig. 21-3): It is rapid, its removal is easier, its strength is generally greater, it provides more effective hemostasis, and it distributes tension evenly along its length. The technique cannot be used over joints, since if one point were to break, the entire stitch would unravel.

To begin a simple continuous stitch, an interrupted stitch is placed at one end of the wound and only the free end of the suture is cut. Suturing is continued in a coil pattern, ensuring that the needle passes perpendicularly across the laceration with each pass. After each pass, the loop is tightened slightly so that tension is equally distributed. To complete the stitch, the final loop is placed just beyond the end of the laceration and the suture is tied with the last loop used as the tail.

Mattress Stitches The horizontal mattress stitch can be used for single-layer closure of laceration that are under tension. It approximates skin edges closely while providing some eversion and de-

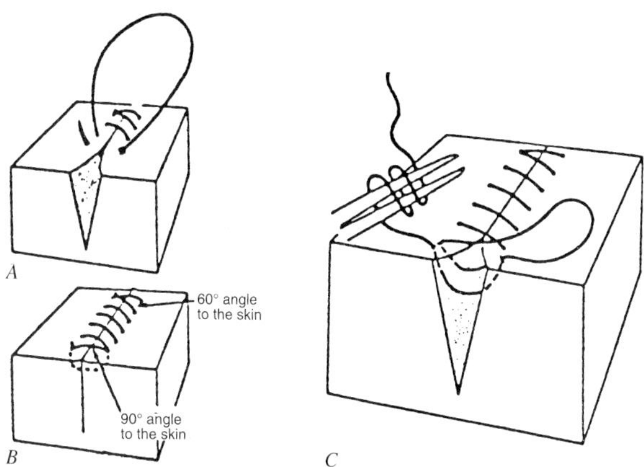

FIG. 21-3 The running suture begins (*A*) with a simple suture at one end of the wound and then runs down the length of the laceration. To complete the repair (*B* and *C*), the suture is knotted to itself. By this technique, the suture lies diagonally above the skin. (From Simon RR, Brenner BE: *Procedures and Techniques in Emergency Medicine,* 2d ed. Baltimore, MD: Williams & Wilkins, 1987, p 302. By permission.)

creases the time needed to suture because 50 percent of knots are tied. A running horizontal mattress suture can be used in areas of the body where loose skin could overlap or invert easily, such as the upper eyelids (Fig. 21-4).

The half-buried horizontal mattress stitch (corner stitch) is the suture of choice for closure of complex wounds with angulated (V-shaped) flaps (Fig. 21-5). The skin is entered and exited directly across from the flap, and the suture loop is coursed within the subcuticular tissue of the flap to maximize blood supply to the tip of the flap.

The vertical mattress stitch is helpful to evert skin edges but causes more ischemia and necrosis within its loop than other stitches. It is useful in areas of the body with little subcutaneous tissue. The stitch begins in the same way as a simple interrupted stitch, but, after the loop is made, the skin is reentered and reexited approximately 1 to 2 mm from the wound edge and the suture is tied. A common technique is to alternate vertical mattress stitches with simple interrupted stitches to close a wound.

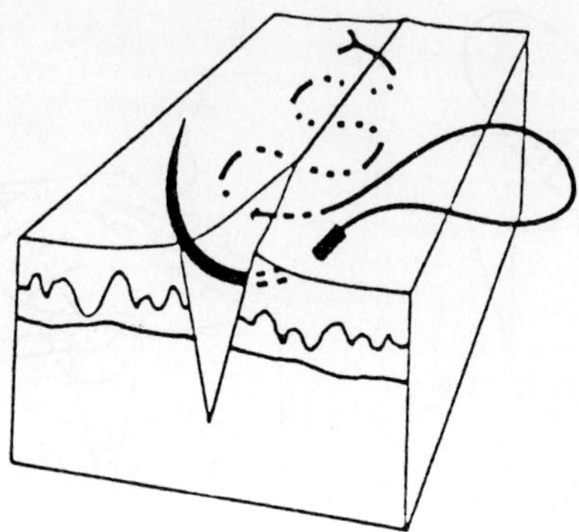

FIG. 21-4 The running horizontal mattress suture. The technique is the same as for a conventional horizontal mattress suture, except that the suture is not cut and tied with each stitch. (From Simon RR, Brenner BE: *Procedures and Techniques in Emergency Medicine,* 2d ed. Baltimore, MD: Williams & Wilkins, 1987, p 307. By permission.)

Secondary Closure

Secondary closure involves allowing wounds to heal by granulation and reepithelialization. It is used to manage ulcerations, drained abscess cavities, deep puncture wounds, older or infected lacerations, and many animal bites. Daily packing is performed with

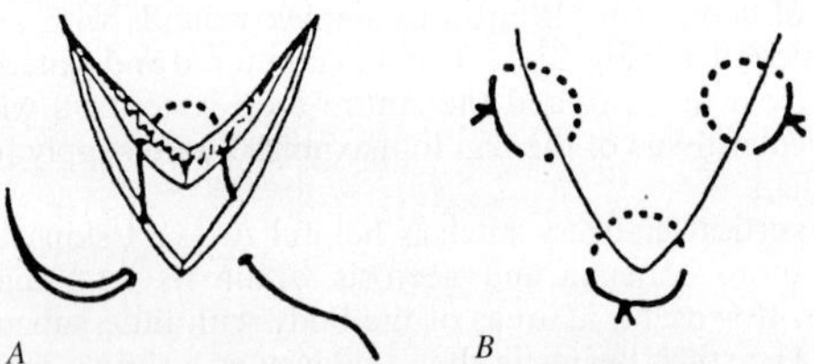

FIG. 21-5 The half-buried horizontal mattress suture. Half of the suture lies beneath the skin, in the subcuticular place (*dashed lines*). (From Simon RR, Brenner BE: *Procedures and Techniques in Emergency Medicine,* 2d ed. Baltimore, MD: Williams & Wilkins, 1987, p 306. By permission.)

saline-soaked gauze or iodoform gauze strips until granulation tissue closes the potential space.

Delayed Primary (Tertiary) Closure

Delayed primary closure with sutures is performed on wounds 3 to 5 days after initial cleansing, debriding, and packing with saline-soaked gauze. Wounds amenable to this form of closure are those that are too contaminated to close primarily but that have not suffered significant tissue loss or devitalization.

Wound Dressing, Drains, and Immobilization

Lacerations heal best in a moist environment, which deters crust formation between the healing edges. Thus, after laceration repair, the skin is cleansed of blood and povidone-iodine and a light coat of antibiotic ointment is applied. Since the antibiotic ointment is used to maintain a moist environment and not for protection against infection, a semiporous nonadherent dressing (Adaptic, Telpha, Xeroform, Vaseline gauze) can be applied to the laceration instead. A second layer of sterile gauze or an adhesive bandage (Band-Aid) is used to cover the ointment or nonadherent dressing. Alternatively, an occlusive or semiocclusive dressing (Op-Site, Tegaderm, DuoDerm, Biobrane) can be used; this reduces the pain associated with dry healing. If there is potential for the formation of a hematoma, a pressure dressing is applied, taking care to avoid compression of the arterial, venous, and lymphatic circulations.

Drains should not be used in sutured wounds. They act as foreign bodies and promote rather than prevent infection. If a wound is considered at high risk for infection, delayed primary closure should be performed rather than suturing and placing a drain in the wound. Drains should also not be used for hemostasis, which is better achieved by proper laceration repair, electrocauterization, and a pressure dressing.

A wound overlying a joint is splinted in the position of function for 7 to 10 days. For children, a bulky dressing will act as a splint and minimize motion at the wound while also preventing the child from tampering with the wound repair; this is especially helpful for hand and foot wounds.

Prophylactic Antibiotics and Tetanus Prophylaxis

More than 90 to 95 percent of wounds treated in the ED heal without complications if given appropriate wound care. There are a few instances, however, in which the use of antibiotics should be considered. Antibiotics are indicated for patients with simple wounds who are prone to infective endocarditis or who have orthopedic prostheses. They should also be given to patients who present with a wound infection due to inappropriate care at home or with wounds that are more than 12 to 24 h old. Antibiotics are also indicated for wounds that are heavily contaminated with feces or saliva; such wounds should also be treated with secondary or delayed primary closure. Extensive intraoral lacerations may benefit from a short course of penicillin or erythromycin. Antibiotic prophylaxis should be considered for any wounds in which there is involvement of cartilage, joint spaces, tendon, or bone. Finally, prophylactic antibiotics should be considered for high-risk wounds (contaminated, devitalized), especially in compromised hosts, such as children with sickle cell disease, diabetes, steroid use, or lymphoma.

When antibiotics are indicated, their effectiveness depends on early administration. The first dose should therefore be given in the ED (preferably within 3 h of the injury), regardless of the route of administration. The choice of antibiotics depends on the type of wound, although most infections are caused by staphylococci and streptococci that are sensitive to penicillinase-resistant penicillins and first-generation cephalosporins or erythromycin for penicillin-allergic patients. Wounds contaminated with saliva generally respond to the same agents. Wounds contaminated with feces require coverage against facultative organisms, coliforms, and obligate anaerobes. Reasonable choices would include second- and third-generation cephalosporins or the combination of clindamycin and an aminoglycoside. For a freshwater-contaminated wound that requires antibiotic coverage, trimethoprim-sulfamethoxazole and parenteral third-generation cephalosporins are effective in children. Generally, 3 to 5 days of oral antibiotics are prescribed for prophylaxis, but no definitive studies have examined the duration of prophylaxis.

Tetanus prophylaxis begins with appropriate wound care. If the wound is tetanus-prone, the child's immunization status is determined (Table 21-2). If the child has a tetanus-prone wound and was not immunized or was only partially immunized or if his or her immunization status is unknown, the child is treated as if he or she has no protection. Human tetanus immune globulin (HTIG) 250 U IM is given, and primary immunization is completed or initiated. If a child has completed primary immunization and has received appropriate boosters, then HTIG is never required. Tables 21-3 and 21-4 summarize tetanus prophylaxis guidelines for children younger than 7 years and those 7 years and older, respectively.

TABLE 21-2 Tetanus-Prone versus Non-Tetanus-Prone Wounds

Tetanus-prone	Non-tetanus-prone
>6–24 h old	<6–24 h old
Deep (>1 cm)	Superficial (≤1 cm)
Contaminated	Clean
Stellate, avulsion, crush, frostbite	Linear, sharp
Retained foreign bodies	No retained foreign bodies
Denervated, ischemic	Neurovascularly intact
Infected	Noninfected

POSTOPERATIVE WOUND CARE AND SUTURE REMOVAL

Successful outcome of traumatic wounds is partly dependent on wound care after discharge from the ED. The patient and parents should be given thorough (preferably written) instructions about care of the wound and what to expect. They should be informed that all wounds of significance heal with scars, regardless of the quality of care. The final appearance of the scar cannot be predicted for 6 to 12 months after the repair. They must also be told about

TABLE 21-3 Tetanus Prophylaxis for Children Younger Than 7 Years

	Non-tetanus-prone wounds		Tetanus-prone wounds	
History of adsorbed tetanus toxoid	DTP[a] (0.5 mL IM)	HTIG (250 U IM)	DTP[a] (0.5 mL IM)	HTIG (250 U IM)
Unknown or less than 3 doses	Yes[b]	No	Yes[b]	Yes
Three or more doses	No[c]	No	No[d]	No

[a] Use DT (diptheria-tetanus vaccine) if pertussis vaccine is contraindicated.

[b] The primary immunization series should be completed.

[c] Yes, if the routine immunization schedule has lapsed.

[d] Yes, if the routine immunization schedule has lapsed or if more than 5 years have passed since the last dose of tetanus toxoid.

Abbreviations: DTP = diphtheria, tetanus, pertussis vaccine; HTIG = human tetanus immune globulin.

Source: From American College of Emergency Physicians: Tetanus immunization recommendations for persons less than 7 years old. *Ann Emerg Med* 16:1183, 1987.

TABLE 21-4 Tetanus Prophylaxis for Children of Age 7 Years and Older

History of adsorbed tetanus toxoid	Non-tetanus-prone wounds		Tetanus-prone wounds	
	Td[a] (0.5 mL IM)	HTIG (250 U IM)	Td[a] (0.5 mL IM)	HTIG (250 U IM)
Unknown or less than 3 doses	Yes[a]	No	Yes[a]	Yes
Three or more doses[b]	No[c]	No	No[d]	No

[a] The primary immunization series should be completed.
[b] If 3 doses of fluid rather than absorbed toxoid are used, give a fourth dose, preferably adsorbed.
[c] Yes, if more than 10 years have passed since the last dose.
[d] Yes, if more than 5 years have passed since the last dose.
Abbreviations: Td = tetanus-diphtheria toxoid; HTIG = human tetanus immune globulin. The primary immunization series should be completed.
Source: From American College of Emergency Physicians: Tetanus immunization recommendations for persons seven years of age and older. *Ann Emerg Med* 15:1111, 1986.

the possibility of infection and that there is always the possibility, despite appropriate management, of a residual foreign body in the wound.

Because lacerations are bridged by epithelial cells within 48 h, the wound is essentially impermeable to the entry of bacteria after 2 days. Instructions should be given to keep the dressing in place and the wound clean and dry for 24 to 48 h. The dressing should be changed only if it becomes soiled or soaked by exudate from the wound. After the initial 1 to 2 days, the dressing may be removed to check for signs of infection, such as erythema, pain, warmth, purulent discharge, excessive edema, or red streaks of lymphangitis. If parental reliability is questionable, the patient should have the wound reexamined in the ED in 2 to 3 days. If there are no signs of infection, the patient or parents are instructed to gently wash the wound daily with soap and water to remove dried blood and exudate. Undiluted hydrogen peroxide should not be used, since it may destroy granulation tissue and newly formed epithelium. Generally, the wound should be protected with a dressing during the first week, with daily dressing changes. Once the dressing is removed, patients and parents should be instructed that sunscreen (SPF 15 or greater) should be applied to the scar for at least 6 months when prolonged exposure to the sun is expected in order to prevent hyperpigmentation of the scar.

Suture removal should be late enough to prevent dehiscence of the wound and early enough to prevent suture track marks and stitch abscesses (Table 21-5). Children both heal and form suture track marks faster than adults and thus need earlier suture removal. After appropriately timed suture removal, skin tape should be applied, since wound contraction and scar widening will continue to occur for several weeks after an injury.

MANAGEMENT OF SELECTED INJURIES

Abrasions

It is generally sufficient to cleanse abrasions and dress them with a nonadherent dressing or antibiotic ointment that can be changed daily after cleaning. Deeper abrasions may be treated similarly to skin-graft donor sites with cleansing and a fine-mesh gauze dressing. It is important to remove any foreign bodies (gravel, dirt, tar, etc.) to avoid infection or tattooing ("road rash"). Anesthesia for the cleansing of abrasions can be difficult, and large abrasions may require general anesthesia or conscious sedation to permit adequate debridement. For smaller areas, topical anesthesia with 2% lidocaine or TAC solution, infiltration of local anesthetic, or nerve blocks can be used. Children with large or deep abrasions should have their wounds reexamined in 2 to 3 days for monitoring of healing.

Scalp Lacerations

The presence of a rich vascular supply and vessels that tend to remain patent when cut are responsible for the profuse bleeding associated with scalp injuries. Usually, the bleeding is halted by rapid suturing. Other methods to control bleeding include the application of direct pressure and infiltration of local anesthetics containing epinephrine into the wound. If these techniques are unsuccessful, Raney scalp clips can be used or larger vessels can be ligated.

Before repairing a scalp wound, a thorough neck and neurologic examination should be completed and the skull palpated for fractures. Examination will reveal fractures more often than will skull radiographs.

The subgaleal layer of connective tissue contains "emissary veins" that drain through vessels of the skull into the venous sinuses within the cranial vault. In scalp wounds that penetrate the galea, bacteria can be carried by these vessels, and a wound infection can result in osteomyelitis, meningitis, or an intracranial abscess. Approximation of galeal lacerations will not only help to control bleeding but also safeguard against the spread of infection.

TABLE 21-5 Suture Repair of Soft Tissue Injuries by Body Location

Location	Anesthetic	Suture material	Type of closure	Suture removal
Scalp	Lidocaine 1% with epinephrine	3-0 or 4-0 nylon[a]; ± 3-0 polyglycolic acid[b] (galea); staples if galea intact	Single tight layer with simple interrupted, vertical mattress, or horizontal mattress for hemostasis; galea requires close approximation, but preferably with single-layer closure	7–10 days
Pinna (ear)	Lidocaine 1% (field block)	5-0 polyglycolic acid[b] (perichondrium); 6-0 nylon[a] (skin)	Simple interrupted; stent dressing	4–6 days
Eyebrow	Lidocaine 1% with epinephrine	4-0 or 5-0 polyglycolic acid[b] and 6-0 nylon[a]	Layered closure	4–5 days
Eyelid	Lidocaine 1%	6-0 nylon[a]	Horizontal mattress	3–5 days
Lip	Lidocaine 1% with epinephrine or mental node block	4-0 or 5-0 polyglycolic acid[b] or (chromic) gut (mucosa); 5-0 polyglycolic[b] (SQ, muscle); 6-0 nylon[a] (skin)	Three layers (mucosa, muscle, skin) if through and through, otherwise two layers	3–5 days

Oral cavity	Lidocaine 1% with epinephrine or field block; sedation may be necessary	4-0 or 5-0 polyglycolic acid[b] or (chromic) gut	Simple interrupted or horizontal mattress	7–8 days or allow to dissolve
Face	Lidocaine 1% with epinephrine or field block	4-0 or 5-0 polyglycolic aicd[b] (SQ); 6-0 nylon[a] (skin)	If full-thickness, layered closure	3–5 days
Neck	Lidocaine 1% with epinephrine	4-0 polyglycolic acid[b] (SQ); 5-0 nylon[a] (skin)	Two-layered closure	4–6 days
Trunk	Lidocaine 1% with epinephrine	4-0 polyglycolic acid[b] (SQ, fat); 4-0 or 5-0 nylon[a] (skin)	Single or layered closure	7–12 days
Extremity	Lidocaine 1% with epinephrine	3-0 or 4-0 polyglycolic acid[b] (SQ, fat, muscle); 4-0 or 5-0 nylon[a] (skin)	Single or layered; splint if over joint	10–14 days (joint); 7–10 days (other)
Hands and feet	Lidocaine 1% (lidocaine 2% or bupivacaine 0.25% for field block)	4-0 or 5-0 nylon[a]	Single-layer closure with simple interrupted or horizontal mattress; Splint if over joint	10–14 days (joint); 7–10 days (other)
Nail beds	Digital nerve block with lidocaine 2% or bupivacaine 0.25%	5-0 polyglycolic acid[b]		Allow to dissolve

[a] Nylon or polypropylene.
[b] Polyglycolic acid (Dexon) or polyglactin (Vicryl).

Although most lacerations involving multiple layers of tissue should be closed in layers, scalp wounds are best closed with a single layer of sutures that incorporates the skin, the subcutaneous fascia, and the galea. Some advocate separate closure of the galea with absorbable suture material; this allows more careful approximation but introduces a foreign body into the wound, thus increasing chances of infection. Superficial scalp lacerations are also amenable to staple closure, which expedites repair and removal.

Forehead Lacerations

In evaluating a forehead laceration, one must consider central nervous system and neck injuries. Lacerations that are limited to the area above the supraorbital rim can be anesthetized with supraorbital and supratrochlear nerve blocks, thus avoiding tissue distortion associated with local infiltration. As with scalp lacerations, one should explore for skull fractures and foreign bodies. The forehead should be closed in layers, beginning with approximation of the frontalis fascia. The layered closure is then continued, taking care to align landmarks, such as forehead furrows.

Eyelid Lacerations

The thin, flexible skin of the eyelid is quite simple to suture. However, it is essential that the emergency physician be aware of injuries that require consultation with an ophthalmologist. A thorough eye examination should be performed whenever there is a laceration of the eyelid or periorbital region. Also, it is vital to ensure that the levator palpebrae muscle and its tendinous attachment to the tarsal plate are intact, or ptosis may result. A laceration to the medial aspect of the lower lid often involves the lacrimal duct, which requires repair by an ophthalmologist. If consultation is not required, lid lacerations are closed in a single layer with 6-0 nonabsorbable suture or fast-absorbing gut, taking care to avoid skin inversion.

Ear Lacerations

Injuries to the ears require expedient cleansing, debridement of devitalized tissue, and coverage of exposed cartilage in order to avoid chondritis. Anesthesia of the external ear is simply accomplished with a field block of the auriculotemporal, greater auricular, and occipital nerves, performed by infiltration at the base of the auricle. Once cleansing and debridement of devitalized tissue is performed, cartilage is approximated using 5-0 absorbable suture material placed through the posterior and anterior perichondrium.

Tension is kept to a minimum to prevent tearing of the cartilage. Next, the posterior skin surface is approximated using 5-0 nonabsorbable suture. Finally, the visible surface of the ear is approximated using 5-0 or 6-0 nonabsorbable suture, ensuring approximation of landmarks such as folds. No cartilage is left exposed. After repair, the ear is dressed with a mastoid compression dressing, including coverage of the anterior and posterior aspects of the auricle. This prevents accumulation of a perichondral hematoma, which can lead to necrosis of cartilage and subsequent deformity ("cauliflower ear").

Lip Lacerations

Lip lacerations are common in the pediatric age group and require careful attention to ensure a good cosmetic result (Fig. 21-6). Prior to beginning repair, the oral mucosa and teeth are inspected for lacerations and trauma. Since local infiltration of anesthetic obscures the lip's landmarks, one may consider performing a mental nerve block for the repair of lower lip lacerations or an infraorbital nerve block for upper lip lacerations. Otherwise, prior to local infiltration of the anesthetic, a thin line of methylene blue can be painted along the vermillion border on each side of the laceration; this can be used as a landmark during repair.

After anesthesia, the wound is cleansed and irrigated in the usual manner, then the first stitch is placed at the vermillion border. If deep sutures are required, the initial stitch is left untied as deep closure proceeds. Through-and-through lip lacerations require three-layer closure. The orbicularis oris muscle is approximated with 4-0 or 5-0 absorbable suture. The mucosa is closed with 5-0 absorbable suture to obtain a tight seal. Finally, after irrigation of the outside surface, the skin is closed with 6-0 nonabsorbable suture material. Four-layer closure, including the subcutaneous layer, can be used to facilitate skin closure. Through-and-through lip lacerations are prone to infection, and prophylaxis with penicillin or erythromycin is recommended.

Fingertip Injuries

In young children, fingers are often injured in doors and windows. Distal fingertip injuries, even complete amputations, heal remarkably well in children. Therapy of distal fingertip amputations consists of a digital block or local infiltration, followed by appropriate cleansing and dressing of the wound with antibiotic ointment or nonadherent gauze; a splint or bulky dressing is used for protection. Frequent wound checks must then be scheduled with a hand surgeon or the ED to watch for infection.

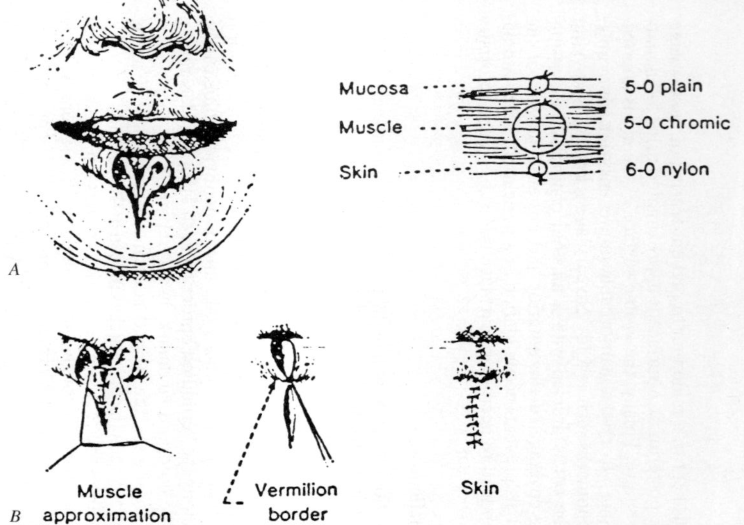

FIG. 21-6 Repair of the lower lip involved in a through-and-through laceration should be by three-layer closure. (From Curtin JW: Basic plastic surgical principles in repair of facial lacerations. *Ill Med J* 129:658, 1966. Reprinted with permission of the Illinois Medical Journal, published by the Illinois State Medical Society. Copyright 1966.)

Prognosis of distal amputations depends on how much of the tip is lost. If the fingernail and nail bed are not involved, prognosis is excellent. If the bone is spared but there is involvement of the nail or nail bed, there may be shortening of the digit. Injuries involving the distal phalanx, especially those at the base of the nail, heal most poorly. More proximal amputations uniformly require consultation with a hand surgeon.

Nail bed lacerations are closed with 6-0 absorbable sutures. The sutures must not be tied too tightly to avoid tearing through tissue. Debridement should be kept to a minimum, and the paronychium and eponychium must be prevented from forming adhesions with the nail bed by packing the space with nonadherent gauze or using the nail itself as a stent after repair of the nail bed. If there is an underlying fracture of the distal phalanx, the finger is splinted and prophylactic antibiotics (cephalosporin or dicloxacillin) are prescribed.

A subungual hematoma is a collection of blood under a fingernail or toenail, usually sustained after a direct blow. If the nail is intact, pressure from the hematoma can cause substantial pain. If the hematoma involves less than 25 to 50 percent of the nail bed, the nail is trephined using one of a number of techniques. The use of electrocautery has most recently been advocated as the simplest, safest, and least painful method to drain a subungual hematoma. Prior to trephination, the nail is cleansed using povidone-iodine; once blood escapes through the nail, the cautery is removed to avoid nail bed damage. The digit is dressed with dry sterile gauze and a splint for protection. For subungual hematomas involving more than 50 percent of the nail bed, there is controversy as to what treatment is best. Nail removal used to be advocated, because the risk of nail bed laceration was thought to be much higher. However, this practice has been questioned as long as the nail and surrounding nail fold are intact.

Puncture Wounds to the Foot

Puncture wounds, most often to the foot, have the potential to result in significant morbidity. Cellulitis, plantar space infections, abscesses, retained foreign bodies, and osteomyelitis can result from a benign-appearing wound.

A reasonable approach to puncture wounds of the foot is to obtain a radiograph to exclude bony involvement, air in the joint spaces, and radioopaque foreign bodies. The wound is anesthetized either locally or with a posterior tibial or sural nerve block, then the puncture site is unroofed, the wound cleansed and debrided, and any foreign bodies removed. The use of prophylactic antibiotics is controversial but should include *Pseudomonas* coverage when feasible, especially if the puncture wound occurs through the sole of a tennis shoe or sneaker. *Pseudomonas aeruginosa* is the most common cause of postpuncture osteomyelitis. Some physicians advocate non-weight bearing for 2 or 3 days. Some advocate non-weight bearing for 3 to 4 days. Follow-up is essential in these injuries.

SPECIAL CATEGORIES OF SOFT TISSUE INJURY

Dental and oral injuries are discussed in Chap. 14. For a discussion of human and animal bites, please refer to Chap. 108. Burns are discussed in Chap. 113.

CONSULTATION GUIDELINES

There are no rules as to what wounds warrant specialist consultation. Those for which consultation should be considered include complex or extensive wounds; wounds with large tissue defects; wounds in which there is tendon, nerve, joint, or critical vessel involvement; lacerations involving the parotid or lacrimal ducts; lacerations of the eyelid tarsal plates; lacerations over fractures; facial lacerations in which cosmetic results are a concern; and wounds about which there is physician uncertainty.

For a more detailed discussion, see Lipton JD: Soft tissue injury and wound repair, chap. 21, p. 138, in *Pediatric Emergency Medicine: A Comprehensive Study Guide.*

Section III
Respiratory Emergencies

22 Emergencies of the Upper Airways

Richard M. Cantor

Acute respiratory emergencies in the pediatric patient are common and may, if improperly treated, result in significant morbidity and mortality. Calm, decisive, and deliberate intervention is mandatory to assure the most effective outcome. The clinician must maintain an awareness of the unique anatomic and physiologic characteristics of the respiratory tract in the growing infant and child. A thorough understanding of the most frequent airway problems encountered in children and the ability to accurately assess the child in respiratory distress are critical in assuring optimal patient care.

PATHOPHYSIOLOGY

The small caliber of the upper airway in children makes it vulnerable to occlusion secondary to a variety of disease processes and results in greater baseline airway resistance. Any process that further narrows the airway will cause an exponential rise in airway resistance and a secondary increase in the work of breathing. As distress is perceived by the child, an increase in respiratory effort will augment turbulence and increase resistance to a greater degree.

Since the young infant is primarily a nose-breather, any degree of obstruction of the nasopharynx may result in significant increase in the work of breathing and present clinically as retractions. The tongue in infants and small children is larger relative to the oropharynx and may occlude the upper airway.

The pediatric trachea is easily distensible due to incomplete closure of semiformed cartilaginous rings. Any maneuver that overextends the neck will contribute to compression of this structure and secondary upper airway obstruction. The cricoid ring

TABLE 22-1 Normal Respiratory Rates

Age	Rate, breaths per minute
Newborn	30–60
Infant (1–6 months)	30–40
Infant (6–12 months)	24–30
1–4 years	20–30
4–6 years	20–25
6–12 years	16–20
>12 years	12–16

represents the narrowest portion of the upper airway and is often the site of occlusion in foreign-body aspiration.

Signs of Distress

Respiratory distress occurs when there is increased work of breathing or increased respiratory rate in order to maintain the respiratory function needed to meet the body's requirements. Respiratory failure ensues when respiratory efforts cannot maintain adequate respiratory function, either oxygenation or ventilation.

Tachypnea (Table 22-1) is the child's most common response to increased respiratory needs. Central stimulation by the medullary respiratory center is predominantly responsible for this physiologic response. Although it is most commonly due to hypoxia and hypercarbia, tachypnea may also be a secondary response to metabolic acidosis, pain, or central nervous system insult.

Infants and children readily utilize accessory muscles as a compensatory mechanism necessary to support the increased work of breathing. Intercostal, subcostal, sub- and suprasternal, and supraclavicular retractions are commonly seen. In addition, if further compromised, the infant and child will demonstrate nasal flaring.

Specific attention must be paid to the child who generates a grunting sound at the end of expiration. This physiologic phenomenon represents closure of the glottis at the end of expiration, which generates additional positive end-expiratory pressure. In many disease states, this is necessary to prevent compromised alveoli from collapsing. Grunting is an ominous sign in the pediatric patient who presents with respiratory distress.

Many infants and children, especially children with upper airway compromise, will assume a "position of comfort," which represents the most adequate anatomical compensation for their disease state. Children with stridor will often assume an upright position, lean forward, and generate their own jaw-thrust maneuver to facilitate opening of the upper airway. Patients with upper airway compromise may also prefer to breathe through an open mouth, which suggests dysphagia with inability to swallow secretions or the general presence of air hunger.

In situations where significant excessive negative intrathoracic pressure is generated, venous return to the heart will increase and left ventricular volume will be compromised. These intracardiac phenomena result in the generation of a pulsus paradoxus of greater than 20 mmHg (normal equals 0 to 10 mmHg). The presence of an elevated pulsus paradoxus correlates well with severe respiratory distress.

Cyanosis is an ominous sign in the pediatric patient. It represents inadequate oxygenation within the pulmonary bed or inadequate oxygen delivery. Cyanosis of respiratory origin tends to be central rather than peripheral. A secondary effect of cyanosis may be the development of somnolence. The most common symptoms and signs of hypoxemia include agitation, irritability, and failure of the young infant to maintain feeding efforts.

By far the most reliable sign of respiratory failure remains the generation of an ineffective respiratory effort by the infant or child and an altered level of consciousness. Auscultation of the chest may reveal decreased air entry, poor breath sounds, and bradypnea as the child progresses towards respiratory failure. Concomitant with hypoxemia in infants is the development of bradycardia. Although bradycardia may also be due to excessive vagal stimulation, hypoxemia should be ruled out in all cases of respiratory distress.

GENERAL MANAGEMENT PRINCIPLES

Any child with respiratory distress requires supplemental oxygen. Humidified oxygen may be delivered in a variety of ways:

Mask with or without rebreather apparatus
Nasal prongs
Face tent
Oxygen hood

Infants and children who feel threatened by the use of frightening equipment may be placed in the mother's arms and receive oxygen by tubing alone (at maximal flow) or by inserting the end of the tubing in a cup.

1. Standardized approach to the patient in mild to moderate distress:
   a. Provide adequate supplemental oxygen.
   b. Allow the child to assume a position of comfort.
   c. Create a comfortable, nonthreatening environment for both parent and child.
   d. Avoid any noxious stimuli in the form of unnecessary procedures.
   e. Maintain normothermia and hydration.
   f. Assess the degree of respiratory distress at presentation and at appropriate intervals thereafter.
2. Arterial blood gases: Measure of Pa_{CO_2}. This provides the clinician with an estimate of alveolar ventilatory sufficiency. The absolute value must be interpreted in relation to the amount of respiratory effort the patient must generate to attain that particular Pa_{CO_2}. Therefore a Pa_{CO_2} of 40, while listed within normal limits in most texts, is less than acceptable when applied to an infant in distress with marked tachypnea. Any degree of fatigue in this patient will promote CO_2 retention and the rapid development of potentially irreversible respiratory failure.

   Measurement of the Pa_{O_2} provides an estimate of alveolar gas exchange and a indication of the balance between tissue perfusion and metabolic demand. Percutaneous oximetry reflects only oxygenation, not the adequacy of ventilation. The use of oximetry should not replace inspection and auscultation in evaluating the pediatric patient in respiratory distress.

   The arterial pH represents the balance between metabolic demand and respiratory expenditure. With metabolic acidosis, the respiratory system is the primary compensatory mechanism for overall balance. In patients with excessive work of breathing, generation of lactate from respiratory musculature may remain uncompensated by hyperventilation, resulting in profound acidemia.
3. Recognize the signs of respiratory failure, including the following:
   a. Decreased level of consciousness (Table 22-2)
   b. Progressive fatigue
   c. Increasing work of breathing and respiratory rate
   d. Poor color (cyanotic, ashen, or gray)
   e. Diaphoresis, retractions, grunting, and flaring
   f. Decreased air movement on auscultation
   g. Hypoventilation or apnea
   h. Acidosis, hypercapnia, or hypoxemia

TABLE 22-2 Assessment of Level of Consciousness

AVPU Scale	
A = Alert	
V = Responsive to verbal stimuli	
P = Responsive to painful stimuli	
U = Unresponsive	
Glasgow coma scale	**Score**
Eye-opening response	
Spontaneous	4
To speech	3
To pain	2
None	1
Verbal response	
Oriented	5
Confused conversation	4
Inappropriate words	3
Incomprehensible sounds	2
None	1
Best upper-limb motor response	
Obeys	6
Localized	5
Withdrawal	4
Abnormal flexion	3
Extensor response	2
None	1

ASSESSMENT AND MANAGEMENT OF SPECIFIC CLINICAL SCENARIOS

Upper Airway Disorders

Stridor, the hallmark of upper airway compromise, results from the generation of inspiratory turbulence as air is forced through a narrowed lumen. Stridor may originate anywhere in the upper airway. In the young infant, stridor is most often the result of a congenital anomaly and often chronic in its presentation.

In the emergency department, the most common causes of acute upper airway obstruction are croup, epiglottitis, and foreign-body obstruction (Table 22-3).

TABLE 22-3 Features of Various Upper Airway Disorders

	Age group	Mode of onset of respiratory distress
Severe tonsillitis	Late preschool or school age	Gradual
Peritonsillar abscess	Usually >8 years	Sudden increase in temperature, toxicity, and distress with unilateral throat pain, "hot-potato speech"
Retropharyngeal abscess	Infancy to 3 years	Fever, toxicity, and distress after preceding URI or pharyngitis
Epiglottitis	2–7 years	Acute onset of hyperpyrexia, with distress, dysphagia, and drooling
Croup	3 months to 3 years	Gradual onset of stridor, barking cough, after mild URI
Foreign-body aspiration	Late infancy to 4 years	Choking episode resulting in immediate or delayed respiratory distress

Abbreviation: URI = upper respiratory infection.

Epiglottitis (Supraglottitis)

Epiglottitis is a true upper airway emergency with life-threatening complications if handled improperly. It may occur at any time of the year and, most importantly, in any age group. Traditionally, it most commonly involves children from 2 to 5 years of age. With the advent of the *Hemophilus influenzae* type b vaccine, the age range has shifted to involve older children. Possible presentations include the following:

1. The acute (several hours) onset of fever, sore throat, and dysphagia with progression to signs of respiratory distress (Table 22-4). The child will often assume a position of comfort consisting of voluntary upper airway posturing (i.e., sitting upright, mouth open, with head, neck, and jaw extension). The voice will be muffled, and stridor, if present, may actually be quite minimal in intensity. The clinician will often note that these

children appear "toxic." In severe cases, airway and swallowing mechanisms may be compromised to such a degree that profound drooling may ensue.

2. Some children will be devoid of any respiratory symptoms. They will, however, complain of a severe sore throat and dysphagia. In the absence of signs of pharyngeal or tonsillar pathology, therefore, epiglottitis must be considered in this subgroup of patients.
3. In patients with crouplike presentations who fail to respond to traditional therapies, the clinician should be alert to the possibility of epiglottitis.
4. Epiglottitis may occur at any age. Up to 25 percent of pediatric cases will be below 2 years of age. Adults will often complain only of a sore throat.

In the past, a vast majority of cases have been caused by *H. influenzae* type b with accompanying bacteremia. Uncommon but reported causative agents include *Streptococcus pneumoniae, Staphylococcus aureus,* and group A beta-hemolytic streptococci. Blood cultures will be positive in 80 to 90 percent of affected individuals.

Factors contributing to airway and ventilatory deterioration include patient fatigue, aspiration of secretions, and sudden laryngospasm. Any and all maneuvers that agitate the child should therefore be avoided, including separation from parents, alteration of optimal airway posture (lying down), fear-inducing events (rectal

TABLE 22-4 Clinical Features of Acute Upper Airway Disorders

	Supraglottic disorders (epiglottitis)	Subglottic disorders (croup)
Stridor	Quiet and wet	Loud
Voice alteration	Muffled	Hoarse
Dysphagia	+	–
Postural preference	+	–
Barky cough	–	+
Fever	++	+
Toxicity	++	–
Trismus	+	–

Abbreviations: – = absent; + = present; ++ = markedly present.

temperatures, blood work, radiographs), and gagging (forcible tongue blade examination of the oral cavity, suctioning).

Radiographs should include anteroposterior (AP) and lateral views of the soft tissues of the neck. Under no circumstances should the child receive these evaluations if they promote agitation and subsequent worsening of stridor and airway compromise. The clinician must be prepared to emergently intubate and ventilate these patients at all times and in all places within the emergency department (ED). In most cases, direct visualization and culture of the epiglottis itself will be performed in the operating suite prior to intubation.

The following management guidelines should be followed to avoid undue morbidity and mortality:

1. Avoid agitating the child in any way.
2. Provide supplemental oxygen in a nonthreatening manner.
3. Allow the patient to assume a position of comfort.
4. Prepare equipment for bag-valve-mask (BVM) ventilation, endotracheal intubation, needle cricothyrotomy, cricothyreotomy, and tracheostomy.
5. Consult an expert in intubation and provision of a surgical airway and alert the operating room (OR).
6. Take the child to the OR for direct visualization of the epiglottis and intubation.
7. If the child suffers a respiratory arrest:
   a. Open the airway.
   b. Attempt BVM ventilation (usually effective).
   c. If unable to ventilate, intubate.
   d. If unable to intubate, perform needle or surgical cricothyroidotomy.
8. Provide appropriate intravenous antibiotics (ampicillin 100 mg/kg every 6 h and cefotaxime 50 mg/kg every 6 h).
9. Provide adequate sedation and restraint postintubation.
10. Transfer the patient to an intensive care unit for further treatment and monitoring.

Croup (Viral Laryngotracheobronchitis)

Laryngotracheobronchitis is a respiratory infection that diffusely affects the upper respiratory tract. This entity accounts for 90 percent of cases of stridor with fever. The subglottic region is most commonly affected, resulting in edematous, inflamed mucosa with a fibrinous exudate. Agents responsible for croup are multiple, including parainfluenza types 1, 2, and 3 (most common); adenovirus; respiratory syncytial virus; and influenza. The seasonal pre-

TABLE 22-5 Clinical Croup Score[a]

	0	1	2
Inspiratory breath sounds	Normal	Harsh with rhonchi	Delayed
Stridor	None	Inspiratory	Inspiratory and expiratory
Cough	None	Hoarse cry	Bark
Retractions and flaring	None	Flaring and suprasternal retractions	As at left plus subcostal and intercostal retractions
Cyanosis	None	In air	In 40% O_2

[a] A score of 4 or more indicates moderately severe airway obstruction. A score of 7 or more, particularly when associated with $Pa_{CO_2} > 45$ and $Pa_{O_2} < 70$ (in room air), indicates impending respiratory failure.

dominance (winter) is related to the epidemiology of the most common causative agents.

Children from 1 to 3 years of age are usually affected. They often present, after several days of nonspecific symptoms of upper respiratory infection, with a characteristic brassy or barking cough that is almost unique to croup (Table 22-4). Inspiratory stridor eventually develops, ranging in severity from mild (only when the child is crying or agitated) to severe (present at rest). Temperatures to 102°F are common in the course of the disease; higher temperatures or the presence of a toxic appearance should alert the clinician to carefully consider other diagnoses, such as atypical epiglottitis or bacterial tracheitis. The usual evolution is a worsening of symptoms for 3 to 5 days followed by resolution over a period of days. The vast majority of children tolerate this common disease without significant morbidity; however, a small percentage may develop complete upper airway obstruction.

A variety of croup scores have been developed that quantify and qualify a constellation of physical findings, assisting the clinician in estimating the severity of subglottic obstruction as mild, moderate, or severe (Table 22-5).

The most common presentation will be the child with mild croup who may be treated as an outpatient if he or she is taking liquids by mouth, is well hydrated, and the physician is comfortable with parent reliability. Cool-mist therapy may be suggested. The classic technique is to fill the bathroom with steam by running a hot shower. The parents can then sit with the child in this home version of a Turkish bath for no more than 30 min at a time. A car ride in the cool night air with the windows slightly open may also diminish the child's symptoms. Follow-up within 24 h should always be arranged if the patient is discharged, with instructions to return if symptoms worsen.

Patients with a mild to moderate croup score can be discharged if they improve with cool, humidified oxygen therapy, they are older than 6 months of age, and the parents are reliable.

Patients with a moderate croup score (stridor at rest) are usually treated as inpatients. The purpose of admission is to provide pharmacologic therapy and to observe the child who may be at risk for progression to airway obstruction. The use of oxygen, cool mist, and racemic epinephrine delivered by nebulizer will usually result in the patient's symptomatic improvement for up to 2 h. The recommended dose of racemic epinephrine is 0.5 mL of a 0.25% solution dissolved in 2.5 mL of normal saline. Peak effects have been demonstrated at 10 to 30 min, with a duration of action lasting up to 2 h. It is important to remember that a child may experience a return to a pretreatment level of obstruction 1 to 2 h after therapy. This phenomenon is inaccurately referred to as *rebound.* Recent data, utilized in patients receiving steroids, have advocated the safe discharge of Vaponefrin recipients after 2 to 3 h of ED observation. Although this is unproved, many believe that a child with severe croup may be successfully carried through the episode with racemic epinephrine therapy as often as every 20 min (as an inpatient), avoiding the need for intubation.

Corticosteroids in higher doses (dexamethasone, 0.6 mg/kg per dose IM) seem to be of benefit in preventing the progression of croup to complete obstruction and may shorten the duration of illness. If corticosteroids are being considered (usually for the moderately or severely obstructed patient), they should be administered as soon as feasible.

If a child has severe croup (score 7 or more); it is prudent to admit that child to an intensive care setting. Treatment with oxygen, mist, racemic epinephrine, and corticosteroids should be initiated as soon as possible in the ED.

Children should be electively intubated for respiratory failure (lethargy, inability to maintain respiratory efforts, $P_{O_2} < 70$ on 100% oxygen or a $P_{CO_2} > 60$), but this decision is best made in the intensive care setting. Children who develop severe upper airway obstruction from this disease do not do so suddenly, but rather progress to it gradually over time. If intubation must be performed in the ED, an endotracheal tube 1 mm smaller than that calculated for age should be utilized to accommodate the subglottic edema and airway narrowing.

The following regimen is suggested for the patient with croup:

1. Avoid agitating the patient, providing humidified oxygen if indicated.
2. Allow the patient to assume a position of comfort (usually in a parent's arms or lap).
3. Initially, provide cool, moist air.
4. If stridor at rest persists (or fatigue or distress is noted), administer aerosolized racemic epinephrine at a dose of 0.5 mL in 2.5 mL normal saline solution. Patients who receive this intervention are candidates for admission, or, at a minimum, observation within the ED for a period of 2 to 4 h.
5. Administer intramuscular or intravenous dexamethasone, 0.6 mg/kg.
6. Intubate if clinically warranted.
7. Upright lateral neck radiographs, if desired, should be reserved for patients without suspicion of epiglottitis, and under close supervision.

Bacterial Tracheitis

Bacterial tracheitis, also referred to as membranous tracheitis, is an infection of the subglottic region. This entity occurs in the same age group as croup; however, these children usually present atypically, with a toxic appearance and high fever. Pus may be produced during spasms of brassy or barking cough. In some cases, the stridor is severe enough to be present during both inspiration and expiration.

Bacterial tracheitis represents a true upper airway emergency since, as with supraglottitis, progression to full airway obstruction is possible. It is not prudent to attempt to differentiate this entity from supraglottitis prior to obtaining a definitive airway in the operating room. Upon intubation, a normal epiglottis combined with the presence of pus, inflammation, and in some cases a pseudomembrane in the subglottic region confirms the diagnosis. Meticulous endotracheal tube suctioning in a pediatric intensive care unit (PICU) setting will usually maintain airway patency. Cultures most commonly grow *S. aureus,* but *Streptococcus, H. influenzae,* and *Pneumococcus* are possible. Antibiotic therapy should be provided using either IV ceftriaxone, 100 mg/kg/day given in 1 or 2 doses, or oxacillin, 150 mg/kg per day, *and* chloramphenicol, 100 mg/kg/day divided into 4 doses.

Retropharyngeal Abscess

Retropharyngeal abscesses are seen predominantly in children below 3 years of age secondary to suppurative cervical lymphadenopathy. Older children may present with this entity, in many instances following penetrating trauma to the posterior oropharynx. Common organisms include group A beta-hemolytic streptococci and *S. aureus.* Symptoms include high fever, muffled voice, difficulty swallowing, drooling, and, less frequently, inspiratory stridor. Dysphagia and drooling are more frequent findings than actual upper airway compromise.

Children with retropharyngeal abscesses can present with a stiff neck and be initially diagnosed as having meningitis. The presentation may also mimic supraglottitis when inspiratory stridor is present. Therefore, it is acceptable to make this diagnosis in the OR on direct visualization.

A high index of suspicion must be maintained to accurately identify the child with a retropharyngeal abscess. Clinically, the diagnosis may be made by noting a swelling of the wall of the posterior pharynx. Given the overlap in presentation with supraglottitis, even if the diagnosis is suspected, it is prudent first to obtain a lateral neck film that will demonstrate swelling of the prevertebral soft tissue at the level of the pharynx and a normal epiglottis and aryepiglottic folds. Attempts to visualize the oral cavity and posterior pharyngeal wall may be made in an older cooperative child as long as agitation does not ensue. In most suspected cases, computed tomography of the neck will identify any soft tissue swelling.

Definitive therapy involves intraoperative drainage of the-abscess after securing the airway by endotracheal intubation. Children with cellulitis but no collection of pus should be treated with antibiotics. Airway management for severe or complete upper airway obstruction should include endotracheal intubation under direct visualization (to avoid rupture of the abscess). In children with partial airway obstruction who do not demonstrate signs of respiratory failure, meticulous observation in a PICU is acceptable. Antibiotics must cover the common organisms (*S. aureus, Streptococcus*, and anaerobes). The recommended regimen is IV penicillin, 100,000 units/kg/day, *and* cefazolin, 100 mg/kg/day.

Peritonsillar Abscess

Peritonsillar abscesses usually affect children over the age of 8 years. They are the most common deep infections of the head and neck, usually representing complications of bacterial tonsillitis or, in some cases, a superinfection of an existent Epstein-Barr infection. Most are polymicrobial in origin, including group A streptococci (predominant), *Peptostreptococcus, Fusobacterium*, and other mouth flora, including anaerobes.

Historically these patients present with increasing dysphagia and ipsilateral ear pain, with progression to trismus, dysarthria, and toxicity. Drooling is common. Patients will often have a "hot-potato" phonation, representing splitting of the palatine muscles during normal speech.

The pharynx will be erythematous with unilateral tonsillar swelling, which in some cases may displace the uvula towards the unaffected side. Fluctuance may confirm the presence of underlying purulent fluid. Reactive cervical adenopathy is common.

The complete blood count will demonstrate elevated white blood cells. Throat cultures (superficial) should be obtained in all cases. Direct tonsillar needle aspiration should be performed by an experienced otolaryngologist, after adequte sedation/analgesia has been administered. Serological testing for Epstein-Barr virus should be performed as well.

Most patients require admission for drainage, intravenous hydration, and antibiotics (nafcillin or a third-generation cephalosporin). Rarely, selected individuals may be discharged from the ED after careful follow-up is arranged.

Foreign-Body Obstruction

Most foreign-body aspirations occur in children below 5 years of age, with 65 percent of deaths affecting infants below 1 year of age. Common offending agents are foods (peanuts, hard candies, frankfurters) and items commonly found in the home (disk batteries, coins, marbles). Symptoms range from mild (cough only) to full-blown upper airway obstruction. It is imperative that the clinician maintain a high index of suspicion relative to the possibility of foreign-body aspiration, especially in the afebrile child with a sudden onset of symptoms. In over 50 percent of cases, there is no history of foreign-body ingestion or a choking spell.

Most patients will present with symptoms of partial obstruction. Evaluation should include AP and lateral views of the upper airway extending from the nasopharynx to the carina. More extensive radiographic investigations include inspiratory and expiratory chest radiographs or bilateral decubital views. Both maneuvers will demonstrate the failure of the affected hemithorax to lose volume as a result of positioning. These examinations are of great value in diagnosing foreign bodies that are radiolucent. A high index of suspicion must be maintained in all suspected cases. Esophageal foreign bodies, if positioned at the thoracic inlet or carina, can impede the upper airway and cause symptoms and signs of airway obstruction.

Foreign body obstruction should be managed as follows:

1. Acute complete obstruction
   a. Children < 1 year: four back blows followed by chest thrusts.
   b. Children > 1 year: repetitive abdominal thrusts.
   c. If the preceding steps are unsuccessful, utilize Magill forceps under direct laryngoscopy in an attempt to remove the foreign body.
   d. If the preceding step is unsuccessful, attempt vigorous BVM ventilation in preparation for bronchoscopy.
2. Incomplete obstruction (phonation, coughing present)
   a. Provide supplemental oxygen.
   b. Allow the position of comfort, avoid noxious stimuli.
   c. Arrange for controlled airway evaluation in the OR.

For a more detailed discussion, see Cantor RM: Emergencies of the Upper Airways, chap. 22, p. 137, in *Pediatric Emergency Medicine: A Comprehensive Study Guide.*

---

23 Asthma

Kathleen Connors

Asthma affects at least 5 percent of the population of the United States and accounts for 1 to 5 percent of all emergency department (ED) visits. Half of these patients will require admission. From 1980 to 1987, the prevalence of asthma increased 29 percent, with the largest increase in the 5- to 14-year-old age group. The increase was most marked among black teenage boys. During the same period, both the hospitalization rate and the death rate due to asthma have also significantly increased (4.5 and 6.2 percent per year, respectively).

ETIOLOGY/PATHOPHYSIOLOGY

Asthma is an intermittent, reversible obstructive airway disease. The major mechanisms thought to contribute to the pathophysiology of asthma are increased airway responsiveness, inflammation, mucus production, and submucosal edema. Airway responsiveness is defined as the ease with which airways narrow in response to various nonallergic stimuli. These stimuli include inhaled pharmacologic agents, such as histamine and methacholine, and physical stimuli, such as exercise. The critical role of airway inflammation in both the development of obstruction and the degree of hyperresponsiveness has only recently been appreciated. Increased mucus production and submucosal edema add to the obstruction that occurs secondary to bronchospasm and inflammation.

There are several differences in the anatomy and physiology of a child compared to those of an adult that make children more prone to obstruction and more vulnerable to respiratory failure. The peripheral airways are smaller and thus offer greater resistance to airflow. Infants do not possess the collateral channels for ventilation that are present in older children and adults. In infancy, the diaphragm is the primary muscle of respiration. Any degree of abdominal distension will provide significant interference to diaphragmatic function and lead to secondary ventilatory insufficiency. The infantile diaphragm possesses muscle fibers that are more prone to fatigue. The chest wall of the pediatric patient is more compliant, preventing adequate stabilization during periods of increased respiratory distress.

CLINICAL PRESENTATION

A family history of asthma, atopy, or allergic disease is common. A recent history of an upper respiratory infection or exposure to a specific trigger is usually obtained. The initial history in a child with an acute asthma attack should include the patient's (or parents') perception of the severity of the attack, precipitating factors, history of past attacks, medications (last doses, recent changes), and duration of symptoms.

Physical examination should start with a general assessment of the patient's degree of distress. Important clues are as follows:

Alertness
Anxiety
Fluid status
General health
Positioning
Ability to speak
Presence of cyanosis

The patient's inability to lie down is significantly correlated with poor vital signs, arterial blood gases, and spirometry. Inability to speak was correlated in one study with hypoxia and a decreased peak flow rate. Vital signs may also have some prognostic value. Fever may point to a more complicated course and significant underlying disease. Increased pulse rate may be a sign of hypoxia.

Pulsus paradoxus (a drop in systolic blood pressure of 10 mmHg or more with inspiration) has been thought to correlate with a worsening status, but its usefulness has been questioned. Increased respiratory rates are usually seen in asthmatic exacerbations, but respiratory rate may decrease with fatigue in severe asthma. The lung examination may reveal a number of findings, including diffuse wheezing. Wheezing results from turbulent airflow and occurs first on expiration alone, then progresses to both inspiration and expiration. The wheezing may be localized and may shift in location with time, as the relative degree of obstruction may vary with location and time. If airway obstruction is severe, there will be little airflow and the chest may be quiet. Thus wheezing is not a reliable indicator of the degree of obstruction. Lung examination may also reveal diffuse or localized rales or a persistent cough with a clear lung examination. Air trapping due to occlusion of small airways leads to hyperinflation of the chest, making it a less efficient muscle of inspiration and forcing the use of accessory muscles. The use of accessory muscles is a more reliable indicator of degree of obstruction.

LABORATORY AND RADIOGRAPHIC FINDINGS

Typical chest radiographic findings are hyperinflation, peribronchial cuffing, and areas of subsegmental atelectasis. These findings are nonspecific and usually add little to the clinical assessment. Chest radiographs have been shown to change the course of treatment in only 10 percent of asthmatics. Specific indications for a chest radiograph in a known asthmatic patient include clinical suspicion of consolidation, effusion, pneumothorax, or impending respiratory failure. Children with first-time wheezing need a chest radiograph to exclude other causes of wheezing (Table 23-1).

Spirometry can be used to assess a patient's degree of respiratory compromise. However, many children are not able to cooperate for spirometry. The simplest spirometry test, peak expiratory flow rate (PEFR), can usually be done in children above 5 years of age.

Oximetry is another tool that helps to assess severity. It correlates with ventilation-perfusion mismatching and thus with degree of obstruction. An initial oxygen saturation of less than 91 percent was correlated with need for admission in one study. A rise in oxygen saturation with treatment was not a determinant of outcome.

Blood gases may help assess the status of severe asthmatics. Hypoxia will be present early because of the ventilation-perfusion mismatching. P_{CO_2} will be decreased early in the disease secondary to compensatory hyperventilation. As the obstruction pro-

TABLE 23-1 Differential Diagnosis in a Wheezing Infant

Bronchiolitis
Foreign-body aspiration
Immune deficiency
Immotile cilia
Bronchopulmonary dysplasia
Cystic fibrosis
Pneumonia
Anaphylaxis
Extrinsic airway compression
Vascular rings
Mediastinal masses
Aspiration
Congestive heart failure

gresses, the number of alveoli being adequately ventilated and perfused decreases and CO_2 retention occurs. Thus a "normal" or slightly elevated P_{CO_2} in a patient with an asthma exacerbation may be a sign of muscle fatigue and impending respiratory failure. Eventually the hypoxia and hypercapnia lead to acidosis.

TREATMENT

Adrenergic bronchodilators remain the first line of emergency treatment of asthma. Bronchodilation is produced by stimulation of $beta_2$ adrenoreceptors, which mediate an increase in cyclic AMP via the enzyme adenyl cyclase. Side effects are typical of sympathomimetic agents and are dose-related. They include tachycardia, tremors, palpitations, hypertension, anxiety, headache, and nausea. Newer agents are more selective for the $beta_2$ receptors. Older agents (isoetharine, metaproterenol) stimulate $beta_1$ and $beta_2$ receptors, resulting, at least theoretically, in more undesirable side effects. Table 23-2 lists the most commonly used sympathomimetic agents, their available forms for administration, their duration of action, and relative $beta_2$ selectivity. Epinephrine is available as a subcutaneous injection, which was used frequently, especially in children, even after aerosols were available. It is more toxic and no more effective than inhalation of a $beta_2$-selective drug. Parenteral administration (0.01 mL/kg up to 0.3 mL of the 1:1000 solution SC)

TABLE 23-2 Comparison of Adrenergic Agents

Agent	Available Forms[a]	Selectivity	Duration, h
Epinephrine	IV, SQ	alpha, beta	1–2
Albuterol	aer, PO	$\beta_2 \gg \beta_1$	4
Terbutaline	aer, PO, SQ, IV	$\beta_2 > \beta_1$	4–6
Isoetharine	aer	$\beta_2 > \beta_1$	1½–3
Metaproterenol	aer, PO	$\beta_2 > \beta_1$	1–5
Isoproterenol	aer, IV	β_1, β_2	1–3

IV = intravenous; SQ = subcutaneous; aer = aerosol; PO = per oral.

should be reserved for those patients who are unable to generate adequate tidal volume to deliver aerosolized drug to the bronchial tree. Subcutaneous terbutaline (0.01 mg/kg up to 0.25 mg), which is more beta$_2$-specific, may be used as an alternative. Inhaled epinephrine, which is available without a prescription, is much shorter-acting than other inhaled beta agonists. Isoproterenol is available as an intravenous preparation, and in the past was used to treat very severe asthma. However, it can cause significant cardiac toxicity, especially in hypoxic patients. Intravenous albuterol or continuous nebulized albuterol was shown to be just as effective and have fewer side effects. Therefore isoproterenol is no longer recommended as a treatment for asthma. Albuterol and terbutaline have a more prolonged duration of action than the other beta-adrenergic agents. Albuterol is the most commonly used adrenergic agent in this country because it combines a long duration of action with beta$_2$ selectivity. It is available in oral and aerosol preparations. Doses of up to 0.15 mg/kg/20 min in severe asthmatics or 0.3 mg/kg/h in moderate asthmatics have been demonstrated to be safe and more effective than lower doses. Since so much of the drug escapes into the atmosphere (see below), especially when being delivered to very young children, many physicians will administer "unit doses" (usually 2.5 or 5 mg albuterol/3 mL NS) to all patients regardless of size. Continuous nebulization of albuterol at initial rates of greater than 3 mg/kg/h has also been shown to be safe and effective. The frequency of aerosols or rate of continuous nebulization should be guided by repeat assessments of the patient's clinical status and not by any set protocol. Although terbutaline is available only in an injectable form, this solution can be used for nebulization. However, it is not FDA-approved for this use and offers no advantage over albuterol.

Aerosol therapy is the most commonly used and recommended form of administration of these agents. It is as effective as subcutaneous epinephrine and more effective than oral therapy. There are two main methods of delivering aerosolized medications. Numerous studies suggest comparable efficacy of metered-dose inhalers and jet nebulization. Metered-dose inhalers (MDIs) are less expensive and more convenient but require a cooperative (usually older) patient who understands the appropriate technique of administration. One method for enabling younger children to use an MDI more effectively is the use of an aerochamber or spacer, which provides a reservoir of particles for inspiration and requires less coordination of MDI activation with inhalation. Advantages of jet nebulization include lack of need for precise timing of inhalation and the psychological factor that the patient is getting therapy that he or she does not receive at home. Particles generated by aerosolization vary in size. Only those in the 1- to 5-μm range are deposited in the lower airways and thus are useful as drug vehicles. These represent only 10 percent of the output from an MDI and 1 to 5 percent from a jet nebulizer. The rest of the particles escape into the room or are dissolved in mucous membranes and swallowed. Low flow rates and greater breath-holding periods optimize drug deposition in the lower airways. Oxygen flow rates of 6 to 7 L/min are recommended.

Although beta agonists remain the first line of treatment for acute asthmatic exacerbations, their role in chronic disease is being questioned. Some are concerned that their use has contributed to fatal epidemics in asthmatics around the world and an increase in asthma mortality. Regular use of beta agonists may be associated with poorer control than when they are used only as needed, and prospective studies have shown that long-term therapy with beta agonists does not decrease airway responsiveness.

Atropine was the first drug used as a bronchodilator. It decreases the influence of cholinergic nerve endings on bronchial tone and dilates the airways.

Ipratropium bromide (Atrovent) is a quaternary amine that fits into the category of anticholinergic agents. It has a slower onset but longer duration of action than beta agonists. It is effective in patients with chronic obstructive pulmonary disease (COPD), where cholinergic tone is very high, but is less effective in asthma. It is reportedly more effective if combined with albuterol. Side effects include dry mouth and metallic taste. The use of aerosolized ipratropium or atropine should be considered in patients responding poorly to beta-agonist therapy.

Once a mainstay in the treatment of acute bronchospastic disease, theophylline/aminophylline has recently been relegated to a second- or third-line role. These methylxanthines are not believed to increase bronchodilation in patients treated maximally with beta agonists. Side effects include tachycardia, arrhythmias, nausea, vomiting, headaches, dizziness, and nervousness.

Multiple studies have demonstrated the effectiveness of glucocorticoids in the treatment of asthma. Benefits that have been demonstrated include rate of improvement measured by clinical scores and pulmonary function studies, increased rate of improvement, decreased duration of symptoms, decreased hospitalization rates, decreased relapse rates, and decreased need for beta agonists.

Glucocorticoids may be inappropriately withheld from asthmatic patients because of the belief that their effects are delayed, the belief that they need to be given intravenously, or fear of side effects. However, these concerns are unwarranted. A number of studies have shown that glucocorticoid benefit can occur promptly enough to affect the patient's disposition from the ED. Oral and parenteral glucocorticoids are known to be equally efficacious. Following a short course of glucocorticoid therapy, adrenal suppression is minimal and clinically insignificant. Glucocorticoid bursts for 5 days or less, if done no more than four times per year, do not require tapering. In the ED, 2 mg/kg of prednisone or an equivalent dose of another glucocorticoid should be given as an initial bolus, followed by 2 mg/kg/day of prednisone. Some suggest a single daily dose given at 7 or 8 A.M. to coincide with the surge in endogenous cortisol production and to minimize adrenal suppression. However, divided doses are sometimes used to minimize gastrointestinal upset. They are most effective if started within 24 h of the onset of symptoms. The use of inhaled glucocorticoids is encouraged for chronic treatment at home in moderately severe asthmatics. They are available as MDI only. Side effects are minimal.

Other therapies that should be considered in all patients with asthma include oxygen and fluids. Asthmatic patients are often dehydrated due to decreased intake or vomiting and may require intravenous fluids.

Indications for intubation include the following:

Decreased level of consciousness
Apnea
Exhaustion
Rising Pa_{CO_2} after treatment
$Pa_{O_2} < 60$ mmHg
$pH < 7.2$

An asthmatic may not immediately improve with intubation, since intubation does nothing to change lower airway obstruction and, in addition, puts the patient at risk for serious complications. In intubating an asthmatic patient, the largest-diameter tube appropriate for the patient's size is used to avoid increasing resistance even further. Although sedation is normally contraindicated in patients with asthma, sedation and paralysis may be indicated to avoid barotrauma, which can result if the child struggles during passage of the endotracheal tube. A modified rapid sequence induction should be used. The dissociative anesthetic ketamine is known to have bronchodilatory properties and therefore may be a good choice for a sedative. Paralysis with succinylcholine may increase secretions but is not contraindicated. Pancuronium is thought to have bronchodilatory properties; however, its long duration of action outweighs this benefit. Intubated patients with asthma may also require sedation and paralysis to maintain effective ventilation. They require a long expiratory time to avoid air trapping due to airway obstruction. Intubated asthmatic patients need to be watched carefully for the development of pneumothorax or pneumomediastinum.

DISPOSITION/OUTCOME

The decision to admit or discharge a patient from the ED after treatment for asthma can be difficult. Studies have shown that there is a high relapse rate for patients discharged after treatment, and many patients return to the ED requiring further therapy or hospitalization. Numerous studies have been published attempting to establish objective criteria for admission. Clinical examination and scoring systems perform poorly in identifying patients requiring hospital admission. Various spirometric parameters have also been proposed but have not proved to have adequate sensitivity. To date, no objective criteria have been shown to be uniformly helpful in making this decision.

The recent increase in mortality from asthma has led to studies investigating who is most at risk. The following risk factors have been identified:

Previous intubation
Two or more hospitalizations in the last year
Three or more ED visits in the last year
Use of systemic glucocorticoids

For a more detailed discussion, see Connors K: Asthma, chap. 23, p. 165, in *Pediatric Emergency Medicine: A Comprehensive Study Guide.*

24 Bronchiolitis

Kathleen Connors

Bronchiolitis is a disease of the very young and occurs almost exclusively in children below 2 years of age.

ETIOLOGY

The most common etiology of bronchiolitis is respiratory syncytial virus (RSV), present in up to 75 percent of infants admitted to the hospital with bronchiolitis. Other viruses that are known to cause bronchiolitis are parainfluenza, influenza, mumps, adenovirus, echovirus, and rhinovirus. *Mycoplasma pneumoniae* and *Chlamydia trachomatis* have also been associated with bronchiolitis.

PATHOPHYSIOLOGY

Infection produces inflammation of the bronchiolar epithelium, which leads to necrosis, sloughing, and lumenal obstruction. Sloughed ciliated epithelium is replaced by cuboidal cells without cilia. Increased mucus production and edema contribute further to airway obstruction. The absence of ciliated epithelium prevents adequate mobilization of secretions and debris. The obstruction is not uniform throughout the lungs. This leads to ventilation-perfusion mismatching, resultant hypoxia, and compensatory hyperventilation. If the obstruction is severe, hypercapnia may occur. Distal to the obstructed bronchiole, air trapping or atelectasis may occur.

CLINICAL PRESENTATION

Typically, a child with bronchiolitis will have a prodrome of an upper respiratory tract infection. There will often be a family or contact history of upper respiratory tract infection.

On physical examination, hyperventilation, as a compensatory response for hypoxia secondary to the ventilation-perfusion mismatching, is common. Respiratory rates of 70 to 90/min or greater are not uncommon. Flaring of the nasal alae and use of intercostal muscles may also be present. Respirations are shallow because of persistent distension of the lungs by the trapped air. Wheezing, prolonged expiration, and musical rales are common. The chest is often hyperexpanded and hyperresonant due to the air trapping. The liver and spleen may be displaced downward because of the hyperinflation and flattening of the diaphragm. Thoracoabdominal asynchrony may be present with breathing and correlates with the degree of obstruction. Fever is present in two-thirds of children with bronchiolitis. Despite these findings, the patient often has a nontoxic appearance.

Respiratory fatigue may occur, since the bronchiolitic infant may increase the work of breathing up to sixfold. Apnea is not uncommon (18 to 20 percent of those hospitalized with RSV bronchiolitis), especially in very young and premature infants. Hospitalized patients should be placed on a cardiac/apnea monitor and watched carefully for apneic episodes.

LABORATORY AND RADIOGRAPHIC FINDINGS

A chest radiograph will reveal hyperinflation in the majority of patients with bronchiolitis. Peribronchial cuffing (thickening of the bronchiole walls) will be seen in about half. There may be areas of subsegmental atelectasis, which can be difficult to differentiate from pneumonia. A chest radiograph is often useful in ruling out the other disease processes in the differential of bronchiolitis. The white blood cell count is usually within the normal range. Viral cultures will usually reveal an etiologic agent. Rapid tests (complement fixation or indirect immunofluorescent antibody testing) for RSV are available in many institutions and may be useful in confirming the diagnosis. Hypoxia is common, and the patient should have oxygen saturations assessed with a pulse oximeter. Hypercarbia will be present in those with more severe obstruction. Respiratory rates greater than 60/min correlate well with CO_2 retention on blood gases.

DIFFERENTIAL DIAGNOSIS

The differential diagnosis for bronchiolitis is essentially the same as for asthma. Bronchiolitis may be very difficult to differentiate from infantile asthma. Response to bronchodilators does not exclude bronchiolitis, since many children with bronchiolitis will have some degree of bronchospasm. Since bronchiolitis most commonly occurs in infancy, particular attention should be paid to other processes that may present in infancy. Congenital heart disease, cystic fibrosis, vascular rings, and other congenital anomalies may all mimic the findings of bronchiolitis. Infants and toddlers are particularly prone to foreign-body aspiration, which must be considered in a wheezing infant.

TREATMENT

Since most children with bronchiolitis will have some degree of hypoxia, monitoring of oximetry and provision of oxygen, if needed, is important. Many of these children will have difficulty drinking secondary to their increased work of breathing, and intravenous hydration should be considered if the patient cannot take adequate oral fluids. However, these patients are also at increased risk for the development of pulmonary edema if they are overhydrated. Fluids in excess of the patient's estimated deficit plus maintenance should be avoided.

No significant benefit has been demonstrated from routine antibiotic usage. In the severely ill patient, a broad-spectrum antibiotic such as cefotaxime may be warranted to cover for the possibility of a bacterial superinfection until this is ruled out by appropriate cultures.

The association between bronchiolitis and the development of asthma, a disease in which glucocorticoids clearly are of benefit, has led some physicians to advocate their use in bronchiolitis. Currently, they are not recommended for routine therapy by most authors.

Bronchodilators produce clinical improvement in many patients with bronchiolitis. A number of recent studies have demonstrated the safety and efficacy of albuterol in the initial treatment of infants with bronchiolitis. Many believe that aggressive albuterol nebulization therapy is advantageous and should be utilized in children requiring admission.

The role of ribavirin in the treatment of RSV bronchiolitis remains controversial. Currently the American Academy of Pediatrics recommends ribavirin therapy for "high-risk" infants with known RSV bronchiolitis (Table 24-1). Ribavirin is given as a continuous aerosol for 3 to 5 days as inpatient therapy.

Of infants hospitalized for bronchiolitis, 2 to 5 percent will go on to develop respiratory failure and require mechanical support. There are no absolute criteria for endotracheal intubation. Suggested indications include P_{CO_2} greater than 60 to 65 torr, recurrent apneic spells, decreasing mental status, and hypoxia despite O_2 therapy. Once intubated, these infants have many of the same problems that intubated asthmatics have and are at risk for air trapping and the development of air leaks. There have been reports of the successful use of nasal or endotracheal continuous positive airway pressure (CPAP) in treating patients with bronchiolitis as a means of avoiding mechanical ventilation and its complications. Recently, there have been reports of successful management of severe bronchiolitis with extracorporeal membrane oxygenation (ECMO) in patients unresponsive to conventional therapy.

DISPOSITION/OUTCOME

Bronchiolitis is a short-lived, self-limited disease lasting a few days. Most patients do not require admission. Follow-up within 24 h is

TABLE 24-1 American Academy of Pediatrics Recommendations for Ribavirin Therapy

1. Infants at high risk for severe or complicated respiratory syncytial virus (RSV) infection. This includes infants with complicated congenital heart disease, bronchopulmonary disease, cystic fibrosis, and other chronic lung conditions; premature infants; children with immunodeficiency, especially those with acquired immunodeficiency syndrome or severe combined immunodeficiency disease; recent transplant recipients; and those undergoing chemotherapy for malignancy.
2. Infants hospitalized with RSV lower tract disease who are severely ill (e.g., $Pa_{O_2} < 65$ mmHg, increasing P_{CO_2}).
3. All patients mechanically ventilated for RSV infection.
4. Those hospitalized with RSV who are at risk for progression to severe disease (below 6 weeks of age) or those in whom prolonged illness might be particularly detrimental to an underlying condition (e.g., neurologic disease, metabolic disease, multiple congenital anomalies).

Source: Adapted from Committee of Infectious Diseases. Ribavirin therapy of RSV. *Pediatrics* 92:501, 1993. With permission.

recommended for those who are discharged. Children with a history of prematurity, congenital heart disease, bronchopulmonary disease, underlying lung disease, or compromised immune function are at the highest risk for morbidity and mortality and should be admitted.

Up to 50 percent of infants with RSV bronchiolitis will go on to have recurrent wheezing. The only factor shown to increase the likelihood of subsequent wheezing is a family history of asthma or atopy.

For a more detailed discussion, see Connors K: Bronchiolitis, chap. 24, p. 173, in *Pediatric Emergency Medicine: A Comprehensive Study Guide.*

25 Pneumonia

Kathleen Connors

Pneumonia is an inflammation of the lung tissue, most commonly caused by an infection and demonstrated by pulmonary infiltrates on a chest radiograph.

ETIOLOGY

Many infectious agents can cause pneumonia. The predominant pathogens that cause pneumonia in infants and children are dependent on the age of the patient, the vaccination status, the presence of underlying disease, attendance in day care, and exposure history. Cases of pneumonia due to a particular agent often occur in clusters, so it is helpful to be aware of recent outbreaks in your locale. Table 25-1 summarizes the most common etiologic agents of pneumonia by age groups in normal, healthy children. The majority (60 to 90 percent) of cases of pneumonia are nonbacterial in origin.

The immediate newborn period is the only time when bacterial infections are the most common cause of pneumonia. The majority of infections in this age group are caused by aspiration of the organisms that colonize the mother's genital tract during labor and delivery.

PATHOPHYSIOLOGY

A majority of pneumonias are acquired through aspiration of infective particles. A number of mechanisms normally help protect the lung from infection. Alterations in any of these protective mechanisms may predispose a child to the development of pneumonia. In a child without any predisposing abnormalities, access to the lung is gained by the infectious particles through alterations in the normal anatomic and physiologic defenses. This most commonly occurs secondary to a viral infection of the upper respiratory tract. Less commonly, bacterial and certain viral pneumonias may be acquired through hematogenous spread from either a localized source of generalized bacteremia or viremia.

Once in the lung parenchyma, bacteria cause an acute inflammatory response that includes exudation of fluid, deposition of fibrin, and infiltration of alveoli with polymorphonuclear leukocytes, followed by macrophages.

CLINICAL PRESENTATION

Symptoms and signs of pneumonia vary with the patient's age, the specific pathogen, and the severity of the disease. The typical history in an older child includes fever, pleuritic chest pain, dyspnea, increased sputum production, and tachypnea. However, in very young children, these classic symptoms may be absent. Pneumonia usually presents as part of a sepsis syndrome in the newborn, and nonspecific symptoms may be due to pneumonia in an infant. These symptoms may include fever without a localizing source, apnea, poor feeding, abdominal pain, vomiting or diarrhea, hypo-

TABLE 25-1 Common Etiologies of Pneumonia

Age	Viral agents	Bacterial agents	Other
Birth to 2 weeks	CMV, HSV, rubella	Group B strep, *E. coli* and other coliforms, *L. monocytogenes*	
2 weeks to 2 months	RSV, parainfluenza, adenovirus, influenza, EBV	*S. pneumoniae* *S. aureus* *H. influenza*	*C. trachomatis*
2 months to 3 years	RSV, parainfluenza, adenovirus, influenza, EBV	*S. pneumoniae* *H. influenza* *S. aureus*	
3 years to 12 years	Influenza, adenovirus, parainfluenza, EBV	*S. pneumoniae* *M. pneumoniae*	
13 years to 19 years	Same	*M. pneumoniae* *S. pneumoniae*	*C. pneumoniae*

thermia, grunting, bradycardia, lethargy, or shock. In children below 3 months of age, apnea is a presenting symptom of viral pneumonia.

The history may also give clues as to the etiologic agent. Viral pneumonia is often preceded by upper respiratory symptoms and may be associated with an exanthem. The onset of lower tract symptoms, primarily tachypnea, is usually gradual. Bacterial pneumonia may also be preceded by a viral upper respiratory infection. However, the onset of lower tract symptoms is usually more sudden in a bacterial pneumonia. Fever, often accompanied by chills, is almost always present. Occasionally, pleuritic involvement produces pain with respiratory effort. The parents may report that the child has been lethargic and eating less than usual. Pneumonia due to *Staphylococcus aureus* is notorious for being particularly rapid in progression of symptoms. A history of chlamydial infection in the mother during pregnancy or conjunctivitis (present in 50 percent of cases) suggests *Chlamydia trachomatis* pneumonia in the infant. Pneumonia caused by *Mycoplasma pneumoniae* is usually seen in adolescents. The presentation is usually insidious and often includes a complaint of sore throat. Mycoplasmal infections generally present with a gradual onset of malaise, fever, and headache. Cough usually begins 3 to 5 days after the onset of illness and is present in as many as 98 percent of cases. Patients with underlying disorders such as sickle cell anemia seem to develop more severe disease.

As with the history, the findings on physical examination will vary with age, specific etiology, and severity of infection. Tachypnea is the most frequent sign of pneumonia in children. However, it is also a very nonspecific symptom and may occur secondary to fever, anxiety, metabolic disease, cardiac disease, or other respiratory problems. Auscultation of the lungs may reveal localized rales, wheezing, or decreased air entry in the affected area. However, auscultatory findings are less reliable in children below 1 year of age. Transmission of breath sounds throughout the chest makes localization difficult. In younger children, decreased breath sounds rather than rales are often heard, as the involved areas tend to be ventilated poorly. Grunting respirations may also be present. Dullness to percussion is a less common finding. With lower lobe pneumonias, abdominal distension and pain may be present secondary to a paralytic ileus. The degree of respiratory compromise should be estimated by the patient's mental status, use of accessory muscles, retractions, nasal flaring, splinting, and the presence or absence of cyanosis.

The physical examination may also give clues as to the etiology of a pneumonia. Children with viral pneumonia are more likely to have diffuse findings on chest examination and will often have a component of airway disease producing wheezing, prolonged expiration, and hyperinflation. Patients with bacterial pneumonia are more likely to have localized findings on chest examination, but again, this may not be true for young infants. Patients with bacterial pneumonia also tend to appear relatively toxic and are almost always febrile. An infant with chlamydial infection is usually afebrile and has a distinct staccato cough; there are diffuse rales on auscultation. These infants rarely appear systematically ill. Mycoplasmal infection may produce a sore throat in addition to fever and a nonproductive, hacking cough. The child usually appears nontoxic. Rales will be present in 75 percent of patients. A variable rash (urticarial, erythema multiforme, papular, or vesicular) is present in about 10 percent of patients.

LABORATORY AND RADIOGRAPHIC FINDINGS

Although an occasional patient with pneumonia who is dehydrated may have a clear radiograph, the chest radiograph confirms or denies the diagnosis of pneumonia in most cases. Chest radiographic findings, like the clinical presentation, will vary with the etiologic agent, age, and underlying health of the child. Viral pneumonias tend to appear as diffuse interstitial infiltrates, frequently with hyperinflation, peribronchial thickening, and areas of atelectasis. The gram-negative bacteria that cause newborn pneumonias tend to be very destructive and result in pneumatocele formation. *Streptococcus pneumoniae* and *Haemophilus influenzae* type B (HIB) typically cause lobar or segmental consolidations. Pneumatocele formation or a combination of pneumothorax and empyema is highly suggestive of *S. aureus* infection. *Chlamydia trachomatis* infections usually lead to hyperexpansion and diffuse alveolar or perihilar interstitial infiltrates. Radiographic patterns for *M. pneumoniae* are variable. Lower lobe streaky or patchy infiltrates are the most common findings, but many other patterns are possible, including lobar infiltrates in 10 to 25 percent of cases. Chest radiographs may also identify complications of pneumonia, such as pleural effusions, pneumatoceles, and pneumothoraxes.

In patients with bacterial pneumonia, blood cultures are positive 10 to 30 percent of the time. In pneumococcal disease, they are positive only about 10 percent of the time. *Haemophilus influenzae* type B, *S. aureus*, and group A streptococcal disease have an even higher incidence (up to 90 percent for HIB) of positive blood cultures. Sputum cultures may also help in identifying the causative organism but may be difficult to obtain from children below 8 years of age. Cultures of the nasopharynx for viral pathogens,

Chlamydia, and *Mycoplasma* will often reveal the etiologic agent in patients with pneumonias caused by these organisms. Since time is required to culture the organisms, these tests are less helpful to the emergency physician. However, these tests may be more helpful in the long-term management of the child and should be considered if the test is available and the disease is clinically suspected. Rapid antigen tests exist for a number of viruses but, again, are not widely available on a stat basis except for the tests used to detect respiratory syncytial virus (RSV) (see Chap. 24).

The white blood cell count (WBC) is usually elevated, with a left shift in bacterial pneumonia, most notably in pneumococcal disease. Typically, viral pneumonias will produce lymphocytosis. However, it is not unusual for viral pneumonia to initially provoke a significant polymorphonuclear cell response. In patients with mycoplasmal pneumonia, the total WBC and differential is normal, but the erythrocyte sedimentation rate (ESR) may be elevated. The exception is children with sickle cell disease or other hemoglobinopathies, where leukemoid reactions may occur. Chlamydial infections or parasitic infections may produce eosinophilia. Blood may also be tested for cold agglutinins, which may be positive in 72 to 92 percent of patients with *M. pneumoniae* infection. However, they also may be present in viral infections and are less consistently positive in young children.

A pulse oximetry measurement is indicated in all patients with pneumonia. Arterial blood gases may help assess a patient with impending respiratory failure.

DIFFERENTIAL DIAGNOSIS

Initially, it is important to differentiate pneumonia from noninfectious pulmonary conditions, such as congestive heart failure, atelectasis, primary and metastatic tumors, and congenital abnormalities, such as pulmonary hypoplasia or congenital lobar emphysema.

TREATMENT

All patients should be assessed for hypoxia and oxygen provided if necessary. Additional respiratory support is provided as dictated by the patient's clinical condition. Fluid status is assessed and hydration provided if needed.

Most children with pneumonia can be managed as outpatients. If a bacterial etiology is suspected, the patient is placed on an appropriate antibiotic. An antibiotic is chosen on the basis of the considerations discussed above regarding the most likely etiologic organisms based on the age and clinical presentation of the patient.

TABLE 25-2 Empiric Parenteral Antibiotic Therapy for Pneumonia

Age	Agent(s)	Alternatives
0 to 1 month	Ampicillin + aminoglycoside	Ampicillin + cefotaxime
1 month to 3 months	Ampicillin + cefotaxime	
3 months to 5 years	Cephalosporin (cefuroxime, cefotaxime, ceftriaxone, ceftazidime)	Ampicillin + chloramphenicol[a]
>5 years	Penicillin	Ampicillin, cephalosporin[a,b]

[a] If patient's course suggests *S. aureus* infection, consider addition of an antistaphylococcal agent.

[b] Consider the addition of erythromycin if patient's course suggests *M. pneumoniae*.

If viral pneumonia is suspected, no specific antibiotic therapy is warranted. Symptomatic treatment should include fever control and hydration. If the patient has prominent symptoms of reactive airway disease (as in bronchiolitis), bronchodilator therapy should be considered. In RSV pneumonia, ribavirin therapy should be considered, utilizing the guidelines discussed for bronchiolitis.

Intravenous antibiotics are administered to patients requiring admission for suspected bacterial pneumonia. Empiric coverage should be guided predominantly by the age of the patient (Table 25-2). In the newborn, ampicillin (150 to 300 mg/kg/day every 6 to 8 h) in combination with either an aminoglycoside (gentamicin 2.5 mg/kg/dose every 8 to 12 h) or third-generation cephalosporin (cefotaxime, 100 to 150 mg/kg/day every 6 to 8 h) is preferred. The ampicillin provides coverage against *Listeria* and *Enterococcus* species. In children over 3 months of age, a cephalosporin alone (cefuroxime, cefotaxime, ceftriaxone) is sufficient. In children who are unresponsive to this therapy or with a suggestive clinical presentation, mycoplasmal and chlamydial infections should be considered. Appropriate coverage includes erythromycin, or tetracycline in children over 9 years of age. If the clinical presentation is suspicious for staphylococcal disease, then appropriate coverage (nafcillin 150 mg/kg/day every 6 h) should be added.

The duration of therapy varies with the clinical response, predisposing host factors, and suppurative complications. For most uncomplicated cases, 7 to 10 days of antimicrobial treatment should suffice. Parenteral therapy, if initiated, should be continued until clinical improvement occurs. Routine follow-up radiographs are not necessary if the patient improves clinically.

DISPOSITION/OUTCOME

The majority of children with pneumonia can be managed as outpatients. Suggested criteria for admission include hypoxia, respiratory distress, toxic appearance, dehydration, age less than 3 months, impaired immune function, and infections unresponsive to oral therapy. The presence of underlying disease and the ability of the caregivers to provide care for the child should also be considered. Age less than 1 year or the finding of a pleural effusion or pneumatocele suggests a pathogen other than *S. pneumoniae* (particularly HIB or *S. aureus*). These infections can be rapidly progressive and are not well tolerated, so strong consideration should be given to hospitalizing these patients. All children discharged with a diagnosis of pneumonia should have clinical follow-up arranged within 24 h.

Most viral pneumonias will resolve spontaneously without specific therapy. Complications are similar to those for bronchiolitis and include dehydration, bronchiolitis obliterans, and apnea. Indications for admitting patients with RSV pneumonia are the same as those for RSV bronchiolitis (see Chap. 24).

Uncomplicated bacterial pneumonia usually responds rapidly to antibiotic therapy. Delay in improvement or a worsening condition after therapy has begun should prompt an evaluation for possible complications. Complications of bacterial pneumonia include pleural effusions, empyemas, pneumothorax, pneumatoceles, dehydration, and development of additional infectious foci.

For a more detailed discussion, see Connors K: Pneumonia, chap. 25, p. 176, in *Pediatric Emergency Medicine: A Comprehensive Study Guide.*

---

26 Pertussis

Kathleen Connors

Pertussis is seen most commonly in infants below 6 months of age but can be seen in any age group. It was a leading cause of morbidity and mortality in children prior to the widespread use of the diphtheria-tetanus-pertussis (DPT) vaccine, which became available in the 1950s. Over the next 30 years, the number of reported cases fell dramatically, to a nadir of about 1000 cases per year in the 1970s; however, in the past decade there has been a fourfold increase in the incidence of pertussis in this country.

Pertussis is an infection of the respiratory tract produced by *Bordetella pertussis. Bordetella pertussis* is spread by respiratory droplet transmission. Following inhalation, *B. pertussis* organisms attach to the epithelial cells of the respiratory tract. Multiplication of the bacteria leads to infiltration of the mucosa with inflammatory cells. Inflammatory debris in the lumen of the bronchi and peribronchial lymphoid hyperplasia obstruct the smaller airways, causing atelectasis. Attack rates in susceptible household contacts approach 100 percent. The incubation period ranges from 7 to 14 days.

CLINICAL PRESENTATION

The disease has three stages. The initial or catarrhal stage is characterized by upper respiratory tract symptoms and lasts 7 to 10 days. This is followed by a paroxysmal phase, characterized by episodic bouts of staccato cough, lasting 2 to 4 weeks. Infants in the paroxysmal phase of *B. pertussis* infection will have a history of intermittent coughing spells, often followed by posttussive emesis and sometimes associated with cyanosis. The paroxysms are often provoked by feeding or exertion and can be elicited by using a tongue blade to examine the throat. The cough is staccato in nature, allowing little or no inspiration between coughs. At the termination of a paroxysm, a prolonged slow inspiration occurs. Inspiration through a partially closed glottis produces the characteristic whoop. However, this feature is often absent in infants. In the convalescent stage, the symptoms gradually wane.

LABORATORY AND RADIOGRAPHIC FINDINGS

Cultures of the nasopharynx may reveal the organism. Fluorescent antibody testing is currently the most utilized confirmatory test but has a low sensitivity and poor predictive value. Pertussis generally produces extreme leukocytosis (20,000 to 50,000), with a predominance of lymphocytes.

This may not occur in infants below 6 months of age. Radiographs in patients with *B. pertussis* infection may demonstrate a shaggy right heart border or may be normal.

DIAGNOSIS

The diagnosis of pertussis is best made through a sensitive history and physical examination coupled with the clinician's awareness of its possible existence. During outbreaks of pertussis, a cough lasting for 14 days or more can be considered a case. For a sporadic diagnosis, the patient must meet the cough criterion and also have paroxysms, whoop, or posttussive emesis. It is important to remember that many cases are atypical, especially in infants or children who have been partially immunized. In such cases, laboratory testing may be helpful.

TREATMENT

The mainstay of treatment is supportive therapy. Infants may become hypoxic during paroxysms and benefit from the administration of humidified oxygen. They may also become dehydrated due to inability to feed and will benefit from intravenous fluids.

Erythromycin is considered to be the most effective antibiotic. However, unless it is started early, it does not modify the course of the disease. Erythromycin is recommended for use in patient contacts. The recommended dose is 40 to 50 mg/kg/day in four divided doses for 14 days. In contacts below 7 years of age who have not received the four-dose primary vaccination series, a dose of DPT should be administered.

DISPOSITION/OUTCOME

Bordetella pertussis infections can be complicated by apnea, seizures, encephalopathy, and secondary bacterial pneumonia. The incidence of these complications and death due to pertussis infection is greater in infants below 1 year of age. Infants below 1 year of age must be admitted and placed on a cardiorespiratory/apnea monitor.

For a more detailed discussion, see Connors K: Pertussis, chap. 26, p. 181, in *Pediatric Emergency Medicine: A Comprehensive Study Guide.*

---

27 Bronchopulmonary Dysplasia

Kathleen Connors

As the care of neonates with respiratory failure becomes more aggressive and more successful, the incidence of chronic lung disease in infants is increasing. The overall rate of bronchopulmonary dysplasia (BPD) is about 15 percent for premature infants requiring mechanical ventilation. The incidence is dependent on birth weight, exceeding 50 percent in infants less than 750 g at birth and 40 percent for infants between 750 and 1000 g. In addition to weight, male sex and white race are risk factors for the development of BPD.

Bronchopulmonary dysplasia is a chronic lung disease of infancy that follows neonatal lung disease. The original insult may be hyaline membrane disease, apnea, persistent fetal circulation, complex congenital heart disease, or any illness requiring prolonged mechanical ventilation in the neonate. Children with residual lung disease after the neonatal period (28 days of age) are said to have BPD. The lung disease may be characterized by respiratory distress, a supplemental oxygen requirement, or significant radiologic and blood gas abnormalities. Oxygen requirement at 36 weeks corrected postgestational age has been shown to be an excellent predictor of the development of BPD.

ETIOLOGY/PATHOPHYSIOLOGY

The pathogenesis of BPD is complex and not yet fully understood. Mechanical ventilation has been implicated as a causative agent. However, some infants who never receive mechanical ventilation go on to develop the clinical syndrome of BPD. Some infants may be genetically predisposed to the development of BPD. The major host susceptibility factor associated with BPD is immature lungs secondary to prematurity. Decreased numbers of alveoli and airways as well as increased distensibility of the airways may predispose premature infants to barotrauma during mechanical ventilation. Immaturity is also associated with a defect in the antioxidant defense system and a decrease in plasma proteinase inhibitors.

CLINICAL PRESENTATION

The clinical spectrum of infants with chronic lung disease ranges from mild, asymptomatic disease to crippling cardiopulmonary dysfunction. Patients who are likely to present to the emergency department (ED) are those that have been discharged home from the neonatal intensive care unit (NICU), typically at about 3 to 6 months of age. These children are often on home oxygen, bronchodilators, apnea monitors, and other medications. They will present to the ED with an exacerbation of their chronic lung disease, most often secondary to a viral upper respiratory infection. Parents may describe increased respiratory distress, poor feeding, lethargy or irritability, and an increased oxygen requirement.

On physical examination, infants with chronic lung disease will usually be small for their age and have hyperinflated chests. They will have tachypnea, rales, wheezes, or areas of decreased breath sounds.

LABORATORY AND RADIOGRAPHIC FINDINGS

A chest radiograph will reveal variable degrees of hyperinflation with areas of "scarring." Comparison with old films is required to differentiate these areas from acute processes.

Oximetry should be checked on all patients with BPD. Blood gas results can be helpful in assessing the more severely symptomatic patient. The results should be interpreted in light of the baseline level of hypoxia and usual need for oxygen therapy.

DIFFERENTIAL DIAGNOSIS

Signs and symptoms of an exacerbation may overlap considerably with those of pneumonia, asthma, or bronchiolitis. Often these problems are coexistent and are the cause of the exacerbation.

TREATMENT

The treatment of an exacerbation in a patient with BPD is mainly supportive. Oxygen is provided if indicated. The patient's fluid status is assessed, and intravenous fluids are provided if indicated. Mechanical ventilation may be necessary for recurrent apneic spells [most commonly with respiratory syncytial virus (RSV) infections], worsening hypercarbia, or refractory hypoxemia.

Bronchodilators are often effective in these patients and should be used in a similar fashion as for asthma. Glucocorticoids are also thought to be effective. Diuretics have been shown to improve lung function and survival in some patients.

OUTCOME/DISPOSITION

Children with BPD often have a very fragile respiratory status and can become very sick with relatively minor insults. Indications for inpatient management include increased respiratory distress, increasing hypoxia or hypercarbia, or new pulmonary infiltrates. Patients with BPD and RSV infections are at high risk for complications of RSV, are candidates for ribavirin administration, and must be hospitalized. It is important to remember that the home care of these children requires a tremendous amount of work on the part of the parents or other caretakers even when the child is not acutely ill. Parents may not be able to cope with an exacerbation. This factor should be considered in making a decision to discharge a patient for home care.

For a more detailed discussion, see Connors K: Bronchopulmonary dysplasia, chap. 27, p. 183, in *Pediatric Emergency Medicine: A Comprehensive Study Guide.*

28 Cystic Fibrosis

Kathleen Connors

Cystic fibrosis (CF) is the most common lethal inherited disease among Caucasians in the United States. It is inherited as an autosomal recessive condition. It occurs in approximately 1 in 2500 and 1 in 17,000 live births in whites and blacks, respectively.

Cystic fibrosis is a generalized defect in all of the exocrine gland secretions. Most patients with CF have the classic triad of manifestations: (1) chronic pulmonary disease, (2) malabsorption, and (3) elevated content of electrolytes in sweat. There can be considerable individual variation in the severity and course of the disease.

PATHOPHYSIOLOGY

The primary pathology is in the exocrine glands. There is a failure to secrete chloride and secondarily sodium and water and an excess reabsorption of sodium by the apical membranes of the epithelium. The channels that conduct sodium and chloride ions across the membrane are present and functional, but there is altered regulation of their activity. The result of this abnormality is increased salt and water reabsorption from surface secretions.

The ion translocation abnormality works in reverse for the sweat gland ducts. The sweat of patients with CF contains a high concentration of chloride. This forms the basis for the most important diagnostic test for CF, the qualitative pilocarpine iontophoresis sweat test.

Clinically, the patients are noted to have abnormalities in clearing mucous secretions, a paucity of water in mucous secretions, an elevated salt content in sweat and other serous secretions, and chronic infections of the respiratory tract. The chronic mucus plugging and infection lead to hyperinflation, bronchiectasis, and atelectasis. Eventually most CF patients die of respiratory failure complicated by cor pulmonale.

The exocrine glands of the pancreas produce viscous, low-volume, bicarbonate- and enzyme-deficient secretions. Abnormal intestinal mucins and biliary tract secretions have also been implicated in the intestinal malabsorption and obstruction seen in CF.

CLINICAL PRESENTATION

Failure to thrive with a history of chronic respiratory or gastrointestinal problems is the most typical presentation. The diagnosis should be considered in any case of failure to thrive, atypical asthma (especially with clubbing, bronchiectasis, or purulent sputum), recurrent respiratory infections, or chronic diarrhea. Hypoproteinemia may develop in those with prominent malabsorption. Malabsorption may also lead to symptoms of vitamin deficiencies. A hemorrhagic diathesis secondary to vitamin K deficiency has been described. Patients with clinical findings suggestive of CF should be referred for diagnostic evaluation.

Patients with known CF may present to the emergency department (ED) with a variety of acute complications. The most common of these is a pulmonary exacerbation. Patients will often present following an upper respiratory infection. Chest examination will reveal diffuse rales, rhonchi, or wheezing. Pneumothoraxes are not unusual in patients with CF and should be considered in any patient with an acute deterioration. Many patients with CF will have intermittent blood-streaked sputum; this is usually not clinically significant. However, significant hemoptysis (30 to 60 mL) can result from erosion of a bronchial vessel. Less commonly, patients with CF will cough up blood from bleeding esophageal varices secondary to advanced cirrhosis. Many patients with CF will develop pulmonary hypertension and right ventricular hypertrophy as a result of their chronic lung disease. Congestive heart failure can develop during a respiratory exacerbation.

Acute nonpulmonary complications of CF include meconium ileus, rectal prolapse, intestinal obstruction, and electrolyte abnormalities. A neonate with meconium ileus will usually have a history of having passed no stool or only a small amount of meconium stool. On physical examination, these patients will have a distended abdomen. They may also have visible peristaltic waves or a palpable abdominal mass. Intestinal obstruction secondary to inability to pass the dry, abnormal stool can also occur in older children with CF and is sometimes called meconium ileus equivalent. Like a meconium ileus, these fecal masses can lead to complications, including volvulus, intussusception, or intestinal perforation. Rectal prolapse is associated with CF and is most commonly seen in children below 3 years of age.

LABORATORY AND RADIOGRAPHIC FINDINGS

A quantitative pilocarpine iontophoresis sweat (sweat chloride) test should be part of the diagnostic evaluation, and any patient with suspected CF should be referred for an evaluation including this test.

In patients with known CF with a pulmonary exacerbation, sputum cultures should be obtained to help guide future antibiotic therapy. Past sputum culture results can be helpful in guiding initial therapy. Blood cultures to rule out bacteremia may be indicated in febrile or toxic-appearing patients.

Electrolyte determination will usually reveal low serum sodium and chloride levels. Bicarbonate levels and serum pH are usually elevated. These abnormalities represent renal compensation for the increased salt loss in the sweat. Dehydration and symptomatic electrolyte deficiencies can occur, especially in periods of hot weather. Patients with significant hemoptysis should have blood sent for a hematocrit, type and crossmatch, and prothrombin time. Oximetry should be checked in any patient with increased pulmonary symptoms. Blood gas determinations may be useful in managing a patient with respiratory failure.

Typical radiographic findings of a patient with CF include diffuse peribronchial thickening, hyperinflation, and variable fluffy infiltrates. It is often helpful to compare current films with previous ones in patients with acute exacerbations. Radiographic studies may be helpful in diagnosing the acute complications of CF. Patients with a sudden change in pulmonary condition should have a chest radiograph to rule out a pneumothorax. Patients with cor pulmonale will have a large heart (as opposed to the narrow heart usually seen in patients with CF) and prominent pulmonary vasculature. Patients with meconium ileus or meconium ileus equivalent will have dilated loops of bowel on an abdominal film. A bubbly granular density in the lower abdomen, representing the meconium or fecal mass, may also be seen.

TREATMENT

The ED physician may be called upon to manage the acute complications of CF. The most common of these will be pulmonary exacerbations. Therapy is aimed at relieving the mucous plugging and obstruction and treating infection. Oxygen should be administered if indicated by pulse oximetry or blood gas. Bronchodilators are often effective in patients with CF and should be used in those who respond clinically. The patient's recent sputum culture and sensitivity results may be helpful in choosing initial antibiotics. If these results are unavailable, empiric therapy should be aimed at the two most common organisms seen in these patients, which are *Staphylococcus aureus* and *Pseudomonas aeruginosa*; empiric antibiotic therapy is also recommended. Chest physiotherapy may be helpful. A pneumothorax that is greater than 10 percent of the area of the hemithorax should be treated with tube thoracostomy. Tension pneumothoraxes should be treated with needle aspiration followed by tube thoracostomy.

Significant hemoptysis (greater than 30 to 60 mL) is an indication for inpatient observation. Vitamin K is indicated if the prothrombin time is prolonged. If bleeding persists, guidelines for replacement are the same as those for bleeding from other sources. Massive hemoptysis (greater than 300 mL) may compromise the airway; ligation or embolization of the bleeding vessel should be attempted with the help of a bronchoscopist or thoracic surgeon.

Cor pulmonale may require treatment with oxygen and diuretics in addition to treatment for the underlying pulmonary disease. Patients with CF and respiratory failure are very difficult to manage. They do not respond as well to mechanical ventilation and have even more complications than patients with other forms of chronic obstructive pulmonary disease. In general, patients in whom respiratory failure is precipitated by an acute insult such as a viral pneumonia or episode of status asthmaticus and whose baseline pulmonary function was good should be considered for mechanical ventilation. In patients who have experienced a steady progressive decline in pulmonary function despite adequate medical therapy, mechanical ventilation is not indicated.

In patients with uncomplicated meconium ileus or meconium ileus equivalent, saline or meglumine diatrizoate (Gastrografin) enemas may relieve the obstruction. Laparotomy is indicated if there are signs of perforation, volvulus, or intussusception or if the medical management is unsuccessful. Patients presenting with dehydration and electrolyte abnormalities should be rehydrated with isotonic saline. Serum electrolytes should be measured frequently to guide fluid therapy.

For a more detailed discussion, see Connors K: Cystic Fibrosis, chap. 28, p. 185, in *Pediatric Emergency Medicine: A Comprehensive Study Guide*.

Section IV
Cardiovascular Emergencies

29 Principles and Structural Aspects of Heart Disease

William C. Toepper

In the fetus, there are several mechanisms to divert blood away from the nonfunctioning pulmonary circulation. Pulmonary arteriolar hypertrophy leads to an increase in pulmonary vascular resistance. The patent foramen ovale results in equalization of right and left ventricular pressures, and there is shunting of blood from pulmonary artery to aorta via the patent ductus arteriosus. Placental blood flow is also directly routed into the fetal systemic circulation via the patent ductus venosus.

At birth, dramatic changes in oxygen saturation and chest wall expansion allow for a decrease in pulmonary vascular resistance and an increase in pulmonary blood flow, left atrial return, and closure of the foramen ovale. Increased oxygen saturation works to close the ductus arteriosus through prostaglandin mediators. All mechanisms result in an increase in pulmonary blood flow and therefore oxygenation, ventilation, perfusion, and a healthy baby.

While this transition generally goes smoothly, even subtle changes in pressure, flow, or saturation due to valvular or structural anomalies can result in a sick child. The newborn's cardiac output compensatory mechanisms are less developed than those of the adult. The neonatal myocardium has proportionately fewer contractile elements, resulting in a heavier reliance on rate for cardiac output. The neonatal myocardium also has an underdeveloped autonomic nervous system, so that less adrenergic responsiveness is seen.

CLINICAL EVALUATION

Cardiac symptoms in children are quite different from those in adults. Poor feeding and failure to thrive are probably the most sensitive and reliable symptoms, but they are very nonspecific. Other features such as lethargy, tachypnea, and frequent respiratory infections in conjunction with an abnormal cardiac examination may suggest or confirm heart disease. The older child will generally present with more "adultlike" symptoms.

The examination begins with the overall impression of the child. In the most fulminant situation, the baby's color and general appearance may be the most important part of the evaluation:

- Pink → congestive heart failure, L→R shunt
- Blue → cyanotic heart disease, R→L shunt
- Gray → outflow obstruction, systemic hypoperfusion, and shock

Of course most children will not present in extremis, and additional physical findings will assist in identifying the pathology. Tachypnea and tachycardia may be out of proportion to the general appearance of the child. Fever may help differentiate infectious processes from structural lesions of the heart. Blood pressure should be evaluated with the proper-sized cuff and compared in both upper extremities and one or both lower extremities. Other important examination features include an assessment of hydration status, general skin and mucosal color, palpation and auscultation of the precordium, auscultation of the lungs, a survey for organomegaly, and a description of pulses in all four extremities.

Congestive heart failure is common and presents with tachypnea, hyperactive precordium, chest congestion, and hepatomegaly. Peripheral edema and neck vein distension will not be seen. Auscultation of the heart may reveal a gallop rhythm or a murmur.

Another common presentation is that of the well-appearing child with a murmur. Pathologic murmurs can be distinguished from benign ones by characterizing the grade, the length, and the location within the cardiac cycle. Nonpathologic murmurs tend to be low-grade and short, and occur early in systole. Pulses, blood pressure, characterization of S1 and S2, electrocardiogram, and chest radiograph are normal. Pathologic murmurs tend to be louder and longer; their location in the cardiac cycle may give a clue as to their etiology. Short, loud midsystolic ejection murmurs are associated with stenotic lesions and are heard best at the left or right second intercostal space. Holosystolic murmurs suggest regurgitant lesions such as mitral or tricuspid regurgitation or the regurgitation through a ventricular septal defect. Diastolic murmurs suggest aortic or pulmonic regurgitation or mitral or tricuspid stenosis. It is important to remember that valve anatomy may be normal, and the harsh sound may be secondary to a relative stenosis from left-to-right shunting and increased flow. Finally, continuous murmurs may have several etiologies, the classic being the machinery murmur of the patent ductus arteriosus (PDA). Bounding pulses may help in the diagnosis of PDA. Absent or

TABLE 29-1 Normal Heart Rate Ranges

Age	Heart rate, beats/min
Newborn	80–180
1 week to 3 months	80–160
3 months to 2 years	80–150
2 years to 10 years	60–110
10 years to adult	50–90

Source: From Gewitz MH, Vetter VL: Cardiac emergencies, in Fleischer GR, Ludwig S (eds): *Pediatric Emergency Medicine*. Baltimore, MD: Williams and Wilkins, 1993, p 546. Used by permission.

diminished lower extremity pulses in the setting of a continuous murmur characterize coarctation of the aorta.

Principles of interpretation of the electrocardiogram (ECG) include the following:

- The ECG is most often used to evaluate chamber size and conduction disturbances. Ischemic changes are rare.
- Fetal and neonatal right-sided forces (i.e., right axis deviation and right ventricular hypertrophy) will take on adult form by age 3 to 4 years.
- Heart rates are faster than in adults, and sinus bradycardia must be recognized in the sick infant (Table 29-1).
- QRS axis and intervals differ from those of adults (Tables 29-2 and 29-3).
- Right bundle branch block is common; left bundle branch block is rare.

TABLE 29-2 Duration of ECG Intervals (Values in Seconds)

	P-R limits		**QRS limits**		**QTc limits**	
Age	Lower	Upper	Lower	Upper	Lower	Upper
0–7 days	0.08	0.12	0.04	0.10	0.34	0.54
7–30 days	0.08	0.12	0.04	0.07	0.30	0.50
1–3 months	0.08	0.16	0.05	0.08	0.32	0.47
3–6 months	0.08	0.12	0.05	0.08	0.35	0.46
6–12 months	0.08	0.14	0.04	0.08	0.31	0.49
1–3 years	0.08	0.16	0.04	0.08	0.34	0.43

Source: Modified from Dittmer DS, Grebe RM: *Handbook of Circulation*. Philadelphia: Saunders, 1959, p 141.

TABLE 29-3 Age-Specific QRS Axis (Frontal Plane)

Age	Range	Mean
1–7 days	80–160	125
1–4 weeks	60–160	110
1–3 months	40–120	80
3–6 months	20–80	65
6–12 months	0–100	65
1–3 years	20–100	55
3–8 years	40–80	60
8–16 years	20–80	65

Source: From Hakim SN, Toepper WC: Cardiac disease in children, in Rosen R, Barkin RM (eds): *Emergency Medicine: Concepts and Clinical Practice II.* St. Louis, MO: Mosby-Year Book, 1992, p 546. Used by permission.

CONGENITAL HEART DISEASE

Left-to-Right Shunt

The patient with a left-to-right shunt presents in mild to severe congestive heart failure. The severity will depend on the level of the shunt, the pressure differential between the affected chambers or vessels, and the overall hydration and health of the child. For example, the atrial septal defect (ASD) is characterized by a small pressure gradient between the left and right atria. As pulmonary vascular resistance decreases in the early neonatal period, the gradient increases, resulting in increased flow to the right side of the heart and pulmonary congestion. Shunting is usually minimal, and the presentation will be subtle. The murmur across the ASD may be very soft. One is more likely to appreciate a systolic murmur of relative pulmonic stenosis, caused by the increased flow across the pulmonic valve. Radiographic findings include enlarged right heart chambers. The ECG will demonstrate a predominance of right-sided forces. Since flow across the shunt can be minimal, some patients will remain asymptomatic until late childhood, when pulmonary hypertension emerges.

In contrast, the ventricular septal defect (VSD) is characterized by larger pressure gradients between the affected chambers and a more dramatic presentation. As pulmonary vascular resistance decreases, shunting begins. The size of the defect is crucial in predicting the clinical course. In small VSDs, most resistance to flow is met at the defect, where flow is minimal. The murmur is subtle. In these cases, diagnosis is important in the prevention of bacterial endocarditis. In moderate-sized defects, flow is greater, murmurs are louder, and right-sided hypertrophy and increased pulmonary blood flow dominate. In large VSDs, the right and left ventricles hypertrophy, yielding biventricular failure. Ultimately, right ventricular pressure may exceed left ventricular pressure, the shunt can reverse, and the cyanosis of Eisenmenger's disease can become apparent.

Other left-to-right shunts include the PDA, which usually presents in the neonatal intensive care unit, and endocardial cushion defects (atrioventricular canal). Endocardial cushion defects are more common in children with Down syndrome than in other children and are characterized by septal and valvular (atrioventricular) defects. The ECG can be diagnostic through the demonstration of an extreme rightward (northwest) axis.

Right-to-Left Shunt

The patient with cyanotic congenital heart disease or right-to-left shunting will present initially with cyanosis, which may be difficult to distinguish from that of primary respiratory disease. Central cyanosis caused by right-to-left shunting is suspected in the presence of cyanotic mucosa and a deterioration during crying episodes (greater cardiac demand). This is in contrast to central cyanosis caused by respiratory illness, which is characterized by respiratory distress and an improvement during crying (alveolar recruitment). The provision of 100% oxygen will usually differentiate respiratory from cardiac cyanosis, since no amount of pulmonary oxygen tension will override the mixing that occurs in a right-to-left shunt.

The classic right-to-left shunt, tetralogy of Fallot (TOF), is characterized by right ventricular obstruction, right ventricular hypertrophy, ventricular septal defect, and overriding aorta. Shunting occurs through the VSD. The chest radiograph will reveal a "boot-shaped" heart and *decreased* pulmonary blood flow. This is in contrast to the other major cyanotic lesion, transposition of the great vessels (TGV), which is characterized by *increased* pulmonary blood flow. In TGV, the right and left sides of the heart are autonomous and life is supported by venous mixing at the level of the VSD or arterial shunting between the pulmonary artery and aorta through the PDA. Patency of the ductus may be crucial and initial administration of prostaglandin (PGE_1) at 0.1 μg/kg may be lifesaving.

There are many other causes of complex cyanotic heart disease, and information obtained from the parent or patient's cardiologist is vital. Most parents will be able to provide baseline oxygen saturation or hemoglobin values. If cardiology input is delayed, several principles may help in the management of these children. Increased right-to-left shunting can be caused either by an *increase* in pulmonary vascular resistance (intercurrent respiratory illness) or by a *decrease* in systemic vascular resistance (hypotension, fever, dehydration). Specific therapy should be aimed at the cause of the change in resistance. The "tet spell," a unique cause of increased pulmonary vascular resistance in the patient with TOF, is caused by obstruction at the level of the pulmonary artery. Management includes placement of the infant in the knee-chest position or allowing the older child to maintain a squat position, reassurance, and administration of intravenous fluid and oxygen. Pharmacologic intervention is often required and includes morphine sulfate (0.05 mg/kg IV or IM), propranolol (0.1 to 0.2 mg/kg IV), or phenylephrine (5 μg/kg IV followed by 0.5 to 2 μg/kg/min) to increase systemic vascular resistance.

Another cause of worsening cyanosis is obstruction of a surgical shunt that was placed to aid in mixing, such as a Blalock-Taussig shunt. If a shunt malfunction is suspected, careful auscultation for the absence of a baseline murmur can be confirmatory; prompt echocardiographic and cardiologic consultation are mandatory.

Left Ventricular Outflow Obstruction

The presentation of left ventricular outflow obstruction, or the "gray baby," is distinguished from congestive heart failure or cyanosis by its dramatic, fulminant course and potentially poor outcome. In these infants, systemic blood flow is dependent on contribution from the patent ductus arteriosus. When the ductus closes, cardiac output and perfusion decrease, and the patient presents in profound shock. Examples include hypoplastic left heart syndrome and severe coarctation of the aorta. Any infant who presents in the first week of life with decreased perfusion, hypotension, or acidosis should be considered a candidate for PGE_1 administration. The prostaglandin is begun at 0.1 μg/kg/min and then decreased to half that dose as the clinical situation improves. Results can be dramatic. The child must be monitored for apnea and hypotension. Some advocate prophylactic intubation if long transport times are anticipated.

One less dramatic form of left-sided outlet obstruction, congenital aortic stenosis (AS), may be asymptomatic or may present with fatigue, exertional dyspnea, or chest pain. The most severe form will present with exertional syncope. Diagnosis is suspected in the presence of a loud systolic murmur, best heard at the base, which radiates into the neck. Diastolic murmurs suggest aortic regurgitation from long-standing disease. Treatment consists of valvectomy or replacement and is dependent on the severity of left ventricular strain and the presence of symptoms.

Coarctation of the aorta (COA), also characterized by left-sided outflow obstruction, may present in infancy as fulminant shock but is more likely to present with congestive heart failure or cyanosis. Presentation features depend on the level of the coarctation (preductal vs. postductal), the patency of the ductus, and the presence of septal defects. Most children who present in infancy will display additional anomalies. Presentation will often be delayed until adolescence. The diagnosis is suspected when elevated blood pressure is discovered. Lower extremity pulses and blood pressure are usually weak or absent. Left ventricular hypertrophy is characteristic, and the diastolic murmur of aortic regurgitation may be found. Collateral circulation above and below the obstruction causes posterior rib notching. Making the diagnosis is crucial, since sequelae from acute and chronic hypertension can be deadly. Surgical correction can be curative if performed prior to end-organ damage from long-standing hypertension.

ACKNOWLEDGMENT

The author wishes to thank Dr. William Meadow, Attending Physician, University of Chicago Hospitals and Clinics and Wyler Children's Hospital.

For a more detailed discussion, see Toepper WC: Principles and structural aspects of heart disease, chap. 29, p. 189, in *Pediatric Emergency Medicine: A Comprehensive Study Guide.*

---

30 Congestive and Inflammatory Diseases of the Heart

William C. Toepper / Joilo Barbosa

CONGESTIVE HEART FAILURE

Congestive heart failure (CHF), the physiologic state in which cardiac output is unable to meet the metabolic demands of the tissues, is broadly defined and encompasses many different etiolo-

TABLE 30-1 Etiologic Basis of Congestive Heart Failure

Preload (volume overload)
Left-to-right shunt: VSD, PDA, AV fistula, etc.
Anemia: iron deficiency, sickle cell, thalassemia
Iatrogenic
Afterload (increased SVR)
Congenital: coarctation of the aorta, aortic stenosis
Systemic hypertension
Contractility
Inflammatory: infectious (viral, bacterial, fungal), rheumatic (ARF, early Kawasaki, SLE)
Toxic: digoxin, Ca^{2+} channel/beta blockers, cocaine
Traumatic: cardiac tamponade, myocardial contusion
Neoplasm: atrial myxoma, leukemic infiltration
Metabolic: electrolyte abnormality, hypothyroidism
Dysrhythmia
Bradyarrhythmia: inadequate cardiac output
Tachyrhythmia: insufficient end-diastolic filling

gies. Management approaches will vary depending on the specific cause (Table 30-1).

Cardiac output is determined by four factors: preload (volume), afterload (systemic vascular resistance), intrinsic contractility, and rate. Inadequacy of any of these determinants may result in poor cardiac output. In infants, this is manifest as irritability, poor feeding, lethargy, or failure to thrive. Volume overload may present insidiously, with symptoms typical of a respiratory tract infection. The lack of fever and rhinorrhea may help differentiate the two. The physical examination reveals tachycardia and tachypnea out of proportion to the symptoms. More specific signs include a hyperactive precordium with gallop rhythm, hepatomegaly, or rales. Peripheral edema and neck vein distension are noted only in the older child. The chest radiograph may reveal cardiomegaly, increased pulmonary vascular markings, interstitial infiltrate, or pulmonary edema. The electrocardiogram may reveal nonspecific ST and T-wave changes; echocardiography may be diagnostic. The child in severe or refractory congestive heart failure may require pulmonary arterial catheterization to determine which factor (preload, afterload, contractility, or rate) is most responsible or most responsive to manipulation.

When possible, therapy for congestive heart failure is directed toward the specific cause of failure. Often the cause is multifactorial or difficult to distinguish, and therapy must be empiric. Supportive therapy includes the provision of comfort, sedation, supplemental oxygen, and placement of an intravenous line to relieve the child of the work of feeding. Pharmacologic therapy is directed toward specific defects. Management is summarized in Fig. 30-1.

The child in moderate to severe congestive heart failure will require admission to the intensive care unit or transfer to a pediatric tertiary care facility. Intubation and inotropic support may be required. Intubation will provide both a higher percentage of oxygen and positive end-expiratory pressure (PEEP). The choice of pressors is best made in conjunction with the pediatric cardiologist. The myocardial response to pharmacologic agents in neonates is very different from that seen in adults. The negative inotropic effect of calcium channel blockers is a vivid example.

Dopamine in low doses (2 to 5 μg/kg/min) acts to dilate renal and splanchnic blood vessels, resulting in increased urine output. Higher doses (5 to 20 μg/kg/min) will increase rate and contractility and can act as a potent vasoconstrictor, increasing blood pressure. In contrast, dobutamine works primarily as a positive inotrope with little peripheral effect. Epinephrine and norepinephrine are used to augment systemic vascular resistance (Table 30-2).

When cardiogenic shock is coupled with an increase in systemic vascular resistance, as with severe myocarditis, a weakened myocardium pumps ineffectively against increased afterload. Afterload reduction with vasodilator therapy may be indicated (Table 30-3). Acutely, sodium nitroprusside is the agent of choice, as it has both venodilator and arteriolar dilator effects. It can be started in very low doses and is easily titratable. Less acutely, angiotensin converting enzyme (ACE) inhibitors can be very effective in reducing afterload in children. Only oral forms are now available, but intravenous agents may soon be approved.

Finally, there is increasing experience with the use of intraaortic balloon pumps, extracorporeal membrane oxygenation (ECMO), and ventricular assist devices in the child. These highly technical advances may be lifesaving in the child with fulminant congestive heart failure who is refractory to conventional intensive support. Many children will proceed to chronic debilitating congestive heart failure or cardiomyopathy and ultimately require cardiac transplantation.

MYOCARDITIS/PERICARDITIS

Both myocarditis and pericarditis can be subtle in their early presentation, and diagnosis is often missed. Inflammatory diseases of the myocardium and pericardium are difficult to distinguish from other infectious or pulmonary diseases. Presenting complaints may

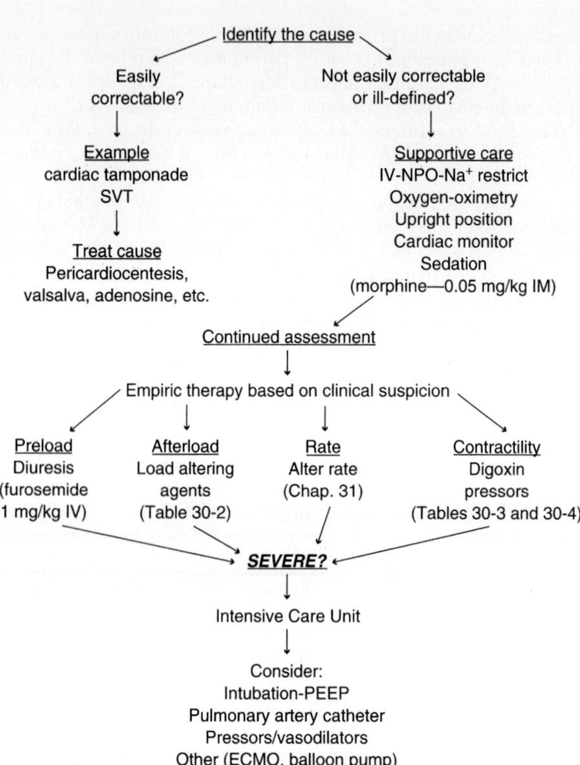

FIG. 30-1 Management of congestive heart failure.

TABLE 30-2 Inotropic Agents: Dosage and Pharmacologic Effects

Drug	Dose	Increase HR	Increase Contractility	Increase Afterload	Vasodilate
Dopamine	1–5 μg/kg/min	1+	1+	0	Renal
	6–20 μg/kg/min	2–3+	3+	1–3+	0
Dobutamine	2–10 μg/kg/min	1+	3+	0	1+
Epinephrine	0.05–1 μg/kg/min	3+	3+	0–3+ (dose-dependent)	0–2+ (dose-dependent)
Norepinephrine	0.05–0.5 μg/kg/min	2+	3+	4+	0

TABLE 30-3 Load-Altering Agents

Drug	Dose	Comments
Nitroprusside	0.5–8 μg/kg/min IV	Cyanide toxicity
Captopril	Infants: 0.5–6 mg/kg/day PO q6–12h Children: 12.5 mg/dose q12h	Neutropenia, cough, proteinuria
Nitroglycerin	0.5–20 μg/kg/min IV, up to 60 μg/kg/min	Use not well established in children

include cough, wheezing, congestion, fever, or tachypnea. Certain subtle clues may suggest a cardiac diagnosis. Bronchospasm that responds poorly to conventional therapy may be an indicator of early myocarditis. Assessment of wheezing in the febrile child or in a child without a history of asthma should include a chest radiograph looking for cardiomegaly or pulmonary congestion. Other signs and symptoms include poor feeding, persistent tachypnea, hypoxia, and grunting. The presence of a murmur, gallop rhythm, rales, or organomegaly, coupled with electrocardiographic (ECG) or chest radiographic changes, may confirm the diagnosis.

The etiologies of myocarditis and pericarditis overlap and include viral pathogens (enterovirus, varicella, mumps), bacteria (*Haemophilus influenzae, Corynebacterium diphtheriae, Mycobacterium tuberculosis*), rickettsiae, fungi, and parasites. Myocarditis associated with the human immunodeficiency virus (HIV) may affect up to 50 percent of patients at time of death. The etiology is nuclear and is not always related to a specific opportunistic pathogen. Other inflammatory etiologies include acute rheumatic fever and Lyme disease. Noninfectious etiologies include collagen vascular disease, neoplasm, and toxic agents.

Primary pericarditis in the older child follows a much more benign course than that of myocarditis. Classic presenting features of pericarditis include pleuritic or positional chest pain, abdominal pain, friction rub, dyspnea, fever, and tachycardia. The ECG can be diagnostic, with diffuse ST-segment elevation and PR depression. Low voltage and electrical alternans help confirm the diagnosis of significant effusion. Cardiac tamponade is rare but should be considered when heart sounds are distant, there is pulsus paradoxus, or jugular venous distension is found. Tamponade results from either excessive effusion or a thickened, constrictive pericardium; it is rarely associated with viral disease. Children with large effusions or hemodynamic compromise are candidates for both diagnostic and therapeutic pericardiocentesis. Antibiotics are inadequate as sole treatment for purulent effusions; drainage procedures should be performed.

Treatment for uncomplicated pericarditis is supportive and directed toward treating the organism, toxin, or metabolic derangement. Inflammation and pain can be treated with nonsteroidal anti-inflammatory drugs. Consultation with a cardiologist and hospitalization are advised. Occasionally, admission to an intensive care setting is necessary; however, most cases will follow a benign course.

Myocarditis, on the other hand, has a 35 percent mortality rate. Physical findings include a gallop rhythm, hyperactive precordium, hepatomegaly, or muscle and joint tenderness. The presentation

TABLE 30-4 Dosage Guidelines for Digoxin

Age and Weight	Acute Digitalization	Maintenance
Premature infant	TDD[a]: 10–20 μg/kg IV[b]	4 μg/kg q12h IV
Full-term infant	TDD[a]: 30 μg/kg IV	4–5 μg/kg q12h IV
1 month–12 months	TDD[a]: 35 μg/kg IV	5–10 μg/kg q12h IV
>12 months[c]	TDD[a]: 40 μg/kg IV	5–10 μg/kg q12h IV

[a] TDD (total digitalizing dose) = daily dose, 1/2 given initially, then 1/4 given at 8 h, and 1/4 given at 16 h.
[b] PO dose is approximately 20 percent greater than IV dose.
[c] Children over 20 kg, TDD = 1–2 mg IV over 48 h.

is often more fulminant with profound congestive heart failure (CHF), cardiogenic shock, acidosis, or syncope secondary to dysrhythmia. Chest radiograph may demonstrate cardiomegaly. Pulmonary vascular congestion is an indicator of an extremely poor prognosis (50 percent mortality). Other negative prognostic indicators include acute onset of CHF, cardiac index <3 L/min, and a "northwest axis" on ECG. More common ECG findings include diffuse nonspecific ST and T-wave changes and rhythm disturbances, such as atrioventricular (AV) block or ventricular ectopy. Ectopy signals diffuse myocardial involvement and a high risk of sudden death. Arterial blood gas determination, blood cultures, tuberculosis testing, and acute viral serologies may help guide management. Emergent echocardiography should be considered. The definitive diagnostic procedure, right-sided endocardial biopsy, may be indicated in severe cases.

Initial management strategies are aimed at the treatment of CHF (see above). Invasive monitoring should be considered. Digoxin is used only with great caution, as it is known to potentiate dysrhythmias (Table 30-4). Dysrhythmias should be aggressively treated. Meticulous treatment of acid-base derangements, metabolic abnormalities, renal failure, and secondary infectious sequelae may be lifesaving. Controversy exists over the use of glucocorticoids and other immunosuppressants; discussion with a pediatric cardiologist is mandatory. Reports of success using the intraaortic balloon pump or extracorporeal membrane oxygenation have been described. One-half of survivors will exhibit chronic cardiac dysfunction, and many will require transplantation.

ENDOCARDITIS

Acute or subacute bacterial endocarditis in children is most often associated with congenital heart disease (30 to 40 percent). As technology and life expectancy improve, an increase in the incidence of endocarditis in children can be expected. Association with central venous catheters or with the use of drugs in the adolescent has been noted. Seeding occurs via dental caries, skin infections, and manipulation of the airway, gastrointestinal tract, or genitourinary tract. The most common offenders are *Staphylococcus aureus* (39 percent), coagulase-negative staphylococci (11 percent), strep species (22 percent), and *Candida.*

The diagnosis of endocarditis is suspected in the at-risk patient by the presence of unexplained fever, weakness, myalgia, and arthralgia. A new murmur is present in less than 50 percent of cases. Other findings may include CHF secondary to valvular insufficiency, petechiae, or new neurologic findings. Adult cutaneous hallmarks such as Janeway lesions or Osler nodes are rare. Blood culture will identify the organism in 90 percent of cases. Other supportive findings include leukocytosis, positive acute-phase reactants, anemia, hematuria, and pulmonary infiltrates (suggestive of septic emboli). The echocardiogram may not be very sensitive, with up to a 50 percent false-negative rate in children with complex congenital heart disease. American Heart Association guidelines for the prophylaxis of endocarditis are outlined in Tables 30-5, 30-6, and 30-7.

After microbiologic confirmation, antibiotic therapy is directed toward the specific organism. Bacteremia will persist in some patients despite appropriate antibiotics, and surgical vegetectomy or valve replacement may be indicated. Other sequelae for which surgery may be required include recurrent embolization, severe valvular failure, recalcitrant arrhythmia, and myocardial abscess. Pulmonary or neurologic emboli are dependent on the site of the vegetation and the presence of intracardiac shunting. Overall, endocarditis carries a 21 percent mortality.

KAWASAKI DISEASE

Kawasaki disease, a diffuse vasculitis of unknown etiology, was first described in Japan in the early 1970s. A comprehensive discussion of Kawasaki syndrome is presented in Chap. 46.

The cardiac complications of Kawasaki disease occur in two phases. In the early stage, approximately 25 percent of patients will have a diffuse but mild form of myocarditis. This stage occurs during the acute febrile period and is characterized by tachycardia, gallop rhythm, or nonspecific ST and T-wave changes. Small pericardial effusions occur. The myocarditis is usually mild and self-resolving; therapy is supportive. The second stage, coronary artery dilatation, usually peaks between 2 and 4 weeks into the illness

TABLE 30-5 Cardiac Conditions Associated with Endocarditis

Endocarditis Prophylaxis Recommended
- High-risk category
  - Prosthetic cardiac valves, including bioprosthetic and homograft valves
  - Previous bacterial endocarditis
  - Complex cyanotic congenital heart disease (e.g., single ventricle states, transposition of the great arteries, tetralogy of Fallot)
  - Surgically constructed systemic pulmonary shunts or conduits
- Moderate-risk category
  - Most other congenital cardiac malformations (other than above and below)
  - Acquired valvar dysfunction (e.g., rheumatic heart disease)
  - Hypertrophic cardiomyopathy
  - Mitral valve prolapse with valvar regurgitation and/or thickened leaflets

Endocarditis Prophylaxis Not Recommended
- Negligible-risk category (no greater risk than the general population)
  - Isolated secundum atrial septal defect
  - Surgical repair of atrial septal defect, ventricular septal defect, or patent ductus arteriosus (without residua beyond 6 months)
  - Previous coronary artery bypass graft surgery
  - Mitral valve prolapse without valvar regurgitation
  - Physiologic, functional, or innocent heart murmurs
  - Previous Kawasaki disease without valvar dysfunction
  - Previous rheumatic fever without valvar dysfunction
  - Cardiac pacemakers (intravascular and epicardial) and implanted defibrillators

Source: Adapted from Dajani AS, Taubert KA, Wilson W, et al: Prevention of bacterial endocarditis: Recommendations by the American Heart Association. *JAMA* 277:1794, 1997. Copyright 1997, American Medical Association. Used by permission.

but has been described as early as 6 days into the febrile illness. It is seen in 20 to 29 percent of all Kawasaki patients. Significant risk factors include male gender, age below 1 year, fever lasting longer than 14 days, early myocarditis, anemia, white blood cell count above 30,000, elevated erythrocyte sedimentation rate (ESR), prolonged elevation of C-reactive protein (CRP), and the presence of noncardiac aneurysms (renal, axillary, iliac). The overall mortality of 0.4 percent in Kawasaki disease can be attributed almost entirely to aneurysm formation. Echocardiography is the study of choice for detecting aneurysms. "Great aneurysms" (those greater than 8 mm) are likely to cause ischemia. Some 50 percent of all aneurysms will resolve spontaneously, but others will persist

TABLE 30-6 Endocarditis Prophylaxis Recommendations for Procedures[a]

Dental
Extractions
Implants and reimplantation of avulsed teeth
Initial placement of orthodontic bands
Intraligamentary local anesthetic injections
Periodontal procedures
Prophylactic cleaning of teeth
Root canal instrumentation
Subgingival placement of antibiotic fibers or strips
Respiratory tract
Rigid bronchoscopy
Surgery involving respiratory mucosa
Tonsillectomy/adenoidectomy
Gastrointestinal tract
Biliary tract surgery
Endoscopic retrograde cholangiography
Esophageal stricture dilation
Sclerotherapy for esophageal varices
Surgery involving intestinal mucosa
Genitourinary
Cystoscopy
Prostatic surgery
Urethral dilation

[a] This table includes selected procedures and is not meant to be all-inclusive.

Source: Adapted from Dajani AS, Taubert KA, Wilson W, et al: Prevention of bacterial endocarditis: Recommendations by the American Heart Association. *JAMA* 277:1794, 1997. Copyright 1997, American Medical Association. Used by permission.

and result in ischemia, infarction, rupture, or sudden death. Clinical and laboratory diagnostic criteria are featured in Table 30-8.

Early high-dose aspirin therapy is recommended for Kawasaki patients during the acute phase of the illness. Initially, 100 mg/kg/day divided every 6 h for 2 weeks is suggested, followed by doses of 3 to 5 mg/kg/day given once in the morning until the platelet count has normalized. Glucocorticoids have not been shown to be helpful. Intravenous gamma globulin has emerged as the most useful agent in the prevention of aneurysm formation. There is increasing evidence that a single bolus of 2 g/kg, given over 12 h within 10 days of the onset of illness, is most protective.

TABLE 30-7 Endocarditis Prophylaxis Regimens

Situation	Agent	Regimen
	Dental, Oral, Respiratory Tract, or Esophageal Procedures	
Standard general prophylaxis	Amoxicillin	50 mg/kg orally 1 h before procedure
Unable to take oral medications	Ampicillin	50 mg/kg IM or IV within 30 min of starting procedure
Allergic to penicillin	Clindamycin	20 mg/kg orally 1 h before procedure
	or	
	Cephalexin or cefadroxil[a]	50 mg/kg orally 1 h before procedure
	or	
	Azithromycin or clarithromycin	15 mg/kg orally 1 h before procedure
Allergic to penicillin and unable to take oral medications	Clindamycin	20 mg/kg IV within 30 min of starting procedure
	or	
	Cefazolin	25 mg/kg IM or IV within 30 min of starting procedure

	Genitourinary or Gastrointestinal (Excluding Esophageal) Procedures	
High-risk patients	Ampicillin plus Gentamicin	50 mg/kg IM or IV (not to exceed 2.0 g) and 25 mg/kg IM or IV 6 h later (or amoxicillin 25 mg/kg orally 6 h later) 1.5 mg/kg within 30 min of starting procedure
High-risk patients allergic to ampicillin/amoxicillin	Vancomycin plus Gentamicin	20 mg/kg IV over 1–2 h, completed within 30 min of starting procedure 1.5 mg/kg IV/IM within 30 min of starting procedure
Moderate-risk patients	Amoxicillin or Ampicillin	50 mg/kg orally 1 h before procedure 50 mg/kg IM/IV within 30 min of starting procedure
Moderate-risk patients allergic to ampicillin/amoxicillin	Vancomycin	20 mg/kg IV over 1–2 h, completed within 30 min of starting procedure

[a] Cephalosporins should not be used in individuals with immediate-type hypersensitivity reaction (urticaria, angioedema, or anaphylaxis) to penicillins.

Source: Adapted from Dajani AS, Taubert KA, Wilson W, et al: Prevention of bacterial endocarditis: Recommendations by the American Heart Association. *JAMA* 277:1794, 1997. Copyright 1997, American Medical Association. Used by permission.

TABLE 30-8 Clinical and Laboratory Features of Kawasaki Disease

Diagnostic criteria (principal clinical findings[a])

- Fever of at least 5 days' duration[b]
- Presence of four of the following principal features
  - Changes in extremities
  - Polymorphous exanthem
  - Bilateral conjunctival injection
  - Changes in the lips and oral cavity
  - Cervial lymphadenopathy
- Exclusion of other diseases with similar findings

Other clinical and laboratory findings

- Cardiac findings
  - Pancarditis in early stages of disease
  - Coronary artery abnormalities, usually beyond 10 days of onset of illness
- Noncardiac findings
  - *Musculoskeletal system*
    - Arthritis, arthralgia
  - *Gastrointestinal tract*
    - Diarrhea, vomiting
    - Abdominal pain
    - Hepatic dysfunction
    - Hydrops of the gallbladder
  - *Central nervous system*
    - Extreme irritability
    - Aseptic meningitis
  - *Respiratory tract*
    - Preceding respiratory illness
    - Otitis media
    - Pulmonary infiltrates
  - *Other findings*
    - Testicular swelling
    - Peripheral gangrene
    - Aneurysms of medium-sized noncoronary arteries

Laboratory findings

- Neutrophilia with immature forms
- Elevated erythrocyte sedimentation rate
- Positive C-reactive protein
- Anemia
- Hypoalbuminemia
- Thrombocytosis
- Proteinuria
- Sterile pyuria
- Elevated serum transaminases

[a] Patients with fever and fewer than four principal clinical features can be diagnosed as having Kawasaki disease when coronary disease is detected by two-dimensional echocardiography or coronary angiography.

[b] Many experts believe that, in the presence of classic features, the diagnosis of Kawasaki disease can be made by experienced practitioners before the fifth day of fever.

If diagnosis is delayed or evidence of inflammation or cardiac involvement persists after day 10, gamma globulin may still be of some benefit.

ACUTE RHEUMATIC FEVER

Carditis associated with acute rheumatic fever differs from other forms of myocarditis in its predilection for valve involvement. The acute phase of rheumatic fever presents 2 to 3 weeks after a group A streptococcal illness (Table 30-9). Typically, carditis follows arthritis and can involve all three layers of the heart. A relatively benign acute phase can be followed by severe valvular insufficiency. Mitral valve involvement is most common and is suspected in the presence of a systolic high-pitched, blowing regurgitant murmur, apical in origin, radiating to the axilla, and lasting long into systole. Regurgitant aortic valve involvement is characterized by a high-pitched, blowing middiastolic murmur, located at the base and radiating into the neck. Other cardiac findings include tachycardia, gallop rhythm, pericardial rub, or CHF. Electrocardiography may demonstrate PR prolongation, other conduction system delays, left ventricular hypertrophy, or dysrhythmia. Echocardiography is helpful only in following the clinical course of a

TABLE 30-9 Guidelines for the Diagnosis of Initial Attack of Rheumatic Fever (Jones Criteria, 1992 Update)[a]

Major manifestations	Minor manifestations
Carditis	Clinical findings
Polyarthritis	Arthralgia
Chorea	Fever
Erythema marginatum	Laboratory findings
Subcutaneous nodules	Elevated acute-phase reactants (erythrocyte sedimentation rate, C-reactive protein)
	Prolonged PR interval
Supporting evidence of antecedent group A streptococcal infection	
Positive throat culture or rapid streptococcal antigen test	
Elevated or rising streptococcal antibody titer	

[a] If supported by evidence of a preceding group A streptococcal infection, the presence of two major manifestations or of one major and two minor manifestations indicates a high probability of acute rheumatic fever.

confirmed case of rheumatic carditis, as subclinical cardiac involvement is not considered in the diagnostic criteria.

Treatment during the acute inflammatory phase of the illness includes hospitalization and bed rest, followed by cardiac rehabilitation. High-dose aspirin is used after the diagnosis is confirmed, and penicillin or erythromycin is given to eradicate any streptococci. Glucocorticoids are controversial, but may have a role in the treatment of carditis or chorea.

CHEST PAIN IN CHILDREN AND ADOLESCENTS

Although chest pain in the pediatric patient is relatively common, it is most often benign. If the pain is cardiac in origin, the disease process is generally less serious than that of adults with the same complaint. Most cases can be attributed to musculoskeletal, pulmonary, traumatic, gastrointestinal, toxicologic, and psychogenic factors. Up to one-third of these patients may have no obvious underlying pathology. Only 4 percent have a cardiac etiology, which may include myocarditis, pericarditis, structural abnormalities, and coronary arteritis.

Upon initial evaluation, it is important to determine how symptoms have developed. Myocarditis-associated chest pain is accompanied by cough, shortness of breath, malaise, and fatigue. Pericarditis presents as sharp substernal pain that worsens with inspiration and is relieved by sitting in a forward-leaning position. With significant pericardial effusion, the patient may also present with neck vein distension, pulsus paradoxus, and decreased heart sounds. Physical findings include a scratchy pericardial rub that may disappear with the onset of pericardial effusion.

The complaint of chest pain accompanied by a new murmur is characteristic of either aortic stenosis or hypertrophic obstructive cardiomyopathy. In such cases the patient has a fixed cardiac output and may have signs of myocardial ischemia, dyspnea, and syncope following exercise. The ECG frequently demonstrates left ventricular enlargement or ST and T-wave abnormalities. These patients should be referred to a pediatric cardiologist as soon as possible.

Although this is extremely rare, a small subset of teens and younger adults are at risk for premature atherosclerosis or other causes of myocardial ischemia. Risk factors include a history of Kawasaki disease and cocaine abuse. Premature-onset atherosclerotic disease is associated with familial hyperlipidemia and hypercholesterolemia, collagen vascular disease, and the chronic use of glucocorticoids. Diagnostic and therapeutic approaches are similar to those for adults.

ACKNOWLEDGMENT

The authors wish to thank Dr. Aaron Zucker, Attending Physician, University of Chicago Hospitals and Clinics and Wyler Children's Hospital.

EDITOR'S NOTE

Table 30-5, Table 30-6, and Table 30-7 are from Dajani AS, Taubert KA, Wilson W, et al: Prevention of bacterial endocarditis: Recommendations by the American Heart Association. *JAMA* 1997, 277: 1794–1801. Copyright ©1997, American Medical Association. Used by permission from the American Heart Association. They are based on Recommendations from the American Heart Association.

For a more detailed discussion, see Toepper WC, Barbosa J: Congestive and inflammatory disease of the heart, chap. 30, p. 194, in *Pediatric Emergency Medicine: A Comprehensive Study Guide.*

31 Dysrhythmias

William C. Toepper

Disorders of rate and rhythm in the pediatric population are better tolerated and follow a more benign clinical course than those in adults. The underlying mechanism, treatment, and ultimate prognosis of the pediatric dysrhythmia are more dependent on the structural aspects of the heart and its conduction system and less dependent on preexisting coronary artery disease.

Dysrhythmias can occur in the absence of underlying congenital heart disease or other structural lesions, and conditions such as hypoxia, electrolyte imbalance, toxin exposure, or inflammatory disease must be ruled out. Echocardiography to evaluate for structural abnormalities is almost always indicated.

Age is an important consideration in the child with dysrhythmia. Some cases of ventricular tachycardia or accelerated junctional tachycardia disappear with growth of the child. In contrast, certain conduction problems may worsen with age. The ventricular rate in third-degree heart block may be adequate for the 2-month-old infant but will rarely provide the cardiac output needed for the 12-year-old child. Age will also be a factor in the clinical presentation of the dysrhythmia. The infant, unable to verbalize, may present with poor feeding, tachypnea, irritability, or signs of a low-output state. The older child will more often present with specific symptoms such as syncope, chest pain, or palpitations.

In the initial emergency management of dysrhythmias, the precise recognition of the rhythm is less important than the ability to classify the rhythm by rate, width of complex, and stability. Knowledge of normal heart rates and blood pressures in children aids in establishing stability. Finally, precise knowledge of the natural history of common pediatric rhythm disturbances is imperative to prevent an overly aggressive approach to what may be a benign condition.

SLOW RATES

Sinus Bradycardia

Sinus bradycardia is almost always a secondary manifestation of a serious underlying disease state or a normal physiologic variant. The clinical picture is of utmost importance. Life-threatening conditions such as severe hypoxemia, hypothyroidism, or increased intracranial pressure must be considered. Sinus bradycardia is a common manifestation of cardiac toxicity due to calcium channel blocker, beta blocker, or digoxin overdose. Treatment is aimed at correction of the underlying condition. For structural cardiac disease, atropine (0.02 mg/kg) should be administered in the unstable or poorly perfused child. For ischemic/hypoxic bradycardia, epinephrine 0.1 mg/kg is recommended.

First- and Second-Degree Atrioventricular Block

First-degree atrioventricular (AV) block has no functional significance in children unless it is a marker of a pathologic state, such as digitalis toxicity or acute rheumatic fever. Mobitz type I second-degree AV block can be a normal variant; however, Mobitz type II block always warrants a noninvasive workup, which can include echocardiography, 24-h Holter monitor, and treadmill testing.

Congenital Complete Atrioventricular Block

Congenital complete AV block, or electrical dissociation of the atria and the ventricles, is usually associated with congenital heart disease (AV canal, ventricular inversion syndromes) or gestational exposure to maternal antibodies, such as those associated with collagen vascular diseases. The QRS complexes occur independent of the P wave and are generally narrow. The His pacemaker rate is usually 50 to 80 beats/min and is under the influence of both the parasympathetic and sympathetic nervous systems. Treatment of the newborn with congenital complete AV block consists of the control of congestive heart failure (CHF), temporary pharmacologic therapy with atropine or isoproterenol, and permanent epicardial pacing. Temporary pacing may be achieved by using a specialized external pacing unit or through the placement of a transvenous unit through a femoral, subclavian, or umbilical vein.

Acquired Complete AV Block

Complete or third-degree AV block is most frequently associated with myocarditis, endocarditis, rheumatic fever, cardiac muscle diseases, or tumor. The QRS complex is usually wide. Treatment is similar to that of congenital block. When the patient presents with syncope, he or she must be paced immediately to prevent sudden death. Complete heart block can also be seen in postoperative patients. While usually transient, it can persist or present years after surgery.

Pacemakers in Children

Transvenous placement may be employed in children as young as 4 years of age, and epicardial units can be implanted in children less than 2 kg. While right ventricular demand pacing has been most commonly used, the availability of synchronous AV pacing has resulted in greater cardiac outputs, a greater response to reflex physiologic mechanisms, and a possible reduction in the incidence of supraventricular and ventricular tachycardia. Units can be programmed to sense, demand, or inhibit at the atrial or ventricular level. In addition, antitachycardia pacemakers and implantable internal defibrillators are being employed in older pediatric patients.

If pacemaker malfunction is suspected, a chest radiograph should be obtained to look for wire fracture or lead displacement. These events are rare, however, and most malfunctions are managed through the use of an external reprogrammer. Any patient with evidence of pacemaker malfunction should be admitted to the hospital if the problem cannot be resolved in the emergency department. Placement of a temporary transvenous pacemaker is rarely necessary.

FAST RATES

Supraventricular Tachycardia

By far the most common dysrhythmia seen in the pediatric age group is supraventricular tachycardia (SVT), which may occur in all age groups but is most common in infancy. Presentation in infancy is characterized by poor feeding, rapid breathing, or irritability. The infant may appear very ill and be misdiagnosed with sepsis. In some 50 percent of infants with SVT, no underlying cause can be found. In another 20 percent, SVT is associated with fever, infection, or drug exposure. In the remaining 30 percent, SVT is associated with congenital heart disease.

The basis of SVT is usually a reentry phenomenon, which can originate from within the AV node (classic SVT) or by way of accessory pathways [Wolff-Parkinson-White (WPW) syndrome or Lown-Ganong-Levine syndrome]. The identification of the mechanism is therapeutically helpful, as medicines known to act specifically within the AV node or accessory pathway are then preferentially chosen.

The diagnosis of SVT is suspected in the child who presents with a heart rate between 200 and 300 beats/min. Congestive heart failure is common. P waves may be present on the electrocardiogram (ECG), and narrow QRS complexes can be abnormally directed. Wide-complex tachycardia is presumed to be ventricular in origin, since SVT with aberration is extremely rare in children.

Initial management of the highly unstable patient begins with immediate synchronized cardioversion at 0.5 J/kg, increasing up to 2 J/kg as needed. If cardioversion is unsuccessful, esophageal overdrive pacing or medical management may be initiated. Once the patient is cardioverted, the patient should be digitalized.

In the stable patient, vagal manipulation should be attempted by application of an ice bag to the face, covering it from the nose to the top of the forehead for 15 to 20 s; the ice bag is then removed for 10 s and the process repeated several times. Ocular pressure is to be condemned, and Valsalva techniques such as the placement of a nasogastric tube are discouraged. Failure of vagal manipulation is common, and medical management is often necessary. Adenosine has revolutionized the care of adults with reentrant SVT, and numerous reports of its use in children have been published. An initial loading dose of 0.1 mg/kg followed by doses of up to 0.3 mg/kg are recommended. Side effects (headache, flushing, chest pain, sinus bradycardia with long pauses, hypotension) are transient. Recurrence of SVT is not uncommon.

The more traditional approach to the infant with stable SVT has been digitalization (see Table 30-4, Chap. 30). Digitalis requires hours for conversion. Other methods should be considered if stability is in question. If electrical therapy is eventually indicated, there is a greater risk of subsequent ventricular fibrillation in the patient who is on digitalis. In this situation, lidocaine, 1 mg/kg, is administered prior to elective cardioversion, and cardioversion is carried out with the lowest effective energy dose.

The child over 1 year of age with a narrow-complex tachycardia who fails adenosine may respond to intravenous verapamil provided that blood pressure is adequate. Intravenous verapamil should never be given to children less than 1 year of age because of its association with severe hypotension and sudden death. Verapamil is given slowly as a 0.1-mg/kg bolus. If hypotension occurs, calcium chloride at 10 mg/kg with a saline bolus should be administered rapidly. The patient's clinical and electrocardiographic status must be carefully monitored because of the negative inotropic effect of calcium channel blockers.

If the above measures fail or tachycardia resumes, conversion with procainamide may be the safest alternative in the well-compensated infant or child. Because of its utility in converting ventricular tachycardia, it is an excellent choice when one is unable to discern the origin of the tachycardia. It is given as a 5- to 15-mg/kg bolus over 20 to 30 min, and hypotension can result.

Finally, in extremely critical situations when cardioversion or medications fail, continuous esophageal or right atrial overdrive pacing at approximately 300 beats/min may be effective. The resultant ventricular rate of 150 (2:1 block) may allow for adequate ventricular filling and improved cardiac output. This mode of therapy should never be utilized without the guidance of an experienced pediatric cardiologist.

When cardioverted, approximately 25 percent of children with SVT will display ECG characteristics consistent with the WPW syndrome. This includes an abnormally short PR interval, a prolonged QRS duration, and the presence of a delta wave (slurring of the initial portion of the QRS complex). Primary conduction is thought to occur through the AV node, with retrograde conduction through an accessory pathway. Digoxin can shorten the refractory period in the bypass tract and enhance conduction in the accessory pathway, leading to a rapid ventricular response and ventricular fibrillation. If the diagnosis of WPW syndrome is known or suspected, an electrophysiologic study to determine the most effective agent is suggested. Propranolol may be preferred. It slows conduction through the AV node without having any significant effect on the accessory pathway. Any child with newly treated WPW syndrome should be hospitalized during the initiation and early phase of therapy.

Finally, the occurrence of SVT secondary to increased automaticity is extremely rare in children and can be difficult to manage. If it is associated with digitalis toxicity, treatment should be aimed at neutralization of its effects by the use of digitalis-directed antibodies. If these are contraindicated or unavailable, ectopy may be reduced with lidocaine, phenytoin, or magnesium.

Atrial Flutter/Fibrillation

Atrial flutter and fibrillation in children is most often associated with either congenital heart disease, rheumatic fever, or dilated cardiomyopathy. Atrial flutter and fibrillation are both exceedingly rare in children yet must be considered in those with long-standing heart disease. Atrial flutter rates typically range from 200 to 500 beats/min. In unstable patients, immediate cardioversion is the therapy of choice, starting with 0.5 J/kg of direct current. Overdrive pacing at rates 10 to 20 beats/min faster than the atrial flutter rate may also be effective.

In stable patients, digitalization can be used to slow ventricular rates. The goal is the elimination of all flutter activity because of the four times greater incidence of sudden death in patients who continue to experience episodes of atrial flutter in the presence of congenital heart disease. Elective cardioversion is frequently required. Care must be taken in patients with long-standing atrial disease, as the sinus node may also be quite diseased. Upon termination of atrial flutter, a resultant slow junctional rate or even asystole may arise; backup pacing must be available. Children probably do not require anticoagulation prior to termination of atrial flutter. Refractory cases necessitate surgical correction or palliation of the underlying congenital defect. Surgical ablation of bypass tracts may be successful.

Premature Ventricular Contractions

The presence of premature ventricular contractions (PVCs) in the infant and young child is rare. Unifocal PVCs begin to appear in normal, healthy children during adolescence. The patient is generally asymptomatic and usually has a normal physical examination, chest radiograph, and resting ECG. Twenty-four-hour Holter monitoring will help define and quantify the extra beats. If PVCs diminish during exercise or stress testing, they are most likely benign and require no therapy. In the setting of the diseased heart (myocarditis, cardiomyopathy, congenital or postoperative hearts), treatment aimed at suppression of the ventricular ectopy is desirable, as a small but significant incidence of sudden death has been reported. Treatment includes correction of electrolyte abnormalities or suppression with lidocaine, procainamide, or phenytoin, depending on the clinical situation.

Ventricular Tachycardia

Idiopathic ventricular tachycardia is occasionally encountered in a child who is completely asymptomatic and has an otherwise normal heart. Underlying causes include cardiomyopathy, digoxin toxicity, intracardiac tumor, mitral valve prolapse, or the prolonged Q-T syndrome. Ventricular tachycardia in the presence of heart disease holds a much poorer prognosis than that of idiopathic ventricular tachycardia. Idiopathic asymptomatic ventricular tachycardia is usually left untreated. New data suggest that up to 50 percent of children with ventricular ectopy and structurally normal hearts may have subclinical cardiomyopathy or myocarditis and may benefit from immunosuppression. Symptomatic children (syncope, chest pain) may require electrophysiologic studies to refine the diagnosis or to guide therapy.

Ventricular tachycardia in the newborn or infant can present with narrow complexes and appear supraventricular in origin. The presence of AV dissociation or fusion beats may help differentiate the two. If the diagnosis is in question and the patient is unstable, synchronized cardioversion at 0.5 J/kg will convert either ventricular or supraventricular tachycardia. In children, stable ventricular tachycardia that requires therapy should be treated with lidocaine. The initial 1-mg/kg bolus is then followed by 0.5 mg/kg at 10 to 15 min and a maintenance drip of 0.01 to 0.05 mg/kg/min. Procainamide at 15 mg/kg IV can also be used but must be administered over 20 to 60 min, time permitting. If the patient is stable and the origin of the rhythm is unclear, procainamide is useful, as it also acts to slow AV nodal conduction. Other alternatives include phenytoin 15 mg/kg over 1 h (especially in the setting of digitalis toxicity) or bretylium 5 mg/kg IV.

Ventricular Fibrillation

As in adults, the treatment of ventricular fibrillation in children is immediate defibrillation. The initial dose of 2 J/kg can then be doubled if necessary. Correction of precipitating factors (e.g., acidosis, hypoxia, metabolic derangements) can aid in the conversion to a perfusing rhythm.

OTHER CARDIAC CONDITIONS ASSOCIATED WITH DYSRHYTHMIAS

Prolonged Q-T Syndrome

The association of syncope, sudden death, and a prolonged Q-T interval was first described in 1959. Congenital prolonged Q-T syndrome is characterized by paroxysmal episodes of ventricular tachycardia and torsade de pointes. The tachycardia can be emotionally induced or stress-related and can progress to ventricular fibrillation and sudden death. Q-T prolongation can also be associated with type IA antiarrhythmics, other drugs, anorexia nervosa, bulimia, and electrolyte derangements. The corrected Q-T interval adjusts for rate, and that which exceeds 0.44 s is considered a sign of delayed repolarization.

Treatment is aimed at correction of any toxic or metabolic derangements. Reports of the utility of magnesium sulfate in the setting of refractory torsade de pointes are promising. Known or suspected congenital Q-T syndrome should be treated with beta blockers, as beta blockade is thought to control the rushes of sympathetic activity responsible for the dysrhythmia. It is crucial to maintain adequate beta blockade at all times, as death has been reported after isolated missed doses of propranolol. Adjunctive therapy may include phenytoin or phenobarbital. Success has also been achieved surgically with left-sided cervicothoracic ganglionectomy or sympathectomy, implantable overdrive pacemakers, and internal defibrillators. Mortality from untreated congenital prolonged Q-T syndrome approaches 80 percent.

Hypertrophic Cardiomyopathy

Hypertrophic cardiomyopathy often presents in adolescence but can occur in patients of all ages. The patient may present with chest pain, dyspnea, syncope, or sudden death; mortality may be as high as 4 percent if it is left untreated. The cause of sudden death is multifactorial and includes the hemodynamic consequences of anatomic and electrophysiologic defects. Supraventricular arrhythmias predominate, but significant ventricular dysrhythmias may also be present and are associated with sudden death. Antiarrhythmics such as propranolol or amiodarone may be helpful. Septal myectomy may be necessary, although patients are not uniformly protected from sudden death by this procedure.

Mitral Valve Prolapse

Most children with mitral valve prolapse (MVP) will do quite well, but MVP has been associated with dysrhythmia and sudden death in both children and adults. Most pediatric dysrhythmias are relatively benign and include frequent and multifocal PVCs, type I second-degree AV block, paroxysmal atrial tachycardia, and brief episodes of ventricular tachycardia. Some children will need treatment for recurrent chest pain or dysrhythmia. Endocarditis prophylaxis must be remembered in children with mitral valve prolapse with regurgitation.

ACKNOWLEDGMENT

The author wishes to thank Dr. Suchinta Hakim, Attending Physician, Hinsdale Hospital, Hinsdale, Illinois.

For a more detailed discussion, see Toepper WC: Dysrhythmias, chap. 31, p. 203, in *Pediatric Emergency Medicine: A Comprehensive Study Guide.*

32 Peripheral Vascular Disease

William C. Toepper / Joilo Barbosa

HYPERTENSION

Normal blood pressures in children are age-dependent. Children whose accurately taken blood pressures are above the 95th percentile are considered hypertensive (Table 32-1).

Upon initial presentation, the diagnosis of hypertension should be based on the measurement of blood pressures in both arms and at least one leg. Special attention to cuff size is imperative. The bladder of the cuff should nearly encircle the arm without overlapping, and the cuff width should be at least two-thirds of the length of the upper arm. The fourth Korotkoff sound (muffling) should be used for diastolic pressure determination in children below the age of 13. Ideally the child should be in a comfortable seated position; the infant should be lying down and quiet. Feeding, sucking, and upright positioning can cause a falsely elevated blood pressure reading in infants. If auscultation is difficult, Doppler or oscillometric methods should be used. Repeated measurements must be made over a period of weeks or months before essential hypertension is diagnosed.

Etiology

While essential hypertension has no specific underlying pathology, many factors contribute to the development and maintenance of this chronic disease. Included are obesity, high-sodium/low-potassium diets, stress, and heredity. Children of hypertensive parents are known to have an abnormal elevation of blood pressure in

TABLE 32-1 Classification of Hypertension by Age Group

Age group	Significant hypertension[a]	Severe hypertension[b]
Newborns (0–7 days)	Systolic BP ≥96	Systolic BP ≥106
Newborns (8–30 days)	Systolic BP ≥104	Systolic BP ≥110
Infants (<2 years)	Systolic BP ≥112 Diastolic BP ≥74	Systolic BP ≥118 Diastolic BP ≥82
Children (3–5 years)	Systolic BP ≥116 Diastolic BP ≥76	Systolic BP ≥124 Diastolic BP ≥84
Children (6–9 years)	Systolic BP ≥122 Diastolic BP ≥78	Systolic BP ≥130 Diastolic BP ≥86
Children (10–12 years)	Systolic BP ≥126 Diastolic BP ≥82	Systolic BP ≥134 Diastolic BP ≥90
Adolescents (13–15 years)	Systolic BP ≥136 Diastolic BP ≥86	Systolic BP ≥144 Diastolic BP ≥92
Adolescents (16–18 years)	Systolic BP ≥142 Diastolic BP ≥92	Systolic BP ≥150 Diastolic BP ≥98

[a] BP persistently between 95th and 99th percentile.

[b] BP persistently above 99th percentile.

Source: Adapted with permission from the Task Force on Blood Pressure Control in Children: Report of the Second Task Force on Blood Pressure Control in Children. *Pediatrics* 79:1, 1987.

response to stress and to have higher levels of urinary catecholamine metabolites and dietary sodium intake.

Acute hypertension in children and adolescents is most commonly associated with an underlying disease state (Table 32-2). Some 80 to 90 percent of cases are caused by renal parenchymal diseases, renovascular anomalies, or coarctation of the aorta. In newborns, secondary hypertension is frequently associated with renal artery obstruction secondary to umbilical artery catheter thrombosis.

Clinical Manifestations

Infant and neonatal indicators of acute hypertension are vague and nonspecific (poor feeding, restlessness, irritability, and vomiting). In children, the signs and symptoms tend to occur late and are related to the development of hypertensive encephalopathy. These include headache, dizziness, visual changes, nausea, vomiting, altered level of consciousness, cranial nerve palsies, and seizures. In younger children, the onset of congestive heart failure

TABLE 32-2 Causes of Hypertension in Children

Drugs and poisons	**Central and autonomic nervous system**
Cocaine	Increased intracranial pressure
Oral contraceptives	Familial dysautonomia
Sympathomimetic agents	Encephalitis
Amphetamines	**Cardiovascular**
Phencyclidine	Coarctation of the aorta
Corticosteroids	Renal artery lesions
Cyclosporine	Renal vein thrombosis
Glycyrrhizic acid (licorice)	Umbilical artery catheterization
Heavy metals (lead, mercury, cadmium, thallium)	Aortic insufficiency
Antihypertensive medication withdrawal (clonidine, methyldopa, propranolol)	**Metabolic**
Vitamins D and A intoxication	Hypercalcemia
Renal	Hypernatremia
Acute glomerulonephritis	Porphyria
Poststreptococcal	**Miscellaneous**
Henoch-Schönlein purpura	Systemic lupus erythematosus
Chronic glomerulonephritis	Immobilization
Hemolytic-uremic syndrome	Bronchopulmonary dysplasia
Acute tubular necrosis	Preeclampsia
Congenital malformations	**Essential hypertension**
Polycystic kidneys	
Endocrine	
Pheochromocytoma	
Neuroblastoma	
Adrenogenital disease	
Cushing syndrome	
Hyperaldosteronism	
Hyperthyroidism	
Hyperparathyroidism	

may be the first sign of hypertension. Any infant with unexplained seizure should be assessed for acute hypertension during the initial evaluation. In secondary hypertension, signs and symptoms may suggest the underlying cause.

Assessment

A detailed history including growth and feeding patterns, irritability, and symptoms of hypertensive encephalopathy is required. Family history and a meticulous physical examination follows. In the physical examination, it is important to palpate the abdomen for masses, auscultate for bruits, palpate peripheral pulses for symmetry, and perform a funduscopic examination. Initial diagnostic studies should include complete blood count, electrolytes, blood urea nitrogen, creatinine, uric acid, chest radiograph, electrocardiogram (ECG), and echocardiogram. If the patient is severely hypertensive, immediate hospitalization for aggressive control of the blood pressure and the initiation of diagnostic studies is warranted. Studies may include renal ultrasound, quantification of urine catecholamines, renal flow studies, or the selective catheterization of renal veins for plasma renin levels.

Management

The management of mild hypertension in children begins with a discussion of life-style changes such as the prevention of obesity, the role of exercise, and the benefits of a low-sodium diet. Other efforts include limitation of alcohol and tobacco use in the home and the employment of a low-fat, low-cholesterol diet for all members of the family. The need to initiate pharmacological therapy in the emergency department (ED) is rare, and acute reduction in blood pressure can result in symptomatic hypotension.

The child who presents with an acutely elevated blood pressure or evidence of target organ injury requires prompt control (Table 32-3). Table 32-4 lists agents that are useful for both hypertensive emergencies and urgencies. In those children with acutely elevated

TABLE 32-3 Therapy

Indications for nonpharmacologic intervention
Systolic and/or diastolic BP ≥ 90th percentile
Indications for initiation of antihypertensive drugs
Significant diastolic hypertension (see Table 32-1)
Evidence of target-organ injury
Symptoms or signs related to elevated BP
Use of parenteral therapy (usually vasodilators such as nitroprusside, diazoxide, or hydralazine) is indicated in acute severe hypertension, such as occurs with acute glomerulonephritis, hemolytic-uremic syndrome, or head injuries, which are often associated with symptoms and increased risk of target-organ damage
Therapeutic goals
Diastolic BP < 90th percentile
Minimal side effects
Use of the least amount of drug necessary to effectively reduce BP
High degree of patient compliance

Source: Adapted from the Task Force on Blood Pressure Control in Children: Report of the Second Task Force on Blood Pressure Control in Children. *Pediatrics* 79:1, 1987. Used by permission.

TABLE 32-4 Drugs Used in Pediatric Hypertensive Crises

Nitroprusside	1–8 μg/kg/min IV
Labetalol	0.2–2 mg/kg IV
Diazoxide	1–5 mg/kg IV
Nifedipine	0.25–0.5 mg/kg PO

blood pressure but no evidence of end-organ injury (hypertensive urgency), oral agents may be used to slowly reduce blood pressure over 24 to 48 h. Hospitalization is recommended in any child presenting with either hypertensive emergency or urgency.

The most commonly used chronic antihypertensives are listed in Table 32-5.

TABLE 32-5 Pharmacologic Management of Hypertension in Children

	Initial dose, mg/kg/dose	Maximum/day, mg/kg	Frequency
ACE inhibitors			
Captopril	0.5–2	6	bid–tid
Enalapril	0.01–0.03	1	bid
Calcium channel blockers			
Nifedipine	0.5	1	qid–tid
Verapamil	2–4	6	tid
Diltiazem	1	4	qid–tid
Diuretics			
Hydrochlorothiazide	0.5	4	qd
Furosemide	1	8	qd
Spironolactone	1	3	qid–qd
Alpha-adrenergic agents			
Prazosin	0.01	0.5	tid–bid
Clonidine	0.005	0.03	bid
Beta blockers			
Propranolol	0.5	8	bid
Metoprolol	1	5	tid–bid
Atenolol	0.5	8	qd
Alpha- and beta-adrenergic agents			
Labetalol	2	10	tid–bid
Vasodilators			
Hydralazine	0.5	5	qid–qd
Minoxidil	0.1	1.5	bid–qd

THROMBOEMBOLIC DISEASE

Virchow's triad (increased viscosity, decreased flow, and disruption of endothelial integrity), the classic description of the physiologic state that allows for pathologic clotting, can apply to children and adolescents as well as adults. The phenomenon is rare, yet autopsy studies suggest that thromboembolic disease is present but often undetected in children. The increasing use of indwelling catheters and other technological advances that prolong life suggests that thromboembolic events will increase in frequency. Major risk factors for thromboembolic disease are listed in Table 32-6.

Deep Vein Thrombosis in Children

Deep vein thrombosis (DVT) in children is most often related to the use of indwelling catheters. Thus, DVT can occur in lower and upper extremities as well as proximal thoracic veins. Spontaneous DVT is more rare and is most often related to severe underlying illness: postsurgical states, cancer, nephrotic syndrome, ulcerative colitis, or systemic infection. Spontaneous DVT can occur in the well individual and is related to congenital protein deficiency. Minor trauma and the use of oral contraceptives may predispose the adolescent with even trivial deficiencies to DVT.

Swelling is the most reliable clinical sign in the at-risk child. The limb may also be tender, warm, and red. Preceding trauma may not necessarily be severe. The iliofemoral vein is most often

TABLE 32-6 Major Risk Factors for Thromboembolic Disease

Adolescents	Children	Adults
Oral contraceptives	Hydrocephalus	Oral contraceptives
Trauma	Trauma	Trauma
Elective abortion	Congenital heart disease	Pregnancy
Surgery	Infection	Surgery
Prolonged immobilization	Neoplasia	Neoplasia
Collagen vascular disease	Prolonged immobilization	Heart disease
Intravenous drug abuse	Surgery	Collagen vascular disease
Rheumatic heart disease	Dehydration	Protein S deficiency
Dehydration	Protein S deficiency	
Obesity		
Renal transplantation		
Protein S deficiency		

affected, although extension into the vena cava or thrombosis of the upper extremity can occur. Venography is considered the study of choice. Noninvasive studies in adults, particularly Doppler ultrasound flow studies, are approaching the sensitivity of venography and may be utilized in children, especially when venography is contraindicated or unavailable. Investigation into the possibility of a congenital hypercoagulable state may also be required.

Treatment for acute DVT begins with anticoagulation. Heparin is started at 75 U/kg, followed by continuous infusion at 22 U/kg/h. Adjustments are made to maintain the partial thromboplastin time (PTT) at 1.5 to 2 times baseline. Oral anticoagulation with warfarin follows immediately. Initial single daily dosing at 0.2 mg/kg is modified to maintain the prothrombin time at twice normal or an INR value between 2 and 3. Data on pediatric thrombolytic use and on selected arterial administration may allow future use in deep vein thrombosis. Greenfield filter placement may be considered in those children who have failed anticoagulation or in whom anticoagulation or thrombolysis are contraindicated. Long-term maintenance consists of the use of warfarin sodium for up to 6 months.

Pulmonary Embolism

Pulmonary embolism (PE) is also underrecognized in children and adolescents. The incidence in pediatric autopsies appears to be around 4 percent, or 1 in 1000 hospital admissions. Approximately one-third of these are thought to have contributed significantly to death.

Pulmonary emboli in children are almost always associated with a disruption of endothelial integrity. The disruption is usually proximal and stems from the use of central venous catheters or ventriculoatrial shunts in the patient with hydrocephalus and from congenital heart disease with endocarditis. In contrast to adults, only 42 percent of PEs in children are associated with peripheral DVT. Emboli need not be massive to cause serious problems in children, as catheter-associated pulmonary hypertension from chronic seeding is also devastating. Disease patterns in adolescents are similar to those in adults.

Presenting symptoms include pleuritic chest pain (84 percent), dyspnea (58 percent), cough (47 percent), and hemoptysis (32 percent). Objective findings include relative hypoxia ($P_{O_2} <$ 80 percent), abnormal chest radiograph (50 percent), tachypnea (42 percent), or fever (32 percent). A classic presentation is rare in children, and no clinical marker is completely predictive. Clinical suspicion is based on a combination of risk factors and clinical findings.

The ventilation/perfusion scan is safe in children and probably underutilized. There are few data on the interpretation of low- or medium-probability scans in children, and if doubt exists, pulmonary arteriography should be considered. Angiography is considered safer than the misuse of heparin, a drug known for causing iatrogenic mishaps.

Management strategy begins with prophylaxis of high-risk patients. In children with a previous history of thromboembolic disease, strong family histories of hypercoagulability, VA shunts, dilated cardiomyopathy, or indwelling catheters, PE should be considered. Inpatients should be started on minidose heparin at 1 U/kg/h. When PE is proven or highly suspected, heparin should be initiated, adjusting to prolong the PTT by 1 1/2 to 2 1/2 times. Warfarin is begun immediately and should be continued for at least 2 months. As in DVT, thrombolytics are showing promise, and Greenfield filters may be necessary in those children with contraindications to anticoagulation.

ACKNOWLEDGMENT

The authors wish to thank Ms. Laura Ruth, Ms. Rose Sturghill-Bradford, and Ms. Mary Richardson for their complete and unqualified support in the preparation of this manuscript.

For a more detailed discussion, see Toepper WC, Barbosa J: Peripheral vascular disease, chap. 32, p. 208, in *Pediatric Emergency Medicine: A Comprehensive Study Guide.*

SECTION V
NEUROLOGIC EMERGENCIES

33 Age-Specific Neurologic Examination

Susan Fuchs

The neurologic evaluation of an infant or child can be more difficult than that of an adult. Very young patients cannot follow directions, and, most importantly, the pediatric nervous system is an evolving organ in which many findings are age-related.

HISTORY

The history focuses on the major symptom, its duration, factors that exacerbate the problem, and associated complaints. Pertinent facts regarding pregnancy and delivery are solicited. The developmental history includes the age when the child reached certain milestones, including rolling over, sitting without support, standing, climbing, and running. A brief history regarding language development may be helpful. It may be useful to compare the patient's development with that of other siblings, which is often information that the parent can easily recall. Review of the family history is important, as several neurodegenerative disorders are transmitted as recessive genes, while other disorders—such as seizures and migraine headaches—are often found in family members.

GENERAL PHYSICAL EXAMINATION

The physical examination includes height, weight, and head circumference, all of which are plotted on growth curves and compared to norms. Heart rate, respiratory rate, and blood pressure are evaluated. The general appearance of the child is important to note, as are obvious dysmorphic features. Cutaneous lesions such as café au lait spots, depigmentation, or angiomas are clues to phakomatoses. The presence of an unusual body odor may be a clue to a metabolic disorder.

NEUROLOGIC EXAMINATION

A quick mental status examination is performed. If the child has an altered mental status, a quick assessment is performed using the APVU system (Table 8-9, Chap. 8). A more formal infant Glasgow Coma Scale (GCS) has been developed to assess younger patients (see Table 8-8, Chap. 8).

After assessing the child's mental status, the neurological evaluation continues with examination of the skull, looking for macrocephaly, microcephaly, or craniosynostosis. Palpation of the fontanelles for size as well as pulsations can reveal increased intracranial pressure. With the child standing, auscultation of the skull—listening over both globes, mastoid region, and temporal fossa—may reveal abnormal intracranial bruits that are heard with angiomas, hydrocephalus, and some tumors. While many normal children have bruits, those that are especially loud or accompanied by a thrill indicate pathology. Transillumination over the frontal and occipital regions is done in a darkened room and may provide evidence of hydrocephalus, hydrancephaly, or Dandy-Walker cysts.

The evaluation of specific neurologic functions begins with the cranial nerves. The function of cranial nerve I is smell. The olfactory nerve is not functional in the newborn, where its role is performed by the fifth nerve. Cranial nerve II is tested by using visual acuity charts or, in an infant, by offering objects to grab. While doing this, the examiner can also assess the visual fields by bringing the objects slowly into the field of vision and noting when the infant's head or eyes turn to the object. Pupillary response to light is an indication of an intact second nerve, as this requires reception by the second nerve and outflow from the third nerve. A fundoscopic examination is performed, noting the disk, retina, and macula. Of note, the blink reflex does not appear until 3 to 4 months of age. The function of cranial nerves III, IV, and VI is evaluated by observing the size of the pupils, the eye position at rest, and the integrity of the extraocular muscles. A penlight or a toy can be moved across six positions of gaze, with the mother holding the child's head still, covering each eye in turn if necessary.

Abnormalities that may be detected include lateral and downward deviation of an affected eye with third-nerve paralysis, medial deviation with sixth-nerve involvement, strabismus secondary to muscular imbalance, and nystagmus. Cranial nerve V is assessed by asking the patient to open and then close the mouth, which involves use of the temporalis and masseter muscles. Trigeminal nerve lesions will result in deviation of the jaw to the affected side. The corneal reflex is another way to test this nerve. Cranial nerve VII is assessed by asking the child to smile or show his or her teeth and to close the eyes tightly against resistance. Upper motor neuron disorders affecting cranial nerve VII spare the upper part of the face, which receives innervation from both sides of the brain, while lower motor neuron produces both upper and lower facial weakness. Cranial nerve VIII is roughly evaluated by ringing a bell or set of keys and watching the infant or child turn to the sound. The use of a tuning fork is usually not required. Vestibular function can be roughly evaluated by having a child "spin like a top" in both directions and looking for nystagmus. Evaluation of phonation and the gag reflex test cranial nerves IX and X, and watching the position of the tongue at rest and when extended tests cranial nerve XII. With a lesion of cranial nerve XII, the tongue deviates to the affected side. Cranial nerve XI supplies the sternocleidomastoid and trapezius muscles, which can be tested by evaluating the patient's ability to rotate the head and shrug the shoulders.

After mental status and cranial nerves are tested, the child is evaluated for the presence of motor weakness. Observing the child walk or run provides clues regarding which muscle groups require formal testing. Pronator drift is performed by having the child raise his or her arms above the head with hands facing each other or outward with palms up and their eyes closed. A positive drift is hyperpronation of the hand or movement of the weak side downward. To test weakness of the lower extremities, the child is asked to lie on his or her stomach and maintain the knees in a bent position.

Testing coordination involves assessing cerebellar function and may be difficult to accomplish in young children. Although some may be able to perform finger-to-nose testing, it may be possible only to have the patient reach for an object and watch for a tremor or overreaching. Rapid pronation-supination of the hand, repeated tapping of the examiner's hand ("high fives"), or tapping the foot can help define pyramidal or extrapyramidal lesions. The tandem-gait (heel to toe) walk is often difficult for the child to comprehend and can be difficult to interpret.

The Romberg test is commonly used to evaluate cerebellar function, but is also useful for sensation. The child is asked to stand with feet together, arms crossed in front of the body. If the child cannot do this, there is a cerebellar problem. If this task is performed, the child is asked to close his or her eyes. If the child has trouble with balance or feeling the feet on the floor, a posterior column lesion or peripheral neuropathy is likely.

TABLE 33-1 Normal Reflexes

Reflex	Appearance	Disappearance, months
Moro	Birth	1–3
Palmar grasp	Birth	4
Plantar grasp	Birth	8–15
Root response	Birth	3–4

There are many primitive reflexes present at birth that disappear as the child grows. In certain neurologic diseases, these reflexes persist and are markers of pathology (see Table 33-1). Standard deep tendon reflexes are relatively easy to evaluate, provided that the child is cooperative or can be distracted. These include the biceps, triceps, radial, patellar, and ankle reflexes. One side is compared to another. Clonus is an exaggerated movement that indicates increased reflex excitability. Sustained ankle clonus is abnormal, but several beats may be normal in some children. The Babinski reflex involves stimulating the plantar surface of the foot from the heel along the lateral border of the sole crossing over the distal end of the metatarsals to the big toe. A positive response is dorsiflexion of the big toe with separation (fanning) of the other toes; it indicates pyramidal tract pathology. However, a positive Babinski can be seen in most normal 1-year-olds and may persist until $2\frac{1}{2}$ years of age.

For a more detailed discussion, see Fuchs S: Age-specific neurologic examination, chap. 33, p. 217, in *Pediatric Emergency Medicine: A Comprehensive Study Guide.*

34 Altered Mental Status and Coma

Susan Fuchs

The term *altered mental status* refers to an aberration in a patient's level of consciousness. It always implies serious pathology. More precise terminology describes the degree of altered mental status:

- *Lethargy* is a state of reduced wakefulness in which the patient displays disinterest in the environment, but remains easily arousable and can communicate.
- *Delirium* is a condition characterized by disorientation, delusions, or hallucinations.
- *Obtundation* is severe blunting of alertness with a decreased response to stimuli.
- *Stupor* exists when the patient can be aroused only by extremely vigorous stimulation.
- *Coma* occurs when a profound reduction in neuronal function results in unresponsiveness to sensory stimuli. It is the most severe form of altered mental status. Coma is further categorized depending on the area of the brain affected.

Several scoring systems exist that permit reproducible assessment of the degree of altered mental status by health care providers. The most widely used score is the Glasgow Coma Scale (GCS), which scores three responses: eye opening, best verbal response, and best motor response. The GCS has been modified so that it can be applied to infants (Table 8-8, Chap. 8).

PATHOPHYSIOLOGY

In general, patients with altered mental status have suffered a diffuse insult to the brain. In patients with no history of trauma, metabolic abnormalities and toxic ingestions are common. In children, infectious etiologies such as meningitis or encephalitis are likely. The more severe the insult, the greater the alteration in mental status.

For coma to occur, the underlying abnormality must involve damage either to both cerebral hemispheres or to the ascending reticular activating system, which plays a fundamental role in arousal.

Coma can result from structural damage, infectious processes, metabolic derangements, toxic ingestions, and inadequate cerebral perfusion. Metabolic, infectious, and toxic etiologies tend to produce diffuse but symmetric deficits. Structural lesions result in focal deficits that progress in a predictable pattern. Supratentorial lesions produce focal findings that progress in a rostral-caudal fashion, while infratentorial lesions result in brainstem dysfunction followed by a sudden onset of coma, cranial nerve palsies, and respiratory disturbances. The causes of coma are listed in Table 34-1, and many of these are included in the mnemonic "tips from the vowels."

TABLE 34-1 Etiology of Altered Mental Status[a]

Trauma	Metabolic
Hemorrhage	Hypoglycemia
Child abuse	Hyperglycemia (DKA)
Tumor	Hyponatremia
Infection	Hypernatremia
Meningitis	Reye's syndrome
Encephalitis	Uremia
Brain abscess	Hypothyroid
Subdural empyema	Hyperthyroid
Poisoning/Intoxication	Addison's disease
Alcohol	Inborn errors
Opiates	Other
Narcotics	Hypoxia
Sedatives	Ischemia/infarction
Salicylates	Intussusception
Carbon monoxide	Hypothermia
Lead	Hydrocephalus
Psychogenic	
Epilepsy	

[a] Tips from the vowels (AEIOU)
T: Trauma/Tumor
I: Insulin (hypoglycemia)/Intussusception/Inborn error of metabolism
P: Poisoning/Psychogenic
S: Shock
A: Alcohol/Abuse
E: Epilepsy/Encephalopathy
I: Infection
O: Opiates
U: Uremia/Metabolic

HISTORY

The history of a patient with altered mental status focuses on identifying the underlying abnormality. Events prior to the onset of mental status changes are elicited, including prior headache, febrile illness, trauma, and drug ingestion. Associated symptoms such as vomiting, diarrhea, or respiratory difficulties are important clues. Past medical history—including diabetes, seizure disorder, or underlying heart or kidney disease—is sought. A prior history of similar episodes may imply an underlying metabolic abnormality.

PHYSICAL EXAMINATION

The physical examination focuses on assessing the degree of neurologic impairment and localizing the lesion responsible for the patient's altered mental status. Particular attention is paid to the vital signs, including temperature.

Examination of the head includes palpation for hematoma or fracture, evaluation of the position of the eyes, reactivity of the pupils, and a fundoscopic exam. The ears and nose are examined for evidence of bleeding, and the neck is examined for evidence of tenderness or rigidity. In an infant, palpation of the anterior fontanelle for fullness, depression, or pulsations can provide quick information about intracranial pressure.

The skin is examined for jaundice, petechiae, or purpura. The chest is auscultated for signs of respiratory pathology. The abdominal examination is especially important in infants, where intussusception is a potential cause of altered mental status.

The general neurologic evaluation focuses on an exact description of the patient's mental status. The cranial nerves and motor function of the extremities are assessed for potentially localizing findings. The biceps, triceps, patellar, and Achilles reflexes are tested for strength and symmetry, and the patient is evaluated for the presence of a Babinski response, which indicates an upper motor neuron lesion.

For patients in coma, the area of the brain involved can be localized by examination of body position, pupil size and reactivity, respiratory pattern, and spontaneous and induced eye movements.

In decorticate posturing, the arms are flexed and the legs extended. This position implies dysfunction of the cerebral hemispheres. Decerebrate posturing is characterized by extension of both upper and lower extremities, which may occur as a response to pain. It implies a lesion at the level of the midbrain. In the event of uncal herniation, decerebrate posturing can be unilateral. Flaccid paralysis implies a diffuse lesion involving both hemispheres and the brainstem.

The patient's respiratory pattern is another clue to the nature of coma. Consistent hyperventilation can occur as compensation for a metabolic acidosis. It can also occur in lesions of the midbrain and lower pons. Cheyne-Stokes respiration is characterized by periods of tachypnea followed by apnea. It signifies a bilateral hemispheric abnormality with an intact brainstem. In some cases it implies impending temporal lobe herniation. Ataxic breathing is characterized by an irregular rate and depth; it can occur with lesions at the level of the pons and medulla.

Examination of the pupils is essential. Small, reactive pupils imply metabolic lesions affecting the cerebral hemispheres or a lesion in the medulla. Pinpoint, nonreactive pupils can result from a metabolic derangement or a lesion in the lower pons. Midposition and fixed pupils imply a lesion in the midbrain or upper pons. In the presence of coma, a unilateral dilated pupil can imply third-nerve compression from uncal herniation. In the late phase of herniation, the pupil is nonreactive. Bilateral fixed pupils can imply tectal herniation and can be seen in severe hypothermia.

Reflex eye movements help to delineate a brainstem lesion. Tests include the oculocephalic ("doll's-eye") reflex and the oculovestibular (caloric) response. To test the oculocephalic reflex, the head is passively moved from side to side. When brainstem function is intact, the eyes move together toward the side opposite that to which the head is turned. Lesions of the cerebral hemispheres have intact horizontal doll's-eye reflexes, while in lesions of the midbrain and upper pons, this reflex is impaired. In lesions of the lower pons and medulla, it is absent.

The oculovestibular response is evaluated by elevating the patient's head to 30° and irrigating one or both ear canals with cold water. In normal patients, irrigation produces deviation of the eyes toward the irrigated ear, with compensatory nystagmus. A normal response implies a relatively intact brainstem.

LABORATORY TESTING

All patients with altered mental status should have a bedside glucose determination and a plasma glucose drawn. Other studies include complete blood count with differential and platelets, electrolytes, calcium, blood urea nitrogen, creatinine, and urinalysis. In some cases, an arterial blood gas and serum ammonia are indicated. Patients who may be victims of an ingestion require a toxicology screen. If infection is suspected, cultures are obtained from the blood, urine, and cerebrospinal fluid. Lumbar puncture is withheld until increased intracranial pressure is excluded.

Radiographic examination of the cervical spine is performed if there is any suspicion of trauma. If physical examination findings suggest a structural lesion, suspected herniation, or increased intracranial pressure, a computed tomography (CT) scan is performed.

THERAPY

The first priority in the emergency department management of a patient with altered mental status is stabilization of the airway. Intubation is required in patients with altered mental status who have lost protective airway reflexes. Intubation is also indicated in patients with evidence of critically increased intracranial pressure (ICP).

All patients receive oxygen, naloxone, and—if hypoglycemia is suspected—0.5 to 1.0 g/kg of glucose. Patients who are hypotensive are resuscitated with crystalloid. Fluids are titrated carefully in patients who may have increased intracranial pressure, since overaggressive hydration can precipitate herniation. Hypotension is avoided, since it can result in cerebral hypoperfusion and ischemia.

Hyperventilation produces vasoconstriction of the cerebral arteries and is the primary treatment for increased ICP. The P_{CO_2} is not reduced below 20 torr because severe vasoconstriction and cerebral ischemia can result. Mannitol or furosemide may be useful adjuncts to hyperventilation in patients with severely increased ICP.

DISPOSITION

Patients with significant alteration in mental status are best managed in an intensive care unit. For patients with milder disease, the decision to admit to the hospital or discharge from the emergency department largely depends on the etiology of the problem.

SPECIAL CONSIDERATIONS

There are several causes of altered mental status and coma that are characteristic of the pediatric population and deserve special mention.

Lead Encephalopathy

Lead toxicity is a consideration in the differential diagnosis of any child with profoundly altered mental status or coma. Lead encephalopathy can be associated with increased ICP and seizures. Patients with lead encephalopathy often have a history of pica, and parents may have noted abdominal pain, constipation, and vomiting prior to the development of encephalopathy.

Intussusception

Although intussusception commonly presents with episodes of intermittent abdominal pain and vomiting, there is a "neurologic presentation" in which the child manifests a depressed level of consciousness that can range from lethargy to obtundation. The overall appearance of the patient can mimic shock. In some cases the abdominal examination may reveal a mass, and rectal examination may reveal heme positive or "currant jelly stools."

Reye's Syndrome

Reye's syndrome is characterized by the acute onset of encephalopathy, often developing about 2 weeks following a viral infection. The exact pathophysiology is unknown but may involve the interaction of salicylates and certain viruses, especially influenza and varicella. Most cases occur in children less than 12 to 13 years of age.

The syndrome begins with unremitting vomiting and can progress from lethargy to disorientation, combativeness, and, in severe cases, coma. The encephalopathy is characterized by increased intracranial pressure, which at high levels can lead to cardiovascular and respiratory instability and often death. It is increased intracranial pressure that appears to be the predominant factor in influencing outcome. In infants, vomiting may be less prominent; unlike the situation in older patients, seizures are common.

The encephalopathy is associated with elevated liver function tests, and serum ammonia is generally three times normal. Characteristically, serum bilirubin is only slightly elevated and jaundice is absent. Hypoglycemia is common in infants and in patients with severe encephalopathy.

A system has been developed that categorizes Reye's syndrome in five stages of severity, according to the degree of encephalopathy. Stage 1 is characterized by lethargy, with an otherwise normal neurologic examination, and stage 2 by stupor or combativeness, with inappropriate verbal response. Stages 3 to 5 are characterized by increasing degrees of coma. In stage 2 the patient's response to pain is purposeful, while in stage 3 the response to pain is decorticate.

If the diagnosis of Reye's syndrome is entertained, aggressive management is indicated. To avoid overhydration and worsening of cerebral edema, intravenous fluids are administered at or slightly below maintenance requirements. Hypoglycemic patients may require 10% dextrose or 25% dextrose. Patients who are unarousable to voice or light pain are candidates for elective intubation and hyperventilation. In practice, this occurs at stage 2. Mannitol or furosemide may be required for control of intracranial pressure. In some cases, barbiturate coma and decompressive craniotomy have been utilized. The need for a liver biopsy to confirm the diagnosis is controversial.

Patients with stage 1 disease usually recover completely. Surviving patients with more severe encephalopathy can suffer permanent neuropsychiatric impairment.

Inborn Errors of Metabolism

There are numerous inborn errors of metabolism that can present early in life, with vomiting, seizures, and altered mental status. Some can result in metabolic acidosis. Others are not associated with metabolic acidosis. Laboratory diagnosis requires examination of urine and plasma for amino acids, organic acids, and carnitine.

Ketotic Hypoglycemia

Ketotic hypoglycemia occurs in young children, generally between 18 months and 5 years of age. It accounts for up to 50 percent of cases of recurrent hypoglycemia in children.

Attacks are often associated with intercurrent illness and often occur in the morning. Ketonuria is generally present. Patients respond to the administration of glucose but not to glucagon. Children tend to "outgrow" the syndrome.

Nonketotic Hypoglycemia

When a normal child is hypoglycemic, ketones are formed. If ketones are not present, there may be a defect in fatty acid oxidation or hyperinsulinism, which can be secondary to a lesion such as nesidioblastosis or islet cell adenoma. In children with recurrent hypoglycemia who do not have ketonuria, evaluation includes urinalysis for organic acids and insulin levels. Referral to an endocrinologist is indicated.

Congenital Adrenal Hyperplasia

In a child with congenital adrenal hyperplasia, hypoglycemia may result from the absence of cortisol. The constellation of symptoms such as lethargy, vomiting, dehydration, and altered mental status suggest this disorder. Virilization may or may not occur. Emergent treatment includes intravenous fluid therapy with saline and glucocorticoid administration.

For a more detailed discussion, see Fuchs S: Altered mental status and coma, chap. 34, p. 220, in *Pediatric Emergency Medicine: A Comprehensive Study Guide.*

35 Seizures

Susan Fuchs

A seizure results from a paroxysmal electrical discharge of neurons within the brain. Epilepsy is defined as two or more unprovoked seizures.

CLASSIFICATION

Seizures are classified as partial or general. Partial seizures are subdivided into partial simple seizures, in which there is no impairment in consciousness; complex partial seizures, in which consciousness is impaired; and partial seizures that evolve into generalized seizures. Generalized seizures are categorized as convulsive or nonconvulsive.

Simple partial seizures can have motor manifestations that remain focal or that spread (march) to other motor groups. They can also occur without motor involvement but with complex somatosensory symptoms, autonomic symptoms, or behavioral manifestations. In general, simple partial seizures involve one cerebral hemisphere.

A predominant aspect of complex partial seizures is the presence of psychomotor automatisms, which occur during the seizure and for which the patient is amnestic. They can include such activities as chewing or swallowing, gestures such as clapping, or repetitive verbalizations. Postictal disorientation is a feature of psychomotor automatisms. Complex partial seizures can be simple at their onset, with alteration in consciousness developing as the seizure progresses, or can begin with alteration of consciousness. Abnormalities in complex partial seizures can be unilateral or bilateral.

Generalized seizures involve both hemispheres of the brain and are classified as convulsive or nonconvulsive. Absence, or petit mal, seizures are nonconvulsive and are characterized by an abrupt and brief loss of awareness (<15 s), which may include staring or eye blinking, without postictal confusion.

There are multiple manifestations of generalized seizures characterized by convulsions. Myoclonic or minor motor seizures consist of unilateral or bilateral muscle contractions. The old classification of grand mal seizures encompasses three distinct types of seizures: Clonic seizures are characterized by rhythmic jerking and flexor spasms of muscles, tonic seizures by sustained muscle contraction resulting in rigidity, and tonic-clonic seizures by a combination of both. Atonic seizures involve a loss of muscle tone, which causes the child to fall to the floor.

There are several distinct types of epilepsy that occur only in children. Benign childhood epilepsy, also known as rolandic epilepsy, has an onset between 3 and 13 years of age, often occurs upon awakening, and consists of facial movements, grimacing, and vocalizations. Diagnosis is based upon finding centrotemporal spikes on an electroencephalogram (EEG). West syndrome involves infantile spasms characterized by sudden tonic contractions of the extremities, head, and trunk. The classic EEG finding is hypsarrhythmia. Lennox-Gastaut syndrome has its onset at 1 to 8 years of age and consists of multiple seizure types.

Neonatal seizures, febrile seizures, and status epilepticus are special syndromes and are discussed in detail in the following sections.

THE FIRST SEIZURE AND RECURRENT SEIZURES

A majority of children who present to the emergency department with seizures have suffered from a febrile convulsion or an exacerbation of a known seizure disorder. However, on occasion a patient may have experienced a first nonfebrile seizure or may be experiencing recurrent manifestations of an atypical, undiagnosed seizure disorder. Aside from fever, the most common causes of seizures in children include infections, trauma, toxic exposures, and failure to take prescribed anticonvulsants. In addition, childhood seizures are often idiopathic. A more thorough list is included in Table 35-1.

TABLE 35-1 Etiology of Childhood Seizures

Infections	Vascular
Meningitis	Intracranial hematoma
Meningoencephalitis	Embolism
Brain abscess	Infarction
	Hypertensive encephalopathy
Trauma	Tumor
Hemorrhage: epidural, subdural	
Posttraumatic	Psychologic
	Hyperventilation
Intoxication	Breath-holding spells
Lead	
Cocaine	Congenital
PCP	Malformations
Amphetamine	Birth asphyxia
Aspirin	Neurocutaneous syndromes
Carbon monoxide	
Theophylline	Other
	S/P DPT immunization
Drug withdrawal (anticonvulsants)	
	Seizure disorder
Metabolic	Noncompliance
Hypoglycemia	Inadequate drug level
Hyponatremia	
Hypernatremia	
Hypocalcemia	
Hypomagnesemia	
Inborn errors of metabolism	

History

In a patient with a suspected seizure, it is necessary to elicit detailed information regarding the episode itself as well as preceding events. A clear description of the patient's level of consciousness during the episode, memory of the event, and any postictal phenomena are important in categorizing the seizure. Abnormal motor movements are noted and characterized as localized or general. Information regarding abnormal eye movements, facial grimacing, lip movements, and urinary or fecal incontinence is elicited. It is important to document the duration of the episode. Patients are questioned regarding the presence of any associated aura or somatosensory manifestations, such as visual or auditory hallucinations. A history of fever, trauma, prior seizures, drug use or withdrawal, underlying medical disorders, perinatal problems, developmental milestones, and seizures in family members will help direct further evaluation.

Physical Examination

If the child is actively seizing, stabilization and treatment are priorities. However, most children will have stopped seizing by the time of evaluation, and a thorough physical examination is required. Complete vital signs—including temperature, heart rate, respiratory rate, and blood pressure—are obtained. Determining the child's level of consciousness is important. The head circumference is measured in a young infant to detect micro- or macrocephaly, and the head is palpated in any child with trauma to detect hematomas or skull fractures. Examination of the eyes includes an assessment of pupillary reactivity, establishing whether gaze is conjugate or disconjugate, and a fundoscopic examination to detect papilledema or retinal hemorrhages. The presence or absence of meningismus and photophobia is documented.

A thorough neurologic examination is performed. In some patients, examination may reveal Todd's paresis, a transient paralysis that can follow a seizure. It is usually unilateral and may involve both the face and the extremities. The skin should be examined for petechiae, café au lait spots, and adenoma sebaceum.

Laboratory Evaluation

A bedside glucose check is performed on all patients to detect hypoglycemia. Other laboratory studies are based upon the type of seizure and likely etiologies, but will usually include a complete blood count, electrolytes, and glucose. Calcium, magnesium, phosphorus, and toxicology screens are obtained if they are clinically indicated, as are more complicated studies such as lead level and urine amino acids. If the child has been on antiseizure medication, a drug level is obtained.

For febrile patients, the etiology of the fever should be investigated. A lumbar puncture is performed in any patient suspected of having a central nervous system infection. However, if there are focal findings on physical examination or suspicions of a mass lesion, the lumbar puncture is delayed pending computed tomography (CT) of the brain.

Radiologic Evaluation

For most patients with a generalized seizure, no focal findings on physical examination, and no history of trauma, there is little use for a CT scan. Neuroimaging should be reserved for those with a focal seizure, an abnormal neurologic examination, a suspected intracranial mass lesion, or infection. Magnetic resonance imaging (MRI) is preferable over CT, as small tumors, hamartomas, or temporal lobe lesions are better seen. If trauma is suspected, a CT scan is performed.

Electroencephalogram

An EEG is best performed a few days to weeks after the seizure. An abnormal EEG is the most important predictor of seizure recurrence. A normal EEG does not rule out a seizure disorder.

Disposition

Any child who experiences a first focal seizure or who has an abnormal neurologic examination is admitted to the hospital. A child with a first generalized seizure does not necessarily need to be admitted and, depending upon the type of seizure and etiology, may not require treatment until an EEG is performed.

It is important to stress to parents that there is no evidence that a single seizure damages the brain. There is no way to absolutely predict seizure recurrence. However, it is more likely when there is an underlying neurologic problem or an abnormal EEG. Other risk factors include a partial seizure, a family history of seizures, prior febrile seizures, and the presence of Todd's paresis after a seizure.

The decision to initiate therapy should be made in conjunction with a pediatric neurologist. Treatment depends on the type of seizure (Table 35-2).

TABLE 35-2 Choice of Anticonvulsant

Seizure type	Drugs of choice (in order of preference)
Absence	Ethosuximide (Zarontin) 20–40 mg/kg/day bid Valproic acid (Depakene) or divalproex (Depakote) 10–60 mg/kg/day bid or qid Clonazepam (Klonopin) 0.05–0.3 mg/kg/day bid/qid
Atonic	Valproic acid, clonazepam, ethosuximide
Myoclonic	Valproic acid, clonazepam
Partial	Carbamazepine (Tegretol) 10–40 mg/kg/day bid or qid, phenytoin (Dilantin) 4–8 mg/kg/day bid Valproic acid, phenobarbital 2–8 mg/kg/day qd/bid, primidone (Mysoline) 12–25 mg/kg/day bid/qid
Generalized, tonic-clonic	Carbamazepine, phenytoin, phenobarbital, primidone, valproic acid
Infantile spasms	ACTH, prednisone

NEONATAL SEIZURES

These are seizures that occur during the first 28 days of life, although most occur shortly after birth. Because the cerebral cortex is immature, seizures in neonates can be extremely subtle, consisting only of lip smacking, eye deviation, or apnea. Motor activity can appear normal.

Neonatal seizures are commonly related to perinatal asphyxia; metabolic abnormalities, especially hypoglycemia and hypocalcemia; central nervous system infections; and perinatal hemorrhage. Central nervous system infections in neonates can also present with seizures. Less commonly, seizures are related to inherited metatabolic abnormalities. These defects often become apparent after the infant begins feeding and usually cause lethargy, vomiting, and poor feeding as well as seizures. A rare cause of refractory seizures in neonates is inherited pyridoxine deficiency (Table 35-3).

History

Information obtained in neonates with seizures includes the gestational age of the patient, maternal infections or drug use during pregnancy, maternal fever during labor, premature rupture of membranes, the duration of labor, and the method of delivery.

Any complications during delivery are noted, especially perinatal asphyxia. Feeding pattern and the type of formula are important for a child who has a seizure after 3 days of age, when inherited metabolic defects become more likely.

Laboratory Evaluation

Bedside glucose determination and levels of serum glucose, electrolytes, calcium, and magnesium are obtained. In most instances, a lumbar puncture for bacterial and viral cultures, cell count, protein, glucose, and Gram stain is performed as soon as possible. In patients in whom an inherited metabolic defect is considered, serum ammonia is measured, as are serum and urine amino acids. Some inherited defects are associated with a metabolic acidosis; therefore, an arterial blood gas is indicated. Cranial ultrasound or CT can be useful to diagnose hemorrhages.

Treatment

The initial treatment is aimed at securing an adequate airway and ensuring oxygenation. If hypoglycemia (<30 mg/dL) is found,

TABLE 35-3 Causes of Neonatal Seizures

Hypoxia/anoxia (intrauterine or perinatal)
Cerebral ischemia (secondary to hypoxia/anoxia)
Hemorrhage
Subarachnoid (birth trauma)
Subdural (birth trauma)
Intraventricular/intracerebral (prematurity)
Infection
Meningitis: group B streptococci, *E. coli*
Meningoencephalitis: herpes, cytomegalovirus, toxoplasmosis
Metabolic
Hypoglycemia (esp. first day of life)
Hypocalcemia (days 3–14)
Pyridoxine (vit B_6) deficiency
Drug withdrawal: narcotics
Inborn errors of metabolism (days 4–7)
Aminoacidurias: maple syrup urine disease, phenylketonuria
Urea cycle defects: citrullinemia
Organic acidurias: proprionic acidemia
Structural anomalies: lissencephaly
Hereditary disorders: tuberous sclerosis

10 mL/kg of 10% dextrose (D10) is administered intravenously, followed by an infusion of D10. Phenobarbital (10 to 20 mg/kg IV) is the drug of choice for neonatal seizures, with phenytoin (10 to 15 mg/kg) the second choice. In refractory seizures, pyridoxine (50 to 100 mg IV) is indicated to treat the potential for pyridoxine-dependent seizures. Other metabolic abnormalities such as hypocalcemia (<7 mg/dL) and hypomagnesemia are corrected. Hypomagnesemia may be made worse by giving calcium.

FEBRILE SEIZURES

A febrile seizure is a seizure caused by a fever. Febrile seizures occur in patients between 6 months and 5 years of age. Most febrile seizures are self-limited, generalized, and brief, lasting less than 15 min, in which case they are classified as simple. A complex or atypical febrile seizure lasts more than 15 min, occurs more than once in a 24-h period, or has a focal component. Following a febrile seizure, children will usually have a postictal period during which they are lethargic, irritable, or confused.

Approximately 3 to 4 percent of all children will experience a febrile seizure. These seizures occur most commonly in children below 2 years of age. Some 25 to 30 percent of children who have one febrile seizure will have a recurrence. The rate of recurrence is increased if the first seizure occurs in a child below 1 year of age. Recurrence is most likely in the first 6 to 12 months after the first seizure. Risk factors that correlate with an increased risk of subsequent epilepsy include a prolonged or unilateral seizure, a prior neurologic deficit, and a family history of epilepsy.

The seizure usually occurs during the early phase of the infectious illness. Commonly implicated etiologies include upper respiratory tract infections, pharyngitis, otitis, pneumonia, gastroenteritis, urinary tract infections, and roseola. Febrile seizures can also occur after immunizations.

The history should focus on the presence of a preceding febrile illness. A description of the seizure and its duration are obtained from a witness. Preexisting neurologic abnormalities, developmental delay, and a family history of seizures are obtained.

In most cases, the seizure will have terminated upon arrival in the emergency department (ED), but the child may still be postictal. In a febrile seizure, the neurologic examination is normal. If a neurologic deficit exists, another etiology for the fever should be considered.

Laboratory Evaluation

A bedside glucose determination is done on all patients. If no source of fever has been determined by physical examination, a blood culture, urinalysis, and urine culture may be helpful. Electrolytes, calcium, and glucose are usually normal but may be useful if the history is compatible with an electrolyte imbalance. The greatest controversy surrounds the need to perform a lumbar puncture in a child who has had a febrile convulsion. A child over 18 months who is nontoxic, has a normal mental status, and has no evidence of neck pain or stiffness does not require a lumbar puncture. In a child who is still postictal or noncommunicative, detecting meningismus may be difficult. In this situation, a lumbar puncture is indicated.

Other studies such as skull radiographs, CT scan, and even EEG are rarely helpful.

Therapy

The initial management of the patient with a febrile seizure includes stabilizing the airway and assuring adequate oxygenation. If the seizure persists for more than 10 min, anticonvulsant therapy is indicated.

Acetaminophen 15 mg/kg PO or PR or ibuprofen 10 mg/kg PO is administered to reduce the fever.

Controversy still exists regarding further therapy for febrile seizures, although a majority favor no treatment. The benign nature of these seizures and the low risk of recurrence outweigh the benefits of the medications used due to their side effects. Parental reassurance and education regarding the benign nature of febrile seizures and the low risk of subsequent epilepsy are part of the discharge instructions, along with encouragement to begin antipyretic therapy early in the course of subsequent febrile illnesses.

STATUS EPILEPTICUS

Status epilepticus is a seizure lasting more than 30 min or two or more seizures without recovery of consciousness in between. It can present in several forms, including convulsive, nonconvulsive, and repeated partial seizures without impaired consciousness.

Etiologies for status epilepticus overlap those for a first seizure and include central nervous system infection, medication change or noncompliance in children on anticonvulsant therapy, head trauma, hypoxia, metabolic disorders, toxic ingestions, tumor, vascular lesions, and progressive neurologic disorders.

Initial therapy consists of meticulous attention to maintaining patency of the airway and adequacy of oxygenation and ventilation.

Head positioning, using the chin lift and jaw thrust, may open the airway, and an oral or nasal airway can be inserted. High-flow oxygen is administered to all patients via face mask or bag-valve-mask, and cardiac status and pulse oximetry are monitored continuously. Intubation may be necessary to oxygenate and ventilate the patient adequately. In addition, when administering anticonvulsants, especially benzodiazepines, intubation may be necessary because of respiratory depression.

After intravenous access is obtained, a bedside glucose determination is performed, and blood is drawn for complete blood count, electrolytes, blood urea nitrogen, glucose, calcium, and magnesium. In patients on anticonvulsant therapy, drug levels are obtained, and in some patients a toxicology screen may be indicated. If the glucose is <60 mg/dL, 0.5 to 1.0 g/kg of dextrose is given as 2 to 4 mL/kg of D_{25} or 1 to 2 mL/kg of D_{50}. If vascular access cannot be obtained, intraosseous access is an acceptable alternative in children below 6 years of age.

Drug therapy requires a clear plan for prompt administration of anticonvulsants in adequate doses, with attention to side effects such as hypoventilation or apnea. Benzodiazepines are effective for the treatment of an actively seizing patient. Lorazepam (Ativan) has an onset of action of 5 to 10 min and a relatively long half-life of 12 to 24 h. Side effects, while less frequent and of shorter duration than those of diazepam, include respiratory depression and sedation. The dose is 0.05 to 0.01 mg/kg, up to 8 mg. Diazepam (Valium) is useful for control of seizures. It has an onset of action of 1 to 3 min, but its half-life of 15 to 20 min means that repeated doses are often required. The dose is 0.1 to 0.3 mg/kg administered slowly by IV push. Side effects include respiratory depression, hypotension, sedation, and cardiac arrest. Diazepam can also be given rectally, using the intravenous formulation in a dose of 0.5 mg/kg for the first dose and 0.25 mg/kg for any subsequent dose, to a maximum of 20 mg. With rectal administration the onset of action is usually within 5 min. Midazolam is a benzodiazepine that is rapidly absorbed after intramuscular injection; it is an alternative to other benzodiazepines when it is impossible to obtain intravenous or intraosseous access. The dose is 0.2 mg/kg.

Because benzodiazepines are not useful for long-term seizure control, the administration of a long-acting antiseizure medication is indicated after seizures are controlled with benzodiazepines. Phenytoin (Dilantin), when given intravenously, has rapid brain deposition but takes longer to control the seizure than a benzodiazepine (10 to 30 min). The loading dose is 20 mg/kg, which must be given slowly—at 50 mg/min in adults or 1 mg/kg/min in children weighing less than 50 kg. Side effects include hypotension and cardiac conduction disturbances (widened QT interval and arrhythmias), which, if they occur, should prompt a slower infusion or stoppage of the medication. Dilantin will precipitate in glucose solutions, so it should be given directly into the vein or in saline. Long-term seizure control can be accomplished by repeating half of the initial dose in 2 to 3 h (IV or PO) and then continuing the medication on a bid schedule (4 to 8 mg/kg), following serum levels. Phosphenytoin is an alternative to Dilantin.

Phenobarbital is still a useful drug for treating status epilepticus, and it remains the drug of choice for neonatal seizures. Peak brain levels are reached in 20 to 60 min, and its duration of action is longer than 48 h. The loading dose is 20 mg/kg IV given slowly (100 mg/min). Side effects include respiratory depression (additive with benzodiazepines on board), sedation, and occasionally hypotension. If seizures stop before the entire loading dose is given, the remainder can be given intravenously or even orally within 1 to 2 h. Long-term therapy can be initiated in 24 h using 2 to 8 mg/kg/day given twice a day, monitoring drug levels to avoid oversedation.

If status persists after one dose of a benzodiazepine followed by phenytoin or phenobarbital, an additional dose of benzodiazepine can be given. If the seizure persists, if phenytoin was given, phenobarbital can be administered (or vice versa). In such cases, the risk of apnea is high, so assisted ventilation and possibly intubation may be required.

For refractory status, pentobarbital, phenobarbital, or paraldehyde can be used. Paraldehyde is given rectally, 0.3 to 0.5 mg/kg diluted 1:1 in vegetable oil, which can be repeated in 20 min. It should not be given intramuscularly because absorption is less reliable and it results in sterile abscesses. Pentobarbital is given as a loading dose of 5 to 20 mg/kg IV followed by an infusion of 0.5 to 3 mg/kg/h to keep the level between 20 and 50 μg/mL and produce cessation of epileptic activity. Vasopressors are often needed with pentobarbital coma, and the patient should be weaned off of the infusion to determine if status has stopped. Phenobarbital can also be used to stop refractory status by giving boluses of 5 to 10 mg/kg every 20 min until the seizure stops or hypotension develops.

Therapy of nonconvulsive status epilepticus is similar to that of convulsive status, using a benzodiazepine or phenytoin. For absence status, a benzodiazepine can be followed by oral or nasogastric ethosuximide, valproic acid, or clonazepam (*both* valproic acid and clonazepam should not be given). Valproic acid can also be given rectally—20 mg/kg of the liquid formulation.

Disposition

Any child who has received lorazepam or a long-acting anticonvulsant medication should be admitted to the hospital. Since diazepam is short-acting, admission decisions can be individualized if no other drugs have been given. Intensive care admission is obviously needed for any child still in status, requiring assisted or mechanical ventilation, or in whom the evaluation has revealed an etiology requiring close monitoring.

For a more detailed discussion, see Fuchs S: Seizures, chap. 35, p. 225, in *Pediatric Emergency Medicine: A Comprehensive Study Guide.*

---

36 Syncope

Susan Fuchs

Syncope refers to a sudden and transient loss of consciousness. Unlike in the adult population, where syncope often results from malignant cardiac arrythmias, in the pediatric population it is often secondary to autonomic dysfunction, and is therefore discussed in this section.

PATHOPHYSIOLOGY

Syncope always results from momentarily inadequate delivery of oxygen and glucose to the brain. There are multiple possible etiologies. Syncope can result from inadequate cardiac output, which can be secondary to obstruction of blood flow, or to an arrythmia. It can also result from inappropriate autonomic compensation for the normal decline in blood pressure that occurs on rising from a sitting or supine position. Respiratory disturbances, especially hyperventilation that results in hypocapnia, can also cause syncope.

HISTORY

The first component in the evaluation of a patient with syncope is determining that momentary loss of consciousness actually occurred. In patients who did indeed lose consciousness, the events antecedent to the syncopal episode are elicited. Information concerning a sudden change in posture, emotional excitement, respiratory difficulty, palpitations, and any history of trauma is essential.

A past history of syncope is sought, as is any history of medication or drug ingestion.

An important consideration in any patient with a history of loss of consciousness is the possibility that the patient may have suffered a seizure. Syncope is generally not associated with myoclonic activity or a postictal period.

PHYSICAL EXAMINATION

The physical examination focuses upon assessing the hemodynamic stability of the patient. Particular attention is paid to vital signs, especially to pulse and orthostatic blood pressure. A positive "tilt test" is a decrease in systolic blood pressure by 20 mmHg accompanied by an initial elevation in heart rate (20 beats per minute), which can be followed rapidly by bradycardia and syncope. The patient's mental status is carefully evaluated and a full neurologic examination performed.

In all patients, a careful cardiac examination is indicated. The regularity of the pulse is noted, as is the quality of the peripheral pulses. The heart is auscultated carefully to detect the presence of a murmer that may indicate congenital heart disease, especially aortic stenosis. The quality and presence of all peripheral pulses are evaluated. Diminished pulses in the lower extremities can imply a coarctation of the aorta.

LABORATORY STUDIES

The laboratory studies indicated in a pediatric patient with a history of syncope are guided by the history and physical. In a patient with a history of fasting or diabetes, a blood glucose is indicated. In the presence of pallor or a history of blood loss, a hemoglobin is obtained. Electrolyte abnormalities are an uncommon cause of syncope, but if an arrhythmia is suspected, serum potassium, calcium, and magnesium are measured. Other studies including arterial blood gas, toxicology screening, and pregnancy testing may be indicated in certain clinical scenarios.

In all patients with a history of syncope, a 12-lead electrocardiogram is indicated. This provides information concerning potential conduction defects or other arrhythmias. Special attention is paid to determination of the corrected QT interval (QTc), since prolonged QT syndrome is a cause of syncope in children. If abnormalities are seen or if a cardiac abnormality is strongly suspected, further evaluation will include 24-h ambulatory (Holter) monitoring and cardiology consultation.

SPECIFIC ETIOLOGIES OF SYNCOPE

Autonomic

The causes of syncope are listed in Table 36-1. The most common of these in children is vasodepressor or vasovagal syncope. There

TABLE 36-1 Causes of Syncope

Autonomic causes
Vasodepressor syncope
Excessive vagal tone
Reflex syncope
Orthostatic hypotension
Cardiac causes
Arrhythmias
Supraventricular tachycardias
Atrial flutter
Wolfe-Parkinson-White syndrome
Ventricular tachycardia
Ventricular fibrillation
Conduction disturbances
Atrioventricular block
Prolonged QTc
Sick sinus syndrome
Obstructive lesions
Aortic stenosis
Pulmonic stenosis
Idiopathic hypertrophic subaortic stenosis
Mitral stenosis
Coarctation of the aorta
Tetralogy of Fallot
Anomalous origin of the left coronary artery
Tumors
Other
Myocarditis
Pericarditis
Cardiac tamponade
Cardiomyopathy
Noncardiac causes
Metabolic causes
Hypoglycemia
Hypocalcemia
Hypomagnesemia
Toxic
Seizures
Psychogenic causes
Hyperventilation
Hysteria

is a sudden, brief loss of consciousness due to vasodilatation and decreased peripheral resistance, hypotension, bradycardia, and decreased cerebral blood flow. It is often precipitated by sudden emotional stress. Patients may have symptoms such as blurred vision, dizziness, nausea, or pallor. This is what is commonly referred to as a "simple faint." Placing the person in a supine position with the head down usually results in improvement.

Another autonomic cause of syncope is excess vagal tone, which can imitate cardiac causes of syncope. Children who exhibit excess vagal tone will have a low resting heart rate, junctional rhythms, and depressed sinoatrial node function. Exercise can increase vagal tone and lead to syncope. Therefore, a history of syncope during exercise should prompt a full evaluation to rule out cardiac etiologies. Orthostatic hypotension can result from an aberrant autonomic response; it is characterized by an initial rise in heart rate followed by bradycardia or a period of asystole and then syncope. Some centers evaluate children with repetitive syncope with "tilt-table testing," which attempts to reproduce the abnormal bradycardia that occurs on moving from a supine to an upright position.

Breath-holding spells can also result in transient loss of consciousness. They tend to occur in toddlers and are almost always associated with some episode that angers or frustrates the child and results in crying. The child then stops breathing, becomes cyanotic, and loses consciousness. Recovery is rapid, and children outgrow the problem.

Reflex syncope is due to a disturbance in the usual sequence of increased vascular resistance, heart rate, and contractility in response to decreased blood flow to the heart. Included in this category are cough, micturition, and carotid sinus syncope.

Cardiac Causes

It is important to exclude cardiac syncope, since it can result in sudden death. Arrhythmias that result in a heart rate that is too fast or too slow can cause a decrease in cardiac output and lead to decreased cerebral perfusion. Included in this are supraventricular tachycardias, Wolff-Parkinson-White syndrome, ventricular tachycardia, sick sinus syndrome (may occur after cardiac surgery), and long QT syndrome. If a cardiac etiology is suspected, admission for cardiac monitoring should be considered.

Obstructive lesions that can cause syncope include aortic stenosis, idiopathic hypertrophic subaortic stenosis (IHSS), and tetralogy of Fallot. Acquired lesions such as cardiac tumors, myocarditis, pericarditis, cardiac tamponade, and cardiomyopathy can also result in syncope.

Functional or Psychological Syncope

Psychological causes of syncope include hyperventilation and hysteria. Hyperventilation results in cerebral vasoconstriction and decreased cerebral blood flow. The patient may complain of shortness of breath and numb fingers before syncope ensues. Hysterical syncope occurs when the patient mimics a loss of consciousness. No abnormalities of heart rate, blood pressure, or skin color are detected, and clues regarding surrounding events may point to the correct diagnosis.

TREATMENT

While the majority of children will not require specific therapy, treatment should be based upon the etiology and frequency of syncopal episodes. A child with hypoglycemia requires glucose, one with anemia may benefit from intravenous fluids while a work-up for the etiology is ongoing. If a cardiac etiology is suspected, depending upon the urgency of the situation, further studies could be performed on an inpatient or outpatient basis, but activity restrictions may be needed while awaiting evaluation. Treatment of a child with orthostatic syncope with betablockers or mineralocorticoids should await the results of formal testing. If a neurologic etiology is suspected, treatment with anticonvulsive medications should be based upon neurologic consultation. If the emergency department evaluation and work-up is negative and the likely etiology is a simple faint, reassurance may be all that is needed. If specific precipitating events were determined, avoidance of these can diminish the occurrence of syncopal events.

DISPOSITION

The majority of patients with syncope will be able to be discharged from the emergency department with appropriate follow-up. Those who require admission are those with a cardiac origin that requires urgent evaluation: arrhythmias (SVT, atrial flutter, ventricular tachycardia or fibrillation), conduction abnormalities (third-degree atrioventricular block, sick sinus syndrome), or newly diagnosed or worsening of obstructive lesions (aortic stenosis, pulmonic stenosis, IHSS).

For a more detailed discussion, see Fuchs S: Syncope, chap. 36, p. 232, in *Pediatric Emergency Medicine: A Comprehensive Study Guide*.

37 Ataxia

Susan Fuchs

Ataxia is a disorder of intentional movement, characterized by impaired balance and coordination. It can variably affect the trunk or extremities. Ataxia of the extremities can result in a wide-based gait, or it can cause dysmetria, which is the tendency of the limbs to overshoot a target.

PATHOPHYSIOLOGY

Ataxia can result from damage to the peripheral nerves, spinal cord, cerebellum, or cerebral hemispheres. Lesions of the cerebellum can be further categorized as affecting the hemispheres, which results in limb ataxia, or the midline vermis, which causes truncal ataxia. Lesions in a single cerebellar hemisphere cause ipsilateral limb manifestations. Damage to the spinal cord can cause ataxia when the patient stands with eyes closed; this is referred to as a Romberg sign.

Metabolic and systemic disorders can also cause ataxia. One of the most common etiologies is drug intoxication, especially with alcohol or phenytoin. Enterovirus and Epstein-Barr virus infections can cause ataxia, as can infection with *Neisseria meningitidis.*

EVALUATION

True ataxia must be distinguished from similar neurologic manifestations. Vestibular disorders can result in vertigo, a sensation of abnormal movement or spinning that can cause a severe gait disturbance, nausea, and vomiting. Vertigo is often accompanied by nystagmus. Myopathies can be confused with ataxia, as can peripheral neuropathies. Chorea is a disorder characterized by involuntary movements and incoordination. It is distinguished from ataxia in that it occurs at rest, while ataxia manifests itself during intentional movement.

Tests that evaluate cerebellar function include finger-to-nose, heel-to-shin, and the assessment of rapid alternating movements. The inability to perform rapid alternating movements is termed dysdiadochokinesia. Patients with ataxia may have a wide-based gait and difficulty ambulating, especially with lesions of the posterior columns.

For diagnostic purposes, it is useful to categorize ataxia as acute, intermittent, or chronic. Chronic ataxia is further categorized as progressive or nonprogressive (Table 37-1).

ACUTE ATAXIA

Acute ataxia generally has an onset of less than 24 h. Drug toxicity and infections are the most common etiologies.

In a patient with acute ataxia, the history and physical examination focus on excluding acute infectious etiologies, such as meningitis or encephalitis; lesions that result in increased intracranial pressure, such as hemorrhage and tumors; and toxic ingestions. Central nervous system infections are usually characterized by fever, headache, and often mental status changes. The physical examination may reveal neck stiffness. Lesions that cause increased intracranial pressure are associated with headache and vomiting, and the physical examination may reveal papilledema. In cases of cerebellar hemorrhage, the onset of ataxia is extremely sudden, while with posterior fossa tumors the history will usually reveal a more protracted process. Toxic ingestions are likely in patients on anticon-

TABLE 37-1 Causes of Ataxia

Acute	Chronic
Postinfectious	Progressive
Acute cerebellar	Tumor
Polymyoclonus/opisthotonus	Abscess
Posttraumatic	Hydrocephalus
Hematoma	Degenerative
Mass	Intermittent
Intoxication	Migraine
Infection	Seizures
Meningitis	Metabolic
Encephalitis	Multiple sclerosis
Polyneuritis	Nonprogressive
Posterior fossa tumors	Cerebral palsy
	Sequelae of:
	Head trauma
	Lead poisoning
	Cerebellar malformations
	Dandy-Walker
	Agenesis
	Hypoplasia

vulsants and are especially common in toddlers. Acute ataxia can also occur after head trauma, as the result of a cerebellar hemorrhage or basilar skull fracture.

Any ataxic patient in whom an acute infectious process is considered requires a lumbar puncture. It is imperative that, prior to a lumbar puncture, increased intracranial pressure be excluded by computed tomography (CT) of the brain. In any patient in whom an ingestion is implicated, a toxicology screen is indicated.

Certain causes of acute ataxia are almost unique to the pediatric population and deserve special mention. A common cause of ataxia in children below 10 years of age is *acute cerebellar ataxia.* The onset of ataxia is insidious and predominantly affects the gait, although dysmetria, nystagmus, and dysarthria can occur. Acute cerebellar ataxia is thought to be a postinfectious phenomenon and often occurs 2 weeks after a viral illness. Ataxia has been reported after infection with varicella, influenza, mumps, echovirus 6, coxsackie B virus, and other viruses. It is a self-limited illness with an excellent prognosis. Acute cerebellar ataxia is a diagnosis of exclusion.

Polymyoclonus-opsoclonus is another cause of acute ataxia. This syndrome occurs in association with occult neuroblastoma and occasionally as a postinfectious phenomenon. It is differentiated from acute cerebellar ataxia by its association with opsoclonus, which describes rapid, chaotic conjugate eye movements, occurring in association with severe myoclonic jerks of the limbs and trunk or head.

Guillain-Barré syndrome can also present with ataxia, although the associated findings of areflexia and, in the Miller-Fisher variant, opthalmoplegia distinguish it from acute cerebellar ataxia.

CHRONIC INTERMITTENT ATAXIA

Chronic intermittent or recurrent ataxia occurs as acute episodes that are similar in nature. In children, the most common cause of intermittent ataxia is a migraine headache that involves the basilar artery. Besides ataxia, associated symptoms include blurred vision, visual field deficits, vertigo, and headache.

Partial complex seizures can also cause intermittent ataxia but are often associated with alteration of consciousness and possibly characteristic motor manifestations.

Rarely, inborn errors of metabolism result in intermittent ataxia. These include maple syrup urine disease, Hartnup disease, ornithine transcarbamylase deficiency, and carboxylase deficiencies.

CHRONIC PROGRESSIVE ATAXIA

Chronic progressive ataxia has an insidious onset and progresses slowly over weeks to months. The differential diagnosis consists of brain tumors, hydrocephalus, and neurodegenerative disorders.

The combination of ataxia, headache, irritability, and vomiting in a child below 6 years of age is characteristic of a medulloblastoma. Cerebellar astrocytomas are located in the cerebellar hemispheres and cause ipsilateral limb ataxia, headache, and double vision. They occur most commonly in school-aged children. Brainstem gliomas present with ataxia and are often accompanied by cranial nerve palsies or spasticity. In some cases, posterior fossa tumors have a relatively acute presentation.

Hydrocephalus, whether congenital or acquired, can cause ataxia. It is often accompanied by headache and vomiting, and can be associated with increased intracranial pressure. Neurodegenerative diseases are a group of inherited disorders that can cause spinocerebellar degeneration and progressive ataxia. These include Refsum disease and abetalipoproteinemia, which are treatable by diet, and Friedreich's ataxia, which is not.

Patients with progressive ataxia require an aggressive evaluation in the emergency department. Computed tomography of the brain is indicated in any patient with signs of a mass lesion or hydrocephalus. Many of these patients are candidates for an emergency ventricular shunt. In patients with signs of increased intracranial pressure, fluid therapy is restricted to two-thirds of maintanance requirements. Patients with suspected neurodegenerative diseases are referred to a pediatric neurologist.

CHRONIC NONPROGRESSIVE ATAXIA

Chronic nonprogressive ataxia may be a sequela of head trauma, meningitis, or lead poisoning. It can also result from congenital malformations, such as cerebellar agenesis or hypoplasia or the Chiari type I malformation (herniation of the cerebellar tonsils into the foramen magnum).

The emergency department evaluation of chronic nonprogressive ataxia consists of assuring, by a careful history and physical examination, that the problem is indeed stable. Patients with an unknown diagnosis may benefit from CT scanning or magnetic resonance imaging of the brain.

For a more detailed discussion, see Fuchs S: Ataxia, chap. 37, p. 235, in *Pediatric Emergency Medicine: A Comprehensive Study Guide.*

38 Weakness

Susan Fuchs

Weakness is a chief complaint that encompasses a vast differential diagnosis that can involve any organ system. This chapter focuses on weakness arising from neuromuscular disorders.

PATHOPHYSIOLOGY

Terms that are applied to neuromuscular disorders include *paresis,* which implies a complete or partial weakness, and *paralysis,* which is a loss of function. *Paraplegia* is paralysis of the lower half of the body, while *quadraplegia* involves all limbs. Both usually result from a spinal cord lesion. *Hemiplegia,* involving one side of the body, generally results from a lesion in the brain.

Abnormalities of the neuromuscular system are further classified as arising from an upper motor neuron unit or a lower motor neuron unit. Diseases of the upper motor neuron usually present with asymmetrical weakness that is contralateral to the lesion, with associated hyperreflexia and increased muscle tone. Diseases of the lower motor neuron present with symmetrical weakness involving specific muscle groups, with associated findings of decreased muscle tone and depressed reflexes. Atrophy and fasciculations may be present.

Involvement of bulbar muscles is manifested by cranial nerve findings, facial muscle weakness, and chewing or swallowing difficulties. It can occur in both upper and lower motor neuron disorders.

Another possibility in the patient presenting with weakness is a myopathy or neuropathy. Myopathies are disorders of muscle that can be inflammatory or congenital. Inflammatory myopathies usually involve proximal muscles and are often associated with muscle pain or tenderness. Reflexes become decreased late in the disease. Congenital myopathies tend to involve specific muscle groups and can present at birth with hypotonia or in older children with progressive weakness. Neuropathies are disorders of nerves and tend to produce more prominent distal muscle weakness, hypoesthesias or paresthesias, and decreased reflexes.

DIAGNOSIS

History

It is vital to distinguish between acute and chronic disorders, since this information will direct the remainder of the work-up. Weakness is described as focal or general. Focal weakness is further characterized as proximal or distal. The rate of progression of symptoms is characterized as acute, which implies minutes to hours; subacute, meaning hours to days; and slowly progressive, which involves a prolonged period of time. Acute onset or rapid progression implies spinal cord compression or a vascular event involving the spinal cord or brain. Subacute progression can be due to infection, inflammation, or tumor. Slowly progressive symptoms imply a chronic or congenital disorder. The loss of developmental milestones implies a degenerative disorder.

The patient and parents are questioned regarding recent illness, fever, headache, neck or back pain, and loss of bowel or bladder function. A history of recent trauma to the head or neck and the presence of underlying medical problems is sought. Prior episodes of weakness may point to an intermittent metabolic problem. A family history of weakness suggests a congenital disorder. A history of exposure to drugs or heavy metals suggests poisoning. A pertinent travel history is indicated, since weakness can occur in tick paralysis or black widow spider bites.

Physical Examination

The vital signs are assessed, with particular attention to respiratory rate and effort. Many neuromuscular disorders are associated with a risk of respiratory failure and warrant repeated examination of the patient's respiratory status. Blood pressure and pulse are carefully monitored, since some neuromuscular disorders, such as Guillain-Barré syndrome, are associated with autonomic instability.

The patient's general appearance is noted, with attention to general muscular development and the presence of kyphosis, scoliosis, or lordosis, which suggests a congenital disorder. Lack of facial expression, a snarl, or a slack jaw suggests myasthenia gravis. Ptosis can be due to myasthenia or myotonic dystrophy. Gross inspection of the muscles is performed, noting the presence of wasting, fasciculations, or hypertrophy.

The specific neurologic examination includes an evaluation of the cranial nerves. If possible, the optic fundus is examined and the visual fields are assessed. In patients old enough to cooperate, motor strength in the extremities is evaluated on a scale of 1 to 5:

0 = Total lack of contraction
1 = Trace contraction
2 = Active contraction without gravity
3 = Movement against gravity
4 = Movement against resistance
5 = Normal motor strength

Infants may be difficult to examine, but those with normal tone will not slide through an examiner's hands and will actively kick both legs against the resistance of the bed. Older children can be asked to walk on their toes and heels. The ability to walk on the heels but not the toes suggests intraspinal pathology.

Deep tendon reflexes at the knees, ankles, elbows, and wrists are elicited. Hyperreflexia or sustained clonus indicates an upper motor neuron lesion, while absent or decreased reflexes imply a problem in a lower motor distribution. Other reflexes noted include the anal wink, abdominal, and cremasteric responses.

Touch and pain are evaluated by assessing soft versus sharp stimulation and two-point discrimination. Position sense is assessed by asking the child to indicate the direction in which an examiner moves one of the child's fingers or toes. Temperature sensation can be assessed by the use of a cold stethoscope or by touching the child with cold or warm water.

An abnormality of touch and position on one side and pain and temperature on the other suggests a cord lesion. The unilateral loss of all sensations suggests a lesion at the level of the brain. A stocking-and-glove distribution of sensory loss suggests a peripheral neuropathy.

Laboratory Evaluation

The laboratory evaluation is based upon the provisional diagnosis. Generally, a complete blood count, serum electrolytes, and magnesium are indicated. Serum creatinine is elevated in children with active inflammatory myopathies. Urine is assessed for the presence of myoglobin and, in selected cases, is used for toxicology screening.

In patients with a suspected spinal cord lesion, radiographs are indicated. Any patient suspected of having a developing lesion of the spinal cord requires evaluation by magnetic resonance imaging (MRI) or contrast myelography. If neither is available, computed tomography (CT) of the spine may be helpful.

In patients with suspected central nervous system lesions, CT of the brain is indicated. Selected patients may require a lumbar puncture.

Electromyography and nerve conduction studies are indicated if lower motor neuron disease is suspected.

SPECIFIC CAUSES OF WEAKNESS

Guillain-Barré Syndrome

Also known as acute inflammatory demyelinating polyradiculoneuropathy, Guillain-Barré syndrome occurs in both children and adults. It is thought to result from an immune response to an antecedent viral infection that triggers demyelination of nerve roots and peripheral nerves. The syndrome often starts with nonspecific muscular pain, most often in the thighs. The pain is followed by weakness, which is most often symmetric and distal. Weakness progresses upward and, in some cases, can result in total paralysis within 24 h. Cranial nerve involvement is common. Deep tendon reflexes are usually absent, but plantar responses remain downgoing. Autonomic involvement can produce labile changes in blood pressure and bowel and bladder incontinence. The degree of weakness and the rate of progression of disease vary considerably from patient to patient. Laboratory findings are generally unrevealing, although the cerebrospinal fluid may reveal albuminocytologic association.

The basic treatment for Guillain-Barré syndrome is supportive care. In some cases, mechanical ventilation is necessary. Attention is given to fluid and electrolyte balance, heart rate, and blood pressure. Steroids and other immunosuppressive agents are of questionable value. Plasmapheresis may shorten the course of disease, as may therapy with intravenous gamma globulin.

Transverse Myelitis

Transverse myelitis is a syndrome characterized by acute dysfunction at a level of the spinal cord. It can occur as an isolated phenomenon or as part of another illness. The onset can be insidious but usually occurs over 24 to 48 h. Patients may initially complain of paresthesias and weakness of the lower extremities. Progressive weakness usually results, and a sensory level is established, most commonly in the thoracic spine. Flaccid paralysis and decreased reflexes are characteristic early in the process but are later followed by increased muscle tone.

In a patient with signs of a rapidly advancing spinal cord lesion, it is imperative to exclude a treatable mass lesion that could be compressing the cord, such as an epidural abscess or hemorrhage. This is done by MRI or contrast myelography.

Most patients with transverse myelitis recover some function. Corticosteroids may benefit some patients.

Tick Paralysis

Tick paralysis is caused by a neurotoxin from the Rocky Mountain wood tick (*Dermacentor andersoni*) or the eastern dog tick (*Dermacentor variabilis*). The tick produces a neurotoxin that prevents liberation of acetylcholine at neuromuscular junctions. Small children are likely victims. Several days after the tick attaches, the patient begins to experience ataxia and difficulty walking. If the tick is not removed, flaccid paralysis and death can result. Removal of the tick is curative.

Botulism

Infection with *Clostridium botulinum* can produce three neurological diseases. Symptoms result from a toxin generated from spores of the bacteria that inhibits release of acetylcholine at the prejunction of terminal nerve fibers.

Food-borne botulism results from ingestion of toxin contained in improperly canned foods. Diarrhea and vomiting are followed by neurologic symptoms, including cranial nerve dysfunction. Blurred vision, dysarthria, and diplopia can occur and can be followed by weakness of the extremities. Mucous membranes of the mouth and pharynx may be dry. Deep tendon reflexes may be weak or absent. Antitoxin may be effective in food-borne botulism.

Wound botulism results from infection of a contaminated wound. Clinically, it is usually indistinguishable from food-borne botulism. Treatment includes wound debridement and antibiotic therapy. Antitoxin may also be useful.

Infant botulism is caused by colonization of the intestinal tract by spores of *C. botulinum,* which release toxin that is systemically absorbed. It has been related to the ingestion of contaminated honey. A prominent manifestation in affected infants is constipation. When the disease is severe, the infant can develop difficulty sucking and swallowing and may become hypotonic. Symmetrical paralysis can develop, with involvement of cranial nerves. Diagnosis is confirmed by isolating the toxin in the infant's stool. Electromyography is also useful. The management of infant botulism is supportive and may require mechanical ventilation. Treatment with antitoxin and antibiotics does not seem to be of benefit.

Myasthenia Gravis

The term *myasthenia gravis* comprises a group of diseases characterized by easy fatigability of muscles. Most commonly, it is associated with antiacetylcholine receptor antibodies that destroy the postsynaptic membrane of the myoneural junction, resulting in decreased transmission of nerve impulses. In children, the striated muscles innervated by the cranial nerves are particularly affected. The diagnosis is established by demonstrating improvement in muscle strength after administration of the anticholinesterase edrophonium (Tensilon). The three basic categories of myasthenia gravis in the pediatric population are the transient neonatal variety, the persistent neonatal form, and juvenile myasthenia gravis.

Neonatal transient myasthenia gravis occurs in infants born to mothers with the disease and is caused by maternal antiacetylcholine receptor antibodies that cross the placenta. It affects 10 to 15 percent of infants whose mothers have myasthenia gravis. In its severe form, it can cause problems with sucking and swallowing as well as ventilatory insufficiency. Treatment is with neostigmine or pyridostigmine. The disease usually improves in 4 to 6 weeks.

Persistent neonatal myasthenia gravis may be autoimmune in nature or of a hereditary variety. Symptoms usually appear on the first day of life and, in more severe cases, include ptosis, swallowing difficulties, and respiratory insufficiency. In less severe cases, the onset can be insidious and clinical manifestations of muscle weakness more subtle. Symptoms may be severe enough to require nasogastric feeding and ventilatory support. Pharmacologic therapy is with anticholinesterase agents.

Juvenile myasthenia gravis is similar to that seen in adults. It commonly has its onset at around 10 years of age. Ptosis, opthalmoplegia, and weakness of other facial muscles are common. Symmetrical limb weakness is usually present, though focal weakness of the ocular muscles can occur. The disease tends to become worse throughout the day. Both remissions and exacerbations are common, and up to 50 percent of children may develop seizures. The primary treatment is with anticholinesterase agents. In refractory or severe cases, immunosuppressive agents, plasmapheresis, or thymectomy may be necessary. Erythromycin therapy can exacerbate symptoms and is avoided.

Myasthenic Crisis

Occasionally, exacerbations of symptoms can occur that result in profound weakness, difficulty swallowing secretions, and respiratory insufficiency. This can be associated with antibiotic therapy, central nervous system depressants, antiarrythmics, or hypokalemia. Patients with myasthenic crisis will usually respond to a challenge with edrophonium. If a myasthenic crisis is suspected, the patient is admitted for monitoring of respiratory status.

Cholinergic Crisis

Patients with myasthenia gravis can also suffer from overdose of anticholinesterase medications, which can provoke cholinergic crisis. Unfortunately, the symptoms of cholinergic excess are similar to those of a myasthenic crisis. In both, increasing weakness is the predominant finding. Patients suffering a cholinergic crisis may also have associated vomiting, diarrhea, and hypersalivation. In patients with obvious, severe cholinergic excess, atropine may be useful in drying airway secretions. However, in most cases, it will be difficult to distinguish between a cholinergic crisis and an exacerbation of myasthenia; therefore, hospital admission and close observation are indicated.

Bell's Palsy

Bell's palsy is a condition that results in unilateral facial weakness. In severe cases, there can be total paralysis of the facial muscles. It is thought to result from swelling and edema of cranial nerve VII—the facial nerve—most commonly as it traverses the facial canal within the temporal bone. As such, it is a peripheral neuropathy, and the distribution of the weakness reflects the territory innervated by the facial nerve. The nerve has motor, sensory, and autonomic functions and, in addition to supplying the muscles of the face, innervates the lacrimal and salivary glands as well as the anterior two-thirds of the tongue. In most cases, Bell's palsy is idiopathic. Certain conditions are associated with unilateral facial weakness, including viral infections, otitis media, Lyme disease, and temporal bone trauma.

Symptoms may begin with ear pain, which is followed by the development of facial weakness, characterized by a drooping mouth and inability to close the eye on the affected side. In some cases, lacrimation and taste are impaired. Inability to close the mouth can make eating and drinking difficult.

The lesion is defined as a peripheral neuropathy, as opposed to a lesion of the central nervous system, by the fact that Bell's palsy affects the muscles of the forehead on the side of the lesion. In a lesion of the central nervous system, the forehead is spared, because it receives innervation from both sides of the brain. A lesion in one cerebral hemisphere will cause weakness confined to the lower part of the face. Laboratory studies are usually normal.

The prognosis of Bell's palsy is generally good, with recovery usually beginning in 2 to 4 weeks. Steroid therapy may be beneficial if started early in the course of the illness. Treatment includes lubricating solutions for the eye on the affected side to maintain moisture of the cornea. Patients with inability to close the eye may require patching. In young children, opthalmologic consultation may be advisable.

Myopathies

Myopathies are diseases that affect skeletal muscle. They are a relatively uncommon cause of weakness in children, and in the majority of cases a child affected with a myopathy will present to the emergency department with a known diagnosis. Many myopathies are congenital, although some result from spontaneous mutations.

Muscular Dystrophies

Muscular dystrophies are disorders associated with progressive degeneration of muscle, resulting in relentlessly increasing weakness. There are many different types of muscular dystrophy that vary in their mode of inheritance, age of onset, the muscles involved, progression of disease, and ultimate outcome. The most common is Duchenne muscular dystrophy, usually an X-linked recessive disorder. Clinical manifestations usually become apparent at about age 3, when patients begin to develop weakness of the hip girdle and shoulder muscles. Patients may have difficulty standing and rise from all fours by placing their hands on the thighs and pushing up (Gower's sign). In the later stages, cardiomyopathy is common, and scoliosis can result in pulmonary insufficiency. Survival beyond early adulthood is rare.

Periodic Paralysis

Periodic paralysis is an example of a metabolic myopathy that results in muscle weakness without involvement of the central or peripheral nervous system. The disease is primarily autosomal dominant. There are three varieties, characterized by associated hypokalemia, hyperkalemia, and normokalemia.

Episodes of hypokalemic periodic paralysis have their onset during the first or second decade of life. They are often precipitated by excitement or ingestion of a carbohydrate meal. Paralysis often begins proximally and spreads distally. The patient may be areflexic. The episode can last many hours. Attacks tend to decrease with age. Serum potassium during an attack is usually decreased when compared to a baseline value. Treatment with potassium during an attack may be helpful. Long-term therapy with acetazolamide may reduce the number of attacks. Severely affected patients can develop permanent muscle weakness.

Hyperkalemic periodic paralysis is also an autosomal dominant condition associated with intermittent attacks beginning in the first or second decade of life. Attacks can be provoked by periods of rest following heavy exertion. Weakness can develop rapidly and last for hours. The respiratory muscles are usually spared. Some patients develop myotonia during attacks. The serum potassium is elevated above baseline values, though the degree of hyperkalemia varies. In severe cases, standard therapy for malignant hyperkalemia is indicated. As in patients with hypokalemic periodic paralysis, chronic weakness can develop. Treatment with acetazolamide may also be beneficial.

Normokalemic periodic paralysis can be provoked by exposure to cold, activity, and alcohol. The serum potassium does not change during an attack. Treatment with sodium during an attack may mitigate weakness.

DISPOSITION

The disposition of a patient with weakness depends on the degree of disability and the nature of the underlying problem. In any patient in whom the development of respiratory compromise is a possibility, hospital admission and close observation are recommended.

For a more detailed discussion, see Fuchs S: Weakness, chap. 38, p. 238, in *Pediatric Emergency Medicine: A Comprehensive Study Guide.*

---

39 Headache

Susan Fuchs

As many as 75 percent of children experience a headache by the age of 15. Headaches can be classified as organic, vascular, functional, or psychological and as due to structures other than the calvarium or its contents.

ORGANIC CAUSES

Organic headaches usually result from increased intracranial pressure or from an inflammatory process. An acute headache with a neurologic deficit, headache accompanied by a fever and neck stiffness, or a chronically progressive headache all indicate an organic disorder.

Causes of increased intracranial pressure include brain tumors, hydrocephalus, hypertensive encephalopathy, pseudotumor cerebri, and both spontaneous and traumatic hemorrhage. Infectious etiologies include meningitis, encephalitis, and brain abscesses.

Brain Tumors and Hydrocephalus

Headaches associated with these disorders are often progressive; are made worse by lying down, coughing, or sneezing; and may be worse in the morning. Increased intracranial pressure is often present. Papilledema is often found on fundoscopic examination. A neurologic examination may reveal ataxia with a cerebellar tumor, or cranial nerve findings with hydrocephalus. Diagnosis is made by computed tomography (CT) scan.

Pseudotumor Cerebri

Pseudotumor cerebri is a condition associated with increased intracranial pressure in the absence of a mass lesion or other obvious etiology. It is associated with high doses of vitamin A and is especially common in obese adolescent females. Patients may have papilledema. The CT scan may reveal small ventricles and an enlarged cisterna magna. Lumbar puncture will reveal an opening pressure greater than 20 cm H_2O, with normal protein, glucose, and cell count. Therapy includes serial lumbar punctures to relieve acute symptoms and acetazolamide to reduce the formation of cerebrospinal fluid.

Hypertensive Encephalopathy

Severe elevation in blood pressure can cause headache and, if untreated, can result in the development of encephalopathy and seizures. This should be suspected in a patient with a severe headache whose diastolic blood pressure is greater than the 95th percentile for age. In young children, the development of hypertension is often secondary to fulminant glomerulonephritis. In severe cases, hypertension can result in cardiac dysfunction.

The blood pressure is checked in all extremities to evaluate the potential for coarctation of the aorta. The laboratory evaluation includes urinalysis to look for blood, protein, or casts, serum electrolytes, blood urea nitrogen, and creatinine.

Acute therapy in the emergency department is individualized, based upon the degree of hypertension and the underlying disorder. Patients with encephalopathy and seizures require rapid reduction of blood pressure with an agent such as nitroprusside.

Acute Hemorrhage

The child presenting with a severe headache of sudden onset, with or without neck or back pain, may have suffered an intracranial hemorrhage. The patient's mental status can range from normal to coma. Focal findings may or may not be present. Spontaneous intracranial hemorrhage usually results from either a ruptured aneurysm or an arteriovenous malformation. It can also occur in association with coagulopathies. The diagnosis and management are further discussed in Chap. 42.

Meningitis/Encephalitis/Brain Abscess

The association of headache with a fever and stiff neck implies an infectious etiology, such as meningitis, encephalitis, or brain abscess. If there are no focal findings or signs of increased intracranial pressure on physical examination, a lumbar puncture is performed. If there are focal neurologic abnormalities or signs of increased intracranial pressure, a brain abscess is possible, and a CT scan of the brain is performed prior to a lumbar puncture to avoid herniation. Management depends upon the specific diagnosis.

VASCULAR HEADACHES

Migraine headaches are due to vasoconstriction followed by vasodilatation of cerebral blood vessels. There is a positive family history in 70 to 90 percent of cases. Males are more commonly affected until puberty, when females become more predisposed.

Migraines tend to be recurrent. The headache tends to be unilateral, throbbing, or pulsating; is often associated with nausea and vomiting; and is relieved with sleep. Migraines are classified as classic, common, and complex.

A classic migraine headache is preceded by an aura. Visual symptoms include scotomas, blurring, and abnormalities in the perception of lights. Somatosensory disturbances may consist of abnormal smells and distorted perception of images. The aura can be very brief or may last for up to an hour. It is followed by the patient's typical headache.

The common migraine is most common in children. It is differentiated from the classic migraine by the lack of a definable aura. However, the child will often complain of malaise or nausea prior to the onset of the headache.

A complex migraine is associated with transient neurologic disturbances, which include opthalmoplegia and hemiparesis. The deficits resolve spontaneously.

A vascular headache that is common in childhood is the basilar artery migraine, which results in ataxia and vertigo, at times accompanied by visual disturbances. "Confusional" migraines can cause an altered level of consciousness. The "Alice in Wonderland" syndrome is a migraine variant that results in distortion of spatial relationships.

The emergency department treatment of migraines consists primarily of providing analgesia during the acute attack. Long-term management can consist of vasoconstricting agents such as caffeine and ergotamines. In some cases, propanolol has been of benefit.

FUNCTIONAL HEADACHES

Muscle Contraction (Tension) Headache

Muscle contraction headaches tend to be chronic and nonprogressive in nature, with the pain described as bandlike, bilateral, or generalized. There is no accompanying aura, and nausea is rare. Tension headaches can last for days or weeks but do not interfere with normal activities.

Muscle contraction headaches are managed with analgesics, such as acetaminophen and ibuprofen. Reassuring the family that the problem is not organic and advising the patient to avoid precipitating factors such as stress are important parts of therapy. In some cases, treatment with amitriptyline is of benefit.

Psychogenic Headaches

Psychogenic headaches tend to be chronic and nonprogressive and are characterized by vague complaints and nonspecific symptoms. They may result from stress, adjustment reactions, conversion reactions, depression, and malingering.

OTHER CAUSES

Included in this group are problems that originate outside the calvarium but that can result in headache, either directly or through referred pain. They include sinusitis, dental abscess, pharyngitis, temporomandibular joint abnormalities, and ophthalmologic problems. Toxic exposures, especially carbon monoxide, can also cause headache.

For a more detailed discussion, see Fuchs S: Headache, chap. 39, p. 244, in *Pediatric Emergency Medicine: A Comprehensive Study Guide.*

40 Hydrocephalus

Susan Fuchs

Hydrocephalus is the excess accumulation of cerebrospinal fluid (CSF). The excess fluid results in swelling of the lateral ventricles and, in most cases, elevated intracranial pressure. A blockage of CSF at any point from its formation in the lateral ventricles to its absorption in the arachnoid villi can result in hydrocephalus.

Hydrocephalus is classified as noncommunicating or communicating. In the noncommunicating form, obstruction blocks the flow of CSF from the lateral ventricles to the point at which it is absorbed into the circulation. Ventriculomegaly occurs rostral to the site of obstruction. Common etiologies of obstruction include aqueductal stenosis, tumors, and congenital malformations, such as Dandy-Walker syndrome. Communicating hydrocephalus is characterized by decreased absorption of CSF. It is most often due to subarachnoid hemorrhage, meningitis, or elevated CSF protein.

CLINICAL PRESENTATION

The clinical presentation of hydrocephalus depends on the age of the patient and the rate at which it develops. Infants with hydrocephalus are often diagnosed when a head circumference disproportionate to age or splitting of the cranial sutures is found during a routine examination. The unfused sutures of the infant allow the calvarium to expand. When the limitations of suture expansion are reached, intracranial pressure begins to rise precipitously, and the infant may experience irritability, poor feeding, or other behavioral changes. When intracranial pressure becomes severely elevated, the infant develops vomiting and lethargy, which can signal impending herniation. The physical examination may also reveal a bulging anterior fontanelle and engorged scalp veins. Dysfunction of cranial nerve III may result in loss of upward gaze or the "sundown" sign.

Older children with hydrocephalus will usually complain of headache, which is often progressive in nature, is worst in the morning, awakens the patient from sleep, and is exacerbated by lying down or straining. The child may suffer visual symptoms that are difficult to specify. Gait disturbances can occur, especially ataxia. Like infants, older children develop vomiting as intracranial pressure begins to become severely elevated. Papilledema is a late finding.

MANAGEMENT

In the emergency department, the primary goal of management of the child with hydrocephalus is the assessment and control of elevated intracranial pressure. Patients may be in imminent danger of herniation. Patients who are lethargic on presentation, those with a Glascow Coma Scale score of less than 8, or those who deteriorate in the emergency department are intubated following rapid sequence sedation. Prior to intubation, hyperventilation with a bag-valve-mask device to attain a P_{CO_2} between 24 and 26 torr may reduce intracranial pressure enough to avert herniation. Patients who do not respond to hyperventilation with an improved mental status may benefit from diuretic therapy with mannitol (0.25 to 1 g/kg) or Lasix (1 mg/kg). It is appropriate to elevate the head of the bed to 25 to 30°.

After the patient is stabilized, computed tomography of the brain is performed to define the lesion and plan definite treatment. Therapy usually includes placement of an intraventricular shunt by a neurosurgeon. In dire circumstances, a percutaneous ventricular tap may be performed.

For a more detailed discussion, see Fuchs S: Hydrocephalus, chap. 40, p. 247, in *Pediatric Emergency Medicine: A Comprehensive Study Guide.*

---

41 Cerebral Palsy

Susan Fuchs

Cerebral palsy is a neurologic syndrome associated with a combination of birth asphyxia and prenatal factors. It is fundamentally a disorder of motor function and is often accompanied by intellectual impairment.

CLINICAL PRESENTATION

The major abnormality is of muscle tone. The infant gradually progresses from hypotonia to spasticity. The term *spastic cerebral palsy* refers to several variants, including spastic quadriparesis, spastic diplegia, and spastic hemiplegia.

Spastic quadriparesis is characterized by a generalized increase in muscle tone. The upper extremities are generally more affected, but in severe forms, the child assumes a posture of decerebrate rigidity. Many children have pseudobulbar involvement, resulting in swallowing difficulties and recurrent aspiration. Intellectual impairment is severe, and half have generalized seizures.

Spastic diplegia is characterized by bilateral spasticity, with greater involvement of the lower extremities. As spasticity progresses, flexion of the hips and knees develops, leading to contractures. Other manifestations include convergent strabismus, delayed speech development, and seizure disorders. Intellectual impairment parallels the motor deficit.

Spastic hemiparesis is a unilateral paresis that usually affects the upper extremity more than the lower. Some degree of spasticity and flexion contracture usually results. The extent of functional impairment varies, with fine movements of the hand affected most. Sensory impairment, growth disturbance, and involuntary movements of the affected limbs can occur. In addition, facial weakness, visual disturbances, and focal seizures are common.

Some children develop an extrapyramidal form of cerebral palsy characterized by choreoathetoid movements of the hands and feet. These children tend to have persistence of primitive reflexes, such as the tonic neck and Moro reflexes, to a more significant degree than patients with the spastic form.

COMPLICATIONS

The most common problem concerning the emergency department management of cerebral palsy is the treatment of breakthrough seizures. The management of seizures is discussed in Chap. 35.

Respiratory difficulties are common in patients with cerebral palsy. Chronic aspiration can result in reactive airway disease and, in some patients, chronic hypoxia and hypercarbia. Aspiration pneumonia is common and is often difficult to diagnose in patients whose baseline chest radiographs are abnormal. Most patients with aspiration pneumonia require admission. The management of patients with bronchospasm includes aggressive therapy with bronchodilators.

Many children with cerebral palsy have significant feeding difficulties that require placement of a gastrostomy tube. Malfunction can result in the inability to deliver feedings and medications, which predisposes to dehydration and subtherapeutic levels of anticonvulsants. In cases where the tube needs to be replaced, correct positioning is confirmed by an abdominal radiograph, accompanied by the injection of radioopaque contrast.

Many patients with cerebral palsy who are significantly impaired are not toilet-trained and are vulnerable to urinary tract infections and perineal skin breakdown that can result in cellulitis. All febrile cerebral palsy patients without an obvious source of infection require a urinalysis and urine culture.

While there is no cure for cerebral palsy, an important goal of emergency department management is assuring that the child is receiving adequate overall therapy through a multidisciplinary approach.

For a more detailed discussion, see Fuchs S: Cerebral palsy, chap. 41, p. 249, in *Pediatric Emergency Medicine: A Comprehensive Study Guide.*

---

42 Cerebrovascular Syndromes

Susan Fuchs

Compared with adults, children rarely suffer from cerebral vascular accident (CVA) or stroke. Those CVAs that occur in children are often associated with congenital lesions. Cerebrovascular accidents are either ischemic, and associated with the occlusion of a blood vessel supplying part of the brain, or hemorrhagic, stemming from rupture of a blood vessel and subsequent bleeding into brain tissue.

ISCHEMIC STROKE

Disease states associated with ischemic stroke in children include sickle cell disease, systemic lupus erythematosus, and congenital heart disease. Cerebral thrombosis is especially common in young children with severe cyanotic heart disease and secondary polycythemia. Mitral valve prolapse and bacterial endocarditis are fairly common cardiac lesions associated with embolic stroke.

A common metabolic condition associated with venous thrombosis is severe dehydration, especially when accompanied by hypernatremia. A primary vascular condition associated with recurrent strokes is moyamoya disease, which is characterized by diffuse narrowing of multiple cerebral vessels. It can present with repeated transient ischemic attacks.

A syndrome of sudden onset of stroke in childhood is referred to as *acute infantile hemiplegia*. It is often preceded by a focal seizure, which is followed by unilateral flaccid paralysis. The hemiplegia can mimic Todd paralysis, a transient loss of motor function that follows seizures. The most commonly affected arteries are the internal carotid or middle cerebral. The cause is unknown.

HEMORRHAGIC STROKE

The majority of hemorhagic strokes are due to congenital vascular lesions. These include aneurysms of the middle cerebral artery, vertebrobasilar system, or carotid bifurcation and also arteriovenous malformations (AVMs). In children, AVMs are the most common lesion associated with spontaneous hemorrhage. Hemorrhagic strokes are occasionally associated with systemic diseases, especially coagulopathies. These conditions are summarized in Table 42-1.

DIAGNOSIS

History

The presenting signs and symptoms of a stroke are usually of rapid onset. Patients often suffer sudden collapse or loss of focal neurologic function. A history of recurrent headaches, transient ischemic attacks, or focal seizures may be elicited. Any history of trauma is significant and suggests a hemorrhagic lesion. Adolescents in particular are questioned regarding illicit drug ingestion, particularly cocaine.

Physical Examination

Complete vital signs include temperature and blood pressure. If trauma is suspected, the head and neck are immobilized. A thorough examination includes auscultation over the head, eyes, and carotid arteries, listening for bruits, as well as auscultation of the heart for murmurs or clicks suggestive of valvular disease. The eyes are examined for extraocular movements and pupillary responses, and, if possible, visual field testing is done. The eyes will look toward the lesion if the cerebral hemisphere is involved but away with brainstem involvement. The skin is examined for petechiae, café au lait spots, or neurofibromas.

Neurologic assessment includes determination of degree of weakness, cranial nerve dysfunction, the side affected, and the extent to which the extremities are involved. Involvement of the basal ganglia, thalamus, or cerebral hemispheres can result in aphasia.

Some disorders that can be confused with a stroke include com-

TABLE 42-1 Factors Associated with Strokes in Children

Cardiac
- Cyanotic heart disease
- Rheumatic heart disease
- Bacterial endocarditis
- Arrhythmias
- Cardiomyopathy
- Prosthetic heart valves
- Mitral valve prolapse
- Cocaine

Infection
- Meningitis
- Encephalitis

Vasculopathy
- Moyamoya disease

Systemic disorders
- Systemic lupus erythematosus
- Periarteritis nodosa
- Nephrotic syndrome
- Inflammatory bowel disease

Hematologic disorders
- Sickle cell disease
- Protein S deficiency
- Protein C deficiency
- Antithrombin III deficiency
- Polycythemia
- Hemolytic uremic syndrome
- Thrombotic thrombocytopenic purpura
- Hemophilia
- Disseminated intravascular coagulation
- Idiopathic thrombocytopenia purpura
- Vitamin K deficiency
- Anticoagulation treatment
- Leukemia
- Aplastic anemia

Vascular malformations
- Arteriovenous malformations
- Aneurysms

Trauma
- Head injury
- Carotid dissection
- Intraoral trauma
- Fat embolism

Drugs
- Oral contraceptives
- Antineoplastic agents
- LSD
- Amphetamines
- Cocaine

Metabolic disorders
- Homocystinuria
- Hypoglycemia
- Mitochondrial encephalomyopathy (MELAS)

Neurocutaneous syndromes
- Neurofibromatosis
- Sturge-Weber syndrome
- Tuberous sclerosis

plicated migraines, partial seizures, Todd paralysis, brain tumors, brain abscesses, and subdural hematoma.

Laboratory Evaluation

Baseline laboratory studies include a complete blood count with differential and platelet count, prothrombin time, and partial thromboplastin time. If sickle cell disease is a possibility, a sickle prep and hemoglobin electrophoresis are performed. Further coagulation studies are indicated if hemophilia or other coagulopathies, such as protein S, protein C, or antithrombin III deficiencies, are suspected. Electrolytes, blood urea nitrogen, creatinine, glucose, and sedimentation rate are obtained, as well as urinalysis looking for red cells or protein. Additional studies, such as antinuclear antibodies, drug screens, lipid profile, blood culture, urine culture, and amino acids, are ordered as warranted. Electrocardiography and echocardiography are performed on all children in whom underlying heart disease is suspected.

Imaging studies provide information that will help differentiate an ischemic from a hemorrhagic stroke. A computed tomographic (CT) scan is superior to magnetic resonance imaging (MRI) in detecting acute hemorrhage (<12 h), but MRI is superior in detecting an infarct. The CT scan may also miss small hemorrhages, AVMs, or aneurysms. A useful sequence is a CT without contrast followed by an MRI. When the etiology of the stroke is not clear after imaging studies, an angiogram should be considered.

In patients in whom a hemorrhagic stroke is possible and in whom the CT scan is negative, a lumbar puncture is indicated. Particularly with a small subarachnoid hemorrhage, the CT scan may not reveal blood. The cerebrospinal fluid (CSF) is evaluated for the presence of red blood cells, which, in the absence of a traumatic lumbar puncture, indicate hemorrhage. In some cases of hemorrhage, the CSF may appear xanthochromic. A lumbar puncture is not performed until a CT scan or careful physical examination rules out increased intracranial pressure.

TREATMENT

The key role of the emergency department (ED) is stabilization of the patient's respiratory and cardiovascular status, especially the blood pressure. In the event of an ischemic infarct, a precipitous decline in blood pressure is avoided, since it can worsen cerebral ischemia. If hypotension is present, careful fluid resuscitation and inotropic support may be needed. If there are signs of impending herniation, mannitol (1 g/kg over 20 min) may be required. Specific therapy depends on the etiology of the stroke. In patients with sickle cell disease, exchange transfusion is indicated for ischemic stroke (see Chap. 71). Anticoagulants and steroids both have a role in certain circumstances, but are rarely indicated in the ED.

DISPOSITION

Children who have suffered strokes are admitted to an intensive care setting for close monitoring of blood pressure, fluid status, temperature, and neurologic function.

For a more detailed discussion, see Fuchs S: Cerebrovascular syndromes, chap. 42, p. 251, in *Pediatric Emergency Medicine: A Comprehensive Study Guide.*

SECTION VI
INFECTIOUS EMERGENCIES

43 The Febrile Child

Matthew Wols / Suchinta Hakim

Fever is most often defined as a rectal temperature greater than or equal to 38.0°C (100.4°F). Oral and skin temperatures are lower than rectal temperatures by 0.6°C (1°F) and 1°C (2 to 2.5°F), respectively. Oral temperatures are not recommended in young children, and skin temperatures obtained from the axilla or forehead are unreliable. Tympanic membrane temperatures are lower than rectal temperatures.

Fever most commonly occurs as a response to infection but may be due to immune-mediated or collagen vascular disease and is associated with many malignancies. During infection, moderate fever is probably beneficial, because it enhances host defense reactions. Rapidly rising temperature, however, is associated with febrile convulsions; hyperprexia, defined as a core temperature greater than 41.1°C (106°F) can result in complications such as central nervous system damage and rhabdomyolysis.

About 20 percent of pediatric patients presenting to the emergency department (ED) have fever as a sign or symptom. A vast majority of these patients have benign illnesses that are caused by viruses and are therefore self-limited or result from bacterial infections that are amenable to outpatient therapy. A small percentage of patients suffer from life-threatening infections.

The approach to fever in the pediatric patient is age-dependent. Neonates and young infants are deficient in the ability to localize and neutralize bacterial infections. The exact age groups are arbitrary and are not based on a scientific understanding of the immune response. Rather, the management of the febrile child is based on cumulative clinical experience and a growing body of research that is challenging traditional treatment. The exact age at which the developing immune system reaches adequate maturity is unknown. For example, how is a 3-week-old different from an 8-week-old in its ability to handle bacteremia? It is also important to realize that, while predictable bacterial organisms tend to affect different age groups, there is a significant crossover. For example, pneumococcus is usually associated with infants older than 2 to 3 months of age but can occur in a 1-month-old. Conversely, group B *Streptococcus,* usually a pathogen in neonates, has been reported in a 5-month-old infant.

THE AGE GROUPS

Neonates below 28 days of age are susceptible to organisms from maternal flora, especially group B *Streptococcus* and *Listeria monocytogenes.* They mount febrile responses poorly. The height of the fever does not necessarily correlate with the severity of the illness. Because they localize bacterial infections poorly, any bacterial infection may disseminate and result in serious bacterial infection (SBI).

Infants between 28 days and 2 to 3 months of age constitute the next major category. Environmentally acquired encapsulated organisms become the chief pathogens from this period throughout the rest of childhood. The traditional ED approach to febrile infants in this age group has been an aggressive search for bacterial illness, followed by hospitalization and empiric antibiotic therapy until cultures of blood, cerebrospinal fluid (CSF), and urine were negative. Management now includes an effort to define a group of low-risk patients who may be candidates for outpatient management.

Patients between 3 and 36 months of age constitute the final major category. The immune system has matured to the extent that disseminated infection from a bacterial focus is much less likely. However, up to 5 percent of patients in this age group with temperatures above 39°C who appear well and have no focus of infection on physical examination will have positive blood cultures—occult bacteremia. The management of these patients is a subject of controversy and ongoing investigation.

After 36 months of age, the management of the nonimmunocompromised febrile pediatric patient is similar to that of the healthy adolescent and adult.

PRESENTATION

The history of the present illness is obtained from the person most familiar with the patient, usually the mother. Observation of the infant or toddler during the history provides a wealth of information and may be useful in differentiating the "sick" or "not sick" patient.

Important information includes the time of onset of the fever and the method of taking the temperature. Temperatures measured by a thermometer may be more accurate than a history that the patient "felt warm." Prior treatment is also important, since antipyretic therapy may result in a normal temperature in the patient with a serious febrile illness. Inappropriate treatment, such as bundling a febrile infant or sponging with alcohol, may also be elicited; the caretaker can then be educated on the proper management of fever.

The caretaker is questioned regarding his or her perception of the severity of the patient's illness. Helpful information in neonates and infants includes the patient's level of activity, feeding, and interaction with the environment. In older patients, a history of play activity is helpful. It is important to attempt to elicit a sense of the child's mental status, but it must be remembered that asking about the presence of "irritability" or "lethargy" introduces terminology into the history that may have a different meaning to the caretaker than to the physician.

The history of the patient's general behavior is followed by questions regarding associated symptoms. A large percentage of infectious illnesses in the pediatric patient population involve the respiratory tract. The combination of rhinorrhea, cough, and sore throat suggests upper respiratory involvement. Acute otitis media is often associated with these symptoms. Infection involving the lower respiratory tract is often characterized by a history of coughing, wheezing, or "noisy breathing." In neonates and infants, difficulty in bottle feeding is the equivalent of dyspnea on exertion and implies significant respiratory distress. Especially in infants, overwhelming infection can cause apnea, which parents may perceive as difficulty breathing. It is important to realize that apnea can be intermittent and that the patient may appear stable between episodes.

Gastrointestinal symptoms are also common in the febrile pediatric patient. Vomiting and diarrhea usually indicate an infectious process involving the gastrointestinal tract. However, they can also occur as nonspecific findings in other infections, including otitis media and pyelonephritis, and may occur in association with life-threatening infections such as meningitis and overwhelming sepsis. Frequency and character of the vomitus or stool are important. Stool that contains blood is associated with bacterial enteritis, which in neonates and young infants is a potentially serious infection.

The caretaker may also be aware of skin or musculoskeletal manifestations of the patient's illness. Many infections and inflammatory diseases are associated with rashes, some of which are transient and whose presence may be obtained only by a careful history. Musculoskeletal manifestations of infectious and inflammatory illnesses associated with fever include arthritis, arthralgia, and in some cases a history of refusal to walk or use a limb.

A history of the patient's exposure to an individual with a similar illness is an important clue obtained in the history. Many infectious illnesses are highly contagious and affect multiple members of a household. They range in severity from the benign common cold to serious diseases such as tuberculosis. It is also important to document the patient's immunization history. While immunizations provide significant protection from many deadly diseases, complications associated with them can prompt an ED visit. These include a febrile reaction that often occurs following a diptheria-pertussis-tetanus (DPT) vaccine and a mild measleslike illness, which can occur after immunization with measles-mumps-rubella (MMR) vaccine.

It is also essential to elicit a history of medications used during both the current and any recent febrile illness. In addition to antipyretics, patients may be taking antibiotics either prescribed by a physician or left over from past infectious illness in either the patient or siblings. Inappropriate treatment with antibiotics may mask symptoms of serious disease, as in the case of partially treated meningitis. Knowledge of prior therapy is also necessary in deciding current treatment in such cases as recurrent or resistant otitis media.

PHYSICAL EXAMINATION

It is impossible to overemphasize the importance of the general assessment in guiding the evaluation and management of the pediatric patient. The general assessment is in part a gestalt and results from a combination of observation, experience, and also "clinical judgment." But also, the general assessment should be based on objective information. Neonates and very young infants are difficult to assess, even in the most experienced hands. Attempts to apply reproducible scales of observation to this age group in order to predict the presence of serious bacterial illness have met with mixed results. While it is certain that an "ill-appearing" infant has a relatively high probability of having an SBI, a well appearance does not rule out serious illness.

The most important clinical tool is the mental status, evaluated by observing the patient's interaction with the environment and parents. Older infants and children should recognize their parents and demonstrate curiosity about their surroundings. After 5 to 6 months of age, "stranger anxiety" is appropriate and is not to be construed as irritability. In younger infants, the presence of a social smile is an important finding that implies well-being. In neonates too young to have developed a social smile, the baby's state of alertness and desire to bottle-feed are noted. Virtually all pediatric patients should be consolable. Patients who are inconsolable or appear worse when held or rocked by their parents are truly irritable, which may indicate a central nervous system infection. Anxiousness, listlessness, or lethargy are also signs of serious illness. Noting the quality of a neonate's or infant's cry can also provide adjunctive information regarding the patient's mental status. A strong, lusty cry is normal, while a weak or high-pitched cry may indicate distress.

The patient's hydration and perfusion are also assessed. In a febrile patient in whom peripheral perfusion is diminished but who has no history compatible with fluid loss, septic shock is likely. In practice, most patients with significantly decreased perfusion will have depressed mental status.

Finally, it is important to realize that depressed mental status and signs of impaired perfusion can be intermittent. The cardiovascular system is able to compensate until late in the course of an overwhelming infection. A parent may give a history of an ashen, mottled, or apneic infant at home. Occasionally such patients respond to stimulation alone and may appear relatively well on arrival in the ED. Conversely, a patient who appeared well on arrival in the ED may suddenly appear to decompensate, only to respond in such a way to stimulation or fluid resuscitation that the presence of serious illness is questioned. Any febrile pediatric patient with a history of even a momentary decrease in mental status or perfusion is presumed to have an overwhelming infection.

In the stable febrile patient, the general assessment is followed by search for a cause of the fever. The skin is evaluated for the presence of exanthems, localized erythema, or petechiae.

The examination of the head focuses on the anterior fontanelle. The eyes are evaluated for conjunctival infection or a discharge. Periorbital redness or swelling suggests cellulitis. All pediatric patients require a careful examination of the ears, since otitis media is the most common bacterial infection identified in this age group. The nose is examined for the presence of discharge. The oral cavity is evaluated for the presence of an enanthem, pharyngeal erythema, or tonsillar enlargement or exudate.

The neck is evaluated for adenopathy or other localized swelling. Localized neck swelling can occur in adenitis and with infection of branchial cleft or thyroglossal duct cysts. Neck suppleness should be determined, realizing that it may not be reliable in excluding meningitis.

The chest is evaluated for retractions, which, in the absence of stridor, indicate lower airway pathology. Auscultation may reveal wheezing, found in reactive airway disease and acute bronchiolitis. Rales are infrequently heard in pediatric patients, even in the presence of lobar pneumonia. Percussing the chest while listening with the stethoscope is more sensitive for determining an area of pneumonic consolidation than isolated abnormal breath sounds.

Muffled heart sounds in a febrile patient may indicate a purulent pericardial effusion, while a new or unexplained murmur may indicate infective endocarditis or an inflammatory process such as acute rheumatic fever.

The abdomen is evaluated for tenderness, guarding, or rebound, which may indicate a surgical problem, such as appendicitis. The size of the liver and spleen is evaluated, since many specific infectious illnesses are associated with hepatosplenomegaly.

The extremities are evaluated for erythema or swelling, range of motion, and limp. Both ostemyelitis and septic arthritis are more common in children than in adults, and early diagnosis is imperative to avoid morbidity.

MANAGEMENT

The Septic-Appearing or Toxic Child

The clinical manifestations of sepsis include poor feeding, decreased activity, somnolence, respiratory difficulty, or apnea, or parents may merely complain that the baby "is not acting right." The infant's failure to recognize its parents is an ominous sign that signifies impaired perfusion to the central nervous system. In most patients, there is fever. A small percentage will have a normal temperature or hypothermia. The physical examination may reveal decreased peripheral perfusion, including delayed capillary refill (> 2 s), cool, pale extremities, or diminished peripheral pulses. Blood pressure is an unreliable indicator of sepsis in children. In the initial stages, the blood pressure can be normal, the extremities warm, and the pulses bounding. As shock progresses, perfusion deteriorates. In the final stage, blood pressure falls. There may be tachypnea and tachycardia out of proportion to the degree of fever. Petechiae or purpura are ominious findings that suggest fulminant meningococcemia.

The successful treatment of sepsis is predicted on early recognition. Any potentially septic patient requires careful monitoring and strict attention to the maintenance of airway, breathing, and circulation. In relatively stable patients, supplemental oxygen and maintenance hydration may suffice. In unstable patients, intubation, mechanical ventilation, and aggressive circulatory support—including massive volume resuscitation, invasive monitoring, and the use of pressors—may be necessary. Antibiotic therapy is tailored to the specific situation; in healthy patients, however, it is predicated on age group–related pathogens. The management of septic shock is discussed more thoroughly in Chap. 3.

Febrile Infants Less Than 28 Days Old

The management of the febrile patient less than 28 days old is based on the assumption that the patient's immune system is inherently unable to localize and contain a bacterial infection, that any bacterial infection is therefore serious and potentially life-threatening, and that any febrile patient may suffer from a bacterial illness. Another fundamental assumption is that in this age group, even the most experienced clinician is unable to distinguish the patient in the early stages of sepsis from the patient with a benign febrile illness.

Febrile neonates are examined for a focus of fever. Most patients with a definable cause of fever will have otitis media, soft tissue infection, or evidence of bacterial enteritis, in which case *Salmonella* is a possible etiology. Blood-borne pathogens include group B *Streptococcus, Escherichia coli,* and *Listeria monocytogenes.* It is assumed that even patients with a focus of bacterial infection are bacteremic and have potentially seeded their cerebrospinal fluid (CSF).

The laboratory evaluation of the febrile neonate includes a complete blood count and cultures of the blood, CSF, and urine. It is imperative that the urine culture be obtained by catherization or by suprapubic tap, since a bag specimen is unreliable and can obscure the diagnosis. Patients with diarrhea or a history of bloody or mucoid stools require a stool culture. Stool microscopy is considered significant if there are more than 5 RBCs or WBCs per high-power field.

Treatment of the febrile patient below 28 days of age includes hospitalization and empiric therapy with ampicillin and an aminoglycoside until all cultures are negative.

FEBRILE INFANTS 28 DAYS TO 3 MONTHS OLD

Current data support the following approach to the well-appearing febrile patient between 28 days and 3 months of age. The child is evaluated for a focus of infection. Any bacterial infection is considered to be a serious bacterial infection (SBI). Infants with evidence of infection of the soft tissue, joint, or bone are admitted for appropriate antibiotic therapy. If no source of infection is found, laboratory data are obtained to differentiate the low from high risk infant. Low-risk criteria include a white blood cell (WBC) count between 5000 and 15,000/mm^3, a band count below 1500/

mm^3, a normal urinalysis, a normal CSF, and, in patients with diarrhea, stool microscopy with less than 5 WBCs per high-power field. White blood cells in the stool reflect the potential for *Salmonella* enteritis.

Infants who fulfill the low-risk criteria appear to have a very small probability of having a SBI (< 1 percent). Infants may be discharged from the ED provided that there is close patient follow-up. Empiric therapy with ceftriaxone, 50 mg/kg is begun. Patients receiving ceftriaxone return to the ED in 24 h for a second dose. Infants with positive cultures of the CSF are admitted for inpatient therapy. Those with positive blood cultures are treated on an individual basis.

Low-risk infants may also be discharged without antibiotic treatment. Close follow-up is necessary. Lumbar puncture may not be necessary, because empiric antibiotics are not used. This management option is most often employed by physicians in small practice settings with little laboratory backup and an established family rapport. If reliability is in question, the patient should be admitted.

INFANTS 3 TO 36 MONTHS OF AGE

Fever with a Focus of Infection

Certain focal bacterial infections are associated with bacteremia, including epiglottitis, buccal and periorbital cellulitis, and septic arthritis. The potential for bacteremia always mandates an aggressive workup, including blood cultures and occasionally lumbar puncture.

Other infections associated with bacteremia include those caused by *Staphylococcus aureus* and *Salmonella* enteritis. *Salmonella* enteritis is especially problematic in younger infants, where it can result in disseminated infection.

Fever without a Focus of Infection

This patient presents a true challenge to the ED physician. The major concern is occult bacteremia, which occurs primarily in patients with a temperature of 39°C or greater. Beyond 39°C, there is a direct correlation between the height of the fever and the probability of bacteremia, reported to be between 3 and 11 percent. All socioeconomic groups are equally affected.

The most common cause of occult bacteremia is *Streptococcus pneumoniae,* which accounts for about 85 percent of cases. The second most common is *H. influenzae* type B, which is dramatically decreasing since the introduction of conjugate *H. influenzae* type B (Hib) vaccine. *Neisseria meningitidis* accounts for about 3 percent of cases. The remainder are accounted for by a variety of organisms, including *Salmonella, S. aureus,* and *Streptococcus pyogenes.*

There is no laboratory test that can definitively diagnose bacteremia in the ED. The WBC count has some value as a screening test. The combination of a temperature above 40°C and a WBC > 15,000 mm^3 increases the probability of bacteremia from about 2.6 percent to 11 percent. The erythrocyte sedimentation rate and C-reactive protein have met with limited success and add little to the complete blood count. Urinary tract infections account for up to 7 percent of male patients less than 6 months of age and 8 percent of female infants less than 1 year of age who have fever without focus. Urine culture must be obtained from catheterization or suprapubic aspiration in order to avoid a contaminated culture. This is especially important, since up to 20 percent of pediatric patients with urinary tract infections will have an unremarkable urinalysis.

A lumbar puncture is indicated in any patient who appears toxic or has clinical findings consistent with meningitis. It is important to remember that in young infants, early meningitis can be extremely subtle, and a liberal approach toward lumbar punctures is indicated. This is especially true in the event that outpatient management with empiric antibiotic therapy is anticipated.

Chest x-rays are unlikely to be helpful in febrile pediatric patients without pulmonary findings, such as cough and tachypnea. Stool cultures are likely to be useful only in patients who have bloody diarrhea or more than 5 WBC per high-power field.

The management of the patient between 3 and 36 months of age who has fever without focus is controversial. Untreated bacteremia with *Pneumococcus* has a 6 percent risk of the subsequent development of meningitis. *Haemophilus influenzae,* carries risk of meningitis of up to 26 percent. Other potential secondary infections include septic arthritis, epiglottitis, and facial cellulitis. Although *Neisseria meningitidis* is an infrequent cause of bacteremia, up to half of affected patients develop meningitis or sepsis.

With at least some patients with occult bacteremia developing serious sequelae management algorithms have been devised. Treatment with parenteral antibiotics may be beneficial in preventing the development of meningitis in patients with occult bacteremia as compared with no treatment or treatment with oral antibiotics. Ceftriaxone covers *H. influenzae,* penetrates the CSF, and has a long half-life.

One option in the well-appearing patient with a temperature above 39°C is to obtain a screening complete blood count. If WBC count is above 15,000/mm^3 blood culture is sent. Male infants less than 6 months of age and females less than 2 years of age have a urinalysis and urine culture. Any patient who appears toxic has a lumbar puncture performed. Empiric therapy with ceftriaxone 50 mg/kg IM is then administered. Another potential strategy is to obtain a blood culture on all patients with a temperature above 39°C and initiate empiric therapy with ceftriaxone. This would result in a large number of patients at low risk of bacteremia receiving treatment, because of the lack of a screening WBC.

Patients who have blood cultures positive for *Neisseria* or *H. influenzae* should be recalled to the ED and hospitalized for treatment. If a lumbar puncture was not performed on the initial visit, it should be done on the patient's arrival. Children with a blood culture positive for *Pneumococcus* who are afebrile can receive a second dose of ceftriaxone and a follow-up course of oral penicillin if not resistant. Patients with pneumococcemia who have persistent fever or are ill-appearing require a repeat septic workup and admission for parenteral antibiotics.

Finally, there are some who feel that neither laboratory evaluation nor empiric antibiotic therapy are indicated in well-appearing febrile children with no focus of infection. All agree that regardless of the emergency department treatment, close follow-up is the most important factor in assuring a good outcome.

THE FEBRILE CHILD ABOVE 36 MONTHS OF AGE

Beyond 36 months of age, the immune system of the healthy child has developed to the point where disseminated bacterial infection is rare. Even bacteremic patients very uncommonly seed their meninges or develop full-blown sepsis. An exception to this is meningococcemia, which remains a serious disease throughout adulthood.

The older febrile child is evaluated for a focus of bacterial infection. Ancillary studies are indicated, depending on the clinical scenario. Examples include throat cultures in patients with pharyngitis and chest x-rays in patients with cough or objective pulmonary findings. Urinary tract infections are fairly common in young girls and can at times have somewhat atypical presentations, including vomiting and diarrhea. Thus a urinalysis is occasionally indicated. Blood counts and blood cultures are rarely indicated except in ill-appearing children. The majority of older febrile patients have viral illness and require no workup.

THE TREATMENT OF FEVER

Despite the tremendous frequency of the problem, treating fever remains controversial. While there is no doubt that extremely elevated temperatures (> 41°C) can be deleterious, the vast majority of patients with fever do well, and lowering the body temperature may obviate some of the potentially beneficial effects of fever.

Patients who require aggressive treatment include those with a history of febrile seizures and those who are physiologically unstable.

Pharmacologic therapy of fever consists of acetaminophen and nonsteroidal anti-inflammatory drugs (NSAIDs). Both normalize the temperature set point, by inhibiting prostaglandin synthesis.

Acetaminophen is an effective antipyretic, and is relatively free of side effects. The dose is 10 to 15 mg/kg every 4 h. An advantage of acetaminophen is that children are fairly tolerant of overdose.

Aspirin is also an effective antipyretic, but, due to a possible link with Reye syndrome, it is generally not recommended.

Ibuprofen has been increasingly used as an antipyretic in pediatric patients. It appears to be as effective as acetaminophen, with a slightly longer duration of action. Its use has not been linked to Reye syndrome. The dose is 10 mg/kg every 6 h.

Body temperature can also be reduced by external cooling, which in small children is easily done by bathing. Water temperature should be tepid and not cold enough to induce shivering. Parents should always be informed that sponging with alcohol is dangerous. Bathing or sponging should be combined with pharmacologic therapy.

For a more detailed discussion, see Wols M, Hakim, S: The febrile child, chap. 43, p. 255, in *Pediatric Emergency Medicine: A Comprehensive Study Guide.*

---

44 Meningitis

Steven Lelyveld

The pediatric population, particularly children under 5 years of age, accounts for almost three-quarters of the cases of bacterial meningitis reported each year in the United States. Over one-half of all cases of meningitis are aseptic. Prior to the introduction of the conjugated polysaccharide vaccines against *Haemophilus influenzae* type b (Hib), approximately two-thirds of bacterial cases beyond the neonatal period were caused by Hib, with a peak incidence between 2 months and 5 years. The remainder was divided between *Streptococcus pneumoniae* (20 to 25 percent) and *Neisseria meningitidis* (8 to 10 percent).

For children under 1 month of age, the predominant organisms are group B *Streptococcus, Escherichia coli, Enterococcus,* Hib, and *Listeria monocytogenes.*

Of the viral causes of meningitis, over 80 percent are seasonal enteroviruses, predominantly echovirus and coxsackievirus. Mumps, herpes, varicella, measles, and arboviruses all have been well described as central nervous system (CNS) pathogens.

Data since 1991 have indicated a dramatic decline in invasive Hib disease, with very little change in the incidence of other pathogens. In the 1980s, there were approximately 7000 cases of Hib meningitis per year. In 1994, there were only 313 cases of all invasive Hib disease reported in children under 5 years of age.

DIAGNOSIS

The "classic" symptoms of meningitis include headache, photophobia, stiff neck, change in mental status, bulging fontanelle, nausea, and vomiting (Table 44-1). The Brudzinski sign occurs when the irritated meninges are stretched, with neck flexion caus-

TABLE 44-1 Signs and Symptoms at Presentation

	Percent
Fever	>95
Lethargy	87–95
Vomiting	54–71
URI Symptoms	46–55
Seizures	22–23
Temperature >38.3°C	59–77
Altered mental status	53–78
ENT infection	22–42
Nuchal rigidity	54–59
Brudzinski's sign	10–13
Kernig's sign	9–11
Focal neurologic defect	5–6
Duration of symptoms	0–9 days

Source: Adapted from: Rothrock SG, Green SM, Wren J, et al: Pediatric bacterial meningitis. *Ann Emerg Med* 21:146–152, 1992.

ing the hips and knees to flex involuntarily. The Kernig sign of nerve root irritation is present when the hip is flexed to 90° and the examiner is unable to passively extend the leg fully.

The younger the child, the less obvious the signs and symptoms until late in the course of the disease. The resistance to flexion of the neck in the anteroposterior plane only is one of the most specific signs of meningitis. It is seen in less than 15 percent of children under 18 months of age.

Meningitis may take either an insidious (90 percent) or fulminant (10 percent) course. If insidious, the patient has a high likelihood of presenting to a physician days before diagnosis with a nonspecific illness. The range of duration of illness before diagnosis has been up to 2 weeks, with a median of 36 to 72 h. Such children run the risk of partial treatment.

When the diagnosis of meningitis is made, pretreated children have a lower frequency of fever and altered mental status and a longer duration of symptoms with more vomiting. Other signs and symptoms, as well as mortality, are not significantly different from those of untreated cases.

The more fulminant the course, the worse the prognosis. Both Hib and *Streptococcus pneumoniae* meningitis may be insidious or fulminant. Typically, meningococcal disease presents with a more fulminant course. Concomitant meningococcal bacteremia rapidly progresses to petechiae, purpura fulminans, and cardiovascular collapse. The management of any of the bacterial meningitides may be complicated by the Waterhouse-Friderichsen syndrome of hemorrhage into the adrenal cortex.

DIFFERENTIAL DIAGNOSIS

In the early phases, meningitis may be confused with a simple gastroenteritis, upper respiratory infection, otitis media, or other minor viral syndrome. As the alteration of mental status becomes more severe, the diagnoses of encephalitis, or subarachnoid/subdural hemorrhage with or without direct trauma or abuse, cerebral abscess, or Reye's syndrome must be considered. Toxic ingestions, seizure disorders, diabetic ketoacidosis, hypothyroidism, and other altered metabolic states may be initially confused for meningitis but do not have the same prodrome or fever. The young child with intussuception may present with vomiting, altered mental status, and cardiovascular collapse. Many of these children are evaluated for meningitis before their diagnosis is clear.

MANAGEMENT

When meningitis is suspected, the diagnostic test of choice is the lumbar puncture. However, it is imperative not to neglect the

ABC's (airway, breathing, circulation) while performing diagnostic procedures. Care must be taken to ensure proper oxygenation and cardiovascular stabilization. This is followed by antibiotic administration for the unstable patient. While appropriate parenteral antibiotics may prevent recovery of the organism on culture of cerebrospinal fluid (CSF), other ancillary tests at a later time will clarify the presence of meningitis.

The initial workup includes a complete blood count (CBC), electrolytes, glucose blood urea introgen (BUN), creatinine, and culture of blood. Countercurrent immunoelectrophoresis (CIE) or other bacterial antigen tests are helpful. Patients should be cooled or warmed to normal body temperature as necessary. If there is an alteration in mental status and a rapid test of glucose is unavailable, give dextrose 1 g/kg IV. Seizures must be controlled with a rapid-acting benzodiazepine (lorazepam 0.05 to 0.1 mg/kg/dose; diazepam 0.2 to 0.5 mg/kg/dose) while care is taken to respond to a potential respiratory arrest.

Once it is safe to do so, a lumbar puncture is performed. The expected laboratory data from this fluid is age-related (see Table 44-2).

A low white count with a predominantly mononuclear cell type, with normal glucose and protein, points to a viral etiology. High protein, low sugar, and elevated polymorphonuclear leukocytes (PMNs) point to a bacterial etiology.

Antibiotics are directed to the specific organisms, if known, or to the predominant organisms based on age of the patient.

Newborns are generally treated with a penicillin (ampicillin 100 to 200 mg/kg/day divided into 4 doses), and an aminoglycoside (gentamicin 2.5 mg/kg/dose). Based on local sensitivities, a cephalosporin active against gram-negative bacilli may be substituted for the aminoglycoside.

Infants and children are generally treated with a cephalosporin (ceftriaxone 100 mg/kg IM qd; or cefotaxime 75 mg/kg/dose tid). If the organism is known to be *Streptococcus pneumoniae,* penicillin is currently the drug of choice. However, the emergence of resistant strains has necessitated the use of vancomycin and other drugs.

The role of steroids in the management of meningitis is controversial. When given prior to the antibiotic, the anti-inflammatory effect of dexamethasone (0.15 mg/kg/dose IV q6h for 4 days) decreases intracranial pressure, cerebral edema, and CSF lactate concentrations. Dexamethasone significantly decreases hearing loss and other neurologic sequelae if the meningitis has been caused by Hib. However, these benefits have not been shown for other bacterial pathogens. In fact, the steroid effect may strengthen

TABLE 44-2 Normal CSF Values

	Preterm Infant	Term Infant	Child
Cell count	9 (0–25 WBC/mm^3), 57% PMN	8 (0–22 WBC/mm^3), 61% PMN	0–7 WBC/mm^3, 0% PMN
Glucose	24–63 (mean 50) mg/dL	34–119 (mean 52) mg/dL	40–80 mg/dL
CSF/blood glucose ratio	55–105%	44–128%	50%
Protein	65–150 (mean 115) mg/dL	20–170 (mean 90) mg/dL	5–40 mg/dL

the blood-brain barrier and limit the penetration of intravenously administered antibiotics into the CSF. This is a potential threat, as organisms resistant to penicillin and the cephalosporins emerge. With the decreased incidence of *Haemophilus influenzae* type b disease, the risks of steroids must be weighed carefully before they are given for meningitis of initially unclear bacterial etiology in children.

SEQUELAE

The vast majority of children with aseptic meningitis have a self-limited illness without subsequent problems. In spite of modern antibiotic treatment, the mortality of Hib meningitis is 5 to 10 percent and for *Streptococcus pneumoniae* meningitis, 20 to 40 percent. Up to one-fifth of survivors will have some long-term sequelae. These include mild learning defects, sensorineural hearing loss (10 percent), afebrile seizures (7 percent), and multiple neurologic defects including retardation and blindness (4 percent). Other neurologic defects may be present initially but resolve in a few months. These include transient hemiparesis (11 percent), ataxia (4 percent), cranial nerve palsy (3 percent), and extensor toes (3 percent). Fortunately, if the child is one of the majority of patients who survive their disease without permanent neurologic deficit, the subsequent risk of epilepsy has not been found to be increased over that of the general population.

For a more detailed discussion, see Lelyveld S: Meningitis, chap. 44, p. 263, in *Pediatric Emergency Medicine: A Comprehensive Study Guide.*

45 Toxic Shock Syndrome

Shabnam Jain

Toxic shock syndrome (TSS) is an acute febrile disease associated with a diffuse desquamating erythroderma, vomiting, abdominal pain, diarrhea, myalgia, and nonspecific neurologic abnormalities. It may progress rapidly to hypotension and multisystem dysfunction. The Centers for Disease Control have formulated a case

TABLE 45-1 Toxic Shock Syndrome: Criteria for Diagnosis

Fever:	Temperature ⩾38.9°C
Rash:	Diffuse macular erythroderma Subsequent desquamation, particularly of palms and soles
Hypotension:	Systolic blood pressure ⩽90 mmHg for adults For children <16 years old, systolic blood pressure below the fifth percentile for age Syncope

Involvement of three or more of the following organ systems clinically or by abnormal laboratory tests:

a. Gastrointestinal: Vomiting or diarrhea at onset of illness
b. Muscular: Severe myalgia or CPK greater than twice normal
c. Mucous membranes: Vaginal, conjunctival, or oropharyngeal hyperemia
d. Renal: BUN or serum creatinine greater than twice normal; pyuria in the absence of a urinary tract infection
e. Hematologic: platelet count $< 100{,}000/mm^3$
f. Hepatic: Evidence of hepatitis (total bilirubin, SGOT, or SGPT greater than twice normal)
g. Central nervous system: Disorientation without focal neurologic signs when fever and hypotension are absent

Negative results on the following tests, if obtained:

a. Blood, throat, or CSF culture
b. Serologic tests for Rocky mountain spotted fever, leptospirosis, or measles

definition (Table 45-1). In the absence of a definitive laboratory marker, the strict application of the case definition undoubtedly excludes the subclinical cases.

CLINICAL MANIFESTATIONS

The diagnosis of TSS is based on clinical manifestations (Table 45-1). There is a sudden onset of high fever associated with chills, vomiting, myalgia, dizziness, hypotension, and rash. Additional symptoms include headache, arthralgia, sore throat, abdominal pain, diarrhea, and stiff neck. There may be orthostatic dizziness or syncope. Diarrhea is profuse and watery, and there is protracted vomiting. The skin findings may be dramatic and present as a severe erythroderma and erythema of mucous membranes. The skin rash is diffuse and blanching. It fades within 3 days of its appearance and is followed by full-thickness desquamation.

In general, victims of TSS appear acutely ill. The physical examination may reveal hypotension or orthostatic decrease in systolic blood pressure by 15 mmHg. In the acute stage, which lasts 24 to 48 h, the patient may be agitated, disoriented, or obtunded. Hypermia of the conjunctiva and vagina is seen. Tender edematous external genitalia, diffuse vaginal erythema, scant purulent cervical discharge, and bilateral adnexal tenderness are seen in menstruation related TSS.

Between the fifth and tenth hospital day, a generalized pruritic maculopapular rash develops in about 25 percent of patients. In all cases, a fine generalized desquamation of the skin—with peeling over the soles, fingers, toes, and palms—occurs.

Abnormal laboratory values reflect the multisystem involvement in TSS. No specific laboratory test can make the diagnosis, but there are several frequently found abnormalities. Leukocytosis with an increase in immature forms is frequently seen. Platelet count may be low. Azotemia and abnormal urinary sediment are seen with the development of acute renal failure. Liver function tests frequently show some elevation of liver enzymes and bilirubin. Electrolyte abnormalities are variable. With severe hypotension, the patient may be acidotic. While clotting studies are usually normal or mildly prolonged, a few patients present with clinical evidence of coagulopathy. Cultures of blood, throat, and cerebrospinal fluid may be useful. Vaginal culture should be done, as well as culture from any identifiable focus of infection. Staphylococcis will be cultured from the cervix or vagina of more than 85 percent of patients with menstrual TSS. The majority of the above tests return to normal by 7 to 10 days after the onset of illness.

DIFFERENTIAL DIAGNOSIS

Several other systemic illnesses with fever, rash, diarrhea, myalgias, and multisystem involvement resemble TSS. Kawasaki disease is characterized by fever, conjunctival hyperemia, and erythema of the mucous membranes with desquamation. Although it is clinically similar, Kawasaki syndrome lacks many of the features of TSS, including diffuse myalgia, vomiting, abdominal pain, diarrhea, azotemia, thrombocytopenia, and shock. Kawasaki disease occurs typically in children under 5 years of age.

The clincial picture of staphylococcal scarlet fever is also very similar to that of TSS. Both illnesses are caused by toxin-producing *Staphylococcus.* Pathology specimens or serologic evidence of the exfoliation toxin differentiates the two entities.

Streptococcal scarlet fever is rare after the age of 10 years, and the "sandpaper" rash of scarlet fever is distinct from the macular rash of TSS.

Septic shock must always be considered in the differential diagnosis of TSS. The appearance of a rash and the laboratory abnormalities associated with TSS will aid in distinguishing these two entities.

MANAGEMENT

Management depends on prompt recognition as well as on the identification of the infectious focus. The focus must be drained and foreign material, such as nasal packing or retained tampon, promptly removed. Cultures should be obtained. Antibiotic therapy is not essential for recovery from the acute episode but is also important for eradication of the organism to reduce the recurrence rate. Beta-lactamase-resistant antistaphylococcal antibiotics, such as oxacillin or nafcillin, should be administered. Alternative antibiotics for patients who are allergic to penicillin include clindamycin, erythromycin, rifampin, and trimethoprim/sulfamethoxazole.

The remainder of therapy depends on the severity and extent of symptoms. The most important initial therapy is aggressive volume replacement. Crystalloids or fresh frozen plasma may be used for the management of hypotension, with pressors added if fluids alone are not sufficient.

Continuous monitoring of heart rate, blood pressure, respiratory rate, urinary output, central venous pressure, and pulmonary wedge pressure is required. As volume resuscitation progresses, chest radiographs, blood gases, and electrolytes must be followed. Thrombocytopenia may require platelet transfusions. If acute respiratory distress syndrome (ARDS) occurs, mechanical ventilation will become necessary.

Corticosteroids are recommended but have not conclusively been shown to affect outcome. There is some evidence that methylprednisone, 30 mg/kg, may reduce the severity of the illness if administered early. The majority of patients become afebrile and normotensive within 48 h of hospitalization. The erythema disappears within a few days and the muscle pain and weakness resolve in 7 to 10 days.

RECURRENCES

More than half of the patients not treated with beta-lactamase-resistant antibiotics have recurrences. Most recurrent episodes occur by the second month following the initial episode, on the same day of menses as the prior attack. In the majority of patients, the initial episode is the most severe. The prevention of the first episodes of TSS involves minimizing the use of high-absorbency tampons or the continuous use of tampons and identifying the factors associated with nonmenstrual episodes.

For a more detailed discussion, see Jain S: Toxin shock syndrome, chap. 45, p. 267, in *Pediatric Emergency Medicine: A Comprehensive Study Guide.*

---

46 Kawasaki Syndrome

Shabnam Jain

Kawasaki syndrome or mucocutaneous lymph node syndrome is an acute, self-limited, multisystem disease of unclear etiology. The diagnosis is based entirely on clinical features; there are no pathognomonic laboratory findings.

The disease may occur sporadically or in miniepidemics. In the United States, cases occur throughout the year, with a slight increase in the summer months. The peak incidence is in children 18 to 24 months of age, with 95 percent of cases occurring under the age of 10 years. It is more common in males, who also have a significantly higher mortality rate from this disease.

CLINICAL FINDINGS

Since there are no pathognomonic laboratory findings, the diagnosis is established clinically. Fever and at least four of five other clinical features (Table 46-1) are required in order to establish the diagnosis. However, all symptoms need not be present simultaneously, and they may vary in severity, time of onset, and duration. In addition, cases of atypical or incomplete Kawasaki syndrome are increasingly being reported, particularly in infants younger than six months. The course of the illness has been divided into three phases.

Acute or Febrile Phase

This phase lasts 7 to 15 days and is the period when most diagnostic clinical features are seen.

Fever is universal, often high, and usually sustained. It lasts 7 to 15 days (mean, 12 days) and is associated with extreme irritability. The fever is unresponsive to antibiotics or antipyretics.

TABLE 46-1 Diagnostic Criteria for Kawasaki Syndrome

1. Fever persisting for 5 or more days and
2. At least four of the following five findings:
   a. Bilateral painless bulbar conjunctival injection without exudate
   b. Mucous membrane changes of the upper respiratory tract, including injected dry, fissured lips, oral mucosal and pharyngeal injection, and "strawberry tongue"
   c. Changes in peripheral extremities, including erythema and edema of the hands and feet in the acute phase and periungual and generalized desquamation in the convalescent phase
   d. Polymorphous truncal exanthem
   e. Acute, nonpurulent cervical lymphodermopathy
3. Findings that cannot be explained by some other known disease process

Cervical adenopathy is another early feature. It is typically not very prominent. Involvement of the anterior cervical chain is most common and may be unilateral. The lymphadenopathy is nonsupportive and may disappear rapidly.

Bulbar conjunctivitis is bilateral, nonexudative, and usually quite prominent. It may persist for several weeks.

Mucocutaneous changes include bright red erythema of the lips, with cracking and peeling, a strawberry tongue (similar to that seen in scarlet fever), and hyperemia of the oral mucous membranes.

Cutaneous changes include rash and changes in peripheral extremities. They represent vasculitis of the small blood vessel and perivasculitis of the dermis and subcutaneous tissues. The rash is polymorphous and develops in most children. It may be morbilliform, maculopapular, or scarlatiniform, but vesiculation does not occur. The rash may actually vary in character from place to place in a single child. It is seen mostly on the trunk and may be prominent in the diaper area. It accompanies the fever throughout the entire acute phase of the disease and then gradually disappears.

Changes in the peripheral extremities occur within a few days of onset. There may be edema of the hands, fingers, feet, and toes, with induration of the dorsa of hands and feet and erythema on the palms and soles.

There are many other ancillary features and alternate presentations of Kawasaki disease. In fact, involvement of almost any system can occur. Relatively common at presentation and during the initial course are pneumonitis, tympanitis, diarrhea, meatitis and sterile pyuria, hepatitis, abdominal pain, arthritis, and arthralgias. Central nervous system involvement often presents as extreme irritability or, occasionally, as aseptic meningitis. These other clinical findings, although not diagnostic criteria, are helpful in supporting the diagnosis.

Subacute Phase

The subacute phase lasts approximately 2 to 4 weeks and begins with resolution of fever and elevation of platelet count. It ends with the return of platelet counts to near normal levels.

This phase is dominated by desquamation, which may have already begun before the disappearance of fever. Desquamation is a constant feature of Kawasaki syndrome. It appears first in the periungual region, with peeling underneath the finger- and toenails. It may also be prominent in the diaper area.

Thrombocytosis is another constant feature of the subacute phase, with platelet counts in the range of 500,000 to 3 million/mm^3. Thrombocytosis is rare in the first week of the illness, appears in the second week, peaks in the third week, and returns gradually to normal about a month after onset in uncomplicated illness.

It is during the subacute phase that complications such as coronary artery aneurysms and hydrops of the gallbladder develop.

Recovery or Convalescent Phase

This phase may last months to years. It is during this phase that coronary artery disease may first be recognized.

ANCILLARY DATA

Laboratory findings are nonspecific in Kawasaki syndrome. The complete blood count often shows elevated white blood cells with a left shift. A mild hemolytic anemia may be present. Platelet counts are elevated in the subacute phase but are usually normal in the acute phase. Acute-phase reactants (C-reactive protein and erythrocyte sedimentation rate) are markedly elevated. Urinalysis demonstrates moderate pyuria from urethritis. Bilirubinuria may occur as an early sign of hydrops of the gallbladder.

Chest radiographs may show evidence of pulmonary infiltrates or cardiomegaly. The electrocardiogram may show dysrhythmias, prolonged PR or QT intervals, and nonspecific ST-T wave changes. Two-dimensional echocardiography may demonstrate coronary artery dilatation or aneurysms, pericardial effusion, or decreased contractility.

COMPLICATIONS

Cardiovascular

The most serious manifestation of Kawasaki syndrome is cardiac involvement. This may result in coronary aneurysms, valvular insufficiency, congestive heart failure, myocardial infarction, dysrhythmias, rupture of aneurysms, and pericardial effusion. It usually occurs in the second week of the illness. Almost all of the early deaths and most of the long-term disabilities are related to involvement of the heart. Patients with Kawasaki syndrome have a 20 percent risk of developing coronary aneurysms in the absence of treatment. Those under 1 year of age at the onset of disease are at greater risk.

It is assumed that during the acute febrile phase of the disease, a pancarditis occurs, with a variable number of children developing coronary vasculitis and arthritis, with necrosis of blood vessel walls, aneurysm formation, or thrombosis. Aneurysm of the coronary arteries may be present at onset or begin as early as the second week of the illness. During the subacute phase, these aneurysms reach their peak development and are usually multiple.

Auscultation of the heart reveals gallop rhythms and distant heart sounds in 80 percent of patients. Rarely, a murmur of mitral regurgitation is heard. Cardiomegaly on chest roentgenography is seen in more than 30 percent of patients. Electrocardiographic changes are common and include low-voltage and ST depression in the first week of illness as well as PR promulgation, QTc prolongation, and ST elevation in the second and third weeks. Arrhythmias are rare and temporary.

Echocardiography is the most sensitive technique for delineating proximal coronary aneurysms; its diagnostic sensitivity is 80 to 90 percent. Angiography in selected cases may demonstrate lesions of the peripheral cardiac vessels, including narrowing and infarction. The left coronary artery is more commonly involved, and the proximal parts of the coronary arteries are involved more frequently. Aneurysms may be found in arteries other than the coronaries, including the subclavian, brachial, and axillary.

The most common cause of early death in Kawasaki syndrome is myocardial infarction, occurring in the subacute phase; it has been described in approximately 2.5 percent of reported cases. The child may die from infarction, coronary thrombosis, or rupture of an aneurysm. Late death may occur from coronary occlusive disease, rupture of an aneurysm several years after onset, or small blood vessel disease in the heart.

Hydrops of the Gallbladder

This is an acalculous cholecystitis and has been noted in the second phase of the illness. Hydrops is a self-limiting condition that occurs in 3 percent of patients and is a functional rather than an obstructive distension. These children present with abdominal pain; a soft, palpable mass in the right upper quadrant; and abdominal distension. Bilirubinemia may be an early sign of hydrops. Diagnosis can be made by ultrasonography.

Other Complications

These include iridocyclitis or anterior uveitis (in about 80 percent of patients), mastoiditis, necrotic pharyingitis, renal infarcts, gangrene of the fingers and toes, encephalopathy, and subarachnoid hemorrhage.

MANAGEMENT

All patients with Kawasaki syndrome should be hospitalized immediately for administration of intravenous gamma globulin (IVGG) and aspirin therapy as well as for cardiac evaluation. Routine laboratory tests include a complete blood count with platelets, urinalysis, electrolytes, liver profile, chest radiograph, electrocardiogram, and echocardiogram.

Bed rest, coupled with close cardiac monitoring, is essential. Only by detecting the initial signs of cardiac complications can appropriate critical measures be taken to save the life of a severely affected child.

Early in the course of the illness, IVGG may help to decrease the inflammatory response as well as the incidence of coronary artery aneurysm. The dose of IVGG is 2 g/kg infused over 8 to 12 h as a single dose or 400 mg/kg/day IV for 4 consecutive days.

Aspirin is another important therapeutic modality. Although it does not have an immediate antipyretic effect, aspirin can reduce the height and duration of fever and may serve as an important antithrombotic factor. It is given in a sequential dosage regimen: high-dose (100 mg/kg/day divided into four doses), followed by low-dose (3 to 5 mg/kg/day as a single daily dose). Aspirin is continued until the platelet count has normalized. Salicylate levels should be monitored during therapy.

Corticosteroids are contraindicated in Kawasaki syndrome.

For a more detailed discussion, see Jain S: Kawasaki syndrome, chap. 46, p. 270, in *Pediatric Emergency Medicine: A Comprehensive Study Guide.*

47 Common Parasitic Infestations

Steven Lelyveld

HISTORY

The child's oral exploratory behavior and poor capacity to avoid arthropods place him or her at particular risk for acquiring parasites. Other important factors in the patient's history include camping trips; travel to regions with questionable sanitation and water purification practices or a warm climate; method of food acquisition and preparation; exposure to pets and other animals, both domestic and wild; participation in day care or other confined situations; adolescent drug abuse; homosexual contacts or sexual abuse; and blood transfusions.

SYMPTOMS

The three groups of parasites causing human disease are protozoa, helminths, and arthropods. Helminths are subclassified into nematodes (roundworms), cestodes (flatworms), and trematodes (flukes).

Virtually all organ systems are at risk for infestation, with symptomatology related to the dysfunction induced. Arthropods are predominantly surface dwellers. They cause pruritus and rash. Nematodes and cestodes infest the gut, producing diarrhea, pain, and nutritional derangement. Along with trematodes, the other helminths may migrate to the lungs and solid organs. Protozoa may live in the gut for generations, shedding cysts in the stool. Like helminths, they can also, under proper circumstances, travel throughout the body. Some parasites produce symptoms months to years after the first exposure. In addition, the symptoms produced are dependent on the stage of the parasitic life cycle. Thus, it can be seen that the varied and nonspecific symptoms produced place parasitic infestation on the expanded differential diagnosis of most patients presenting to the emergency department. The challenge to the pediatric emergency physician is, therefore, to be aware of the patterns of worldwide distribution of these organisms and the symptoms they produce. It is important not to overlook this possibility when treating large numbers of patients with common complaints.

NEMATODES (ROUNDWORMS)

Ascaris lumbricoides is the largest human nematode. While it is most commonly found in tropical and subtropical climates, it is present throughout the United States. Upon ingestion, the egg hatches in the small intestine. The larvae burrow through the gut mucosa, enter the bloodstream, and migrate to the lungs. They cause shortness of breath, hemoptysis, eosinophilia, fever, and Löffler's pneumonia as they break through the alveoli, migrate up the bronchial tree, and are swallowed. Maturing to the adult form, *A. lumbricoides* can live freely in the small intestine for up to a year, shedding eggs in the stool. In this stage it may remain asymptomatic or cause gastrointestinal symptoms, including pain, protein malabsorption, biliary duct or bowel obstruction, and appendicitis. While stool testing for ova is diagnostic, serologic hemagglutination and flocculation tests are available. Mebendazole (100 mg bid for 3 days) or pyrantel pamoate (11 mg/kg once; maximum 1 g) is curative. If multiple infestations are present, it is recommended that *Ascaris* be treated first, as treatment of other parasites may stimulate a large worm burden to migrate simultaneously, causing obstruction.

Enterobius vermicularis (pinworm) is present in all parts of the United States. The most common presentation is that of a toddler or small child with anal itch. The egg is oval, approximately 50 by 25 μm in size. It is inhaled or ingested and hatches between the ileum and ascending colon, growing to an adult length of 3 to 10 mm. The adult may live and copulate in the colon for 1 to 2 months. The gravid female migrates to the anus, where it deposits embryonated eggs, usually during early morning hours. When the host stirs, the adult will migrate back into the body, causing symptoms of pruritus ani, dysuria, enuresis, and vaginitis. Scratching and hand-mouth behavior reinoculates the host, and the cycle repeats.

Scotch tape—placed sticky side to perianal skin when the child first awakens and then viewed under low power—is diagnostic. Treatment is with pyrantel pamoate (11 mg/kg) or mebendazole (100 mg). Each drug is given as a single dose, with a repeat given 2 weeks later to remove secondary hatchings.

Trichinella spiralis is found throughout the United States, with increasing prevalence in the Northeast and mid-Atlantic states. While fewer than one hundred cases of clinical disease are reported annually, cysts are found at autopsy in the diaphragms of 4 percent of patients. Current control efforts include laws governing the feeding of swine destined for sale to the public, specifically the heat treatment of garbage used as feed, and recommendations for the preparation of meat in the home.

Digestive enzymes liberate the encysted larvae, which lodge in the duodenum and jejunum, grow, and, within 2 days, mature and copulate. The females give birth to living larvae that bore through the mucosa, become bloodborne, and migrate to striated muscle, heart, lung, and brain. Host defenses produce inflammation at each site. While a classic triad of fever, myalgia, and periorbital edema has been described, symptoms of gastroenteritis, pneumonia, myocarditis, meningitis, and seizures can occur.

While most cases are mild and self-limited, the history and physical—along with elevation of muscle enzymes and eosinophilia—may suggest further investigation. Serologic tests are available from the Centers for Disease Control. Muscle biopsy is confirmative.

Treatment, with aspirin and steroids, is initially aimed at reducing the inflammatory symptoms. Mebendazole (200 to 400 mg tid for 3 days, then 400 to 500 mg tid for 10 days) is indicated for severe disease but may not be effective after encystment.

Strongyloides stercoralis (threadworm) is found in southern Appalachia, Kentucky, and Tennessee. Like the hookworms, it penetrates through the skin, producing pruritus and cutaneous larva migrans. Pulmonary and gastrointestinal symptoms occur as the larvae migrate. The human, however, is a definitive host; it is common for ongoing autoinfection to be slowed by the host's immune response. Immunocompromised patients and the elderly may suffer fatal infestation. The rise in acquired immunodeficiency syndrome (AIDS) has been mirrored by a rise in reported cases of *Strongyloides* infestation. A definitive diagnosis is made by recovering *Strongyloides* in stool, sputum, or duodenal aspirate. Thiabendazole (50 mg/kg/day divided bid, maximum 3 g/day) for 2 days is recommended.

TREMATODES (FLUKES)

Flukes are oval, flat worms with a ventral sucker for nutrition and attachment. Eggs are shed in the stool of definitive hosts, hatch into miracidia, and enter an intermediate host such as a snail or other crustacean, fish, or bird. They develop into cercariae. These cercariae leave the intermediate host to become free-living prior to infesting the definitive host. The intermediate host may also be ingested, releasing this infective form of the parasite. Symptoms are produced as the fluke reaches its destination. *Fasciolopsis buski* infests the gut; *Fasciola hepatica, Opisthorchis* (formerly *Clonorchis*) *sinensis,* and *Schistosoma mansoni* infest the liver; *Schistosoma haematobium,* the bladder; and *Paragonimus westermani* the lung. None of these flukes are endemic in the United States. Praziquantel (75 mg/kg/day divided tid for 1 or 2 days) is recommended.

Of particular interest to the pediatric emergency physician is the avian schistosome *Trichobilharzia ocellata.* Spread by migratory birds to the freshwater lakes of the northern United States, the cercariae cause a dermatitis known as swimmer's itch. The intense reaction produced by host defenses is treated with heat and antipruritics. Severe cases are treated with thiabendazole cream.

CESTODES (FLATWORMS AND TAPEWORMS)

Cestodes attach to the gut of the definitive host with hooks or suckers at the head (scolex), from which grow segmented proglottids. Each proglottid is equipped to produce large volumes of eggs. These eggs, along with terminal proglottids, pass in the stool and are ingested by the intermediate host. The eggs hatch into a larval stage—either *Cysticercus,* cysticercoid, *Coenurus,* or hydatid cyst, depending on the species. Symptoms are produced as these larvae act as space-occupying lesions or cause inflammation. When the intermediate host is ingested by the definitive host, the larvae attach to the intestine and the cycle repeats.

Four cestodes produce the majority of clinical disease seen in the United States: *Taenia solium, Taenia saginatum, Diphyllobothrium latum,* and *Echinococcus granulosus.*

Taenia solium (pork tapeworm) and *Taenia saginatum* (beef tapeworm) are generally asymptomatic, and are diagnosed when a parent brings a proglottid to the emergency department for identification. A history of raw meat consumption may be elicited. Patients occasionally will have gastrointestinal complaints. When *T. solium* enters the *Cysticercus* phase, it may migrate to the heart, brain, breast, eye, skin, or other solid organ. Subcutaneous nodules, visual field defects, focal neurologic findings, acute psychosis, and obstructive hydrocephalus may develop years after infestation. Calcified cysts may be found on plain radiographs, and cysts may be seen as a ring of calcification on computed tomography (CT).

Diphyllobothrium latum (fish tapeworm) is becoming more prevalent with the increased popularity of raw fish. Because *D. latum* absorbs over fifty times more vitamin B_{12} than *Taenia,* it causes pernicious anemia.

Echinococcus granulosus (sheep tapeworm) is found in agricultural countries. Most reported cases are from the southeastern United States. Symptomatology is secondary to hydatid cyst formation with mass effect.

Most tapeworms are treated with praziquantel (5 to 25 mg/kg once). *Echinococcus* infection and cysticercosis respond best to albendazole (15 mg/kg/day divided tid for 28 days).

PROTOZOA

Entamoeba histolytica is a waterborne single-cell organism. It is found in epidemic proportion after heavy rain in areas of suboptimal sanitation and among closely confined populations. In addition to ingestion of contaminated water, it may be spread by direct human contact, both sexually and in breast milk. The majority of patients carry amebas asymptomatically in the cecum and large intestine. Heavy infestations of *E. histolytica* produce a colitislike picture. These patients may present with nausea, vomiting, bloating, pain, bloody diarrhea, and leukocytosis without eosinophilia. The amebas live at the base of large flask-shaped ulcers. When the infection is severe, direct inspection will reveal pseudopolyps of normal tissue on a base of ulcerative disease. *Entamoeba histolytica* has the capacity to invade the blood, causing abscess formation in the liver, lung, brain, and breast. Diagnosis is confirmed with stool specimen or colonoscopic aspiration. Metronidazole (35 to 50 mg/kg/day divided tid for 10 days) followed by iodoquinol (40 mg/kg/day divided tid for 20 days) is recommended to eradicate this infestation.

The flagellate *Giardia lamblia* thrives in the relatively alkaline pH of the duodenum and proximal small bowel. Infestation occurs after ingestion of contaminated water or other fecal-oral behavior. It is commonly found in day-care centers; among travelers, immunocompromised children, and patients with cystic fibrosis; and in association with hepatic or pancreatic disease. Flatulence, nonbloody diarrhea or constipation, abdominal distention, and pain are common symptoms. Fever, weight loss, and fat, carbohydrate, and vitamin malabsorption can occur. While cysts may appear in the stool, it is often necessary to perform duodenal aspiration to confirm the diagnosis. Metronidazole (15 mg/kg/day divided tid for 5 days) is recommended.

In 1993, a total of 1411 cases of malaria were reported to the Centers for Disease Control. Over the past 10 years, the number of cases has remained stable at approximately one thousand per year, one-quarter of which occur in children. Ninety percent of these cases are equally divided between *Plasmodium falciparum* and *Plasmodium vivax*. The remainder are caused by *Plasmodium ovale* and *Plasmodium malariae*. Two-thirds were imported from sub-Saharan Africa. In 1993, three cases of *falciparum* malaria which could not be traced to immigration or travel were reported in New York City. It is felt that these cases might be the first sign of a resurgence of indigenous malaria. Transmission of all forms of malaria is by direct blood innoculum, usually by the *Anopheles* mosquito. It may also be passed transplacentally to the fetus. Following a 1- to 3-week incubation in the liver, *Plasmodium* enters an asexual erythrocytic cycle. *Falciparum*, *vivax*, and *ovale* have a 48-h cycle and have a preference for reticulocytes, while *malariae* has a 72-h cycle and is found in older red blood cells.

These cycles produce the classic periodicity of fever and shaking chills. Headache, diarrhea, cough, altered consciousness, jaundice, and disseminated intravascular coagulation (DIC) leading to cardiovascular collapse can ensue. The mortality rate exceeds 4 percent.

With a high index of suspicion, one looks for the parasite on thick and thin blood smears. *Falciparum* is characterized by a predominance of ring forms within the red blood cells, banana-shaped gametocytes, and the absence of mature trophozoites and schizonts. *Malariae, vivax,* and *ovale* have round gametocytes with mature trophozoites and schizonts on smear.

To prevent infestation in travelers, prophylaxis is recommended beginning 1 week prior to departure and continuing for 4 to 6 weeks after return. Resistance of *P. falciparum* and *P. vivax* to chloroquine is now spreading. If a person is traveling to a sensitive area, chloroquine (5 mg/kg of base, maximum 300 mg) given once a week is recommended. For resistant areas, mefloquine is the drug of choice. Once someone is infected, chloroquine (10 mg/kg of base, maximum 600 mg, followed by 5 mg/kg of base, maximum 300 mg at 6, 24, and 48 h) or quinine sulfate (25 mg/kg/day divided tid for 3 to 7 days) and pyrimethamine-sulfadoxine (number of tablets based on age) given on the last day of quinine is recommended. As *P. vivax* and *P. ovale* tend to relapse, they should, when identified, also be treated with primaquine phosphate (0.3 mg/kg/day for 14 days).

Pneumocystis carinii has a low virulence and is found in latent phase in a large percentage of the American population. When the host is immunocompromised, trophozoites replicate in alveolar spaces and spread through the vascular and lymphatic beds. The patient experiences respiratory distress, fever, and nonproductive cough with limited auscultatory findings. The radiograph may be normal or have symmetric interstitial ground-glass infiltrates in the middle and lower lung fields.

Pneumocystis reactivation occurs in debilitated patients and those with suppressed immune responses. It is found in more than 60 percent of patients with human immunodeficiency virus (HIV) infection. The overall mortality rate in children is 40 percent, rising to 100 percent once radiographic changes occur in untreated non-AIDS patients.

Given the high incidence of asymptomatic carriers, the diagnostic method of choice is silver nitrate–methenamine stain of a lung biopsy specimen in the proper clinical setting. Treatment is with trimethoprim (15 to 20 mg/kg/day) and sulfamethoxazole (75 to 100 mg/kg/day) in three or four divided doses orally or pentamidine (3 to 4 mg/kg/day) intravenously for 2 to 3 weeks.

Cryptosporidium, Isospora belli, and *Toxoplasma gondii* belong to the protozoan subclass Coccidia, which also includes *Plasmodium.* Modes of transmission include direct human contact and ingestion of fecally contaminated food and water. *Toxoplasma* is also transmitted transplacentally, with blood transfusion and organ transplantation. Intermediate hosts include farm animals (*Cryptosporidium*), cats (*Toxoplasma*), and other mammals.

While some children harbor *Cryptosporidium* and *Isospora* asymptomatically, both can cause a secretory, choleralike diarrhea after a 2-week incubation. Large volumes of watery, nonbloody, leukocyte-free stool may produce significant dehydration. Fever, headache, and anorexia are followed by malabsorption of lactose and fat. These symptoms are self-limited and last up to 3 weeks. The oocysts may be shed for an additional month. Immuno-compromised children may manifest infective symptoms of liver, gallbladder, appendix, and lung as well as a reactive arthritis. No toxins have been demonstrated, and the pathogenic mechanism of this spectrum of symptoms is not known. Direct examination of stool with modified Ziehl-Neelsen stain is the diagnostic method of choice. There is no proven antiparasitic cure. Octreotide (300 to 500 μg tid subcutaneously) may control the diarrhea of patients with HIV.

The trophozoites of *Toxoplasma gondii* have a predilection for the brain, heart, and bone, although they can invade any nucleated cell. Approximately 2500 infants are born annually in the United States with congenital disease, 10 percent of whom have the *Toxoplasma* triad of hydrocephalus, chorioretinitis, and intracranial calcification. The long-term prognosis for these children is poor.

Acquired toxoplasmosis in the immune-competent host is asymptomatic but may produce a subclinical reaction in the reticuloendothelial system. In patients with AIDS and other types of immunocompromise, reactivation produces severe central nervous system involvement and dissemination to the heart and lungs. Between 30 and 40 percent of AIDS patients will develop *Toxoplasma* encephalitis or mass lesions of the brain and cranial nerves. The diagnosis is made by antigen detection or by seeing a ring formation on CT with contrast. Prompt treatment with pyrimethamine (2 mg/kg/day for 3 days, then 1 mg/kg/day for 4 weeks) and sulfadiazine (100 to 200 mg/kg/day for 4 weeks) is recommended. However, there is a high fatality rate once *Toxoplasma* becomes reactivated.

ARTHROPODS

The parasites *Pediculus humanus capitis* (head louse), *Pediculus humanus corporis* (body louse), and *Phthirus pubis* (pubic or crab louse) are 1 to 2 mm long. They attach 0.8-mm-long eggs (nits) firmly to hair shafts, close to the skin. Lice are transmitted by direct human contact or the sharing of clothing or other personal articles. They are not transmitted to or from domestic animals and are found on children with proper hygiene. They require a hair-bearing surface, with the adult viable for only 2 days and the nit for 10 days off the host. The most common complaint is itching. *Phthirus pubis* may produce blue-colored macules (maculae ceruleae). A 10-min rinse with 1% permethrin will kill adult lice and most nits. It may, however, exacerbate the pruritus and erythema. It is too toxic to use near the eyes, where petrolatum is recommended to suffocate the lice. Eyelid lice in prepubescent children should alert the physician to the possibility of sexual abuse. Care must be taken to delouse other family members and the child's environment. A spray of permethrin and piperonyl butoxide should be employed on furniture and bedding used in the previous 2 days. Alternatively, objects can be sealed in plastic bags for 2 weeks until all adults and nits are no longer viable. Dead nits can be removed from hair shafts with a fine-toothed comb.

Sarcoptes scabiei (scabies) are transmitted by direct close and prolonged human contact. Scabies will not flourish on other animals. Following a 3- to 6-week incubation, the 200- to 400-μm-long scabies mite burrows between the fingers and toes as well as in the groin, external genitalia, and axillae, depositing eggs in the tunnel as she goes. The itch is worse at night, with infants sleeping poorly and rubbing their hands and feet together. Small red, raised, papules are formed, which may progress to vesicles and pustules. Secondary excoriations are also present. The diagnosis is made clinically. However, one may scrape burrows or papules overlaid with mineral oil and inspect the scrapings for adults, eggs, and excreta for confirmation. A single application of 5% permethrin cream is curative for children over 2 months old. Younger children may be treated with sulfur precipitated in petrolatum. The long incubation period makes treating the entire family advisable. As the parasite lives less than 24 h off the host, environmental decontamination may not be necessary.

For a more detailed discussion, see Lelyveld S: Common parasitic infestations, chap. 47, p. 274, in *Pediatric Emergency Medicine: A Comprehensive Study Guide.*

48 Immunoprophylaxis

Susan Aguila-Mangahas

In the United States, immunization has decreased or practically eliminated many diseases, among them diphtheria, measles, mumps, pertussis, poliomyelitis, congenital and acquired rubella, tetanus, and, recently, *Haemophilus influenzae* type b disease. However, due to the persistence of these diseases in other countries and in some areas of the United States, immunizations should still be continued. It is imperative that physicians keep abreast of developments in the area of immunoprophylaxis. Recently, many public health professionals have advocated that health care providers offer immunizations at every available opportunity, including in the emergency department.

IMMUNIZATION SCHEDULE

The American Academy of Pediatrics and the American Academy of Family Physicians have established a conjoint Advisory Committee on Immunization Practices. Their recommended schedule for childhood immunizations is shown in Table 48-1. The current version of these recommendations eliminates the differences between the former schedules approved by the American Academy of Pediatrics and the Centers for Disease Control.

LAPSED IMMUNIZATIONS

A lapse in the immunization schedule does not require repeating the entire series. If there is a long interval between doses, the next dose should be administered at the next visit as if there had been no interruption. Longer-than-recommended intervals do not reduce the final antibody concentration, but delays unnecessarily put the child at risk for developing the illness. Shorter than recommended intervals, on the other hand, may decrease the antibody response.

HYPERSENSITIVITY TO VACCINE COMPONENTS

There are four types of hypersensitivity reactions. *Allergic reactions to egg-related antigens* are a concern with measles, mumps, rubella, and influenza vaccines, all of which contain small amounts of egg protein. Skin testing is recommended for those with a history of anaphylactic reaction after egg ingestion. Minor reactions or manifestations of allergy to egg are not contraindications to vaccine

TABLE 48-1 Recommended Childhood Immunization Schedule United States, January–December 1998[a]

Age ▶ / Vaccine ▼	Birth	1 Month	2 Months	4 Months	6 Months	12 Months	15 Months	18 Months	4-8 Years	11-12 Years	14-16 Years
Hepatitis B[c,d]	Hep B-1	Hep B-2			Hep B-3					Hep B[d]	
Diphtheria, Tetanus, Pertussis[e]			DTaP or DTP	DTaP or DTP	DTaP or DTP		DTaP or DTP[e]		DTaP or DTP	Td	
H influenzae type b[f]			Hib	Hib	Hib	Hib					
Polio[g]			Polio[g]	Polio	Polio[g]				Polio		
Measles, Mumps, Rubella[h]						MMR			MMR[h]	MMR[h]	
Varicella[i]						Var				Var[i]	

[a] Vaccines[b] are listed under the routinely recommended ages. Bars indicate range of acceptable ages for immunization. Catch-up immunization should be done during any visit when feasible. Shaded ovals indicate vaccines to be assessed and given if necessary during the early adolescent visit.

[b] This schedule indicates the recommended age for routine administration of currently licenced childhood vaccines. Some combination vaccines are available and may be used whenever administration of all components of the vaccine is indicated. Providers should consult the manufacturers' package inserts for detailed recommendations.

[c] ***Infants born to HBsAg-negative mothers*** should receive 2.5 μg of Merck vaccine (Recombivax HB) or 10 μg of SmithKline Beecham (SB) vaccine (Engerix-B). The 2nd dose should be administered at least 1 mo after the 1st dose. The 3rd dose should be given at least 2 mos after the second, but not before 6 mos of age.

Infants born to HBsAg-positive mothers should receive 0.5 mL of hepatitis B immune globulin (HBIG) within 12 hrs of birth, and either 5 μg of Merck vaccine (Recombivax HB) or 10 μg of SB vaccine (Engerix-B) at a separate site. The 2nd dose is recommended at 1–2 mos of age and the 3rd dose at 6 mos of age.

Infants born to mothers whose HBsAg status is unknown should receive either 5 μg of Merck vaccine (Recombivax HB) or 10 μg of SB vaccine (Engerix-B) within 12 hrs of birth. The 2nd dose of vaccine is recommended at 1 mo of age and the 3rd dose at 6 mos of age. Blood should be drawn at the time of delivery to determine the mother's HBsAg status; if it is positive, the infant should receive HBIG as soon as possible (no later than 1 wk of age). The dosage and timming of subsequent vaccine doses should be based upon the mother's HBsAg status.

[d] Children and adolescents who have not been vaccinated against hepatitis B in infancy may begin the series during any visit. Those who have not previously received 3 doses of hepatitis B vaccine should initiate or complete the series during the 11 to 12-year-old visit, and unvaccinated older adolescents should be vaccinated whenever possible. The 2nd dose should be administered at least 1 mo after the 1st dose, and the 3rd dose should be administered at least 4 mos after the 1st dose and at least 2 mos after the 2nd dose.

[e] DTaP (diphtheria and tetanus toxoids and acellular pertussis vaccine) is the preferred vaccine for all doses in the vaccination series, including completion of the series in children who have recieved 1 or more doses of whole-cell DTP vaccine. Whole-cell DTP is an acceptable alternate to DTaP. The 4th dose (DTP or DTaP) may be administered as early as 12 mos of age, provided 6 mos have elapsed since the 3rd dose and if the child is unlikely to return at age 15–18 mos. Td (tetanus and diphtheria toxoids) is recommended at 11–12 years of age if at least 5 years have elapsed since the last dose of DTP, DTaP or DT. Subsequent routine Td boosters are recommended every 10 years.

[f] Three *H influenzae* tybe b (Hib) conjugate vaccines are licensed for infant use. If PRP-OMP (PedvaxHIB[Merck]) is administered at 2 and 4 mos of age, a dose at 6 mos is not required.

[g] Two poliovirus vaccines are currently licensed in the US: inactivated poliovirus vaccine (IPV) and oral poliovirus vaccine (OPV). The following schedules are all acceptable to the ACIP, the AAP, and the AAFP. Parents and providers may choose among these options.

1) 2 doses of IPV followed by 2 doses of OPV.
2) 4 doses of IPV.
3) 4 doses of OPV.

The ACIP recommends 2 doses of IPV at 2 and 4 mos of age followed by 2 doses of OPV at 12–18 mos and 4–6 years of age. IPV is the only poliovirus vaccine recommended for immunocompromised persons and their household contacts.

[h] The 2nd dose of MMR is recommended routinely at 4–6 yrs of age but may be administered during any visit, provided at least 1 mo has elapsed since receipt of the 1st dose and that both doses are administered beginning at or after 12 mos of age. Those who have not *previously* received the second dose should complete the schedule no later than the 11 to 12-years visit.

[i] Susceptible children may receive varicella vaccine (Var) at any visit after the first birthday, and those who lack a reliable history of chickenpox should be immunized during the 11–12-year-old visit. Susceptible children 13 years of age or older should receive 2 doses, at least 1 month apart.

Approved by the Advisory Committee on Immunization Practices (ACIP), the American Academy of Pediatrics (AAP), and the American Academy of Family Physicians (AAFP).

administration and are not an indication for skin testing. *Mercury sensitivity* can occur in some recipients of immune globulins or vaccines. *Antibiotic-induced allergic reactions* can develop in patients receiving inactivated poliovirus vaccine (IPV) and measles-mumps-rubella vaccine (MMR). The former, IPV, contains both streptomycin and neomycin, while the latter, MMR, contains neomycin. If a patient has a history of an anaphylactic reaction to these antibiotics, administration of the vaccine should be deferred. *Hypersensitivity can also develop to some component of the infectious agent or to some other component of the vaccine.*

SPECIAL CIRCUMSTANCES

Fever

While minor illness and fever are not contraindications to the administration of vaccine, children who have moderate to severe febrile illness should have immunization deferred until the febrile illness has resolved.

Preterm Infants

Preterm infants should be immunized on the basis of their chronological age. If the patient is still in the nursery at 2 months of age, the usual immunizations are given with the exception of oral polio vaccine (OPV), which is deferred until the time of discharge. This is done to prevent nosocomial infection. No change in dose of vaccine is needed due to prematurity.

Pregnancy

Pregnancy is a contraindication to the administration of live vaccines except when susceptibility and exposure are highly probable and the disease to be prevented poses a greater threat to the mother or fetus than the vaccine.

Immunodeficient and Immunosuppressed Children

Live bacterial and viral vaccines are contraindicated in patients with immunodeficiency and their household contacts. Although OPV should be avoided for patients and contacts, MMR can be given to household contacts and siblings.

When children have received immunosuppressive therapy, vaccines should not be administered for at least 3 months after the last dose of immunosuppressant.

Children with human immunodeficiency virus (HIV) infection should receive MMR regardless of their clinical status. Pneumococcal vaccine should be given for those 2 years of age or older, while DTP, IPV, and Hib should all be given based on the standard recommended schedule.

Asplenic children are at risk for fulminant bacteremia. Pneumococcal and meningococcal vaccines should be given to asplenic children who are 2 years of age or older, and Hib should be given according to the standard recommended schedule. Antimicrobial prophylaxis is indicated, using oral penicillin V, 125 mg twice daily for children under 5 years of age and 250 mg twice daily for those 5 years old or older.

Seizures

If an infant has had a recent seizure, pertussis immunization should be deferred until a progressive neurologic disorder is excluded or the etiology of the seizure is determined. A family history of seizures is not a contraindication to pertussis or measles vaccine.

SPECIFIC IMMUNIZATION GUIDELINES

Diphtheria/Tetanus/Pertussis Vaccine

This vaccine is administered in a dose of 0.5 mL intramuscularly. Local redness, edema, induration, and tenderness are common. A mild to moderate febrile reaction associated with drowsiness, fretfulness, anorexia, vomiting, and crying may occur. Prolonged crying, for 3 h or more, occurs in approximately 1 percent of vaccinated children. More severe reactions, such as seizures and shocklike state, are rare (1:1750). An allergic rash is not uncommon, but anaphylaxis is very rare. An alternate form of the vaccine, which contains acellular pertussis vaccine (DTaP), is associated with fewer reactions. Contraindications and precautions are listed in Table 48-2 (see also Appendix A, page 868).

Haemophilus Influenzae Type B Vaccine

This vaccine is administered in a dose of 0.5 mL intramuscularly. No vaccine-related side effects have been reported. Children who have invasive *H. influenzae* type b disease at age 24 months or older usually develop a protective immune response. Younger children do not develop a sufficient immune response and remain at risk for the disease. The vaccine should be administered according to the age-appropriate schedule, ignoring any previous immunization.

Hepatitis B Vaccine

Hepatitis B vaccine (HB) dosage guidelines are given in Table 48-3. Adverse reactions include pain at the injection site, fever,

TABLE 48-2. Guide to Contraindications and Precautions to Vaccinations[a]

True Contraindications and Precautions	Not Contraindications (Vaccines May Be Administered)
General for All Vaccines (DTP/DTaP, OPV, IPV, MMR, Hib, Hepatitis B)	
Contraindications	**Not contraindications**
Anaphylactic reaction to a vaccine contraindicates further doses of that vaccine	Mild to moderate local reaction (soreness, redness, swelling) following a dose of an injectable antigen
Anaphylactic reaction to a vaccine constituent contraindicates the use of vaccines containing that substance	Mild acute illness with or without low-grade fever
Moderate or severe illnesses with or without a fever	Current antimicrobial therapy
	Convalescent phase of illnesses
	Prematurity (same dosage and indications as for normal, full-term infants)
	Recent exposure to an infectious disease
	History of penicillin or other nonspecific allergies or family history of such allergies
DTP/DTaP	
Contraindications	**Not contraindications**
Encephalopathy within 7 days of administration of previous dose of DTP	Temperature of <40.5°C (105°F) following a previous dose of DTP
Precautions[b]	Family history of convulsions[c]
Fever of ≥40.5°C (105°F) within 48 h after vaccination with a prior dose of DTP	Family history of sudden infant death syndrome
	Family history of an adverse event following DTP administration

Collapse or shocklike state (hypotonic-hyporesponsive episode) within 48 h of receiving a prior dose of DTP	
Seizures within 3 days of receiving a prior dose of DTP[c]	
Persistent, inconsolable crying lasting ≥3 h within 48 h of receiving a prior dose of DTP	
OPV[d]	
Contraindications	**Not contraindications**
Infection with HIV or a household contact with HIV	Breast-feeding
Known altered immunodeficiency (hematologic and solid tumors; congenital immunodeficiency; and long-term immunosuppressive therapy)	Current antimicrobial therapy
	Diarrhea
Immunodeficient household contact	
Precaution[b]	
Pregnancy	
IPV	
Contraindication	
Anaphylactic reaction to neomycin or streptomycin	
Precaution[b]	
Pregnancy	

(*Continued*)

TABLE 48-2. Guide to Contraindications and Precautions to Vaccinations[a] (*Continued*)

True Contraindications and Precautions	Not Contraindications (Vaccines May Be Administered)
MMR[d]	
	Not contraindications
Contraindications	Tuberculosis or positive PPD skin test
Anaphylactic reactions to egg ingestion and to neomycin[e]	Simultaneous TB skin testing[f]
Pregnancy	Breast-feeding
Known altered immunodeficiency (hematologic and solid tumors; congenital immunodeficiency; and long-term immunosuppressive therapy)	Pregnancy of mother of recipient
	Immunodeficient family member or household contact
Precaution[b]	Infection with HIV
Recent immune globulin administration	Nonanaphylactic reactions to eggs or neomycin
Hib	
Contraindication	**Not a contraindication**
None identified	History of Hib disease
Hepatitis B	
Contraindication	**Not a contraindication**
Anaphylactic reaction to common baker's yeast	Pregnancy

[a] This information is based on the recommendation of the Advisory Committee on Immunization Practices (ACIP) and those of the Committee on Infectious Diseases (Red Book Committee) of the American Academy of Pediatrics (AAP). Sometimes these recommendations vary from those contained in the manufacturer's package inserts. For more detailed information, providers should consult the published recommendations of the ACIP, AAP, and the manufacturer's package inserts.

[b] The events or conditions listed as precautions, although not contraindications, should be carefully reviewed. The benefits and risks of administering a specific vaccine to an individual under the circumstances should be considered. If the risks are believed to outweigh the benefits, the vaccination should be withheld; if the benefits are believed to outweigh the risks (for example, during an outbreak or foreign travel), the vaccination should be administered. Whether and when to administer DTP to children with proven or suspected underlying neurologic disorders should be decided on an individual basis. It is prudent on theoretical grounds to avoid vaccinating pregnant women. However, if immediate protection against poliomyelitis is needed, OPV is preferred, although IPV may be considered if full vaccination can be completed before the anticipated imminent exposure.

[c] Acetaminophen given before administering DTP and thereafter every 4 h for 24 h should be considered for children with a personal or family history of convulsions in siblings or parents.

[d] No data exist to substantiate the theoretical risk of a suboptimal immune response from the administration of OPV and MMR within 30 days of each other.

[e] Persons with a history of anaphylactic reactions following egg ingestion should be vaccinated only with caution. Protocols have been developed for vaccinating such persons and should be consulted. (*J Pediatr* 102:196–199, 1983; *J Pediatr* 113:504–506, 1988.)

[f] Measles vaccination may temporarily suppress tuberculin reactivity. If testing can not be done the day of MMR vaccination, the test should be postponed for 4 to 6 weeks.

Source: Centers for Disease Control: General recommendations on immunization of the Advisory Committee on immunization practices. *MMWR* 43(RR-1): 1994, pp. 24–25.

NOTE: General vaccine specific recommendations are updated regularly in the *Red Book: Report of the Committee on Infectious Diseases, American Academy of Pediatrics*. (See also Appendix A, which appears on page 868.)

TABLE 48-3 Recommended Dosages of Hepatitis B Vaccines[a]

	Vaccine[b,c]			
	Recombivax HB[d]		Energix-B[e,f]	
	Dose: μg	(mL)	Dose: μg	(mL)
Infants of HBsAG-negative mothers and children <11 years	2.5	(0.5)[g]	10	(0.5)
Infants of HBsAg-positive mothers [HBIG (0.5 mL) should also be given]	5	(0.5)[h]	10	(0.5)
Children and adolescents 11 to 19 years	5	(0.5)[h]	20	(1.0)
Adults ≥ 20 years	10	(1.0)[h]	20	(1.0)
Dialysis patients and other immunosuppressed adults	40	(1.0)[i]	40	(2.0)[j]

[a] Heptavax B (available from Merck & Co), a plasma-derived vaccine, is also licensed but no longer produced in the United States.

[b] Vaccines should be stored at 2°C to 8°C. Freezing destroys effectiveness.

[c] Both vaccines are administered in a 3-dose schedule.

[d] Available from Merck & Co.

[e] The Food and Drug Administration has approved this vaccine for use in an optional 4-dose schedule at 0, 1, 2, and 12 months.

[f] Available from SmithKline Beecham.

[g] Pediatric formulation.

[h] Adult formulation.

[i] Special formulation for dialysis patients.

[j] Two 1.0-mL doses given at one site in a 4-dose schedule at 0, 1, 2, and 6-12 months.

Source: Committee on Infectious Diseases, American Academy of Pediatrics: *1997 Red Book,* 24th ed. Elk Grove Village, IL: American Academy of Pediatarics, 1997, p. 252.

and allergic reactions. Allergic reactions are infrequent and anaphylaxis has been reported only in adults. Children in high-risk groups (Table 48-3) and all adolescents should be immunized if not already routinely immunized.

Measles/Mumps/Rubella Vaccine

This vaccine is given in a dose of 0.5 mL subcutaneously. The measles vaccine can produce a high fever that occurs 7 to 12 days after immunization and persists for 1 to 2 days. Febrile convulsions can result. A transient rash occurs in 5 percent of vaccinated children. Transient thrombocytopenia can also occur and, rarely, encephalitis and encephalopathy develop. Allergic reaction to egg protein and hypersensitivity to neomycin are rare complications. Adverse reactions to the mumps vaccine are extremely rare. The rubella vaccine results in a syndrome of rash, fever, and lymphadenopathy, which develops 5 to 12 days after immunization in 5 to 15 percent of vaccinated children. Transient pain in small peripheral joints may develop 7 to 21 days postimmunization.

The MMR vaccine should not be given to pregnant women or to those considering pregnancy within 3 months. If immune globulin has been administered recently, MMR administration should be deferred for 3 months, or longer if a high dose was given. Tuberculosis skin testing may be done on the day of immunization but not for 4 to 6 weeks after immunization.

Poliovirus Vaccine

Oral poliovirus vaccine (OPV) is a live-virus vaccine. An alternate form is available as inactivated poliovirus vaccine (IPV), which is given intramuscularly to immunodeficient patients and their household contacts. Poliovirus vaccination is avoided during pregnancy due to a theoretical potential risk to the fetus. Neither diarrhea nor breast-feeding are contraindications to the use of OPV. Paralysis in vaccinated individuals and their contacts has been reported to occur very rarely (1:6.8 million).

For a more detailed discussion, see Aguila-Mangahas S: Immunoprophylaxis, chap. 48, p. 281, in *Pediatric Emergency Medicine: A Comprehensive Study Guide.*

SECTION VII
GASTROINTESTINAL EMERGENCIES

49 Gastroenteritis

Elizabeth C. Powell / Sally Reynolds

Worldwide, diarrheal diseases are the leading cause of childhood death. In the United States, they result in around 500 deaths per year. Most reported deaths in the United States occur in children below 1 year of age. Viruses cause 80 percent of gastroenteritis in children, with bacteria and parasites accounting for the rest.

ETIOLOGY

Viruses

Most gastroenteritis is caused by rotavirus, enteric adenovirus, Norwalk virus and other calciviruses, or astrovirus. Rotavirus is the most common cause of severe diarrhea. It is most severe in infants. Illness usually begins with fever and vomiting, followed by watery nonbloody diarrhea. Symptoms last 5 to 7 days. Rotavirus occurs during winter months. Enteric adenovirus accounts for 5 to 10 percent of gastroenteritis requiring hospital admission. Ill children have fever and watery diarrhea; respiratory symptoms are rare. The diarrhea lasts 5 to 12 days. The Norwalk virus causes epidemic gastroenteritis in older children during winter months. Illness is short, usually lasting less than 3 days. Fever and myalgia often accompany the gastrointestinal symptoms.

Bacteria

Campylobacter jejuni, *Salmonella* species, *Shigella* species, *Yersinia enterocolitica*, *Clostridium difficile*, and *Aeromonas* are the usual organisms that cause bacterial gastroenteritis in U.S. children. *Escherichia coli* (enterotoxigenic, enteropathogenic, enteroinvasive), the pathogen responsible for most bacterial diarrhea worldwide, is an uncommon cause of diarrhea in the United States. Most infections are spread by contaminated food or water. Infected children usually have fever and blood-streaked or bloody diarrhea.

In young children, *Salmonella* and *Shigella* infections are associated with specific complications. *Salmonella* gastroenteritis is associated with a 5 to 10 percent incidence of bacteremia in infants below 1 year of age. Young infants and children who are immunocompromised or have sickle cell disease are at risk for focal complications from *Salmonella* infection, including pneumonia, meningitis, and osteomyelitis. *Shigella* gastroenteritis is associated with seizures, which may precede diarrhea. *Yersinia* gastroenteritis can cause mesenteric adenitis or terminal ileitis.

Parasites

Giardia lamblia and *Cryptosporidium* also cause diarrhea in U.S. children. *Giardia* is a common pathogen in children attending day care. It is responsible for both acute and chronic diarrhea. It has a high rate of asymptomatic infection, and untreated children can shed cysts for months. *Cryptosporidium* is spread person to person. Transmission is aided by asymptomatic carriers and the organism's resistance to chlorine.

PATHOPHYSIOLOGY

Viral diarrhea is noninflammatory. Infection causes lytic damage to small bowel enterocytes, which results in shortening of the intestinal villi, loss of absorptive surface, and increased bowel motility. Carbohydrate malabsorption produces an osmotic diarrhea. Bacterial infection is either noninflammatory, inflammatory, or penetrating (Table 49-1). In the United States, bacterial diarrhea is usually inflammatory. Bacteria infect the bowel wall, usually in

TABLE 49-1 Etiology of Diarrhea

Noninflammatory (watery)	Inflammatory
Vibrio cholera	*Shigella*
Escherichia coli (enterotoxigenic)	*Salmonella*
Staphylococcal food poisoning	*Campylobacter jejuni*
Clostridium perfringes food poisoning	*Clostridium difficile*
Rotavirus	*E. coli* (invasive)
Enteric Adenovirus	**Penetrating**
Norwalk-like virus	*Salmonella typhi*
Giardia	*Yersinia*
Cryptosporidium	*Campylobacter fetus*

Source: Adapted with permission from Guerrant R et al: Acute infectious diarrhea. I. *Pediatr Infect Dis* 5:353, 1986.

the colon. Noninflammatory bacterial diarrhea involves the small bowel. Parasitic diarrhea is noninflammatory.

HISTORY AND PHYSICAL EXAMINATION

The history is focused on the child's state of hydration and gastrointestinal symptoms. The parent's report of intake and output of both stool and urine is useful to estimate fluid balance. Vomiting and crampy abdominal pain usually accompany the diarrhea. The past history focuses on prior gastrointestinal surgery, inflammatory bowel disease, or current antibiotic use, and solicits information concerning institutional or day care, foreign travel, and diet.

The physical examination is directed toward assessing hydration and distinguishing gastroenteritis from other enteric illnesses. Weight loss, tachycardia, tachypnea (reflecting acidosis), a flat or sunken fontanelle, dry mucous membranes and lack of tears, and decreased skin turgor are all evidence of dehydration (Table 49-2). In gastroenteritis, the abdomen is usually soft and nondistended, and bowel sounds are decreased. Stool is visually inspected for gross blood and is tested for occult blood. Approximately 10 percent of children with gastroenteritis have bloody stools.

DIAGNOSTIC EVALUATION

Most children with uncomplicated gastroenteritis need no laboratory studies. Stool cultures are useful in febrile children with blood in their stools. Routine stool cultures in most hospital laboratories include *C. jejuni, Salmonella,* and *Shigella*. The Rotazyme assay is used to detect rotavirus. It is rarely indicated in managing outpatients. Even with a selective approach, many stool cultures will be negative.

The electrolytes in children with diarrhea and dehydration frequently show abnormal bicarbonate levels (10 to 18 meq/L). Less commonly, serum sodium is abnormal, and the blood urea nitrogen (BUN) may be elevated. In specific situations, a leukocyte count is helpful. Infants less than 3 months old with *Salmonella* enteritis are more likely to have bacteremia when the leukocyte count is greater than 15,000/mm^3. *Shigella* is associated with a normal total leukocyte count but an increased number of band forms. *Campylobacter* and *Yersinia* are also associated with leukocyte counts in the normal range.

TREATMENT

Most children with gastroenteritis are successfully managed with oral solutions as outpatients. Children who are dehydrated or

TABLE 49-2 Clinical Assessment of Severity of Dehydration

Signs and symptoms	Mild dehydration	Moderate dehydration	Severe dehydration
General appearance and condition			
Infants and young children	Thirsty, alert, restless	Thirsty, restless, lethargic but irritable or drowsy	Drowsy, limp, cold, sweaty, cyanotic extremities, may be comatose
Older children and adults	Thirsty, alert, restless	Thirsty, alert, postural hypotension	Cold, sweaty, muscle cramps, cyanotic extremities, conscious
Radial pulse	Normal rate and strength	Rapid and weak	Rapid, sometimes impalpable
Respiration	Normal	Deep, ± rapid	Deep and rapid
Anterior fontanel	Normal	Sunken	Very sunken
Systolic BP	Normal	Normal or low	>90 mmHg; may be unrecordable
Skin elasticity	Pinch retracts immediately	Pinch retracts slowly	Pinch retracts slowly (>2 s)
Eyes	Normal	Sunken	Sunken
Tears	Present	Absent	Absent
Mucous membranes	Moist	Dry	Very dry
Urine flow	Normal	Reduced amount, dark	None for several hours
Body weight loss (%)	4–5	6–9	10 or more
Estimated fluid deficit	40–50	60–90	100–110

Source: Adapted with permission from Behrman RE, Kliegman RM (eds): *Nelson Textbook of Pediatrics*, 14th ed., p 200, 1992.

appear toxic require hospital admission for intravenous therapy. Very young children, children with chronic diseases, and children with chronic malnutrition are managed conservatively.

Oral Therapy

Children estimated to be less than 5 percent dehydrated can usually be managed with oral solutions. Oral intake is restricted for approximately 1 h after the most recent episode of emesis. Fluids thereafter are given slowly, at a rate of 15 mL every 15 min for the first hour. The volume can be doubled every hour if it is tolerated. If the vomiting has already stopped, oral fluids are offered immediately, starting with 30 to 60 mL (1 to 2 oz) of clear liquids every 30 min. The two basic types of oral rehydration solutions differ in sodium concentration. Initial rehydration is done with Rehydralyte, which contains 75 to 90 meq/L of sodium. Pedialyte and Ricelyte contain less sodium (40 to 60 meq/L) and are available for maintenance therapy. Ricelyte contains glucose polymers, which may shorten the duration of diarrhea. For toddlers, juices or Gatorade are acceptable. They should be supplemented with bouillon or soups to provide sodium. Apple and white grape juice contain sorbitol, which can make diarrhea worse. Breast-fed infants should be nursed through the course of their illness.

Solid foods are introduced after 24 h of clear liquids. Foods best tolerated include bananas, applesauce, cereal, rice or noodles, potatoes, and bread. Infants taking formula should drink oral rehydration solutions for 12 to 24 h, after which formula is restarted. Discharge instructions are outlined in Table 49-3.

Intravenous Therapy

Children with moderate to severe dehydration (estimated greater than 5 percent) need intravenous fluids. A bolus of normal saline (20 mL/kg) is given over 20 to 30 min to replace intravascular volume. In healthy children, a second 20-mL/kg bolus of normal saline is indicated if the heart rate remains elevated or perfusion decreased. Electrolytes and a BUN are useful to identify acidosis and sodium abnormalities.

Dehydrated children awaiting admission require ongoing management in the emergency department. The fluid deficit is calculated using the estimated percentage of dehydration. In isotonic dehydration, half of the estimated deficit is given in the first 8 h and the remaining half over the next 16 h. It is essential that maintenance requirements and ongoing losses be added to the volume deficit. An appropriate solution is D_5 0.2*NS* with 20 meq

TABLE 49-3 Parent Instructions

First Day

1. Stop all milk and solid foods for 24 h.
2. Give only clear liquids for 24 h if your child has: Diarrhea without vomiting—feed child 1 to 2 oz of clear liquids every 30 min. Then feed child as much of the liquid as desired every 1–2 h.
   Vomiting alone or vomiting and diarrhea—give child nothing to drink or eat for 1 h. Then feed small amounts (1/2 oz to 1 tblsp) of clear liquids every 15 min and double the amount every hour. Once the child is not vomiting for 2 to 3 h, allow the child to take as much of the clear liquid as desired every 1 to 2 h.
   Clear liquids
   Pedialyte or Ricelyte (best in children younger than 1 year), Gatorade, apple juice (diluted half strength), Seven-up or ginger ale (with the bubbles stirred out), popsicles, clear soup or broth

Second Day

After 24 h of clear liquid, if your child is improving, continue the clear liquids and gradually start to feed milk and solid foods as below:

Infants—full-strength baby formula. The diarrhea may initially increase slightly; as long as the child is drinking well, the formula should be continued. Bananas, applesauce, rice, cereal, and strained carrots may be added.

Children—regular milk may be given. Bananas, applesauce, rice or noodles, mashed potatoes, Jell-o, toast, crackers, lean meats. If better after 48 h, go back to regular diet.

Call your doctor or return to the emergency department if your child is unable to take fluids or looks more ill, if your child has a dry mouth and makes no tears when crying, or if your child has not urinated in 8 h.

KCl/L. The management of dehydration in cases of serum electrolyte abnormalities is discussed in Chap. 56.

Toddlers and older children with mild to moderate dehydration, mild acidosis, and normal sodium values may be discharged from the emergency department after intravenous rehydration if they tolerate oral intake.

Antidiarrheal agents and antiemetics are not recommended in the treatment of infectious gastroenteritis. Bismuth subsalicylate (Pepto-Bismol) may be of modest benefit in reducing the duration of diarrhea. Although phenothiazines reduce emesis, extrapyrimidal reactions limit their usefulness in children.

Antibiotics are used to treat specific bacterial infections. *Salmonella* gastroenteritis is treated with antibiotics in infants younger than 3 months, in children who are immunosuppressed, and in children with sickle cell disease. They are also indicated for severe

TABLE 49-4 Antibiotics for Bacterial Diarrhea

Salmonella	Ampicillin and chloramphenicol or (IV) trimethoprim/ sulfamethoxazole	Treatment of specific high-risk patients or focal infection; prolongs carrier state
Shigella	Trimethoprim/ sulfamethoxazole or ampicillin	Treatment recommended Ampicillin only in susceptible strains
Campylobacter	Erythromycin	Treatment of severe dysentery; shortens excretion
Giardia	Furazolidone	Treat symptomatic infection; furazolidone suspension available
	Quinicrine	Bitter; children tolerate poorly

Source: Adapted with permission from Peter G (ed.): American Academy of Pediatrics Report of the Committee on Infectious Diseases, 22nd ed., 1991.

colitis, focal infection, and bacteremia (see Table 49-4). Recommended antibiotics are ampicillin and chloramphenacol; trimethoprim/sulfamethoxazole is an alternative therapy. Uncomplicated *Salmonella* gastroenteritis in children and in healthy infants older than 3 months does not require antibiotics, as they may prolong the carrier state.

In *Shigella* gastroenteritis, antibiotics are recommended. For susceptible strains, ampicillin is acceptable. If the susceptibility pattern is not known, trimethoprim/sulfamethoxazole is the treatment of choice. In older children, tetracycline is acceptable. Amoxicillin is not effective.

Most *Campylobacter* enteritis will resolve spontaneously. Severe dysentery is treated with erythromycin. In some areas, erythromycin is not effective, and treatment is based on sensitivity testing.

Symptomatic infection with *Giardia* should also be treated. Furazolidone, available in a liquid suspension (50 mg/15 mL), is the most practical drug to use to treat children. Quinacrine hydrochloride is effective but very bitter in taste.

For a more detailed discussion, see Powell EC, Reynolds S: Gastroenteritis, chap. 49, p. 289, in *Pediatric Emergency Medicine: A Comprehensive Study Guide.*

50 Nonsurgical Gastrointestinal Problems

John W. Graneto

ABDOMINAL PAIN

Approximately 20 percent of children will seek attention for abdominal pain sometime during their childhood. The majority of these patients will suffer from medical rather than surgical problems.

History

Patients and the parents are questioned regarding the duration of the pain, its location, its severity, and the character of the discomfort. Persistent, nonremitting pain of more than several hours' duration indicates a high likelihood of a surgical etiology, as does pain that is localized to a specific area. Pain that wakes the patient from sleep almost always indicates organic pathology, which can be surgical or medical. Crampy or colicky pain usually results from the distension of a viscus. It is most commonly due to gastroenteritis but can also be seen in surgical emergencies such as a bowel obstruction or intussusception. Sharp, localized pain is often an indication of peritoneal inflammation, as is seen in appendicitis.

All patients with abdominal pain are questioned about pertinent associated findings, including vomiting, diarrhea, fever, dysuria, and, in females, gynecologic complaints, such as vaginal discharge or bleeding. Patients with recurrent or chronic abdominal pain are questioned regarding associated weight loss, fatigue, arthralgias, melena, or hematochezia, all of which indicate an ongoing inflammatory process. For patients in whom no organic etiology of abdominal pain appears likely, the possibility of a psychosomatic disorder exists.

Physical Findings

The examination of the abdomen includes assessment of bowel sounds, tenderness, guarding, rebound, and distension. The size of the liver and spleen is also noted. Having the parent hold the child on his or her lap can facilitate the evaluation. While this is less than optimal, it allows for a basic assessment that at least can help to exclude an acute surgical emergency.

If there is a history of gastrointestinal bleeding or a surgical emergency is suspected, a rectal examination is indicated, after which the stool is checked for occult blood. Especially in infants, it is imperative that the perianal area be evaluated for the presence of a rectal tear or fissure. In addition, every pediatric patient with abdominal pain requires a genital examination.

In many cases, no laboratory evaluation is indicated. In younger children, however, in whom the history and physical examination are less reliable, laboratory studies can help determine the etiology of the problem. An especially useful test is a urinalysis, since the manifestations of a urinary tract infection in a child can be nonspecific and the physical examination unrevealing. In cases where a surgical problem such as an appendicitis is possible, an elevated leukocyte count can provide inferential evidence that an infectious process is present. In patients with suspected liver disease, a hepatic profile is indicated, and in the rare pediatric patient with suspected pancreatitis, a serum amylase may be helpful. When dehydration is suspected, electrolytes, blood urea nitrogen, and serum creatinine are indicated. In patients with abdominal pain and diarrhea, the stool can be evaluated for red or white blood cells, both of which indicate an inflammatory process usually secondary to bacterial enteritis.

Abdominal radiographs are useful in the patient with a suspected bowel obstruction, and a chest radiograph can exclude pneumonia, which, especially when it involves the right lower lobe, can cause severe abdominal pain.

VOMITING

Vomiting is most commonly a manifestation of a benign, self-limited illness. However, it can indicate a life-threatening process reflecting primary pathology of the gastrointestinal tract, can be secondary to a systemic illness, or can result from a process affecting the central nervous system.

The history begins with distinguishing true vomiting from gastric regurgitation, which is common in neonates and infants. In true vomiting, the patient expels most of the stomach contents. Postprandial emesis is common in patients with acute gastroenteritis but can also indicate a bowel obstruction. Posttussive emesis is common in conditions such as asthma and pertussis. In an infant, projectile emesis raises the suspicion of pyloric stenosis. The presence of bile in the emesis is never "normal" and suggests the possibility of an obstructive lesion, especially in an infant, where it is consistent with malrotation. The presence of blood in the emesis can indicate a gastrointestinal hemorrhage, although true blood must always be distinguished from other substances. The patient and parents are questioned regarding associated gastrointestinal symptoms such as nausea, diarrhea, or constipation. Associated abdominal pain is especially worrisome if it is present in between episodes of vomiting. Other constitutional symptoms to ask about include fever, headache, dysuria, flank pain, and, in females, gynecologic complaints.

The physical examination of the patient with vomiting is similar to that of the patient with abdominal pain. Nongastrointestinal causes of vomiting are excluded, with particular attention paid to the central nervous system. Lethargy, papilledema, and, in infants, splitting of the sutures or a full anterior fontanelle indicate increased intracranial pressure. The abdomen is assessed for the presence of distension, the character of the bowel sounds is evaluated, and the presence of tenderness, guarding, or rebound is noted. In patients in whom a surgical problem is not considered likely and in whom there is no evidence of gastrointestinal hemorrhage, a rectal examination is probably not helpful. However, if a surgical abdomen is considered, a rectal examination is indicated, along with a stool guaiac examination to rule out the presence of blood in the fecal material.

Laboratory studies are not indicated in the majority of patients with vomiting. In patients in whom a surgical process is possible, a complete blood count is indicated. A urinalysis is used to evaluate the possibility of a urinary tract infection, a common cause of vomiting that is notoriously difficult to diagnose clinically. The urine specific gravity is also useful as an indication of the status of the patient's hydration. In patients who appear dehydrated, serum electrolytes, creatinine, and blood urea nitrogen are indicated. In patients with suspected liver disease, a hepatic profile is used to evaluate the presence of hepatitis. In cases where the clinical evaluation supports the presence of a bowel obstruction, abdominal radiographs are indicated.

DIARRHEA

Diarrhea is a significant problem for children presenting to the emergency department, accounting for up to 20 percent of all pediatric outpatient visits and up to 8 percent of all pediatric hospital admissions. The vast majority of patients with diarrhea are suffering from mild, self-limited infectious illness. However, diarrhea can occasionally be the manifestation of an acute life-threatening problem.

The first step in caring for the patient with the complaint of diarrhea is to determine whether there is an abnormality in the pattern of stooling. In general, diarrhea is present if there is an increase in the frequency and a decrease in the consistency of the patient's stools. This can range from a slight increase in the number of stools per day to a fulminant loss of water and electrolytes through the gastrointestinal tract. It is important to distinguish between a previously normal patient with acute diarrhea and a patient with a gastrointestinal illness that can result in chronic constipation and overflow diarrhea, such as Hirschsprung disease or cystic fibrosis (see Chap. 51).

In patients who are found to have true diarrhea, further information is obtained regarding the stool's consistency and color and whether the stool contains blood. The presence of blood usually indicates an infectious etiology, which is often due to a bacterial enteritis. However, life-threatening events can also cause bloody diarrhea. These include intussusception and the hemolytic uremic syndrome. In patients previously treated with antibiotics, pseudomembranous colitis is a consideration. Severe inflammatory bowel disease can also cause bloody diarrhea and can result in life-threatening toxic megacolon. In young infants, *Salmonella* gastroenteritis can cause bloody diarrhea (see Chap. 49).

Patients are questioned regarding associated vomiting, abdominal pain, dysuria, and fever. In young infants, a careful feeding history is obtained. Overfeeding can cause diarrhea, as can formula intolerance. True formula allergy can cause bloody diarrhea but is not life-threatening.

The physical examination of the patient with diarrhea focuses on determining the etiology of the problem and assessing the hydration status of the patient. The presence of fever implies an infectious etiology, which can originate in the gastrointestinal tract or can be a manifestation of another source of infection. The tympanic membranes are evaluated for the presence of otitis media, an often-overlooked cause of diarrhea. The chest is examined to exclude pneumonia. The abdominal examination focuses on excluding a surgical emergency. The character of the bowel sounds and the presence of tenderness, guarding, rebound, or organomegaly are noted. In the presence of bloody diarrhea, an abdominal mass indicates a high probability of an intussusception. If there is any history of bloody diarrhea, the patient appears ill, or the patient is less than 2 to 3 months old with fever and diarrhea, a rectal examination is indicated and the stool is examined for the presence of red and white blood cells.

In nondehydrated patients with mild, nonbloody diarrhea, no laboratory workup is indicated. In ill-appearing patients in whom the etiology of the diarrhea is not known, stool cultures are indicated. A urinalysis may reveal an underlying urinary tract infection, which can have diarrhea as its sole manifestation. In febrile patients with bloody diarrhea, stool is sent for bacterial culture and evaluation for ova and parasites. Neonates with stools positive for white blood cells also have stool cultures performed to rule out *Salmonella.* In patients with bloody diarrhea who are not febrile, it is imperative that a life-threatening process such as intussusception or hemolytic uremic syndrome be excluded. In patients who have been treated with antibiotics, stool is sent for assay of *Clostridium difficile* toxin.

CONSTIPATION

Constipation is a decrease in the frequency of stooling, often associated with a change in the character of the stool. It is a frequent presenting complaint in the pediatric population, especially in neonates. There are few life-threatening diagnostic possibilities in the pediatric patient with constipation.

A detailed history is important to differentiate true from perceived constipation. Symptoms such as grunting, straining, or turning red during defecation do not necessarily imply constipation. Crying during defecation may be associated with a painful anal fissure but normal consistency of the stool. Especially in neonates, it is important to establish the pattern of stooling from birth, since delayed passage of meconium is associated with organic pathology, especially Hirschsprung disease. In infants, a feeding history is important, since a formula change may be associated with a change in bowel habits. It is also important to establish normal growth and development in the infant with constipation, since organic causes of constipation can be associated with failure to thrive. In toddlers and older children, a history of toilet training is sought, since difficulties in making the transition from diapers can result in psychogenic constipation. It is also important to solicit a history of fecal incontinence, or encopresis. Associated symptoms to elicit include lethargy, poor feeding, fever, and vomiting.

The physical examination of the constipated patient focuses on differentiating a systemic etiology from an obstruction of the gastrointestinal tract. The general appearance of the patient is noted in terms of neurologic status and growth and development. Infants are evaluated for the stigmata of hypothyroidism or the cranial nerve palsies of infantile botulism, both of which can cause constipation. The abdomen is evaluated for the presence of bowel sounds and distension. The abdomen is palpated in an attempt to elicit tenderness, which is occasionally present in the left lower quadrant. Constipation should never cause peritoneal findings. A digital rectal examination is performed, along with a stool guaiac test to rule out occult blood. Presence of impacted stool in the rectal vault suggests true constipation. Absence of stool in the rectal vault suggests proximal pathology, such as Hirschsprung disease.

If any abnormality is noted on the physical examination or the history is suggestive of a surgical emergency, an abdominal radiograph is indicated to rule out a bowel obstruction or severe colonic dilatation.

The mainstay of treatment of constipation consists of dietary manipulation to increase fiber and bulk, decrease fat content, and increase total fluid intake. In neonates and young infants, additional feedings of water between feedings may be all that is necessary to break the cycle. A temporary change to a formula low in iron or without iron can result in improvement. Parents of children old enough to take solid foods are encouraged to provide beans, celery, bran, and other high-fiber foods. Juices made from naturally occurring fruits and vegetables are probably helpful. In some cases, cow's milk may be a contributing factor, and a trial of lactose-free milk can be beneficial.

Stool softeners, such as docusate, are generally considered safe for children and may be useful until bowel habits have been reregulated. However, their use does not supersede dietary manipulation. Although not considered a routine treatment, a one-time insertion of a glycerin suppository may be helpful in stimulating a bowel movement in an acutely constipated patient.

In severely impacted patients, a pediatric enema may also provide relief. Recurrent use of these products is not recommended.

The patient with chronic or recurrent constipation presents a difficult problem that is beyond the scope of the emergency physician. Such patients often suffer from serious family pathology and may benefit from referral to a pediatric gastroenterologist or pediatrician familiar with the management of these cases.

GASTROINTESTINAL BLEEDING

Life-threatening gastrointestinal (GI) bleeding in children is uncommon.

For the purposes of evaluation and management, GI hemorrhage is divided into upper GI hemorrhage, occurring proximal to the ligament of Treitz, and lower GI hemorrhage, occurring distal to the ligament of Treitz, most commonly in the colon.

Presentation

Gastrointestinal bleeding can present dramatically as acute hemorrhage that threatens the patient with hemodynamic instability or as a subtle, chronic process that results in chronic anemia. Hematemesis is almost always a manifestation of an upper GI hemorrhage. The blood may be bright red or, if digested by gastric acid, have a coffee-ground appearance. The color of the blood is not indicative of the severity of the hemorrhage, and it is important to note that hematemesis is absent in 20 to 40 percent of patients with upper GI bleeding. The term *melena* refers to the passage of dark, sticky, sweet-smelling stools. While it is difficult to quantitate the rate of blood loss in patients with melena, it usually implies a loss of at least 2 percent of blood volume. Melena usually results from an upper GI hemorrhage. Hematochezia is the passage of bright red blood from the rectum. This usually involves a hemorrhagic process in the lower GI tract. Hematochezia may consist of the passage of pure blood, as can occur with an ulcerated Meckel diverticulum or avulsed juvenile colonic polyp. More commonly, blood is either mixed with the stool, which usually indicates an infectious or inflammatory process, or noted as streaks on the outside of the stool, which is commonly seen in lesions of the anus, such as fissures.

UPPER GASTROINTESTINAL HEMORRHAGE

Etiology

The most common causes of upper GI bleeding in the pediatric patient population are gastritis, esophagitis, duodenal ulcers, and esophageal varices. In newborns, vitamin K deficiency is a common cause of upper GI bleeding.

Gastritis

Gastritis in pediatric patients is often associated with severe physiologic stress, such as trauma, burns, and sepsis. It can also be precipitated by the use of aspirin. The normal buffering capacity of the gastric mucosa is altered in such a way that erosion of the mucosa occurs, mainly in the fundus of the stomach. Abdominal pain is a common presenting complaint, and vomiting can occur. In severe cases, hematemesis or melena can develop, though life-threatening hemorrhage is uncommon. The primary treatment consists of antacids and H_2 blockers.

Ulcer Disease

Peptic ulcer disease in children has somewhat similar manifestations to that in adults, and up to 70 percent of children with ulcers have a family history of ulcer disease. Older children are likely to present with abdominal pain, with or without associated vomiting and nighttime wakening. Preschool children often suffer gastrointestinal bleeding, obstruction, or perforation. Of these, bleeding is the most common symptom. The decreased use of aspirin appears to have reduced the incidence of gastritis and ulcer disease in children. Patients can suffer from chronic low-grade bleeding that results in iron-deficiency anemia, or they may develop life-threatening hemorrhage presenting as hematochezia or melena. Stress ulcers are common in pediatric patients with serious illness, such as sepsis, or after major trauma or extensive burns.

Patients with known chronic ulcer disease are managed with antacids and H_2-blocking agents such as cimetidine and ranitidine. If endoscopy shows an acutely bleeding ulcer, aggressive treatment with antacids to keep the stomach pH above 4.5 is indicated. Sucralfate is a topical agent used to coat ulcers and may be helpful.

Esophageal and Gastric Varices

Varices are associated with intrahepatic and extrahepatic portal venous obstruction, which leads to portal vein hypertension. Extrahepatic portal vein obstruction is usually secondary to catheterization of the umbilical vein or inflammatory omphalitis in the neonatal period. Intrahepatic obstruction is most commonly due to cirrhosis secondary to biliary atresia, which is the most common cause of variceal bleeding. Other causes of cirrhosis are neonatal hepatitis, congenital hepatic fibrosis, and cystic fibrosis. Two-thirds of pediatric patients with portal hypertension suffer hemorrhage before 5 years of age. In rare cases, bleeding varices are the presenting manifestation of underlying portal hypertension. They are the most common cause of life-threatening upper GI hemorrhage in children.

The Newborn

In the newborn, vitamin K deficiency can result in GI hemorrhage, although this problem has been effectively dealt with by the use of prophylactic vitamin K. In some cases, GI hemorrhage occurs for which no cause is found and which usually ceases within 24 h. Maternal blood may be swallowed during delivery and confused with GI bleeding in the newborn. The origin of the blood can be determined by adding sodium hydroxide to the specimen. The newborn's blood will remain pink, since fetal hemoglobin resists alkalinization, while maternal blood will turn brown.

Management of Upper GI Hemorrhage

In all patients with upper GI hemorrhage, it is essential that the hemodynamic status of the patient be established and protected. The evaluation and management of hypovolemic shock is covered in Chap. 3.

Stable patients with a history of hematemesis are evaluated for the possibility of a non-GI source of bleeding. Common sources are nosebleeds and bleeding gums. Occasionally, a severe pharyngitis can produce blood-tinged sputum that is mistaken for hematemesis. All patients with hematemesis or melena are evaluated for the stigmata of chronic liver disease, especially jaundice and hepatosplenomegaly. The skin is examined for signs of bleeding diathesis such as petechiae or purpura.

Laboratory studies include a complete blood count, electrolytes, and a serum blood urea nitrogen and creatinine. A coagulation profile and liver function tests are indicated in all but the most mild cases. Blood is sent for an urgent typing and crossmatch; if liver disease is present, fresh frozen plasma is ordered.

Placement of a nasogastric tube is indicated in all patients with a history of hematemesis or an examination that reveals melena. Gastric contents are evaluated for bright red blood or coffee-ground material, the presence of which confirms an upper GI hemorrhage. A negative nasogastric aspirate does not conclusively rule out a hemorrhage, since up to 16 percent of patients with clear drainage have active bleeding.

If the nasogastric aspirate reveals active bleeding, gastric lavage is indicated. The size of the tube is limited by the size of the nares. The known or suspected presence of varices is not a contraindication to the insertion of a nasogastric tube. There is controversy as to the most effective composition of the lavage fluid. Presently, free water appears to be as safe as normal saline, and fears about inducing water intoxication seem to be exaggerated. The temperature of the water does not appear to influence the outcome. In addition to confirming the presence of an upper GI hemorrhage and stopping the bleeding, nasogastric lavage also clears the stomach of blood, which, in the presence of liver failure, can lead to hyperammonemia and hepatic encephalopathy.

In the vast majority of cases of upper GI hemorrhage due to gastritis, esophagitis, and ulcer disease, lavage will result in cessation or significant slowing of the bleeding. In hemorrhage that results from bleeding varices, bleeding can be brisk and refractory to lavage. In persistent hemorrhage due to esophageal varices, vasopressin in a dose of 0.1 to 0.4 U/min may control the bleeding. Possible side effects include ischemia of the extremities or viscera. Somatostatin is a hypothalamic extract that decreases splenic flow and may be more effective than vasopressin in controlling variceal hemorrhage. Experience in children is limited.

Variceal bleeding refractory to gastric lavage and vasopressin can be controlled by the insertion of a Sengstaken-Blakemore tube into the stomach and esophagus. This instrument has balloons that can be inflated in the proximal stomach and distal esophagus and can tamponade the bleeding. Depending on the site of hemorrhage, the esophageal component, the gastric component, or both may have to be inflated. Accurate placement of the tube is confirmed radiographically. Inflation is usually maintained for at least 12 h.

If a gastroenterologist is available, injection of a sclerosing agent into the varices is useful for stopping an acute hemorrhage and preventing rebleeding. This may be preferable to inserting a Sengstaken-Blakemore tube.

It is vital for all patients with upper GI bleeding to be referred for endoscopy. When performed within 24 h of the onset of bleeding, endoscopy can identify the lesion 90 percent of the time and is therefore superior to barium studies.

LOWER GASTROINTESTINAL BLEEDING

In children, lower GI bleeding is rarely life-threatening, although on occasion it signifies a serious disease process. The sight of blood in a child's stools is always anxiety-provoking and mandates an aggressive attempt at determining a diagnosis.

Etiology

The Newborn

Rectal bleeding in the newborn is uncommon. In the immediate neonatal period, it is possible for swallowed maternal blood to be confused with that of the baby. If a bright red specimen is obtained, the two can be distinguished by the addition of sodium hydroxide, which alters the color of the maternal blood but not that of the newborn.

Necrotizing Enterocolitis

Necrotizing enterocolitis (NEC) is a serious inflammatory condition of the bowel usually associated with significant prematurity. However, up to 10 percent of cases occur in full-term infants. The condition usually occurs within the first 10 days of life. Early symptoms include lethargy, poor feeding, temperature instability, and apnea. Abdominal distension can develop, and, as the disease progresses, either heme-positive stools or grossly bloody stools are seen. Physical examination usually reveals an ill-appearing infant with or without abdominal tenderness. The workup includes a complete blood count, serum electrolytes, and cultures of the blood, urine, and spinal fluid. Abdominal radiographs may reveal air in the bowel wall (pneumatosis intestinalis). The patient is given nothing by mouth, and broad-spectrum antibiotic coverage is initiated. Surgical consultation is indicated (see Chap. 51).

Coagulopathy

Coagulopathy in the newborn is almost always due to vitamin K deficiency, although thrombocytopenia may occasionally occur. The infant may have ecchymoses or petechiae. Vitamin K–induced coagulopathy has become less common since the advent of prophylactic administration of vitamin K at birth. However, any newborn with significant GI bleeding should receive supplemental vitamin K.

Surgical causes of lower GI bleeding in the newborn include Hirschsprung disease and malrotation with volvulus (see Chap. 51).

Infants (1 Month to 2 Years)

Anal Fissures Anal fissures are the most common cause of rectal bleeding in infancy. Patients usually present with blood-streaked stools, pain with bowel movements, and occasionally constipation. The fissure is often visible on inspection of the anus. In some cases, an internal fissure can be diagnosed by inserting a small test tube into the anus, which facilitates visualization of the internal anal ring. A severe fissure or rectal tear raises the question of sexual abuse. Treatment is usually with stool softeners and sitz baths.

Formula Intolerance Intolerance to protein contained in cow's milk or soy-based formulas can result in an enterocolitis that usually presents in infants around 1 month of age. The presentation varies from chronic diarrhea and failure to thrive to grossly bloody stools. Further discussion appears later in this chapter.

Infectious Colitis Infectious colitis is a common cause of lower GI bleeding worldwide (see Chap. 49). It can appear from early infancy through adulthood. Certain bacterial organisms are strongly linked to bloody diarrhea, although viruses can also cause heme-positive stools. Infectious colitis usually presents with vomiting and diarrhea. Patients are often febrile. Older children may complain of colicky abdominal pain, but the abdomen is usually not tender on examination. Microscopic examination of the stools usually reveals red blood cells and polymorphonuclear leukocytes.

Lymphonodular Hyperplasia Lymphonodular hyperplasia is a benign disorder seen in infants and preschoolers. It can be associated with bright red rectal bleeding, which is rarely severe. Diagnosis is made by sigmoidoscopy or air contrast radiography. There is no treatment, and the disorder usually resolves within 3 months of onset.

Meckel Diverticulum Meckel diverticulum is the result of incomplete obliteration of the omphalomesenteric duct, usually located within 10 cm of the ileocecal valve. The condition can result in massive, painless rectal bleeding, obstruction, perforation, and peritonitis, or it may remain totally silent. Rectal bleeding results from acid secreted by ectopic gastric tissue that causes ulceration and erosion of tissue. The diverticulum is confirmed by performing a scan with technetium 99m that identifies ectopic gastric tissue. When symptomatic, the diverticulum is removed surgically.

Preschool (2 to 5 Years)

Juvenile Polyps In preschoolers with painless rectal bleeding, a juvenile polyp is a likely possibility. Juvenile polyps account for 90 percent of all polyps found in children. They are found primarily in children less than 8 years old, with a peak at 3 to 4 years. These polyps have no malignant potential. Rectal bleeding is usually minor, but in some cases it can be severe. Diagnosis is made by colonoscopy, and treatment consists of polypectomy.

School Age (Over 5 Years)

In children over 5 years of age, lower GI bleeding is most commonly the result of an infectious diarrhea. Juvenile polyps can also cause bleeding, although they are more likely to present in younger children. In older children, a major consideration in patients with lower GI bleeding is inflammatory bowel disease.

FORMULA INTOLERANCE AND ALLERGY

Formula intolerance can result from a true allergy to cow's milk protein. Enterocolitis can result and usually presents in infants of about 1 month of age. Bloody diarrhea is characteristic, and vomiting can occur. In older infants, chronic diarrhea and failure to thrive can be seen. Occasionally, significant protein loss and iron-deficiency anemia may be seen. Extragastrointestinal symptoms such as eczema, wheezing, and anaphylaxis can also develop. The incidence of cow's milk allergy may be as high as 8 percent. Some 20 to 30 percent of infants intolerant to cow's milk are also intolerant to soy-based formulas.

The only diagnostic test that may be useful is colonoscopy. It is imperative that bacterial colitis be ruled out. Since infants with formula-induced enterocolitis can have fever, elevated white blood cell counts, fecal leukocytes, and blood-streaked stools, it may be difficult to distinguish formula-induced enterocolitis from an acute infectious problem. Stool cultures will identify pathogens, but results are usually not available for 48 h.

Infants with suspected milk- or soy-induced colitis are treated with a trial diet consisting of elimination of the suspected offending formula. At least 48 h after elimination of the milk, a reintroduction of the antigen will reproduce the symptoms. An antigen challenge is best left to a pediatric allergist or gastroenterologist. Allergic infants are treated with a diet of an elemental formula, such as Nutramagen or Pregestamil.

COLIC

Colic is an imprecise term used to describe a combination of symptoms that occur in infants between the ages of 1 and 4 months, including episodes of excessive crying, fussiness after feeding, and paroxysms of irritability. Infant colic has been reported to occur with an incidence of between 16 and 30 percent. The severity of symptoms varies greatly, and it may be relieved by the passage of stool or gas. Episodes of colic often occur in the evening and can last several hours, resulting in extremely frustrated or worried parents and an emergency department visit. Infants appear well and are afebrile. The etiology of colic is essentially unknown but may be related in some instances to formula intolerance.

In many cases, persistent crying is the only manifestation of colic. It is important to exclude serious causes of inconsolable crying in an infant before making the diagnosis of colic. These include sepsis, meningitis, entrapment of the penis or a digit by a hair, an occult fracture, and incarcerated hernia. Intraabdominal pathology, including intussusception and volvulus, is also ruled out. Other common causes of inconsolable crying include corneal abrasions, anal fissures, and misplaced diaper pins.

Colic is a transient phenomenon. Infants may benefit from rhythmic rocking motions or from the vibration associated with a car ride. Some patients may benefit from a change in formula. Administration of acetaminophen assists with temporary relief of the symptoms of pain in the acute episode. For more persistent problems, simethicone, which reduces intestinal gas, may provide some relief. Sedatives and anticholinergics are not indicated.

GASTROESOPHAGEAL REFLUX

Gastroesophageal reflux (GER) refers to the regurgitation of stomach contents into the esophagus. It is common in young infants due to relatively low tone in the distal esophageal sphincter. Persistent GER is often associated with a hiatal hernia. Untreated, severe long-term GER can result in esophagitis and GI bleeding, recurrent aspiration pneumonia and reactive airway disease, failure to thrive, and iron-deficiency anemia.

Parents frequently seek medical attention because infants "spit up" after feedings. The regurgitated contents are not bile-stained, but they often contain partially digested formula and in severe cases can be bloody. In the emergency department, it is important to distinguish reflux from true vomiting, which in an infant can result from an obstructive lesion. In the majority of cases, an extensive emergency department workup is not indicated. Infants with refractory regurgitation and those with associated symptoms require more extensive evaluation. Studies performed vary, but include barium swallow, esophageal pH monitoring, endoscopy, and scintiscanning with a ^{99}Tc sulfur-colloid-labeled meal.

In most cases, GER resolves with age. In young infants, feeding smaller amounts at more frequent intervals and thickening the formula with cereal may result in an improvement of symptoms. Parents are encouraged to "burp" the baby frequently during feeding. Placing the infant in the prone position at 45 to 60° after feeding may help infants with more severe regurgitation. Medical management includes histamine blocking agents such as ranitidine; bethanechol, which increases gastric motility; and metoclopramide, which increases tone in the lower esophageal sphincter and relaxes pyloric sphincter tone. In older children, symptomatic management includes antacids and sucralfate.

Patients who do not respond to medical management may require surgical intervention, most commonly a Nissan fundoplication, in which the body of the stomach is wrapped around and sutured in front of the esophagus.

GALLBLADDER DISEASE

Diseases of the gallbladder in children are rare. However, certain disorders can predispose children to gallstones, and therefore to cholecystitis. Hemolytic anemias predispose patients to the formation of pigmented stones. Patients with cystic fibrosis also have a relatively high incidence of gallstones, as do patients with ileal Chron's disease.

Cholelithiasis in children presents much as it does in adults. Intermittent, colicky right upper quadrant pain that may radiate to the scapula is characteristic. Vomiting may occur. The presence of nonremitting pain accompanied by fever and leukocytosis indicates the development of cholecystitis. Ultrasonography will demonstrate stones and can define the anatomy of the gallbladder wall and the width of the common bile duct. In most cases, management is expectant, but on occasion cholecystectomy is necessary.

PANCREATITIS

Pancreatitis results when an inflammatory process causes a cascade of events that eventually lead to autodigestion of the pancreatic tissue by various pancreatic enzymes, including lipase, amylase, elastase, and phospholipase. It is uncommon in children, especially before the age of 10 years.

Blunt abdominal trauma is a relatively frequent cause of pancreatitis in children. In some cases the injury may appear relatively trivial, and in some cases it results from child abuse. Viral illnesses, especially mumps, can cause pancreatitis, as can a multitude of drugs. It is also associated with congenital anomalies of the biliary tree and infrequently with gallstones that obstruct the pancreatic duct.

Pancreatitis usually causes epigastric pain, which is constant and may radiate to the back. In many cases, the onset of pain is gradual. Vomiting is usually present. Patients with severe disease or who develop hemorrhagic pancreatitis may be hypotensive. The abdominal examination may reveal tenderness in the epigastrium, but the severity of the patient's pain may be out of proportion to the abdominal findings. Affected children tend to lie still, with their hips slightly flexed. High fever is uncommon.

The laboratory workup includes measurement of liver function tests, a complete blood count, electrolytes, blood urea nitrogen, creatinine, glucose, and calcium. The serum amylase is useful as a screening for pancreatic disease. However, it does not correlate with the severity of illness and can be elevated in diseases other than pancreatitis, including diabetic ketoacidosis and pelvic infections. Somewhat more specific is an elevation in the amylase to creatinine clearance ratio. Serum lipase may also be elevated. An abdominal radiograph may show a sentinel loop sign, localized ileus, blurred psoas margins, or other nonspecific signs. An ultrasound of the pancreas or computed tomography (CT) of the abdomen may be useful.

Therapy consists of fluid resuscitation and maintenance of serum electrolytes. Nasogastric suction may help to diminish pain. Analgesics are usually necessary for pain relief. Most patients with acute pancreatitis recover in a period of days. Complications include the formation of a pancreatic abscess or pseudocyst and the development of pleural effusion.

HEPATITIS

Hepatitis is a common viral illness with clinical manifestions that range from asymptomatic infection to fulminant liver failure. Several distinct viral etiologic agents have been identified.

Hepatitis A

The hepatitis A virus is an RNA virus of the picornavirus group. Transmission in humans is usually via contact with infected fecal material. This is particularly concerning for children who attend day care centers or who are institutionalized. The incubation period is usually 2 to 4 weeks.

The illness associated with hepatitis A infection is usually mild and self-limited. In young children, the infection is frequently asymptomatic and is usually not associated with jaundice. Symptomatic patients usually suffer an acute febrile illness characterized by nausea, anorexia, and fatigability.

Laboratory findings indicate elevation of serum transaminases. Both conjugated and unconjugated fractions of bilirubin are elevated. The erythrocyte sedimentation rate is also elevated. IgM antibody to hepatitis A is usually detectable for 6 to 8 weeks after the illness. IgG develops later and persists for years.

Treatment of hepatitis A is supportive, and most patients recover uneventfully. Hospitalization is indicated in patients who are unable to tolerate oral nutrition. Serum immune globulin is indicated in household contacts of affected patients to prevent the spread of clinical hepatitis. Families are encouraged to promote good hand washing and stool precautions during the course of the illness.

Hepatitis B

Hepatitis B virus (HBV) is a DNA virus with multiple components, including the surface antigen (HBsAg), the core antigen (HBcAg), and the hepatitis B e antigen (HBeAg). It is transmitted through body secretions such as semen, cervical secretions, saliva, and wound exudates. It can also be transmitted by infected blood or blood products, where even a minute quantity can produce active infection. Hepatitis B is a common infection in intravenous drug abusers. Unlike hepatitis A, HBV can also be transmitted from an infected mother to the newborn, perhaps at delivery. About 90 percent of infected newborns become chronic carriers of the infection. The incubation period of HBV is 2 to 5 months. Rarely, HBV results in severe, fulminant hepatitis.

In many patients, especially infants and young children, infection with HBV is asymptomatic. Symptomatic infection produces symptoms similar to those of hepatitis A, with nausea, vomiting, and malaise being common. The course of the illness tends to be less severe but more protracted. Prior to the onset of gastrointestinal symptoms, patients may develop various skin manifestations, including urticaria, and can suffer from arthralgias. Some patients can develop immune-mediated glomerulonephritis. Hepatomegaly or splenomegaly may be present with or without lymphadenopathy. By the time jaundice appears, if it develops at all, the child will probably be afebrile. The classic finding of clay-colored stools may not be present in children.

Laboratory findings reveal elevated serum transaminases and both conjugated and unconjugated bilirubin. Testing for the HBV infection is through a series of serum tests for antigen and antibody detection.

Treatment of HBV infection is supportive. Hospital admission is indicated for patients in whom nausea and vomiting preclude adequate hydration and nutrition and for the rare patient with fulminant hepatitis.

Infection with HBV is now preventable due to the development of a highly effective synthetic vaccine. Passive immunization is possible with hepatitis B immune globulin (HBIG).

Other Types of Hepatitis

Parenterally acquired non-A, non-B hepatitis is now called *hepatitis C.* It is considered a mild infection of insidious onset, manifested by malaise and jaundice. It is more common in adults. The incidence of developing chronic liver disease approaches 50 percent. Blood supplies are routinely screened for hepatitis C. Enterically transmitted non-A, non-B hepatitis is now called *hepatitis E.* Transmission of hepatitis E closely resembles that of hepatitis A. Malaise and jaundice are the usual presenting signs, with arthralgias, fever, and abdominal pain occasionally being associated. There are no serologic markers for hepatitis E, and therefore it is a diagnosis of exclusion.

Hepatitis D virus can multiply only in the presence of hepatitis B. It is usually transmitted parenterally. Infection with hepatitis D results in an increased incidence of chronic liver disease.

FULMINANT HEPATIC FAILURE

Fulminant hepatic failure is a syndrome characterized by severe hepatic dysfunction and encephalopathy. It usually evolves over a period of less than 8 weeks and affects all organ systems. Any infectious cause of hepatitis can result in fulminant hepatic failure, although it is uncommon in hepatitis A. Hepatic failure can also result from toxic exposure, especially from overdose of acetaminophen or ingestion of the mushroom *Amanita phalloides.* Severe shock can result in hepatic necrosis and liver failure. Depending on the etiology, hepatic failure may be reversible or irreversible.

A predominant manifestation of hepatic failure is encephalopathy, which usually begins with lethargy and can progress to confusion and combative behavior. In later stages, coma can develop. Cerebral edema may develop and may result in death. Associated complaints include anorexia, vomiting, and abdominal pain. On abdominal examination, the liver may appear small, and there may be ascites. Tachypnea may be present and results in a respiratory alkalosis. Failure to synthesize liver-dependent coagulation factors results in coagulopathy, which manifests itself clinically in a bleeding diathesis. Laboratory findings reveal elevated transaminases and serum ammonia. The prothrombin time is increased. Serum albumin may be decreased. In the vast majority of cases, serum bilirubin is increased. An exception to this is Reye syndrome, in which the serum bilirubin is usually not significantly elevated. Hyponatremia may be present, but it is usually dilutional. In some patients, renal failure develops.

Management consists of support of respiration, circulation, electrolyte balance, and nutrition, until such time as hepatic regeneration can occur. Hypoglycemia is especially common and may necessitate the administration of $D_{10}W$ or $D_{15}W$. The administration of fresh frozen plasma may help correct the coagulopathy. Gastrointestinal hemorrhage is a potential complication and may be averted by the administration of prophylactic H_2 blockers. Oral lactulose causes watery diarrhea of a low pH, and it may decrease serum ammonia by decreasing its formation by ammonia-forming organisms in the GI tract. Oral neomycin may also decrease the formation of ammonia.

JAUNDICE

Jaundice is the clinical manifestation of hyperbilirubinemia. It is relatively common in newborns, in whom some degree of hyperbilirubinemia is virtually universal. However, the appearance of jaundice beyond the immediate neonatal period is virtually always a manifestation of pathology, and in some instances reflects life-threatening disease.

Unconjugated Hyperbilirubinemia

The Newborn and Young Infant

In the immediate neonatal period, unconjugated hyperbilirubinemia is of great concern largely because of its association with kernicterus, an irreversible neurologic disorder that occurs when unbound bilirubin is deposited in the brain. In its early phases, kernicterus is characterized by lethargy, poor feeding, and, in some cases, opisthotonos. In its full-blown form, it ultimately results in choreoathetosis, extrapyramidal signs, and mental retardation. In full-term newborns, kernicterus is associated with levels of unconjugated serum bilirubin greater than 20 mg/100 mL. In premature infants, lower levels can cause kernicterus. In addition to the danger of kernicterus, the presence of hyperbilirubinemia can signify the presence of serious underlying disease. It is therefore essential that the differential diagnosis be fully considered.

The most common cause of unconjugated hyperbilirubinemia in the neonatal period is *physiologic jaundice.* It is thought to result from increased destruction of red cells and transiently impaired conjugation and excretion. Jaundice becomes visible on the second or third day of life and peaks around the fourth day. The maximum elevation is usually less than 6 mg/100 mL. In premature infants, jaundice both peaks and resolves somewhat later, and peak levels can reach 12 mg/100 mL.

In general, jaundice is more common in breast-fed infants. This may be due in part to substances contained in breast milk that antagonize the conjugation and excretion of bilirubin. Rarely, breast-fed infants can develop elevations of unconjugated bilirubin starting in the first week of life that can reach 15 to 27 mg/100 mL by the second or third week. The hyperbilirubinemia resolves with the cessation of breast-feeding and does not recur when it is resumed. A diagnosis of *breast milk jaundice* assumes that other pathologic causes of hyperbilirubinemia have been considered and eliminated.

Increased hemolysis is the most common cause of unconjugated hyperbilirubinemia in newborn infants that is severe enough to warrant phototherapy or exchange transfusion. It is usually secondary to maternal-fetal blood group incompatibility. Jaundice in infants with hemolysis secondary to blood group incompatibility is usually present in the first 24 h of life. Other causes of hemolysis include congenital diseases such as hereditary spherocytosis and glucose-6-phosphate dehydrogenase deficiency. Severe bruising or cephalohematoma secondary to trauma during delivery can also result in increased metabolism of heme proteins and unconjugated hyperbilirubinemia.

Unconjugated hyperbilirubinemia can also result from a variety of unusual causes. These include hypothyroidism, Down syndrome, and pyloric stenosis. Bacterial infections, including those from the urinary tract, can cause unconjugated hyperbilirubinemia, although there may also be a component of conjugated bilirubin.

Evaluation and Management The evaluation of unconjugated hyperbilirubinemia depends on the time at which jaundice is noted and the rate of rise of bilirubin (guidelines are presented in Appendix B, which appears on page 868). Infants with unconjugated bilirubin greater than 5 to 6 mg/100 mL after 2 to 3 days of life merit investigation. In general, it is useful to evaluate the patient for the presence of a hemolytic anemia by obtaining a complete blood count, reticulocyte count, and Coomb's test. If a bacterial infection is a consideration, cultures of blood, cerebrospinal fluid, and urine are obtained, in addition to a urinalysis. In infants with vomiting, a bowel obstruction must be ruled out. The diagnosis of breast milk jaundice is made after pathologic causes of hyperbilirubinemia are excluded, and serum bilirubin decreases when breast-feeding is stopped.

A majority of newborns with unconjugated hyperbilirubinemia do well with expectant management, with particular attention paid to maintaining adequate hydration. For patients with moderate to severe elevation, phototherapy is the treatment of choice. Indirect hyperbilirubinemia is reduced by exposure to high-intensity light. The criteria for the initiation of phototherapy are not completely clear and vary according to gestational age and birth weight. Premature infants are more susceptible than full-term babies to the neurologic toxicity of bilirubin. In the full-term infant, 20 mg/100 mL of indirect bilirubin is the concentration generally associated with a risk of kernicterus. Exchange transfusion is indicated in full-term infants with values above this, or in infants with rapidly rising serum bilirubin who do not respond to phototherapy.

The Older Child

In the older child, unconjugated hyperbilirubinemia is most likely the result of a hemolytic process or an inherited defect in the conjugation of bilirubin. Hemolytic anemia can be congenital or acquired. The workup for hemolytic anemia includes a complete blood count, reticulocyte count, and a serum haptoglobin. A common genetic defect in conjugation is Gilbert's syndrome, a deficiency in glucuronyl transferase that is associated with normal hepatic function.

Conjugated Hyperbilirubinemia

The Newborn and Infant

Conjugated hyperbilirubinemia is far less common in newborns and young infants than is unconjugated hyperbilirubinemia. It is present when the conjugated fraction of bilirubin exceeds 20 percent of the total. It most commonly occurs secondary to intrahepatic cellular damage and less often due to obstruction of biliary flow. Unlike unconjugated hyperbilirubinemia, conjugated hyperbilirubinemia is always pathologic and requires an accurate diagnosis so that appropriate therapy can be instituted. Most infants with abnormalities that result in conjugated hyperbilirubinemia will present within the first month of life. Since it can be associated with significant hepatocellular damage, the possibility of a coagulopathy is of concern.

Neonatal cholestasis can occur secondary to hepatic injury from a multitude of infectious causes. Cytomegalovirus, rubella, herpes simplex, varicella, coxsackie, and hepatitis B are common viral etiologies. Syphilis and toxoplasmosis are also implicated. Most of these result from intrauterine involvement and are often associated with congenital anomalies and hepatosplenomegaly.

Bacterial sepsis results in conjugated hyperbilirubinemia, although the unconjugated fraction is also usually increased. The mechanism is uncertain, but it may include increased hemolysis. The urinary tract is a common site of infection and can involve gram-negative organisms such as *E. coli.* Jaundice often starts at 3 to 4 days of age, and in some instances can be the only manifestation of infection.

While they are uncommon, a myriad of metabolic abnormalities can result in conjugated hyperbilirubinemia. Included in these are $alpha_1$ antitrypsin deficiency, cystic fibrosis, and galactosemia. Most metabolic disorders will have clinical manifestations other than jaundice that will lead to the diagnosis.

The major extrahepatic cause of conjugated hyperbilirubinemia in infancy is biliary atresia, a syndrome characterized by absence of the bile ducts anywhere between the duodenum and hepatic ducts. The cause of the disorder is unknown, but it appears to be the end result of an inflammatory process. Patients present with jaundice, dark urine, and often acholic stools. Mild hepatomegaly may be present. The evaluation of patients with suspected biliary atresia usually includes a liver biopsy, which may allow it to be distinguished from neonatal hepatitis, a disorder of unknown etiology in which there is diffuse hepatocellular disease and which is also characterized by conjugated hyperbilirubinemia. Depending on the location of the lesion in the bile ducts, surgical anastomosis of the remaining bile ducts to the bowel may be successful. Despite surgery, many of these patients go on to develop cirrhosis and portal hypertension, with associated esophageal varices.

Another cause of extrahepatic biliary obstruction is a choledochal cyst, a congenital saccular dilatation of the common bile duct. It can present with jaundice and a right upper quadrant mass, or with symptoms of cholangitis, including fever and leukocytosis.

Evaluation and Management The evaluation of conjugated hyperbilirubinemia is largely predicated on associated signs and symptoms. A diligent search for antenatal infections is usually indicated, and the possibility of a bacterial infection is excluded by blood, urine, and potentially cerebrospinal fluid cultures. A coagulopathy is excluded by measuring prothrombin time and partial thromboplastin time. Ultrasonography may be useful in excluding a structural abnormality such as a choledochal cyst. Most patients will require referral to a pediatric gastroenterologist for further workup, including a liver biopsy.

The Older Child

Conjugated hyperbilirubinemia in the older child most commonly results from infectious hepatitis. Drug-induced liver injury is also fairly common. Less commonly, genetic or metabolic disorders can present with jaundice and conjugated hyperbilirubinemia. Relatively common metabolic defects include $alpha_1$ antitrypsin deficiency and Wilson disease.

For a more detailed discussion, see John W. Graneto: Nonsurgical gastrointestinal problems, chap. 50, p. 296, in *Pediatric Emergency Medicine: A Comprehensive Study Guide.*

51 Acute Abdominal Conditions That May Require Surgical Intervention

Jonathan Singer

The differential diagnosis gastrointestinal surgical emergencies in the pediatric population is much more limited than in adults. Lesions are also remarkably age-related. A knowledge of the differential diagnosis is important for the emergency physician, especially in the evaluation of the neonate and preverbal child. The most common lesions are discussed under the headings of obstruction, intraabdominal sepsis, foreign body, and megacolon.

THE OBSTRUCTIONS

Malrotation with or without Midgut Volvulus

Malrotation occurs when there is an arrest of the normal embryonic rotation of the intestinal tract. This can result in the bowel, including the vascular supply, being anchored by a narrow pedicle instead of the normal broad-based mesentery. Adhesive bands (Ladd's bands) can cause partial or complete duodenal obstruction. While some patients remain asymptomatic, most develop problems within the first month of life. Neonates classically present with bilious emesis. Symptoms can also include failure to thrive, chronic recurrent abdominal distension, or persistent diarrhea. A volvulus occurs when the midgut twists upon its narrow mesenteric pedicle. Those who sustain a midgut volvulus experience sudden abdominal pain and vomiting. Intestinal ischemia can result in bloody or heme-positive stools. If the volvulus is not recognized within hours, viability of the gut may be compromised.

Plain radiographs of the abdomen may reveal signs of duodenal obstruction but are generally nondiagnostic. The test of choice is the upper gastrointestinal series; it should be performed on all neonates with bilious emesis. The findings of midgut volvulus include obstruction of the duodenum at its third portion and an associated inability to locate the normal ligament of Treitz to the left of the spine. Intestinal obstruction of the descending duodenum just over the right of the spine is pathognomonic.

Obstructed children require intestinal decompression. Patients may require aggressive fluid resuscitation. In selected circumstances, blood replacement may be needed in the preoperative period. Prophylactic antibiotics are preferred in toxic patients. In patients with volvulus, prompt laparotomy is necessary.

Pyloric Stenosis

Pyloric stenosis is the most common cause of intestinal tract obstruction after the first month of life. Affected patients may present as early as 1 week or as late as 3 months of age. The typical infant becomes symptomatic between the second and sixth weeks of life. Males are four times more likely to be affected than females. Symptoms of gastric outlet obstruction are produced by hypertrophy of circular fibers about the pylorus.

The initial symptom of pyloric stenosis is occasional nonprojectile vomiting. Within a week, nonbilious, postprandial, projectile vomiting develops. Anorexia is absent. Stools are generally small and infrequent. Urination may decrease in frequency secondary to dehydration.

The physical examination generally reveals an alert infant with good nutritional status. However, adipose tissue may be reduced and there may be decreased elasticity of the skin, particularly if dehydration is present. The hydration status may be severely compromised if vomiting has been prolonged. Unless significantly electrolyte- or volume-depleted, infants suck eagerly and, if fed, swallow without difficulty. A midabdominal peristaltic wave may be seen prior to the eventual regurgitant event. An epigastric, rounded mass is found in some patients.

A plain abdominal radiograph may demonstrate a dilated stomach but is nondiagnostic. Ultrasonography reveals an elongated and hypertrophied pyloric sphincter, a thickened gastric wall, and retained gastric contents. If ultrasonography is not available, then an upper gastrointestinal study is adequate. Loss of both potassium and hydrogen ion from repetitive vomiting of stomach contents can result in a characteristic hypokalemic, hypochloremic metabolic alkalosis.

The emergency physician should place a nasogastric tube and institute volume and electrolyte replacement in infants determined to have pyloric stenosis. Once a diagnosis is confirmed, surgical intervention with a pyloromyotomy is necessary.

Intussusception

Intussusception is an invagination of a proximal portion of the intestine into a distal adjacent part. More than 60 percent of cases occur in the first year of life, with most of those occurring between the fifth and ninth months. Males are affected twice as often as females, and this difference becomes more pronounced in children over 4 years of age, rising to an 8:1 ratio.

Intussusception classically creates a triad of colicky pain, vomiting, and bloody stools. In a typical case, there is a sudden onset of severe abdominal pain that may last several minutes. After an asymptomatic interval, repeated paroxysms will cause the child to cry out again. The intermittent nature of the pain is a significant clue to the diagnosis. Vomiting may occur either with the initial painful episode or soon after. Concurrent with vomiting, the child typically has several bowel movements, which vary from formed stools to thin liquid. Within 12 to 24 h, mucus, blood, or both may be passed per rectum, creating the classic "currant-jelly" stool.

Unfortunately, the classic triad is found in less than one-third of all patients. Findings are often nonspecific and include anorexia, which is almost universal, and diarrhea, which may be seen in about 7 to 10 percent of cases where there is complete intestinal obstruction and in up to 40 percent of cases where there is partial obstruction. Apathy or listlessness may occasionally be the dominant finding. This altered sensorium with intussusception may be seen in the context of prolonged symptomatology or as the initial complaint.

The general appearance of an affected child may vary from cheerful and interactive to lethargic and poorly perfused. Guarding or distension is uncommon. Bowel sounds may be normal, decreased, or absent. A sausage-shaped mass is found in 60 to 95 percent of cases. Stools may be grossly bloody, or normal-appearing stool may be positive for occult blood. Plain radiographs of the abdomen are unreliable in diagnosing intussusception. Ultrasonography of the abdomen has proved to be an acceptable diagnostic tool.

Nontoxic, hydrated children with a provisional diagnosis of intussusception are given nothing by mouth (placed NPO). Those who appear dehydrated are given intravenous fluid pending serum electrolytes, and a nasogastric tube is inserted. Either an air insufflation or barium enema reduction is performed in the presence of a surgical consultant. Because of the risk of barium peritonitis, attempted reduction with barium enema is contraindicated if there is evidence of intestinal perforation or peritonitis.

Incarcerated Hernias

In children, hernias occur with descending frequency at the umbilicus, inguinal and scrotal regions, midline epigastrium, and lateral border of the rectus sheath. When the contents of the hernia sac cannot be reduced into the peritoneal cavity, strangulation and necrosis of tissues may result. Male children with hernias outnumber female children by an 8:1 to 10:1 ratio. Both sexes have the greatest risk for incarceration during the first 6 months of life. With advancing age, incarceration becomes less likely.

The first symptom of incarceration in infancy is the abrupt onset of irritability. Expressive children indicate crampy abdominal pain that does not necessarily localize to the hernia site. Poor rooting and refusal to feed are seen in infancy shortly after incarceration. Anorexia or nausea may be expressed in older children. Infrequent nonbilious vomiting may rapidly progress to bilious vomiting. If the incarceration is long-standing, feculent vomiting may be seen as the bowel strangulates.

All children with incarceration appear uncomfortable. The abdominal findings vary depending upon the site of incarceration. The omental, reproductive, or intestinal masses are usually nontender and fluctuant at onset. They become firm and tender with passage of time and when viability of the viscus is compromised.

Plain films of the abdomen may reveal partial or complete bowel obstruction. With inguinal hernias, gas-containing soft tissue masses may be noted within the scrotum. Ultrasonography may be useful to discriminate the contents of the incarcerated sac.

Nonoperative reduction of a strangulated hernia can often be achieved by the emergency physician. Greatest success follows a period of withheld oral intake and application of ice to the hernia sac. Sedation is usually necessary. Suspected strangulation or unsuccessful reduction by the emergency physician mandates surgical consultation.

INTRAABDOMINAL SEPSIS

Acute Appendicitis without Perforation

The late elementary school population has the highest incidence of appendicitis in childhood. There is a gradual reduction in frequency in younger children, with a precipitous drop in children below 2 years of age. Acute appendicitis is encountered equally in both sexes. Transmural bacterial invasion of the appendix may begin as an intraluminal infection or result from obstruction of the appendiceal lumen by enlarged lymphatic tissue, intestinal parasites, foreign bodies, or fecalith.

The triad of abdominal pain, vomiting, and low-grade fever is suggestive of appendicitis. Abdominal pain is the first manifestation of the disease. At onset, the pain is epigastric or periumbilical and is described as dull. It later becomes more intense and constant. As the inflammation proceeds to include the parietal peritoneum, pain localizes, in most cases, 3 to 5 cm from the anterior-superior iliac spine on a straight line drawn from that process to the umbilicus (McBurney's point). Pain may radiate to the flank or back. At least one or two episodes of nonbilious vomiting occur in over 90 percent of cases. Temperature elevation is a noted feature in 75 to 80 percent of patients. An inflamed appendix, particularly if retrocecal, may cause fecal urgency, tenesmus, and frequent passage of a small volume of stool. Some 5 to 15 percent of children with an inflamed appendix in proximity to the ureter may experience dysuria. The latter two atypical symptoms are more often clinical features in misdiagnosed cases.

With the exception of low-grade fever, patients with nonperforated appendicitis will have minimal alteration of their vital signs. Some patients may favor the right leg. If the appendix is in a retrocecal position, elevation and extension of the right leg against pressure of the examiner's hand causes pain (iliopsoas sign). When the flexed right thigh is held at right angles to the trunk and internally rotated, hypogastric pain may result (obturator sign). Abdominal distension is absent. Patients may voluntarily guard the entire abdomen or only the right lower quadrant. Exquisite tenderness is often noted directly over McBurney's point. Pressure applied to the descending colon may cause referred pain at McBurney's point (Rovsing's sign). A rectal examination reveals right-lower-quadrant tenderness but no masses.

Radiologic studies and other imaging techniques are not necessary with clear-cut appendicitis. However, various studies may be helpful in an equivocal case. Plain radiographic findings suggestive of appendicitis include protective scoliosis of the lumbar spine, localized air-fluid levels in the region of the cecum and terminal ileum, obliteration of the right properitoneal fat stripe, haziness over the right sacroiliac joint, loss of the right-sided psoas shadow, and fecalith. A contrast enema in which the appendix fails to fill with barium is highly suggestive of appendicitis. In appendicitis, ultrasonography may demonstrate greater than 2-mm thickness or an outer wall-to-wall diameter greater than 6 mm.

In cases of suspected appendicitis, surgical consultation is indicated.

Acute Appendicitis with Perforation

Age is the single most important factor affecting the likelihood of perforation in the course of acute appendicitis. Symptoms in the very young may be misleading. The percentages of patients with perforation at the time of diagnosis are as follows: nearly 100 percent in the first year of life, 94 percent for those below age 2, 60 percent for those below age 6, and 30 to 40 percent for children over 6 years of age. Rapid progression to perforation in as little as 6 to 12 h from onset of symptoms has been described in preschool-aged children.

Classically, patients who perforate experience increasingly severe abdominal pain until the appendix perforates. Pain may then lessen or cease. After the appendix ruptures, a small amount of pus is extruded. In the first year of life, a short, thin omentum has little capacity to wall off infection. Diffuse peritonitis within hours to days is likely. Older children tend to isolate an expanding collection of pus. Children whose appendixes have perforated may encounter vague abdominal complaints for days to weeks after the intraperitoneal event. There may be periods of remission interspersed with exacerbations. The abscesses that develop are most common in the periappendiceal region.

Patients with perforated appendicitis tend to be ill-appearing. Vital signs are abnormal. Tachycardia and fever are common. The temperatures tend to in the range of 39 to 40°C. Extreme tachycardia, hypotension, and altered tissue perfusion may be found with severe dehydration or superimposed sepsis. Patients most often have excruciating abdominal pain. Abdominal distension may be prominent, especially in infancy. Bowel sounds are diminished or absent. Children will voluntarily and involuntarily guard the abdomen. Palpation of the abdomen in any quadrant may be painful. Rebound tenderness is most prominent in the right lower quadrant. Iliopsoas and obturator signs are variable. Rectal tenderness is noted, but a mass is an inconstant finding.

Results of barium enema may mimic an ileocecal intussusception or pathognomically demonstrate extravasation of contrast near the cecum. Ultrasonography, in addition to revealing an enlarged, edematous appendix, may demonstrate a periappendiceal fluid collection. Abdominal computed tomography may assist in localizing an abscess.

The preferred preoperative management of the patient with perforated appendicitis includes 45 to 60° elevation of the head of the bed, nasogastric suction, aggressive hydration, and antibiotics. Urgent surgical consultation is mandatory.

Spontaneous Peritonitis

Spontaneous peritonitis may occur in previously healthy children, but patients with ventriculoperitoneal shunt, splenectomy, and ascites from cirrhosis or nephrosis are at increased risk. The condition tends to occur more often in females and peaks between the ages of 5 and 10 years.

Patients with spontaneous peritonitis have an insidious onset and develop diffuse abdominal pain. The pain does not localize and increases in intensity over hours to days. Nonbilious vomiting, diarrhea, and temperature elevation follow the abdominal pain. Patients are anxious and ill-appearing. Temperature elevations are noted in the 39 to 40.5° C range; tachycardia is prominent. The respirations are rapid and shallow and may be accompanied by a terminal expiratory grunt. Bowel sounds are diminished. The abdomen is diffusely distended and tender, and ascites may be present.

Plain radiographic features of peritonitis include marked gaseous distension of the large and small intestines, in which multiple air-fluid levels may be present. Intestinal loops may become separated, and the more dependent portions become more opaque.

If a spontaneous peritonitis is suspected preoperatively, abdominal paracentesis with Gram stain and culture may obviate the need for exploratory laparotomy. Fluid resuscitation and antibiotic therapy are indicated.

Necrotizing Enterocolitis

Diverse events in the perinatal period may lead to gastric dilatation, functional ileus, and erosive intestinal mucosal injury—all characteristic of necrotizing enterocolitis (NEC). The terminal ileum and colon are the most common sites of histologic changes.

The pathologic findings range from mucosal edema to full-thickness necrosis with perforation. Premature infants who have sustained any of multiple stresses to the cardiovascular system—such as acute blood loss, transient hypotension, and birth asphyxia—or who require central vascular instrumentation are at increased risk for NEC. Most infants are diagnosed prior to their initial hospital discharge.

Necrotizing enterocolitis represents a spectrum of illness that varies from a self-limited, transient process to a potentially fatal disease. Anorexia and gastric distension followed by nonbilious vomiting, abdominal distension, or diarrhea are seen at onset. Hematochezia may develop. Apnea, bradycardia, hypotension, and vascular instability may all occur.

Affected infants are pale and often septic-appearing. Abdominal distension may be generalized, or a single segment of colon may dilate to striking proportions. Abdominal tenderness and guarding are highly variable. Bowel sounds are diminished. Rectal examination reveals grossly bloody stool or seedy stool that is guaiac-positive.

On abdominal flat plate, bowel distension is the most common radiographic finding. The dilatation may occur in an isolated, diseased, unobstructed colonic segment. Alternatively, multiple loops of distal small and large bowel exhibit dilatation, suggesting partial obstruction. Intraluminal air (pneumatosis intestinalis) may be limited to scattered colonic segments or be generalized. Intrahepatic portal vein gas or pneumoperitoneum are ominous findings. Ultrasonography in NEC has proven to be of benefit only to detect and track the passage of air through the portal vein system.

Treatment includes withholding feedings, initiating parenteral nutrition, nasogastric decompression, and parenteral as well as intraluminal antibiotics. In the absence of perforation, obvious peritonitis, and gangrenous bowel, surgery is withheld.

Hirschsprung Disease

Hirschsprung disease is characterized by the absence of intramural ganglion cells. The deficit is usually limited to a segment of bowel in the rectosigmoid region. Relaxation needed to facilitate the onward movement of stool does not occur. This disease is four times more frequent in males than females.

The diagnosis may be suspected within the first few days of birth or not entertained until late childhood. Newborns with aganglionosis may have delayed passage of the first meconium stool. Infants have diminished stool frequency. If the disease remains undiagnosed, the clinical course in the first year of life is one of gradually increasing fecal retention, obstipation, constipation, and sporadic abdominal distension. Diminished appetite and failure to thrive are often noted. Intermittent vomiting and occasional unexplained bouts of nonbloody diarrhea may be encountered.

Examination of the affected child reveals a variable nutritional status. There may be mild to moderate abdominal distension. The abdomen is soft and nontender, and mobile fecal masses may be palpable in the left lower quadrant. Children's underwear is not soiled from overflow, as is typically the case with children who have functional constipation. Rectal examination reveals an empty vault. Withdrawal of the examining finger may result in an explosive release of stool. If the diagnosis is not entertained, patients may precipitously develop a potentially fatal enterocolitis.

Enterocolitis with Hirschsprung disease is more common in the newborn period but can occur at any age. The enterocolitis is characterized by sudden abdominal distension, generalized abdominal discomfort, and explosive diarrhea that rapidly becomes bloody. Temperature elevation, volume depletion, and altered mental status are typically noted. With the most severe cases, a denudation of the intestinal mucosa predisposes to colonic perforation, peritonitis, and gram-negative septicemia.

Diagnostic modalities in chronic constipation include plain abdominal films, barium enema, anal rectal manometry, and pathologic examination of rectal tissue. With aganglionosis, the abdominal flat plate may be normal or demonstrate a dilated colon proximal to the aganglionic segment. Barium enema confirms a normal caliber of the rectum and dilatation of the proximal colon. A cone-shaped transition zone between the two is pathognomonic.

At the time of enterocolitis, plain abdominal radiographs show variable distension of multiple intestinal loops and gas-fluid levels. The sigmoid or descending colon may be massively dilated. Pneumoperitoneum may be present if spontaneous perforation of the colon has occurred.

Emergency department intervention for enterocolitis includes NPO, gastric decompression, a rectal tube, fluid resuscitation, and parenteral antibiotics.

AERODIGESTIVE FOREIGN BODIES

Gastrointestinal Foreign Bodies

The size, configuration, consistency, and chemistry of an ingested object, coupled with the child's age and personal anatomy, determine whether the child remains asymptomatic or develops clinical manifestations. Small (less than 15 to 20 mm), round, oval, and cuboid objects without sharp edges or projections cause the least difficulty. Rigid, elongated slender objects may also traverse the intestinal tract without difficulty but are more inclined to cause complications. Concretions from repeated ingestion of hair or vegetable matter can lead to bezoars. Ingested batteries retained within the esophagus or stomach or lodged in the appendix or a Meckel diverticulum can cause perforation. Children with underlying congenital, anastomotic, or inflammatory diseases of mediastinal structures are at increased risk of gastrointestinal foreign-body impaction. Children below 1 year of age are at increased risk for complications.

Complications of gastrointestinal foreign bodies include obstruction within the gastrointestinal tract and perforation anywhere within the gut. Other gastrointestinal complications include gut fistulization or hemorrhage. Less common but more dangerous are complications of a retained esophageal foreign body, including mediastinitis and erosion into the major vessels.

Foreign bodies typically lodge at the hypopharynx, the thoracic inlet, or the cardioesophageal junction. Patients with a hypopharyngeal foreign body have persistent gagging and pooling of oral secretions. They are unable to swallow or speak. Patients with a foreign body at the aortic arch may localize pain to the area of the sternal notch. They too have dysphagia and drooling, but they lack dysphonia. Foreign bodies retained at the distal esophagus create vague chest discomfort as well as dysphagia and odynophagia. Obstruction lower down in the intestinal tract causes intermittent abdominal pain with or without vomiting. Distal problem sites include the pylorus, the loop of the duodenum, the ligament of Treitz, and the ileocecal valve.

Physical findings are limited when an ingested foreign body has caused isolated obstruction in the gastrointestinal tract. Vital signs are usually normal. The abdomen is generally soft and nontender, and—with the exception of bezoars—there is no mass. Bowel sounds are normal or high-pitched. Metallic foreign bodies have been successfully located with coin detectors; however, the majority are diagnosed by plain radiograph. A lateral neck film is reserved for children with retained esophageal coins.

All patients discharged home from the emergency department need to know the delayed signs and symptoms of retained foreign body in the gastrointestinal tract. Only those with retained esophageal foreign body consistently require immediate intervention. Endoscopy is generally used to remove esophageal foreign bodies, especially batteries with corrosive potential. Very rarely, elective surgical retrieval of an intragastric pointed or elongated foreign body may be necessary.

MEGACOLON

Inflammatory Bowel Disease

Inflammatory bowel disease in late childhood or early adolescence consists of ulcerative colitis (primarily a disease of the rectal and colonic mucosae) and Crohn's disease, a transmural disease primarily but not necessarily restricted to the distal ileum. The risk of acquiring either disease is similar in both sexes. Extraintestinal manifestations such as growth retardation, fever, anemia, arthritis, arthralgia, mouth ulcerations, erythema nodosum, pyogenic gangrenosa, liver dysfunction, and uveitis are common to both disorders and may precede the onset of the gastrointestinal complaints. In most children with these two conditions, the overriding concern is persistent diarrhea followed by the appearance of mucus and blood admixed in the stools. In the majority of cases, the diarrhea begins insidiously, but a small percentage may have an acute, fulminant course, manifesting apparent bacterial sepsis with profuse, bloody diarrhea.

Either as an exacerbation of long-standing disease or as the precipitating event of the disease, patients with both conditions may develop a toxic dilatation of the colon (megacolon). The transverse colon is typically involved. A transmural inflammatory process occurs, and the segment of colon dilates massively. Significant hemorrhage and multiple areas of microperforation may be preludes to peritonitis and overwhelming sepsis.

Patients with megacolon develop fever and experience malaise and anorexia. Abdominal pain will develop over a period of a few hours to a day. Lethargy may develop.

Physical examination is remarkable for toxicity and apparent volume depletion. Temperature elevation and tachycardia are noted. Bowel sounds are diminished. The abdomen is distended, tympanitic, and tender. Guarding and rebound may occur with frank perforation. Rectal examination is painless and reveals no masses, sinuses, or fistulas unless the inflammatory bowel disease has been long-standing. Stool is grossly bloody.

The hallmark radiologic feature of toxic megacolon seen on a supine abdominal film is dilatation of the transverse colon $\geq$6 to 7 cm in diameter. As perforation may complicate megacolon, an upright or decubitus view should be obtained to search for free air. Ultrasonography is more useful following perforation.

Initial treatment for toxic megacolon involves fluid resuscitation, with added albumin or blood as necessary. High-dose corticosteroids are required for patients on maintenance steroids. Pending surgical consultation, a nasogastric tube should be passed and parenteral antibiotics begun.

For a more detailed discussion, see Singer J: Acute abdominal conditions that may require surgical intervention, chap. 51, p. 311, in *Pediatric Emergency Medicine: A Comprehensive Study Guide.*

SECTION VIII
ENDOCRINE AND METABOLIC EMERGENCIES

52 Disorders of Glucose Metabolism

Arlene Mrozowski

DIABETIC KETOACIDOSIS

Diabetic ketoacidosis (DKA) is characterized by hyperglycemia, dehydration, and metabolic acidosis. As the initial presentation of diabetes, DKA is common in young children. In young patients, DKA accounts for 70 percent of diabetes-related deaths.

In DKA, a lack of insulin prohibits intracellular utilization of glucose. The levels of counterregulatory hormones—cortisol, epinephrine, glucagon, and growth hormone—rise. Gluconeogenesis and glycogenolysis occur in the liver. Lipolysis in fatty tissues forms the ketoacids betahydroxybutyrate and acetoacetic acid. The combination of hyperglycemia and ketoacidosis causes a hyperosmolar diuresis that can result in a profound loss of fluids and electrolytes. The combination of ketonemia and hypoperfusion can result in a severe anion gap metabolic acidosis.

Common precipitants of DKA include lack of compliance with insulin, infection, and stress.

The clinical manifestation of DKA depend primarily on the severity of the hyperglycemia and metabolic acidosis and the degree of intravascular volume depletion. Mental status ranges from normal to lethargy and, in severe cases, coma. Virtually all patients have signs of significant dehydration. The metabolic acidosis induces hyperventilation in order to decrease P_{CO_2}. Patients with severe acidosis may demonstrate Kussmaul breathing, characterized by deep, sighing respirations. Some patients may develop vomiting, which can be accompanied by severe abdominal pain.

Laboratory Studies

Laboratory studies include a complete blood count, serum electrolytes and glucose, calcium, phosphorus, and serum acetone. In

DKA, the serum glucose is almost always greater than 300 mg/dL. The patient's urine can also be tested at the bedside for the presence of ketones. The patient's acid-base status is evaluated with an arterial blood gas or venous pH.

During the resuscitation, serum glucose levels are monitored every hour. Serum electrolytes and venous pH are monitored every 2 to 3 h. Urine is monitored for ketones at every void.

Management

The fundamental management of DKA consists of replacing the patient's fluid losses and reversing the fundamental pathophysiology by the administration of exogenous insulin.

Most patients with DKA are at least 5 to 10 percent dehydrated. The initial fluid resuscitation is with either normal saline or Ringer's lactate at a dose of 20 mL/kg. In stable patients, the bolus is given over 1 h; in patients in shock, it is administered as fast as possible. After the initial bolus, the patient's cardiovascular status is reevaluated. If perfusion is not adequate, a second bolus of 20 mL/kg is administered. After the initial resuscitation, rehydration is continued with 0.45*NS*. In patients with extreme hyperosmolarity, some recommend continuing therapy with isotonic fluids until serum osmolarity decreases below 315 mosm/L.

Recommendations for continuing fluid resuscitation vary. Common practice is to replace 50 percent of the estimated deficit over the initial 8 h and the remainder over the next 16 h, though some recommend replacing losses over 36 to 48 h. It has been recommended that fluid not exceed 4 L/m^2/24 h.

As soon as the diagnosis of DKA is made and fluid resuscitation instituted, supplemental insulin is administered. Current recommendations are for continuous infusion, which provides reliable, titratable absorption. An initial bolus is not necessary. The starting dose is 0.1 U/kg/h. The goal of therapy is to decrease the serum glucose by 75 to 100 mg/L/h. When the serum glucose reaches 250 mg/L, 5% glucose is added to the infusing fluid. If the serum glucose is dropping precipitously, 10% glucose is administered. In some cases it may be necessary to decrease the insulin infusion to 0.3 to 0.6 U/kg/h. It is dangerous to completely discontinue the infusion, since this can worsen the ketoacidosis. On occasion, the infusion may need to be increased to 0.15 to 0.2 U/kg/h to lower the serum glucose and reverse the ketosis.

When the serum glucose normalizes, metabolic acidosis resolves, urine ketones clear, and the patient is able to eat and drink, the insulin infusion is discontinued. Subcutaneous insulin is administered 30 min prior to discontinuing the infusion to allow for the transition to the patient's normal insulin usage. Not administering subcutaneous insulin prior to discontinuing the infusion can lead to rebound hyperglycemia and ketoacidosis.

Potassium

Virtually all patients with DKA are potassium-depleted. Depending on multiple factors, including the severity and acuity of acidosis and the degree of dehydration, the initial serum potassium can be low, normal, or high. Both severe hypo- and hyperkalemia can cause life-threatening cardiac arrhythmias. Hypokalemia is most common several hours after rehydration is initiated. Replacement therapy is started once a normal or low serum potassium is assured and urine output is established. The usual dose of potassium is at twice daily maintainance, or 3 to 4 meq/kg/24 h.

Sodium

Laboratory studies do not reflect actual serum sodium, since both the hyperglycemia and the hyperlipidemia of DKA cause factitiously low values. Some of the depleted sodium is replaced during the initial resuscitation with normal saline or Ringer's lactate. During the continuing resuscitation, sodium levels are monitored every 2 to 3 h. As the glucose falls, the serum sodium should rise. A fall in serum sodium during continued fluid resuscitation may indicate excess accumulation of free water and may be a risk factor for the development of cerebral edema.

Phosphate

Phosphate is also depleted during DKA. The benefit of urgent replacement of phosphate during DKA is debatable; however, supplementation is indicated if the serum level is below 2 meq/L. Phosphate can be administered in conjunction with potassium replacement as a potassium salt. For example, an infusion could consist of 20 meq of potassium chloride and 20 meq of potassium phosphate in a liter of 0.45 normal saline.

Bicarbonate

The use of sodium bicarbonate in the treatment of DKA remains extremely controversial. Clinical studies have failed to demonstrate improved outcome in patients treated with supplemental bicarbonate. Its use can be considered in patients with severe acidosis (pH less than 7.1 or serum bicarbonate less than 5 meq/L). Only enough bicarbonate is administered to increase the pH to 7.2. From 1 to 2 meq/kg is administered over 2 h as part of a 0.45 *NS* solution.

Complications of Diabetic Ketoacidosis

Complications in the management of DKA include hypoglycemia, electrolyte imbalance, cardiac arrhythmias, and cerebral edema.

Hypoglycemia often occurs 6 to 8 h after the initiation of therapy. Treatment consists of adjusting the insulin infusion and providing supplemental intravenous and oral glucose.

Hypokalemia is the most common electrolyte abnormality and occurs within several hours of initiation of therapy. Treatment is with supplemental potassium, as discussed above.

Cerebral edema accounts for at least half of DKA-related deaths. It usually occurs as the patient's metabolic parameters are improving and is often heralded clinically by complaints of headache, dizziness, changes in behavior, incontinence, and alterations in pulse and blood pressure, all of which can indicate increased intracranial pressure. It seems to be more common in young diabetics and in cases of new-onset diabetes.

At present, the etiology of cerebral edema is unknown and its occurrence is unpredictable. Factors implicated include a rapid fall in blood glucose, hypoglycemia, excessive administration of fluids, a failure of the serum sodium to rise during treatment, and the use of bicarbonate.

The treatment of cerebral edema consists of hyperventilation, mannitol, and fluid restriction, all of which decrease intracranial pressure. Given the unpredictable nature of cerebral edema, careful attention to neurologic status is mandatory in the treatment of all patients with DKA.

Disposition

All patients presenting with DKA as the initial presentation of diabetes are hospitalized. Patients with severe acidosis are best treated in an intensive care unit, though criteria for this vary among institutions.

Outpatient management of DKA has been advocated for a selected group of patients. This includes those with stable vital signs, the ability to tolerate oral fluids, established physician follow-up, and a competent family setting. If after 3 to 4 h of emergency department treatment the serum pH has risen to 7.35 or greater and the serum bicarbonate is greater than 20 meq/L, the patient is discharged.

HYPOGLYCEMIA

Hypoglycemia is defined as a decrease in the serum glucose level to below 50 mg/dL in children and below 30 mg/dL in neonates.

In children seen in the emergency department, the most common cause of hypoglycemia is an adverse reaction to insulin therapy in a known diabetic.

Signs and Symptoms

Newborns and young infants may be asymptomatic or may manifest nonspecific symptoms such as irritability, pallor, cyanosis, tachycardia, tremors, lethargy, apnea, or seizures. Older children exhibit more classic symptoms of hypoglycemia, including diaphoresis, tachycardia, tremor, anxiety, tachypnea, and weakness. Prolonged hypoglycemia can cause confusion, stupor, ataxia, seizures, and coma. In the early phase, many patients will complain of headache.

Differential Diagnosis

Hypoglycemia secondary to lack of exogenous glucose is common in acutely ill infants and children, since oral intake is often decreased during an acute illness. Deliberate fasting anorexia in an older child may present as hypoglycemia. Ketogenic hypoglycemia is an entity usually seen in underweight males between the ages of 2 and 7 years with a history of low birth weight. It is characterized by episodic bouts of hypoglycemia associated with ketonuria. The pathogenesis is unknown. In the acute phase, patients respond promptly to glucose. Avoidance of prolonged fasting is the only treatment necessary. The disorder is outgrown by late childhood.

Conditions leading to hyperinsulinemia can result in hypoglycemia. This most commonly occurs in a diabetic patient who has taken insulin but does not ingest sufficient calories. Other causes of hyperinsulinemia include islet cell adenomas, neisidioblastosis, and the beta cell hyperplasia of Beckwith-Wiedemann syndrome.

Inborn errors of metabolism can result in hypoglycemia by disrupting endogenous glucose metabolism. These include a wide array of defects in amino acid metabolism, glycogen storage diseases, and enzyme deficiencies in gluconeogenic and glyconeogenic pathways.

Hormonal disorders such as hypopituitarism, hypothyroidism, and adrenal insufficiency can also cause hypoglycemia. Especially in infants, these disorders can be very difficult to diagnose in the emergency department.

Management

A rapid determination of serum glucose is achieved by direct measurement done on an initial venous sample. A urinalysis is sent for measurement of ketones, which if absent indicate hyperinsulinemia or a defect in fatty acid metabolism. The presence of ketones indicates an appropriate stress response to hypoglycemia.

Glucose is administered to symptomatic patients in a dose of 0.5 g/kg/dose. Dextrose 25% in water in a dose of 2 to 4 mL/kg is appropriate therapy. In neonates and preterm infants, dextrose 10% in dose of 1 to 2 mL/kg/dose is used to avoid sudden hyperosmolarity. In older children and adolescents, dextrose 50% at a dose of 1 to 2 mL/kg/dose is used. If hypoglycemia persists, a continuous infusion of $D_{10}W$ or D_5W and 5 mg/kg/min is indicated.

In the event that intravenous access is not possible, glucagon at a dose of 1 mg is given, regardless of the age. It is effective in hyperinsulin-induced hypoglycemia. Glucagon is not indicated in infants that are small for gestational age.

Patients with mild hypoglycemia who are capable of eating or drinking are treated with orange juice or some other age-appropriate source of calories.

Disposition

In cases where the cause of hypoglycemia is not known, hospital admission for further evaluation is indicated. Insulin-dependent diabetics who experience hypoglycemia can be discharged unless they have been experiencing episodes of hypoglycemia that indicate that hospitalization is needed to adjust the insulin dose.

For a more detailed discussion, see Mrozowski A: Disorders of glucose metabolism, chap. 52, p. 321, in *Pediatric Emergency Medicine: A Comprehensive Study Guide.*

53 Adrenal Insufficiency

Elizabeth E. Baumann / Robert L. Rosenfield

Adrenal insufficiency (AI) results from disruption of the hypothalamic-pituitary-adrenal axis at any point in the system. The symptoms of AI result from deficiencies of cortisol (glucocorticoid deficiency) and aldosterone (mineralocorticoid deficiency).

Glucocorticoid deficiency impairs gluconeogenesis and glycogenolysis, resulting in fasting hypoglycemia. It also resets the "osmostat" and causes dilutional hyponatremia via the syndrome of inappropriate secretion of antidiuretic hormone (SIADH). Glucocorticoid deficiency also contributes to dysfunction of the mineralocorticoid system by decreasing the sensitivity of the vascular system to angiotensin II and norepinephrine, resulting in vascular instability.

Aldosterone deficiency results in decreased sodium retention by the kidney, resulting in hyponatremia, hypovolemia, and vascular collapse. In addition, it causes a decreased distal renal tubular exchange of potassium and hydrogen ions for bicarbonate ions, leading to hyperkalemia and acidosis.

Adrenal androgen deficiency is associated with poorly developed sexual hair in pubertal and postpubertal females.

In primary adrenal insufficiency, adrenocorticotropin (ACTH) oversecretion results in hyperpigmentation.

ETIOLOGY

Adrenal insufficiency is classified into primary (adrenocortical failure), secondary (pituitary), or tertiary (hypothalamic) types. Primary adrenal insufficiency results from congenital or acquired adrenal gland dysfunction. Clinical signs and symptoms do not become manifest until at least 90 percent of the adrenocortical tissue from both glands is destroyed. The onset of primary adrenal insufficiency is usually gradual, resulting in vague symptoms of fatigue, anorexia, occasional mild postural hypotension, or polyuria.

The most common cause of primary adrenal insufficiency in infants is congenital adrenal hyperplasia (CAH). The female newborn presents with genital ambiguity secondary to virilization in utero. Hyponatremia, hyperkalemia, natriuresis, and shock typically do not develop until about 7 to 14 days. Boys characteristically present at this time in cardiovascular collapse. 17-Hydroxyprogesterone is usually elevated. Congenital adrenal hypoplasia is a rare cause of primary AI in infancy. Congenital primary AI can also result from adrenal aplasia or hemorrhage associated with a traumatic delivery. A rare form of AI in infancy is the syndrome of familial unresponsiveness to ACTH. The mineralocorticoid system is intact; thus cardiovascular collapse is rare.

Adrenoleukodystrophy (ALD) is a rare cause of childhood primary AI. It is an X-linked recessive familial disorder in which fatty acid accumulation occurs in adrenocortical and neural cells secondary to the inability of peroxisomes to degrade them. It is associated with progressive central demyelination, resulting in blindness, deafness, dementia, quadriparesis, and death.

Acquired causes of primary adrenal insufficiency, less common than congenital disorders, include autoimmune, infectious, infiltrative, hemorrhagic, or ablative disorders.

Autoimmune adrenalitis, which accounts for 80 percent of all cases of acquired primary AI, is often associated with immune destruction of other glands and is encountered in both types of polyglandular autoimmune syndromes.

Acquired adrenal failure can occur secondary to infection of the adrenal gland with tuberculosis or fungi (e.g., coccidiomycosis, blastomycosis, histoplasmosis, and torulosis). Human immunodeficiency virus infection (AIDS) has been reported as a cause of primary AI.

Infiltrative diseases such as sarcoidosis, hemochromatosis, or malignancy may affect the adrenal cortex, leading to destruction.

Primary AI may result from an acute adrenal hemorrhage in fulminating sepsis (Waterhouse-Friderichsen syndrome).

Isolated abnormality of the renin-angiotensin-aldosterone system can lead to isolated hyponatremia, hyperkalemia, and failure to thrive.

Secondary and tertiary adrenal insufficiency result from pituitary or hypothalamic underfunction, respectively. Both result in isolated cortisol deficiency. The mineralocorticoid system is intact, and thus hyperkalemia and shock do not occur. Dilutional hyponatremia may be encountered, however, secondary to SIADH.

Secondary AI also results from any process that interferes with the pituitary's ability to secrete ACTH, such as tumors, craniopharyngioma, infections, infiltrative diseases of the pituitary, lymphocytic hypophysitis, head trauma, or intracranial aneurysms. Isolated ACTH deficiency is rare, and most occurrences are attributable to an autoimmune process. It may occur as an autosomal recessive disorder ("miniature form" of congenital adrenal hypoplasia), in association with cerebral malformation.

Tertiary AI is most commonly caused by withdrawal from chronic administration of glucocorticoid pharmacotherapy, which suppresses the hypothalamic-pituitary-adrenal axis. Hyponatremia and hyperkalemia do not occur.

CLINICAL PRESENTATION

Crisis is typically encountered in a child with newly diagnosed primary AI who has been subjected to the stress of an acute illness. It may occur in a patient with previously established AI who has not increased the prescribed steroid dose appropriately during the stress of an intercurrent illness.

Acute cardiovascular collapse is the most common presentation of AI. In impending AI, patients may complain of anorexia, nausea, vomiting, abdominal pain, weakness, fatigue, or lethargy. Diffuse myalgia and arthralgias may occur. Fever may be present. Hypoglycemia may be the presenting symptom.

Signs of primary AI include hyperpigmentation, most notably in areas exposed to the sun, areas subject to friction, the buccal mucosa, areolae, and anal mucosa. Vitiligo secondary to melanocyte destruction suggests an underlying autoimmune disorder. Moniliasis is associated with the AI of polyglandular autoimmune syndrome type I. Severe or long-standing AI has associated psychiatric abnormalities, including organic brain syndrome, depression, or psychosis.

Laboratory findings in primary AI include hyponatremia, hypochloremia, hyperkalemia, and metabolic acidosis. Urinary sodium excretion is elevated, approaching the osmolarity of serum. An increased blood urea nitrogen (BUN)/creatinine ratio occurs as the result of dehydration. Mild to moderate eosinophilia, lymphocytosis, and anemia are common. The electrocardiographic abnormalities that occur as a result of hyperkalemia include peaked T waves, low P waves, and wide QRS complexes. Low cortisol levels, elevated ACTH levels, low aldosterone, increased plasma renin activity, and low dehydroepiandrosterone-sulfate levels are confirmatory.

In pure glucocorticoid deficiency, as is characteristic of unresponsiveness to or deficiency of ACTH, hypoglycemia is the only finding. Seizures or coma may occur. Shock is a rare finding. Hyperpigmentation does not occur in secondary or tertiary AI. Dilutional hyponatremia may be present secondary to SIADH. If AI is due to hypopituitarism, symptoms and signs of other pituitary hormone deficiencies occur, and there may be central nervous system abnormalities, visual field disturbances, or papilledema.

DIFFERENTIAL DIAGNOSIS

Hyponatremia

Other causes of low serum sodium include excessive intake of free water, diminished water output, sodium deficiency states, and states in which extracellular sodium is redistributed into a "third space." A renal ultrasound may be useful for detecting obstructive nephropathy as the cause of hyponatremia.

Hypoglycemia

The differential diagnosis of substrate-limited hypoglycemia includes growth hormone deficiency and liver disease.

Shock

Two of the most common causes of shock in infants and children are sepsis and hypovolemia secondary to dehydration.

MANAGEMENT

It is critical to recognize adrenal crisis immediately and treat it aggressively.

If sepsis is suspected, blood, urine, and cerebrospinal fluid cultures must be obtained. Then it is advisable to obtain a blood sample in an EDTA (ethylenediaminetetraacetic acid) tube for cortisol and ACTH levels and promptly put it on ice. In addition, one must obtain urine electrolytes, serum electrolytes, glucose, blood urea nitrogen, and creatinine levels, as well as a urinalysis. An aldosterone level and plasma renin activity (also in EDTA tubes, on ice) may prove to be helpful for diagnosis later. If the patient's condition permits, synthetic ACTH (Cosyntropin) 0.15 mg/m^2 is administered to rapidly assess adrenal function by obtaining cortisol levels 30 to 60 min later.

Treatment of individuals in adrenal crisis with steroids should never be delayed inordinately in order to perform diagnostic tests. However, the rapid ACTH test is recommended at first presentation and can be completed in the first 30 to 60 min of treatment while fluid resuscitation is occurring. At the very least, a baseline level of cortisol and ACTH should be obtained in anyone presenting with unexplained shock.

Fluid therapy should begin by giving a 20 mL/kg bolus of 5% dextrose/normal saline rapidly by the intravenous route. After the initial resuscitation, normal saline is usually required at a rate appropriate for severe dehydration. Twice the normal maintenance rate or 200 mL/kg/day for children weighing less than 10 kg and 2250 to 3000 mL/m^2/day for older children is used to replenish sodium stores and to keep up with ongoing losses of salt and water. Input and output must be monitored closely, with close attention to sodium losses in the urine. Hypoglycemia should be treated with boluses of 50% dextrose in water, and 10% glucose should be included in replacement fluids as needed.

Specific treatment requires initiating glucocorticoid therapy with cortisol (hydrocortisone; Solu-Cortef) 50 mg/m^2/dose intravenously every 6 h and cortisone acetate 50 mg/m^2 intramuscularly daily. Mineralocorticoid need not be given in acute adrenal crisis as high-dose hydrocortisone has mineralocorticoid-like action.

Diagnosis and treatment of the underlying stressor should be addressed. Antibiotics should be initiated intravenously if septic shock is suspected.

DISPOSITION

All patients presenting to an emergency department in acute adrenal crisis must be admitted to the hospital for continued parenteral fluid and corticosteroid therapy. After the patient has been stabilized, efforts to further establish the cause of adrenal failure must ensue.

For a more detailed discussion, see Baumann EE, Rosenfield RL: Adrenal insufficiency, chap. 53, p. 325, in *Pediatric Emergency Medicine: A Comprehensive Study Guide.*

54 Hyperthyroidism

Elizabeth E. Baumann / Robert L. Rosenfield

Thyrotoxicosis results from thyroid hormone excess due to either overproduction of thyroid hormone by the thyroid gland itself or administration of exogenous synthetic hormone. Specifically, an increased concentration of serum free thyroid hormone is almost always found in thyrotoxicosis. Occasionally, only blood levels of T_3 are elevated ("T_3 toxicosis"). Why some individuals have few symptoms and others develop the most extreme clinical manifestation of thyroid hormone excess, "thyroid storm," is poorly understood.

Thyroid hormones activate the adrenergic system by inducing beta-adrenergic receptors. Symptoms of sympathetic nervous system overactivity, including hyperthermia, may be present and can be blocked by beta-adrenergic antagonists.

Specific conditions known to precipitate thyroid storm in a patient with hyperthyroidism include thyroid surgery, withdrawal of antithyroid medications, radioiodine therapy, vigorous palpation of a generous goiter, iodinated contrast dyes, or states in which thyroid hormone levels drastically increase. Emotional distress, general surgery, infection, or other conditions in which the patient encounters a high degree of stress may also precipitate storm.

ETIOLOGY

Autoantibodies against the thyrotropin-stimulating hormone (TSH) receptor are usually the cause. These antibodies have thyroid-stimulating activity (TSA). They act at the TSH receptor on thyroid cells and stimulate cAMP production in a manner similar to that of TSH itself.

The most common disorder causing thyrotoxicosis in children, as in adults, is the autoimmune disorder *Grave's disease.* Many patients have a family history of goiter, thyroid dysfunction (hyper- or hypothyroidism), or other autoimmune diseases. Graves' disease is more common in girls than in boys, and its incidence increases with age.

In 5 to 10 percent of thyrotoxicosis, the disorder is due to a variant type of chronic autoimmune thyroiditis called *Hashitoxicosis.* Patients present with goiter without ophthalmopathy.

In an even smaller percentage of patients, subacute thyroiditis can cause thyrotoxicosis due to destruction of thyroid tissue. This process is usually due to viral or granulomatous diseases and is self-limiting.

Autonomously functioning thyroid nodules, typically single (toxic adenoma), are sometimes encountered in children. Multinodular goiters with thyrotoxicosis are unusual in childhood.

Rarely, hyperthyroidism is secondary to TSH oversecretion from a pituitary tumor or to isolated pituitary resistance to negative feedback control by thyroid hormones on a genetic basis. Signs of an intracranial mass may be present with the former. Goiter is present with both.

A less common condition is neonatal thyrotoxicosis. It is caused by transplacental passage of TSA from a mother with Graves' disease to her fetus.

The possibility of a molar pregnancy, which may elaborate a thyroid stimulator, must be considered in adolescent females with thyrotoxicosis in order to guide appropriate therapy. Oversecretion of T_4 from ectopic thyroid tissue lying within a teratoma of the ovary (struma ovarii) can cause thyrotoxicosis.

Administration of iodine-containing medications, such as dyes, to patients with a nodular goiter may induce hyperthyroidism.

Finally, thyrotoxicosis can occur as the result of excess thyroxine or triiodothyronine intake.

CLINICAL PRESENTATION

Children who present with thyrotoxicosis complain of nervousness, palpitations, weight loss, muscle weakness, and fatigue. A history of declining school performance due to a decreased attention span can usually be elicited. Other symptoms include tremulousness, excessive sweating, temperature intolerance, and emotional lability. Gastrointestinal overactivity with symptoms of frequent stools is common. An increased appetite is classically present; however, an apathetic state, including decreased appetite, occasionally occurs. The only symptoms of exophthalmos may be sleeping with the eyes open and a resultant conjunctivitis.

A goiter is the most common physical finding in Graves' disease. The eye signs of Graves' disease are usually subtle in children. Decreased accommodation is more common than exophthalmos. Stare and lid lag are eye signs resulting from sympathetic overactivity. Graves' dermopathy of the shins is uncommon in children.

Signs of sympathetic overactivity are common. These include tremor, brisk deep tendon reflexes, tachycardia, supraventricular tachycardia, flow murmur, overactive precordium, and a widened pulse pressure.

Congestive heart failure (CHF) may occasionally develop due to the inability of cardiac function to meet metabolic demands. Venous pressure is normal. Mitral valve prolapse is common in the absence of CHF.

In thyroid storm, signs and symptoms of thyrotoxicosis are accentuated. Storm is suggested by the following: severe hyperpyrexia, atrial dysrhythmia and CHF, delirium or psychosis, severe gastrointestinal hyperactivity, and hepatic dysfunction with jaundice. A key feature in thyroid storm is a precipitating event, illness, or major stress, which should be sought and identified.

DIFFERENTIAL DIAGNOSIS

Causes of tachydysrhythmias include electrolyte disturbances and cardiac disease. The murmur of mitral valve prolapse along with tremor and fever may suggest rheumatic fever. The patient who is flushed and febrile may appear "toxic," mimicking an acute bacterial infection. Drug ingestions also may mimic the hypermetabolic state seen in thyrotoxicosis. Gastrointestinal hyperactivity may imitate an acute abdomen in thyroid storm.

MANAGEMENT

Treatment of severe thyrotoxicosis or impending thyroid storm is aimed at preventing further thyroid hormone synthesis and secretion, alleviating the acute peripheral effects of excess thyroid hormone if the patient is very symptomatic, and identifying the cause.

Initial laboratory tests should include the measurement of total and free T_4, T_3, and TSH levels. Antithyroid antibody levels help confirm the presence of autoimmune thyroid disease.

Complete blockade of new hormone synthesis can be accomplished by the administration of propylthiouracil (PTU) at a dosage of 175 mg/m^2/day or 4 to 6 mg/kg/day at 6- to 8-h intervals. Alternatively, methimazole or carbimazole may be given at a dosage one-tenth that of PTU. However, PTU is preferred because it also inhibits peripheral conversion of T_4 to T_3.

To block release of thyroid hormone from the gland, inorganic iodine therapy is started 1 h after initiating antithyroid medication is initiated. Iodine is administered as Lugol's solution, 0.1 mg/kg/day orally or by nasogastric tube in orange juice, divided every 8 to 12 h, or as a saturated solution of potassium iodide (SSKI, 10% iodide) in a dose of 1 to 3 drops three times daily. Lithium carbonate can alternatively be used to impair thyroid hormone release in patients with a history of iodine-induced reactions. One must observe for signs of adverse reaction to iodide, such as rash, drug fever, or anaphylactic shock.

Beta-adrenergic antagonists are useful in the management of severe thyrotoxicosis or thyroid storm. They are most clearly indicated for arrhythmia. Propranolol, in addition to its antiadrenergic effects, modestly decreases the conversion of T_4 to T_3. In neonates, it is administered as 2 mg/kg/day orally in four divided doses. In adolescents and adults, 10 to 40 mg every 6 h orally is adequate. Beta-adrenergic blockade must be given cautiously to patients with cardiac failure or asthma or to diabetics who suffer from hypoglycemic unawareness.

Glucocorticoids are indicated in thyroid storm to inhibit peripheral conversion of T_4 to T_3 and for their immunosuppressive effect. Hydrocortisone should be used in stress doses of 50 mg/m^2 IV every 6 h.

If metabolic decompensation has occurred as the result of thyroid storm, management must include a measure to reverse hyperthermia, such as acetaminophen or cooling blankets. Salicylates must be avoided, as they may displace thyroid hormone, worsening the hypermetabolic state. If gastrointestinal and insensible fluid losses are excessive, normal saline, 20 mL/kg, is administered, then the fluid deficit is calculated and replaced in the form of 0.45 normal saline over the next 24 to 48 h. Because hepatic glycogen stores are usually depleted, 5 to 10% dextrose is used in the replacement fluids.

Cardiovascular complications such as arrhythmias and congestive heart failure are treated with antiarrhythmics, digoxin, and diuretics. Finally, the precipitating event causing severe thyrotoxicosis must be sought and treated.

Plasmapheresis has been used for the physical removal of thyroid hormone. This should be reserved for cases of thyroid storm or thyroid poisoning refractory to conventional treatment.

DISPOSITION

Patients who present in severe thyrotoxicosis or thyroid storm and those with cardiovascular compromise should be transported to an intensive care unit. Patients with a milder presentation may be discharged home after baseline thyroid function studies are obtained and propranolol is begun. Specific treatment must be instituted upon obtaining confirmatory laboratory results.

For a more detailed discussion, see Baumann EE, Rosenfield RL: Hyperthyroidism, chap. 54, p. 329, in *Pediatric Emergency Medicine: A Comprehensive Study Guide.*

---

55 Calcium Abnormalities

Elizabeth E. Baumann / Robert L. Rosenfield

Calcium is one of the most abundant and important minerals in the body, with 99 percent of body calcium stored in bone. Of the 1 percent in the circulation, 40 to 45 percent is bound to proteins such as albumin, 5 to 10 percent is complexed with anions such as phosphate and citrate, and 45 to 50 percent is physiologically free and ionized. Calcium is controlled over a narrow range by the interaction of parathyroid thormone (PTH), vitamin D, and calcitonin. These regulate intestinal absorption, skeletal resorption, and renal reabsorption. Close control is essential due to the functions of calcium in the body, including cellular depolarization, muscle excitation and contraction, neurotransmitter release, hormonal secretion, and the function of both leukocytes and platelets.

A serum calcium level includes both ionized and protein-bound calcium, and may need to be corrected for changes in albumin, since approximately half of serum calcium is albumin-bound. For every 1 g/dL decrease in serum albumin, serum calcium is corrected by adding 0.8 mg/dL. Ionized calcium levels have recently become available on a widespread basis to many clinicians.

HYPOCALCEMIA

Normal calcium levels in neonates (24 to 48 h of age) range from 7.0 to 12.0 mg/dL and gradually change to the normal range found in adults, which is 8.4 to 10.2 mg/dL. Serum calcium <7.0 mg/dL constitutes latent tetany and warrants treatment. Calcium levels <6.0 mg/dL indicate impending tetany and prompt institution of emergency department therapy.

Normal phosphate levels are 4.8 to 8.2 mg/dL in the neonate. Phosphate levels then gradually fall throughout childhood. Upon completion of puberty, the levels have fallen to the adult range, 2.7 to 4.7 mg/dL.

Over 99 percent of the body's calcium stores lie in the skeleton. Nearly half of bone calcium is rapidly exchangeable in infants. Thus relatively high replacement doses of calcium are needed during the treatment of hypocalcemic disorders in infancy. Intravascular calcium is partially bound to proteins (primarily albumin) and partially exists in a free, unbound form (ionized calcium). Both the free and bound fractions of calcium normally constitute 45 percent of the circulating calcium; the remaining portion (10 percent) is complexed to bicarbonate, phosphate, or citrate ions. The bioavailable fraction is the serum free calcium.

Blood calcium is routinely measured as total calcium. However, it is the ionized calcium concentration (Ca^{2+}) that is critical. Under normal conditions, one can estimate the Ca^{2+} as approximately one-half the total. In the face of hypoalbuminemia, the total calcium is lower than normal but the ionized fraction is typically normal. One can "correct" the total calcium level by adding to the laboratory value 0.8 mg/dL for every 1.0 g/dL that albumin is below normal. Acidosis causes dissociation of calcium from albumin, thereby causing an increase in free calcium. Alkalosis has the opposite effect. Other factors that alter the fractional binding of calcium to albumin include the free fatty acid concentration and osmolality, as well as the availability of circulating ions that bind free calcium (phosphate and citrate). Blood transfusions, which introduce large amounts of citrate into the blood, or massive cytolysis (postchemotherapy), causing an acute rise in phosphate levels, may lead to significant decreases in ionized calcium levels. In conditions such as these, direct measurement of Ca^{2+} is important.

Pathophysiology/Etiology

Hypocalcemia can be attributed to either hypoparathyroidism, vitamin D deficiency, resistance of target tissues to either parathyroid hormone or vitamin D, or processes that sequester or alter the partitioning of ionized calcium. Causes of hypocalcemia are therefore best categorized by relationships between calcium, phosphate, and PTH levels (Fig. 55-1).

Hypoparathyroidism is characterized by hyperphosphatemia

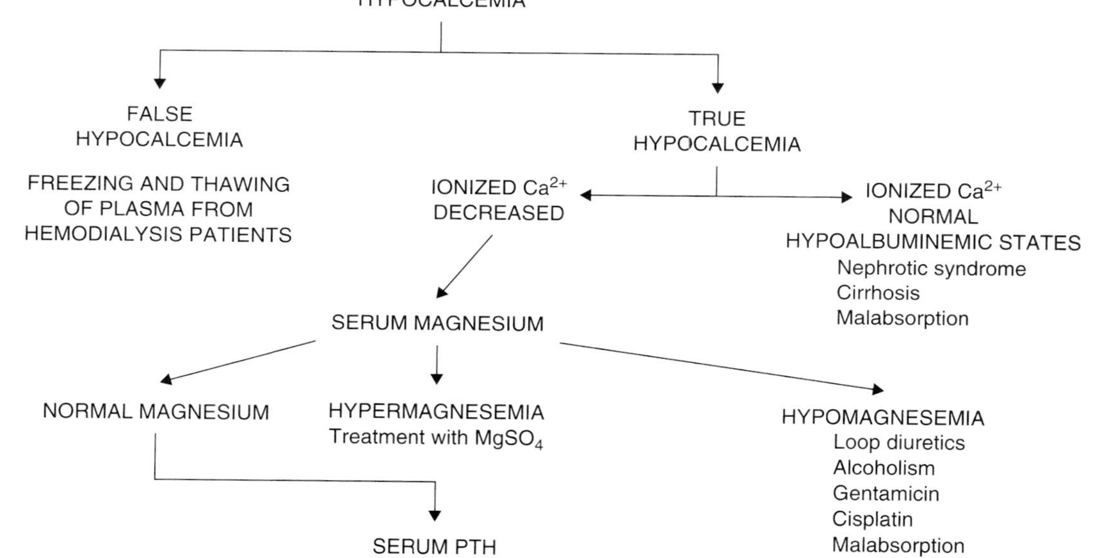

FIG. 55-1 Evaluation of a patient with hypocalcemia. PTH = parathyroid hormone. (From Benabe JE, Martinez-Maldonado M: Disorders of calcium metabolism, Maxwell MH, Kleeman CR, Narins RG (ecs): *Clinical Disorders of Fluid and Electrolyte Metabolism*, 4th ed. New York, McGraw-Hill, 1987, p 773, with permission.)

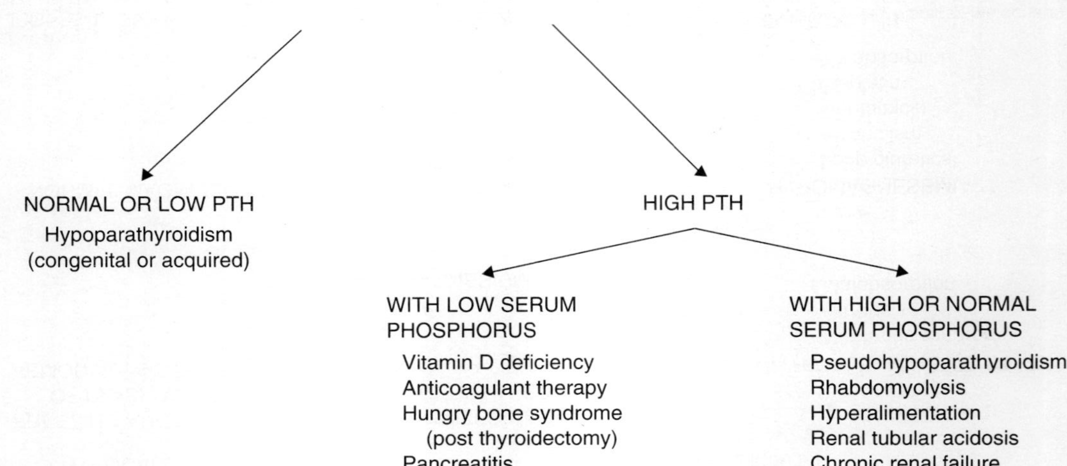

FIG. 55-1 (*continued*)

and hypocalcemia with a serum level of PTH that is disproportionately low for the level of Ca^{2+}. Congenital absence of the parathyroid glands occurs sporadically. DiGeorge syndrome, the most common cause of hypoparathyroidism neonatally, is characterized by various combinations of thymic aplasia, defective cell-mediated immunity, congenital cardiac anomalies, and craniofacial anomalies. Most prevalent in older children is hypoparathyroidism that results from autoimmune destruction of the parathyroid gland. Autoimmune polyglandular syndrome (APS) type I is typically found in childhood and consists of mucocutaneous candidiasis, hypoparathyroidism, and Addison's disease. Less frequently, chronic active hepatitis, malabsorption, alopecia, pernicious anemia, gonadal failure, and thyroid disease may occur. Type II APS predominantly occurs in adults.

Primary hypoparathyroidism may also result from iatrogenically induced parathyroid gland destruction (after thyroidectomy or neck irradiation) or be secondary to infiltrative diseases of the parathyroid glands, such as hemachromatosis or Wilson disease. Hypoparathyroidism is rarely inherited as an X-linked recessive trait, with males affected early in life.

Transient neonatal hypocalcemia (TNH) with hyperphosphatemia occurs in preterm infants and infants of diabetic mothers (IDM) in the first 3 days of life. In the former, hypocalcemia is the result of either hypoparathyroidism (caused by a combination of decreased gland responsiveness to calcium and decreased renal responsiveness to PTH) and/or birth asphyxia leading to increased phosphate levels. In IDM, hypoparathyroidism may be secondary to hypomagnesemia. Transient neonatal hypocalcemia also may begin after 1 week of age in babies fed cow's milk formulas; the high phosphate load is responsible.

In pseudohypoparathyroidism (PHP), the hypocalcemia and hyperphosphatemia resemble primary hypoparathyroidism, but PTH levels are high. End-organ resistance to PTH is the primary abnormality.

Vitamin D deficiency is characterized by hypophosphatemia due to secondary hyperparathyroidism.

The most common abnormality of vitamin D metabolism resulting in hypocalcemia in childhood is vitamin D–deficient rickets. Inadequate exposure to sunlight, dark skin, and breast-feeding without vitamin D supplementation each increase the risk of its development. Characteristic signs of rickets include rachitic rosary, frontal bossing, craniotabes, widening of the wrists, bowed legs, and enlarged fontanelles that are slow to close. Alkaline phosphatase levels are elevated, and, except in the earliest stage of rickets, bone radiographs reveal cupping and fraying of long bone metaphyses. Rickets may also occur in premature infants with very low birth weights due to low calcium and phosphate intake and furosemide diuresis causing calcium loss.

Vitamin D dependency, which requires a supranormal intake of vitamin D, has a number of causes. Malabsorption of fats, as occurs with pancreatic or bile duct obstruction or small bowel disease, increases the requirement for vitamin D. Rickets can result from liver or kidney disease secondary to interference with activating hydroxylations of vitamin D. Anticonvulsants, particularly phenobarbital and phenytoin, by increasing hepatic P450 enzyme activity, cause increased vitamin D turnover, thus lowering 25-hydroxyvitamin D levels and predisposing the individual to rickets. Vitamin D–dependent rickets type I is characterized by low serum calcitriol levels secondary to inefficient 1-alpha-hydroxylation in the kidney. Vitamin D–dependent rickets type II is true vitamin D resistance caused by a mutation of the vitamin D receptor. Blood calcitriol levels are high. This disorder is rare; its signs include alopecia, milia, epidermal cysts, or oligodontia.

Other conditions in which hypocalcemia and secondary hyperparathyroidism may occur include acute pancreatitis, bone tumors, or osteoblastic metastases.

Multiple transfusions with citrated blood and acute rhabdomyolysis may be associated with hypocalcemia. Intravascular infusions of phosphate and impaired renal function with resultant hyperphosphatemia may also cause hypocalcemia.

Gram-negative sepsis and toxic shock syndrome cause hypocalcemia for reasons that are unclear.

Magnesium deficiency may lead to inadequate PTH secretion and end-organ unresponsiveness. Congenital hypomagnesemia may present in the first few weeks of life; it is an autosomal recessive disorder of magnesium absorption.

Symptoms and Signs

Symptoms of hypocalcemia result from neuromuscular irritability. Patients may complain initially of numbmess and tingling of the distal extremities or around the mouth. As hypocalcemia worsens, patients become hyperreflexic or experience muscle cramps and spasms. Tetany causes uncontrolled muscle spasms ("carpal-pedal" spasms) characterized by abnormal flexion of the elbow, wrist, and metacarpophalangeal joints, with adducted thumbs and extended interphalangeal joints. Generalized or focal seizures may follow. Typically the postictal phase is brief. Hoarseness, stridor, or dyspnea may result from laryngospasm or bronchospasm.

Chronic symptoms and signs of hypocalcemia include cataract

formation, dry skin, coarse hair, brittle nails, and dental and enamel hypoplasia.

Examination of the patient will sometimes reveal signs of generalized neuromuscular excitability. To elicit Chvostek's sign, one taps gently on the area of the facial nerve, just anterior to the ear, over the upper portion of the parotid gland. If ipsilateral contraction of the corner of the lip occurs, this signifies neuromuscular irritability. However, Chvostek's sign occurs in 10 percent of normocalcemic individuals. Trousseau's sign, carpal spasm after inflating a blood pressure cuff to a pressure greater than that of the systolic pressure for 3 to 5 min, as well as Chvostek's sign, may be absent in the presence of significant hypocalcemia. Other signs of hypocalcemia include hypotension, bradycardia, and cardiac arrhythmias.

Diagnostic Tests

Electrocardiography is the most rapid means of obtaining confirmatory evidence of hypocalcemia. A prolonged Q_oT_c interval is a sensitive and specific finding.

After documenting hypocalcemia, it is important to obtain a full chemistry screen, including a serum phosphate level, albumin (to rule out hypoalbuminemic states), electrolytes, blood urea nitrogen (BUN), creatinine, liver function studies, and an alkaline phosphatase level. The phosphate level is essential in the differential diagnosis of hypocalcemia. Ionized calcium is not necessary initially but is recommended if it cannot be estimated reliably. The serum magnesium level should be measured if the cause of hypocalcemia is not apparent or if hypomagnesemia is suspected. A serum sample for PTH drawn during the hypocalcemic event, prior to initiation of calcium salts, is necessary for diagnosis. The level of 25(OH)-vitamin D is confirmatory for the diagnosis of vitamin D deficiency; a $1,25(OH)_2D$ level is useful only in the diagnosis of rare forms of rickets. Radiographs of the chest, wrist, and knees should be obtained shortly after stabilization of the patient.

Management

If the calcium level is <7.0 mg/dL, a peripheral intravenous line is established and intravenous calcium is administered immediately; 10% calcium gluconate (calcium gluconate contains 9.4% elemental calcium; 10 mL contains 0.9 g of elemental calcium) is given IV, 200 to 500 mg/kg/24 h in four divided doses, each infused over 1 h. A baseline electrocardiogram is obtained, and the patient is monitored continuously during calcium infusions, as serious cardiac dysfunction can result if intravenous calcium is given too rapidly. The peripheral IV site must be observed carefully and frequently for IV fluid extravasation. Calcium burns can be devastating, resulting in sloughing of the skin. Calcium levels should be monitored frequently.

Intravenous calcitriol (as Calcijex) is initiated at a dosage of 0.125 to 0.25 μg/kg/24 h in two divided doses.

If hypomagnesemia is present, the child is treated with magnesium sulfate (100 mg/mL) IM or IV, 25 to 50 mg/kg/dose every 4 to 6 h for 3 or 4 doses or as needed.

Vitamin D (ergocalciferol) 300,000 U IM should be given within the first 24 h of initiating treatment to avoid prolonged hospitalization. One can anticipate that it will begin to take effect on day 4, with its peak effect on day 7. In the child for whom intravenous calcitriol therapy was initiated, once calcium levels increase to 7 to 8.0 mg/dL, oral calcitriol (Rocaltrol) can be substituted to prevent rebound hypocalcemia while waiting for the ergocalciferol to metabolize to its active form. Older infants and toddlers with vitamin D–deficient rickets require at least 1 to 2 g of oral elemental calcium per day.

Disposition

Hypocalcemic patients must be admitted to the hospital for stabilization of calcium and phosphate levels on intravenous regimens. A Holter monitor and laryngoscope with endotracheal tube must be ordered for the bedside.

HYPERCALCEMIA

Hypercalcemia, defined as a serum calcium above 10.5 mg/dL, is often associated with nonspecific signs and symptoms. When symptomatic, complaints are likely to include constipation, anorexia, nausea, vomiting, abdominal pain, and pancreatitis. Lethargy, depression, confusion, psychosis, or coma may also occur. Nephrolithiasis may occur, and impaired renal concentrating ability may result in polyuria and nocturia.

Laboratory data should include a calcium (ionized if available), complete blood count, serum protein, urinalysis, electrolytes, BUN, and creatinine. A hyperchloremic metabolic acidosis suggests primary hyperparathyroidism. An electrocardiogram may show QT segment shortening, bradycardia, heart block, sinus arrest, and dysrythmias.

Causes of hypercalcemia are diverse (Fig. 55-2). Most cases are due to malignancy or hyperparathyroidism.

For patients with significant symptoms, cardiac changes, or levels

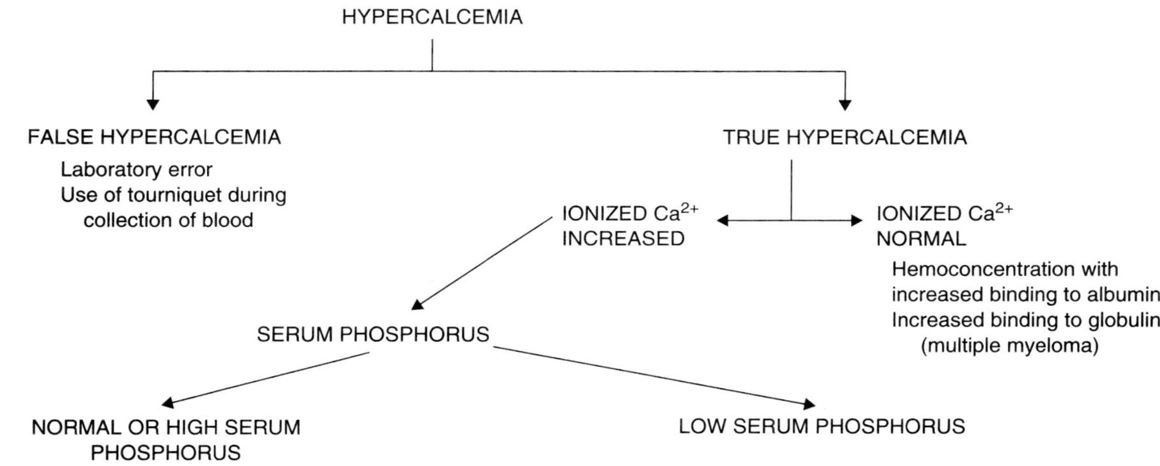

FIG. 55-2 Evaluation of a patient with hypercalcemia. (From Benabe JE, Martinez-Maldonado M: Disorders of calcium metabolism, in Maxwell MH, Kleeman CR, Narins RG (eds): *Clinical Disorders of Fluid and Electrolyte Metabolism*, 4th ed. New York, McGraw-Hill, 1987, p 772, with permission.)

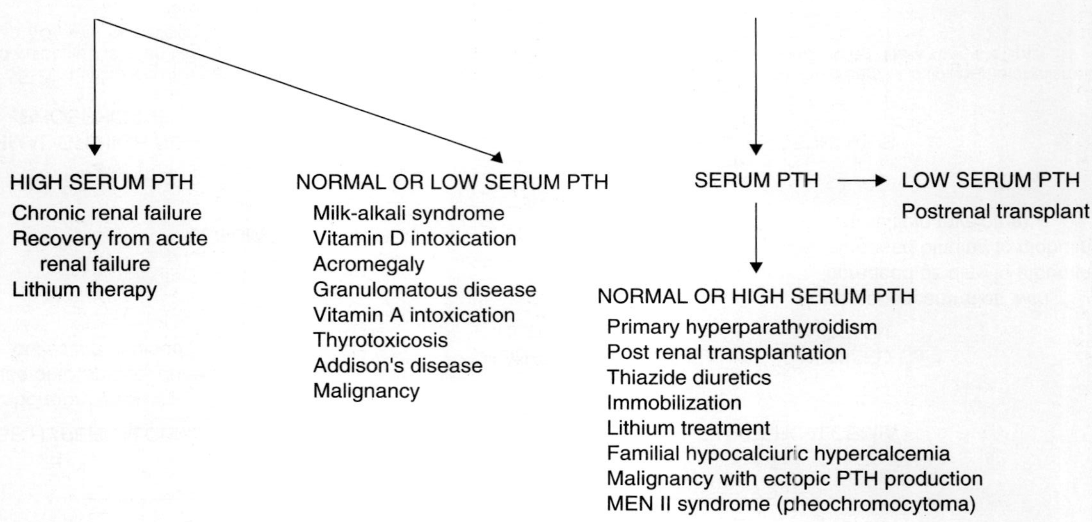

FIG. 55-2 (*continued*)

>14 mg/dL, aggressive therapy should be started in the emergency department. Principles of treatment include ECF expansion, calcium excretion, increased bone storage, and definitive treatment of the underlying cause.

Rapid rehydration with isotonic crystalloid is the first step, with consideration of invasive monitoring with urinary catheter and central venous pressure monitor. With continued hydration, a brisk diuresis using loop diuretics is initiated. Serum calcium levels, along with other electrolytes, must be closely followed. Hemodialysis may be needed in the setting of renal insufficiency or life-threatening symptoms such as cardiac dysrythmias.

Glucocorticoids, with an onset of action in several days, may suppress bone resorption and diminish intestinal absorption. Mithramycin, calcitonin, and the diphosphonates all act to suppress bone resorption, with an onset of 24 h. Intravenous phosphate may result in rapid calcium deposition in soft tissues as well as bone, limiting its clinical utility.

For a more detailed discussion, see Baumann EE, Rosenfield RL: Hypocalcemia, chap. 55, p. 333, and Rudzinski JP, Wolanyk D, Mackey M: Fluids and electrolytes, chap. 56, p. 337, in *Pediatric Emergency Medicine: A Comprehensive Study Guide.*

56 Fluids and Electrolytes

John P. Rudzinski / Dean Wolanyk / Mark Mackey

FLUIDS

Total body water is divided into the intracellular and extracellular compartments, with the extracellular compartment subdivided into intravascular and extravascular compartments. The relative size of these compartments varies with age (Table 56-1).

Body water exists as a complex solution of salts, organic acids, and proteins. The exact composition varies with body compartment (Table 56-2). Water will move between compartments to maintain osmolar equilibration. Osmolarity normally ranges between 280 and 290 mOsm/L and may be estimated by the equation:

$$\text{Osmolarity (mOsm/L)} = 2(\text{sodium}) + \text{BUN}/2.8 + \text{glucose}/18$$

with BUN standing for blood urea nitrogen.

TABLE 56-1 Distribution of Body Water between Extracellular and Intracellular Fluid as a Percent of Body Weight

Age	Total water, %	Extracellular water, %	Intracellular water, %	Extracellular water/ intracellular water
0–1 Day	79.0	43.9	35.1	1.25
1–10 Days	74.0	39.7	34.3	1.14
1–3 Months	72.3	32.2	40.1	0.80
3–6 Months	70.1	30.1	40.0	0.75
6–12 Months	60.4	27.4	33.0	0.83
1–2 Years	58.7	25.6	33.1	0.77
2–3 Years	63.5	26.7	36.8	0.73
3–5 Years	62.2	21.4	40.8	0.52
5–10 Years	61.5	22.0	39.5	0.56
10–16 Years	58.0	18.7	39.3	0.48

Source: As modified from Holliday MA: Body fluid physiology during growth, in Maxwell MH, Kleeman CR (eds): *Clinical Disorders of Fluid and Electrolyte Metabolism*, 2d ed. New York, McGraw-Hill, 1972, p. 544, with permission.

TABLE 56-2 Electrolyte Composition of Body Compartments

Electrolytes	Extracellular fluid (plasma), meq/L	Intracellular fluid (muscle), meq/kg H_2O
Cations		
Sodium	140	±10
Potassium	4	160
Calcium	5	3.3
Magnesium	2	26
Anions		
Chloride	104	±2
Bicarbonate	25	±8
Phosphate	2	95
Sulfate	1	20
Organic acids	6	
Protein	13	55

Source: As modified from Hill LL: Body composition and normal electrolyte concentrations. *Pediatr Clin North Am* 37:244, 1990, with permission.

Fluid Requirements and Losses

Water requirements are directly proportional to body surface area and are predicated on metabolic rate. A child's ratio of surface area to mass is as much as five times greater than that of an adult. In children, a relatively large proportion is lost in the kidney to facilitate the removal of waste products. Other routes of water loss from the body include insensible losses from lungs and skin and losses from fecal excretion. Weight correlates closely with body surface area and can be used to calculate fluid requirements (Table 56-3).

TABLE 56-3 Daily Water Requirements

Weight, kg	Water, mL/kg/day
0–10	100 mL/kg/day
11–20	100 mL/kg/day for first 10 kg plus 50 mL/kg/day for each kilogram above 10 kg
21 and up	100 mL/kg/day for first 10 kg plus 50 mL/kg/day for next 10 kg plus 20 mL/kg/day for each kilogram above 20 kg

DEHYDRATION

Dehydration may result from increased losses, as occurs with vomiting or diarrhea, or from reduced intake. Gastrointestinal loss is the most common cause of dehydration in the child. Another common contributor to dehydration in the child is fever, which increases the metabolic rate and water requirement by 10 percent for each degree (Celsius) elevation. The magnitude of dehydration is divided into mild (water loss < 5 percent of body weight), moderate (water loss 5 to 10 percent to body weight), and severe (water loss > 10 percent of body weight) and can be estimated at the bedside (see Table 49-2).

Treatment of Isotonic Dehydration

Isotonic dehydration occurs when sodium and water are lost in such a proportion that serum sodium and therefore osmolarity remains within normal limits. It is the most common form of dehydration in children.

Resuscitation is aimed at restoring tissue perfusion by increasing intravascular volume with an isotonic fluid bolus, typically 20 mL/kg of lactated Ringer's solution (LR) or 0.9% normal saline (NS). If clinical reassessment shows no improvement in pulse, blood pressure, skin color, capillary refill time, or mental status, the bolus is repeated.

Next, lost water volume is replaced, with half the deficit replaced in the first 8 h of treatment and the remainder replaced over the next 16 h. Commonly, $D_5 0.2NS$ or $D_5 0.45NS$ is used. Potassium can be added to the infusion once the patient begins urinating. It is important to add the patient's daily maintenance requirements to the volume deficit and to include any ongoing losses, such as those from persistent diarrhea. The maintenance requirement can be calculated using the patient's weight (Table 56-3).

SODIUM

Disturbances of Sodium Concentration

It is important to emphasize that total body sodium in both hypernatremia and hyponatremia may be high, low, or normal. It is the amount of total body water relative to total body sodium that determines sodium concentration.

Hypernatremia

Hypernatremia is defined as a serum sodium greater than 150 meq/L. Hypernatremia can occasionally occur via the ingestion of large quantities of salt in excess of what the body can excrete, as seen with the ingestion of improperly diluted infant formula. The most common cause of hypernatremia is loss of free water in excess of sodium loss. This most often occurs from excessive free water loss from diarrhea. Hypovolemic hypernatremia is the most common form of hypernatremia in the pediatric population. Less common causes of hypernatremia are listed in Fig. 56-1. The most common of these is diabetes insipidis (DI), which results either from a deficiency of antidiuretic hormone (central DI) or from functional resistance to antidiuretic hormone at the renal level (nephrogenic DI). With an intact thirst mechanism and a mild deficiency, normal hydration status may be maintained.

Clinical manifestations of hypernatremia depend on the volume status of the patient and both the degree of hyperosmolarity and the rate at which it develops. Central nervous system manifestations include irritability, lethargy, coma, and seizures. Increased extracellular osmolarity in hypernatremia draws water from the intracellular into the extracellular compartment, resulting in a characteristic "doughy skin." The movement of water from the intracellular space and interstitium into the vascular tree can protect blood volume and result in relatively normal pulse and blood pressure despite relatively profound dehydration.

The treatment of hypernatremia is focused on restoration of normal sodium levels in a timely manner. To preserve osmotic equilibrium, brain cells generate "idiogenic osmoles" (also called "organic osmolytes"), which act to increase intracellular osmolarity and thus maintain brain cell volume. The rapid administration of excess hypotonic fluid can result in movement of water from the vascular tree into the relatively hypertonic brain cells, leading to cerebral edema. Thus, the goal is to restore normal sodium slowly—at a rate of 10 to 15 meq/L/24 h. The specific type of fluid used for total body water restoration is somewhat controversial and is probably not as important as the rate at which it is administered. Because intravascular volume tends to be preserved, perfusion is usually adequate and massive volume resuscitation is not usually necessary. If a bolus is necessary, 0.9*NS* is used. Fluid replacement should then be directed toward restoring lost body water over 48 to 72 h, as opposed to 24 h in isotonic dehydration. It is reasonable to begin with $D_5$0.45*NS* and closely follow serum sodium to ensure a gradual reduction. As sodium begins to fall into the normal range, $D_5$0.2 can be substituted. In severe hypernatremia (Na^+ greater than 165 meq/L), it is advisable to consult a pediatric intensivist or nephrologist.

Children with hypernatremia are prone to hyperglycemia and hypocalcemia, and these levels should be monitored.

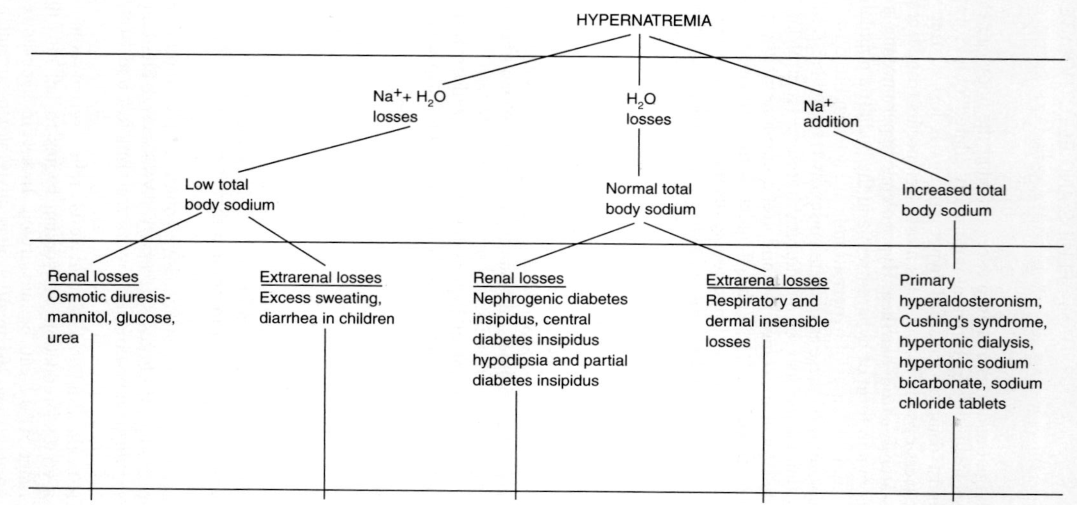
HYPERNATREMIA
$Na^+ + H_2O$ losses
H_2O losses
Na^+ addition
Low total body sodium
Normal total body sodium
Increased total body sodium
Renal losses
Osmotic diuresis-mannitol, glucose, urea
Extrarenal losses
Excess sweating, diarrhea in children
Renal losses
Nephrogenic diabetes insipidus, central diabetes insipidus hypodipsia and partial diabetes insipidus
Extrarenal losses
Respiratory and dermal insensible losses
Primary hyperaldosteronism, Cushing's syndrome, hypertonic dialysis, hypertonic sodium bicarbonate, sodium chloride tablets

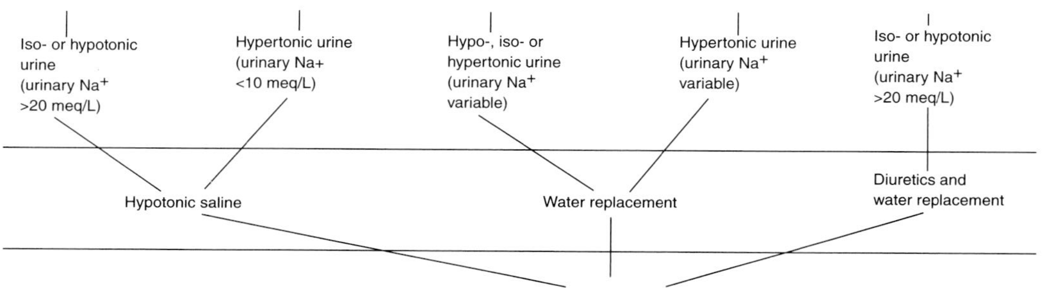

FIG. 56-1 Hypernatremia. (From Berl F, Anderson RJ, McDonald KM, Schrier RW: Clinical disorders of water metabolism. *Kidney Int.* 10:117, 1976, with permission.)

For children with DI, hormonal replacement therapy may be initiated in the emergency department after consultation with an endocrinologist. The drug of choice is desmopressin (DDAVP). This synthetic hormone has been chemically altered in such a way as to increase its antidiuretic effect and diminish its smooth muscle effect. Intranasal vasopressin has a duration of effect of 8 to 20 h and exhibits an antidiuretic effect in 30 to 60 min. The dose is 1.25 to 10 μg once or twice daily.

Hyponatremia

Hyponatremia is defined as a serum sodium concentration less than 130 meq/L and reflects excess body water relative to body sodium. Total body sodium may be increased, normal, or decreased. Hyponatremia may occur as a result of sodium losses, as seen in adrenocortical insufficiency or diarrhea. An excess of free water may also occur, as with congestive heart failure and renal failure or with the syndrome of inappropriate ADH (SIADH) secretion. Potential causes of hyponatremia are listed in Fig. 56-2.

Clinical signs of hyponatremia depend on the absolute level of sodium and the rate at which it drops. Central nervous system manifestations include lethargy, seizures, and coma. Seizures are especially likely to occur with rapid drops in serum sodium, and they usually occur when sodium drops below 120 meq/L.

The rate of correction of serum sodium depends on the clinical status of the patient rather than the absolute value of serum sodium. Gradual correction theoretically allows brain cells time to equilibrate, while a rapid rise in serum sodium can cause neurologic sequelae. The ideal rate of sodium correction has been proposed as no more than 12 meq/L the first day, with a total increase no greater than 18 meq/L in the first 48 h. For severely symptomatic hyponatremia, usually manifested by seizures, 4 to 6 mL/kg of hypertonic 3% saline may be administered. Each 1 mL/kg of 3% saline raises serum sodium by 1 meq/L. The majority of patients with hyponatremia-related seizures will respond to a small bolus of 3% saline.

Most patients with SIADH will respond to fluid restriction to either half normal maintenance or replacement of insensible water losses. The underlying disorder must be addressed.

POTASSIUM

Potassium is the main intracellular fluid (ICF) cation. An intake of 1 to 2 meq/kg/day is recommended for the normal healthy child.

Hyperkalemia

Hyperkalemia (a potassium greater than 5.5 meq/L or greater than 6 meq/L in the newborn) may reflect an increase in total body stores or a shift in concentration between the extracellular fluid (ECF) and intracellular fluid (ICF) compartments. It must be distinguished from pseudohyperkalemia, which can result from prolonged tourniquet use or heel squeezing as well as hemolysis from smaller-gauge needles. Hyperkalemia can occur when potassium is released from cells, as in rhabdomyolysis or in severe burns. Systemic acidosis can increase serum potassium, as hydrogen ion is exchanged with intracellular potassium. As in adults, renal failure is a common cause of hyperkalemia in children.

Most patients with mild hyperkalemia are asymptomatic. As potassium levels increase, muscle weakness may occur. With severe hyperkalemia, cardiac conduction can be affected, since tissue excitability is reduced and conduction velocity slowed. Characteristic ECG changes evolve from peaked T waves to prolongation of the PR interval and then to progressive widening of the QRS complex. Above 8 meq, the P wave gradually disappears, and the "sine wave" pattern occurs as the QRS widens and merges into the T wave (Fig. 56-3); this may rapidly degenerate into asystole or ventricular fibrillation.

Potassium intake should be halted for hyperkalemic patients. This may be all that is required for some patients with mild hyperkalemia. Patients with potassium levels above 7 meq/L or with ECG changes require aggressive intervention to stabilize the cellular membrane, shift potassium intracellularly, and increase potassium excretion.

Membrane stabilization is effected by the administration of calcium, which has an immediate onset and a duration of action of 30 to 60 min. Calcium gluconate, 10%, in a dose of 0.5 to 1.0 mg/kg, may be given over 2 to 5 min with constant ECG monitoring. This may be repeated in 5 min if no effect is noted. An intracellular shift of potassium will result from the administration of sodium bicarbonate, with an onset of action in 5 to 10 min and a duration of up to 2 h; 1 to 2 meq/kg may be administered intravenously over 5 to 10 min. Intravenous glucose and insulin have an onset of action within 30 min which lasts 4 to 6 h. Glucose, 0.5 to 1.0 g/kg, is given, with 1.0 unit of regular insulin administered per 3 g of glucose. Recent reports of beta-agonist agents reducing potassium levels make this is an attractive treatment option, especially while awaiting intravenous access. Nebulized albuterol, in a dose of 2.5 mg for patients <25 kg and 5 mg for patients >25 kg, has been reported to decrease potassium by an average of

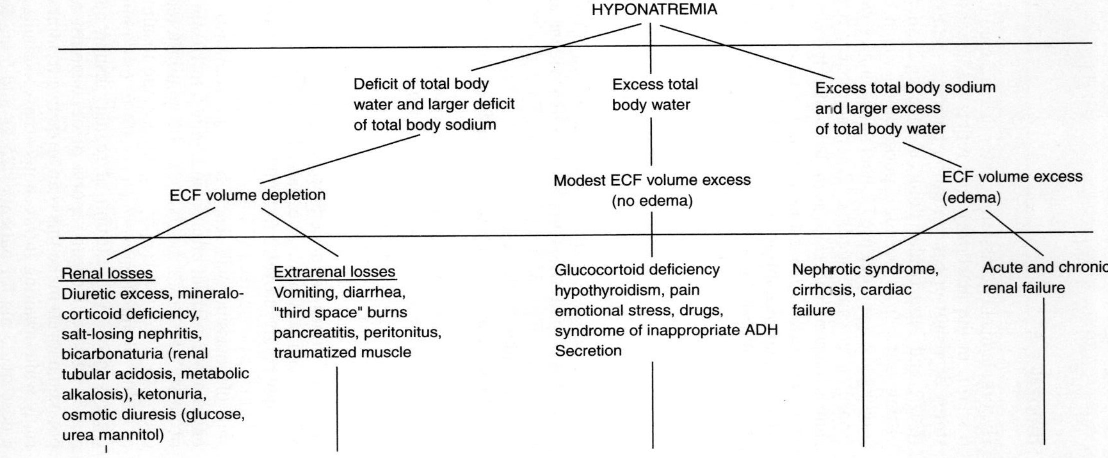
HYPONATREMIA
Deficit of total body water and larger deficit of total body sodium
Excess total body water
Excess total body sodium and larger excess of total body water
ECF volume depletion
Modest ECF volume excess (no edema)
ECF volume excess (edema)
Renal losses
Diuretic excess, mineralo-corticoid deficiency, salt-losing nephritis, bicarbonaturia (renal tubular acidosis, metabolic alkalosis), ketonuria, osmotic diuresis (glucose, urea mannitol)
Extrarenal losses
Vomiting, diarrhea, "third space" burns pancreatitis, peritonitus, traumatized muscle
Glucocortoid deficiency hypothyroidism, pain emotional stress, drugs, syndrome of inappropriate ADH Secretion
Nephrotic syndrome, cirrhosis, cardiac failure
Acute and chronic renal failure

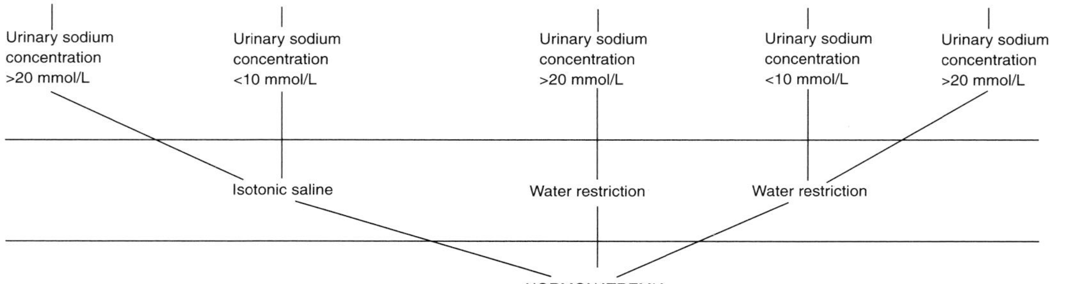

FIG. 56-2 Hyponatremia. (From Berl F, Anderson RJ, McDonald KM, Schrier RW: Clinical disorders of water metabolism. *Kidney Int.* 10:117, 1976, with permission.)

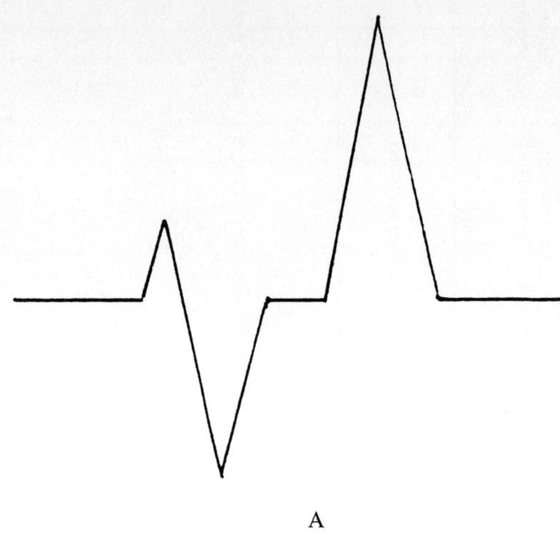

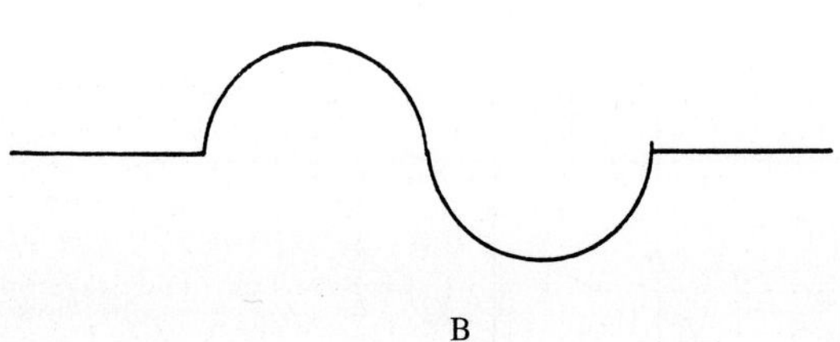

FIG. 56-3 Changes in ECG due to hyperkalemia. *A* Loss of P wave, widening of QRS complex, tall peaked T wave. *B* Sine wave pattern of severe hyperkalemia.

0.61 mmol/L at 30 min without significant toxicity. Though trials have used patients with chronic renal failure, this may be an easily administered and effective treatment for any patient with significant hyperkalemia.

Potassium excretion may be enhanced with loop diuretics such as Lasix, which is administered at 1 mg/kg. Sodium polystyrene sulfonate (Kayexelate) is a resin that exchanges sodium for potassium at a 1:1 ratio. Administration of 1 g/kg will lower potassium by 1.2 meq/L within 4 to 6 h of administration. This may be repeated every 4 to 6 h and may be administered orally or via retention enema. Dialysis will definitively lower potassium levels and should always be considered for severe cases of hyperkalemia.

Hypokalemia

Hypokalemia (potassium < 3.5 meq/L) may result from diminished supply, increased loss, or shifts in relative concentrations between body compartments.

Dietary deficiency can result in hypokalemia, as can renal losses, especially in patients on diuretics. Diarrhea commonly causes hypokalemia in children as a result of gastrointestinal losses. Protracted vomiting or nasogastric tube losses can also result in hypokalemia. A rare cause is hypokalemic periodic paralysis.

Clinical manifestations of hypokalemia are related to its rapidity of onset and degree of severity. Muscle weakness, ileus, areflexia, and autonomic instability can occur. In extreme cases, cardiac dysrhythmias and respiratory insufficiency can ensue.

The ECG can show premature atrial and ventricular beats, ST segment depression, and U waves. Patients on digoxin are especially vulnerable to arrhythmias.

A low serum potassium reflects a large total body deficit. Mild or chronic hypokalemia can be corrected gradually with oral supplementation. Extracellular fluid volume loss will continue to waste potassium and is corrected. Patients with severe hypokalemia may require intravenous potassium. Intravenous potassium should be administered at a rate less than or equal to 0.2 to 0.3 meq/kg/h with a concentration of no more than 40 meq/L. For life-threatening conditions, concentrations of up to 80 meq/L may be given at up to 1.0 meq/kg/h via central venous access with constant ECG monitoring and frequent reassessment.

For a more detailed discussion, see Rudzinski JP, Wolanyk D, Mackey M: Fluids and electrolytes, chap. 56, p. 337, in *Pediatric Emergency Medicine: A Comprehensive Study Guide.*

57 Metabolic Acidosis

Marshall Lewis

The regulation of acid-base balance is a fundamental component of physiology. In clinical practice, acid-base status is reflected in the measurement of pH, which is defined as the negative log of the hydrogen ion. Metabolic acidosis is the most frequent acid-base disturbance encountered in children in the emergency department. It results from an increase in the concentration of hydrogen (H^+) or a decrease in the concentration of bicarbonate (HCO_3^-).

An acid is defined as a proton donor (H^+) and a base as a proton acceptor (B^-). The average child produces 1.5 to 2.5 meq/kg/day of acid, while adults produce about 1 meq/kg/day. The body must also cope with the addition of any nonphysiologic acids. The initial defense is through buffering systems, which accept free H^+ and mitigate severe changes in pH.

The major extracellular buffer mechanism is the bicarbonate–carbonic acid system, described by the equation

$$H^+ + HCO_3^- \leftrightarrow H_2CO_3 \leftrightarrow H_2O + CO_2$$

Since CO_2 is easily dissolved in aqueous solution, the contribution of H_2CO_3 is negligible. Acid-base balance can be described by the equation:

$$pH = 6.1 + \log \frac{[HCO_3^-]}{0.03P_{CO_2}}$$

Systemic acidosis stimulates the respiratory center to increase the excretion of CO_2. The integrity of the bicarbonate–carbonic acid buffer system relies on the ability to maintain an open system for excreting CO_2; thus any factor that impedes ventilation produces a rapid drop in pH. It also depends on the ability of the kidney to resorb HCO_3^- and excrete hydrogen, which is essential in providing chronic compensation. Plasma and intracellular proteins and phosphates are the other major buffering systems of the body. Hemoglobin is an especially important buffer. Bone is another source with a large capacity to buffer excess hydrogen ions.

It is important to recognize that normal values for pH, P_{CO_2}, and HCO_3^- vary during childhood (Table 57-1). These differences are attributed to the relatively higher production of acid secondary to the increased metabolic demands in children and to an inability

TABLE 57-1 Normal Acid-Base Values for Pediatric Patients

Group	pH	P_{CO_2}	tCO_2
Preterm	7.35 ± 0.04	32 ± 3	17.9 ± 2.2
Term	7.34 ± 0.03	37 ± 1	20.2 ± 0.8
Children	7.41 ± 0.04	39 ± 3	25.2 ± 1.6
Male adults	7.39 ± 0.01	41 ± 2	25.2 ± 1.0

Source: Reprinted with permission from Edelman CM (ed): *Pediatric Kidney Disease.* Boston: Little Brown, 1992.

of the developing kidney to excrete acid and resorb bicarbonate. This "normal" tendency toward acidosis may predispose children to more severe disturbances in acid-base balance than adults.

CLINICAL PRESENTATION

The clinical presentation of metabolic acidosis depends on the underlying disease process and the rapidity with which it developed. Because the primary compensatory mechanism is a decrease in P_{CO_2}, tachypnea is a universal finding in the acutely ill patient. Severe alterations in pH affect mental status, and patients may be agitated, lethargic, or, in extreme cases, comatose. Derangements in mental status are especially severe in patients in whom acidosis develops quickly. In situations in which hypovolemia occurs, as in diabetic ketoacidosis, poor perfusion may be present. Common gastrointestinal complaints include nausea, vomiting, and abdominal pain. In patients with chronic, well-compensated metabolic acidosis, the presentation can be insidious, such as failure to thrive.

The presence of acidosis is confirmed by obtaining an arterial blood gas. In addition to confirming acidosis, the arterial gas should demonstrate adequate respiratory compensation. For every 1 meq/L fall in the serum bicarbonate, the P_{CO_2} should decrease 1 to 1.5 mmHg. Serum electrolytes, blood urea nitrogen and creatinine, and serum glucose are also drawn. If an ingestion is suspected, a toxicology screen is indicated.

METABOLIC ACIDOSIS WITH AN ELEVATED ANION GAP

The etiology of metabolic acidosis is aided by calculating the anion gap (AG), which is defined as the difference between the measured serum cations and anions. In practice, sodium is the only cation used in calculating the AG, because the other extracellular cations—potassium, calcium, and magnesium—are present in small

TABLE 57-2 Causes of Anion Gap Acidosis

Lactate
Shock
Anoxia
Ischemia
Diabetic ketoacidosis
Uremia
Toxins
Methanol
Ethylene glycol
Salicylates
Inborn errors of metabolism

quantities. The measured serum anions are chloride and bicarbonate. Thus, the formula for the AG is

$$\text{Sodium} - (\text{chloride} + \text{bicarbonate})$$

The normal AG is between 8 and 16 and represents serum anions other than chloride and bicarbonate, mostly negatively charged plasma proteins. The finding of an elevated AG implies the presence of an endogenously created or an exogenously ingested acid. In children, the most likely causes of acute endogenous production of acid are diabetic ketoacidosis and processes that result in the accumulation of lactic acid, such as hypovolemic or septic shock. Many ingestions can cause metabolic acidosis, especially salicylates and alcohols (Table 57-2).

Another cause of elevated AG acidosis virtually unique to the pediatric patient is inborn errors of metabolism (IEM). While individually these diseases are quite rare, as a group their incidence approaches 1 in 5000 live births. Of the IEMs that cause metabolic acidosis, the most common are methylmalonic, propionic, and isovaleric acidemia. A more complete list is included in Table 57-3. The typical emergency department (ED) presentation is a neonate with vomiting, lethargy, poor feeding, and failure to thrive. Although the diagnosis of a specific IEM is unlikely to be made in the ED, helpful ancillary studies that are readily available include serum lactate, pyruvate, and ammonia.

TREATMENT

The treatment of an elevated anion gap acidosis is predicated on reversing the underlying etiology. Many severely ill patients re-

TABLE 57-3 Inborn Errors of Metabolism Producing Acidosis

Organic acidemias
Methylmalonic acidemia
Propionic acidemia
Isovaleric acidemia
Amino acidurias
Maple syrup urine disease
Citrullinemia
Argininosuccinic aciduria
Glycogen storage disease
Type I
Type III
Fatty acid oxidation defects

Source: From Burton B: Inborn errors of metabolism: the clinical diagnosis in early infancy. *Pediatrics* 79:359, 1987, with permission.

quire aggressive fluid resuscitation. Patients with severe alteration of mental status may require intubation and mechanical ventilation. Controversies focus on the role of bicarbonate therapy as well as that of other buffering agents such as tromethamine (Tham) and Carbicarb (an equimolar solution of $NaHCO_3$ and Na_2CO_3). In practice, therapy with bicarbonate is rarely indicated, especially as a bolus. Therapy with buffering agents may play a role in the postresuscitative phase of asphyxial arrest. The treatment of inborn errors of metabolism is complex and requires consultation with a pediatric endocrinologist.

NON-ANION GAP METABOLIC ACIDOSIS

Metabolic acidosis with a normal or near normal AG results from loss of bicarbonate or failure of the kidney to excrete an appropriate amount of hydrogen ion. A compensatory increase in chloride preserves a normal AG. The clinical presentation is unlikely to be as acute and fulminant as that of metabolic acidosis with an elevated AG.

DIFFERENTIAL DIAGNOSIS

The most common cause of a normal AG acidosis in the pediatric patient is acute diarrhea. Normal intestinal fluid is rich in bicarbonate, which is lost in the stool. Concomitant losses of sodium may decrease the kidney's ability to acidify the urine, exacerbating the acidosis. In the emergency department, many infants appear well hydrated despite electrolyte profiles demonstrating serum bicarbonate between 16 and 20 meq/L. The condition resolves with resolution of the diarrhea. Infants with diarrhea that results in severe dehydration may develop metabolic acidosis accompanied by an increased anion gap.

Another cause of non-AG metabolic acidosis in children is renal tubular acidosis (RTA). The different types of RTA are classified as distal (Type I), proximal (Type II), and type IV, which is associated with hypoaldosteronism. The usual finding is a metabolic acidosis in which hyperchloremia preserves a normal anion gap.

Distal RTA is a defect in the ability of the kidney to acidify urine. Clinically, findings are often subtle, with polyuria, occasional vomiting, mild dehydration, and constipation.

Aside from the non-AG hyperchloremic metabolic acidosis, laboratory values in distal RTA may reveal hyponatremia and hypokalemia. Hypokalemia can be severe enough to result in severe muscle weakness. Most importantly, despite a systemic acidosis, urine pH will typically be 6.5 to 7.5, reflecting the inability to excrete hydrogen.

Proximal RTA can be thought of as a defect in resorbing bicarbonate. Normally, virtually all filtered bicarbonate is resorbed, mostly in the proximal tubules. The specific defect in proximal RTA has not been isolated.

Type IV RTA is associated with hyperkalemia. The disorder is associated with hypoaldosteronism, and in some cases with decreased responsiveness of the distal tubules to aldosterone. Type IV RTA is common in adults and is associated with renal insufficiency, volume contraction, and potassium-sparing drugs.

The fundamental treatment of all types of RTA is directed at maintaining a normal or nearly normal pH. Most patients can be managed with supplemental bicarbonate at a dose of 5 to 10 meq/kg/day. Some patients may require supplemental potassium. Patients with type IV RTA may benefit from therapy with mineralocortocoid. Successful treatment can prevent some of the complications of RTA and permits normal growth and development.

For a more detailed discussion, see Lewis M: Metabolic acidosis, chap. 57, p. 350, in *Pediatric Emergency Medicine: A Comprehensive Study Guide.*

SECTION IX
GENITOURINARY EMERGENCIES

58 Genitourinary Problems

Marianne Gausche

TESTICULAR PAIN/SCROTAL MASSES

The causes of the painful scrotum in the child are varied. The emergency physician must distinguish these causes by considering the age of the patient, the history of symptoms, the physical findings, and results of the diagnostic evaluation. One may separate the causes of scrotal swelling into painful or painless testicular swelling (Table 58-1).

In all cases, the possibility of a surgical emergency must be considered and the evaluation and management proceed accordingly. The emergency physician must maintain a high level of suspicion for testicular torsion as the cause of the scrotal pain and swelling because the consequences of a missed diagnosis can be devastating.

Epididymitis

Signs and Symptoms

A careful history must be obtained, including previous scrotal pain or surgeries; history of trauma, sexual activity, and urinary symptoms; vomiting or fever; and time course for the onset of symptoms. Symptoms in the younger child may be vague and nonspecific. Fever and vomiting may be present, followed by swelling of the epididymis and the hemiscrotum. The caregivers may note scrotal swelling and bring the infant or child in for evaluation. In the older child, the onset is often insidious, with pain isolated to the hemiscrotum and later becoming diffuse. Fever and urinary symptoms may also be present.

Physical examination reveals an erythematous, warm, swollen epididymis, testicle, and scrotum. A careful examination should note that tenderness is more posterior and lateral to the adjacent testis and can be separated from actual testicular tenderness. The

TABLE 58-1 Causes of Scrotal Swelling in Children

Painful	Painless
Epididymitis	Testicular tumor
Testicular torsion	Idiopathic scrotal edema
Torsion of the appendix testis	Henoch-Schönlein purpura
Incarcerated hernia	Inquinal hernia
Idiopathic scrotal edema	Hydrocele
Trauma (testicular rupture)	Varicocele
Scrotal cellulitis or inflammation	Anasarca

Prehn sign, or relief upon elevation of the scrotum, may be present but is not reliable in distinguishing epididymitis from torsion.

Diagnostic Evaluation

The prepubescent child with signs and symptoms of epididymitis is difficult to distinguish from the child with testicular torsion. A urinalysis may be helpful in showing signs of urinary tract infection with increased white cells and bacteria, but pyuria is present in a minority of cases of epididymitis. Because the consequences of a missed testicular torsion are dire, the emergency physician should obtain prompt urologic consultation when the cause of the scrotal pain is unclear. Nuclear medicine imaging or a testicular scan using technetium pertechnetate or color Doppler ultrasonography (US) should be performed on all children in whom the diagnosis of the scrotal swelling is unclear. Both the nuclear scan and the color Doppler US will reveal normal or increased flow to the affected testis if the patient has epididymitis. Once the diagnosis of epididymitis is confirmed, the evaluation includes a urine culture, possibly an intravenous pyelogram (IVP), renal US, and voiding cystourethrogram for the prepubescent child who may have a preexisting urologic abnormality. In the sexually active adolescent, a urethral swab for gonorrhea and chlamydial cultures and blood for VDRL or rapid plasma reagent tests should be sent.

Management

Management is dependent upon the age and toxicity of the child. Children under 1 month of age with associated urinary tract infection should be admitted and receive intravenous antibiotics. This approach should be considered for the infant 3 months of age or younger. Older infants and children under 2 years of age may also require admission, depending on the level of toxicity and associated signs and symptoms.

Inpatient antibiotic therapy should include ampicillin and an aminoglycoside or cefotaxime (Table 58-2). A majority of children can be managed as outpatients. For the non-sexually active child, trimethoprim/sulfamethoxazole (TMP/SMX) is the drug of choice. Prompt urologic consultation and subsequent follow-up is recommended for all of these patients.

Testicular Torsion

Testicular torsion may occur in children of any age, from infancy to adulthood. There is a bimodal distribution of cases in children that peaks during the neonatal period and adolescence. Torsion of the testes is a urologic emergency and results in a significant amount of legal action against emergency physicians for missed diagnosis. The emergency physician must have a high level of suspicion for this diagnosis in any child with complaint of scrotal pain or signs of scrotal swelling on physical examination.

Pathophysiology

The classic description of the anatomic abnormality associated with torsion is the "bell-clapper" deformity, which is often bilateral and causes the testes to have a horizontal lie within the scrotal sac (Fig. 58-1). The testicular attachments to the intrascrotal subcutaneous tissue of the tunica vaginalis are incomplete, allowing the testis and the spermatic cord and associated testicular artery to twist within the scrotal sac. If the torsion is complete, vascular compromise ensues, and eventually the testis will necrose and atrophy. After 12 h of pain, the testicular salvage rate is approximately 20 percent. Generally, patients with symptoms for more than 24 h are unlikely to have a viable testis.

Signs and Symptoms

Patients may report a history of trauma in 5 to 6 percent of cases of torsion, but the absence of a history of trauma should not dissuade the emergency physician from pursuing a diagnosis of torsion. Physical examination often reveals a swollen, tender, and erythematous hemiscrotum. The testis may be high-riding or lying horizontally within the scrotum. Tenderness of the affected testis is diffuse, and the cremasteric reflex may be absent. Elevating the testis will cause further pain (Prehn sign) instead of the relief that can be seen in epididymitis. Associated symptoms of nausea, vomiting, and abdominal or flank pain are common.

TABLE 58-2 Antibiotic Therapy for Epididymitis in Children

Antibiotic	Dose	Route
Outpatient Management		
Non-sexually active		
Trimethoprim/sulfamethoxazole	8–10 mg/kg/24 h	PO bid for 10 days
If allergic to sulfa: amoxicillin or a first-generation cephalosporin		
Sexually active		
Ceftriaxone	125 mg	IM
plus if patient ≥9 years of age tetracycline	500 mg	PO qid for 10 days
plus if patient <9 years of age erythromycin	50 mg/kg/24 h	PO qid for 10 days
Inpatient Management		
Ampicillin	100 mg/kg/24 h	IV q 6 h
plus gentamicin	7.5 mg/kg/24 h	IV q 8 h
or cefotaxime	50–150 mg/kg/24 h	IV q 6 h

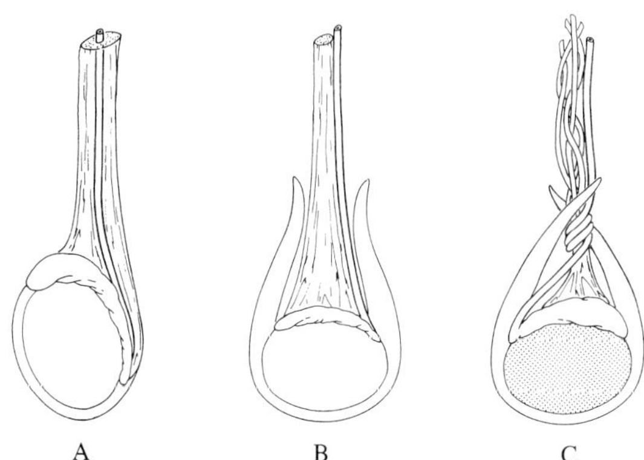

FIG. 58-1 *A.* Normal attachment of tunica vaginalis to the testis. *B.* Abnormal attachment resulting in horizontal lie of the testis. *C.* Resultant torsion of the spermatic cord.

Diagnostic Evaluation

In equivocal cases, a urinalysis should be performed, looking for the signs of urinary tract infection that are sometimes seen in cases of epididymitis. Other laboratory studies such as a complete blood count and chemistries are not helpful and could delay definitive management. Scrotal Doppler for testicular artery flow is rarely helpful because of the high (20 percent) false-positive and false-negative rates. Once the diagnosis of testicular torsion is considered, consultation with a urologist should be obtained. Further diagnostic evaluation is reserved for those patients in whom the diagnosis of torsion is in question and in whom any delay in obtaining studies will not result in increased morbidity.

The nuclear medicine scan with technetium 99m pertechnetate has been the diagnostic test of choice in the past, but many clinicians are opting to evaluate testicular artery flow with color Doppler ultrasonography. Neither test should delay the urologic consultation. The radionuclide testicular scan requires that intravenous access be obtained, which can cause added pain for the child. This test is otherwise simple and fairly rapid (25 min). Testicular scans may not be available 24 h a day in some hospitals, causing delay in management. A unilateral, "cold" defect on the side of the testicular pain indicates lack of blood flow to the testis and indicates possible torsion. Accuracy is excellent and ranges from 86 to 100 percent, but false-positive and false-negative scans occur. Real-time US has been studied in conjunction with scintigraphy and has identified findings suggestive of alternative diagnoses in cases of false-positive scans. In addition, US may identify patients who underwent spontaneous detorsion and had false-negative scans. Sonography alone is useful in the evaluation of many scrotal disorders; however, it may not reliably distinguish between cases of epididymitis and torsion.

Color Doppler US is very accurate in adults, with a reported sensitivity of 86 to 100 percent, a specificity of 100 percent, and accuracy of 97 percent. Color Doppler US involves no radiation exposure and can be performed easily. Prospective studies in small numbers of children demonstrate that while this technique is accurate, there are false-positive studies in the prepubescent child because of the small testis and the low volume of arterial flow. Additional limitations to its general use include the lack of availability of the procedure at all times of the day or night and variability in the experience of the physician interpreting the test. One author recommends the use of scintigraphy in pediatric patients with absence of flow noted on color Doppler US of the testis.

Management

Rapid urologic consultation should be obtained on all patients with suspected torsion. Manual reduction of the torsed testes may be attempted by the emergency physician to reduce the ischemic time while awaiting the arrival of the urologist. The patient is sedated, and the testicle is detorsed by turning it outward toward the thigh. A hand-held Doppler stethoscope may be used to verify the increase in blood flow to the testicle. The patient must then undergo bilateral orchiopexy to avoid recurrence. In all cases of torsion, the affected testicle is untwisted and the contralateral testis is pexed. Orchidectomy of the affected testicle is often recommended. However, leaving the testicle in the scrotum did not result in autosensitization in 17 of 18 patients in one study.

Torsion of the Appendix Testis

Appendixes are common and may occur on the testicle, the spermatic cord, or the epididymis. The hydatid of Morgagni or appendix testis is the most common of the types of vestiges to torse. Torsion of the appendix testis is often difficult to distinguish from torsion of the spermatic cord. Torsion of the appendix testis frequently occurs between 10 and 14 years of age—an age group in which testicular torsion also occurs.

Signs and Symptoms

Signs and symptoms of torsion of the appendix testis may be less severe than those of testicular torsion but may be indistinguishable. Systemic symptoms such as nausea and vomiting are rare, and physical examination may reveal focal tenderness in the upper pole of the testis or diffuse testicular enlargement and pain. A "blue dot" sign is occasionally noted in the young child when the necrotic appendage produces a blue hue under the scrotal skin.

Diagnostic Evaluation

Laboratory evaluation is not helpful and the urinalysis is normal. Testicular scan and color Doppler US are normal or reveal increased flow to the testicle.

Management

Once the diagnosis of torsion of the appendix testis is made, bed rest, urologic follow-up, and analgesia are recommended. Surgical intervention is sometimes indicated in cases in which the diagnosis of testicular torsion cannot be reliably excluded. Most patients are much improved within days, and complications are rare.

Scrotal Trauma and Testicular Trauma

Trauma to the scrotum can occur by many mechanisms, including child abuse. Most often, the mechanism is blunt—a result of play or motor vehicle accident. The resulting injury is scrotal hematoma and, rarely, testicular rupture.

Testicular Rupture

Testicular rupture occurs when the testis is crushed against the bony pelvis. The patient presents with a painful, swollen testis after a traumatic incident. If the mechanism was minor, the possibility of a tumor should be considered, as tumors may rupture after minimal trauma. Bleeding into the scrotum occurs, and the scrotum may be ecchymotic or tense with blood. The testis may be difficult to palpate and may have an irregular border or be ill defined. If testicular rupture is suspected, prompt evaluation of the integrity of the testis by US and urologic consultation are essential. Ultrasound can locate a dislocated testicle which was displaced after major trauma.

TESTICULAR MASSES

Testicular Tumors

Signs and Symptoms

Most often children or adults present with a feeling of fullness, tugging, or increased weight to the scrotum. The patient or the patient's caregivers may have felt a mass. On physical examination, the mass is firm, smooth, or nodular and will not transilluminate. Generally the tumor is painless, but bleeding into the tumor can cause sudden onset of testicular pain or referred pain to the abdomen or flank. A thorough physical examination should be performed, including examination for lymphadenopathy, abdominal mass or hepatosplenomegaly, and gynecomastia.

Diagnostic Evaluation

A urinalysis and a complete blood count are performed. The urine is tested for the presence of human chorionic gonadotropin by a rapid urine pregnancy test. Ultrasound may be performed in cases where the presence of a tumor mass is unclear.

Management

Immediate urologic consultation and prompt biopsy or removal of the mass are necessary to establish tumor type and subsequent treatment options for the patient.

Inguinal Hernia

Inguinal hernia repair is the most common surgery performed on children. It occurs when peritoneal or pelvic contents herniate through a patent processus vaginalis into the scrotal sac. Boys are five times more likely to have an inguinal hernia than girls. Inguinal hernias often present in the first year of life, when the parent notes an intermittent bulge into the scrotal sac when the infant cries or coughs. Some parents report that the infant is fussy. Children may note a pulling feeling or a heaviness in the groin and also note a bulge with increases in intraabdominal pressure. Systemic signs of fever, abdominal pain, and nausea and vomiting should alert the clinician to the possibility of incarceration of the hernia. Other signs of incarceration include a firm, painful, nonreducible mass in the scrotum.

Management

Most reducible inguinal hernias can be referred to a surgeon for repair. Incarcerated hernias can be reduced 85 to 95 percent of the time with firm finger pressure on the internal inguinal ring, analgesics, ice pack to the area, and placing the patient in the Trendelenburg position. If the hernia is reduced easily, then the patient can be discharged home, with close follow-up with a surgeon for definitive repair. Patients with hernias that do not reduce easily but still can be reduced should be admitted for observation and delayed surgical repair. Patients with hernias that remain incarcerated or patients who demonstrate signs of peritonitis or bowel perforation must be taken to the operating room immediately. In these cases, stabilization of the patient and fluid resuscitation should be initiated in the emergency department.

Henoch-Schönlein Purpura

Henoch-Schönlein purpura (HSP) is a systemic vasculitis that often results in abdominal pain, gastrointestinal bleeding, purpuric rash, nephritis, and arthritis. The patient may also complain of testicular pain, scrotal edema and swelling, or purpuric rash on the scrotum. In some cases it is impossible to distinguish HSP from testicular torsion clinically. The physician must then assume that the patient has testicular torsion, consult a urologist, and obtain color Doppler US or scintigraphy. If the diagnostic evaluation is negative and the patient has other features of HSP, surgical exploration may not be necessary.

Hydrocele

A hydrocele is formed from a patent processus vaginalis, which normally regresses to form the tunica vaginalis. The hydrocele may communicate with the peritoneal cavity and be associated with an indirect inguinal hernia. Fluid is noted adjacent to the testis and may result in a swollen and bluish-appearing scrotum. Transillumination of the swelling reveals that the mass is fluid-filled, but it may be difficult to distinguish from indirect inguinal hernia. If the hydrocele becomes or presents as a painful swelling, then the physician must consider intraperitoneal pathology such as a ruptured appendix or testicular torsion as the primary cause. Otherwise a nonpainful hydrocele may be observed for the first 6 months of life for spontaneous resolution. If the hydrocele persists past the first year of life, a patent processus vaginalis is surgically repaired.

Other Causes of Scrotal Pain or Swelling

Other causes of scrotal swelling with and without pain include scrotal cellulitis, idiopathic scrotal edema, and lymphadenitis.

Fournier's Gangrene

Fifty-six cases of Fournier's gangrene in children have been reported. This rare entity of infectious origin, which results in necrotizing fasciitis, may present initially as cellulitis, balanitis, balanoposthitis, or scrotal pain and swelling. The patient may appear relatively nontoxic even when obvious gangrene appears in the perineum. Although staphylococci and streptococci are the most common organisms to be cultured, management includes broad-spectrum antibiotic therapy to cover anaerobic and aerobic gram-positive and gram-negative organisms. Prompt surgical consultation and operative incision and drainage of infected tissue with excision of necrotic tissue is paramount. Generally, the prognosis is better in children than in adults, and more conservative surgical debridement is recommended in children.

PENILE EMERGENCIES

Phimosis

Phimosis occurs when the distal prepuce cannot be retracted over the glans penis. Normally, the prepuce cannot be retracted over the glans in infants, and it should not be forced. With normal growth and stretching of the prepuce, it will become retractable in 90 percent of children by the age of 6 years.

Diagnosis and Management

Phimosis may be noted on routine physical examination or may be reported by parents. Pain and swelling can occur with associated infections of the glans. The urinary stream may, in some cases, be diverted to one side, or the child may present with hematuria.

Physical examination generally establishes the diagnosis; however, examination of the urine for urinary tract infection may be considered.

Reassurance and an explanation of the natural course of this condition to parents is needed. Patients with recurrent balanitis, balanoposthitis, urinary tract infection, or obstruction should be referred to a urologist for circumcision.

Paraphimosis

Paraphimosis is a condition in which the prepuce in the uncircumcised male is retracted over the glans and then cannot be moved into normal position. The prepuce, once retracted over the glans, may swell from venous congestion, preventing movement.

Signs and Symptoms

The patient presents with pain, swelling, and edema of the distal penis and prepuce. The physician must establish whether or not the child has been circumcised; if not, a thorough examination to look for possible hair tourniquets and penile foreign bodies must follow.

Management

The management of this condition focuses on retracting the prepuce back over the head of the glans. Ice packs to the groin are poorly tolerated by most children without anesthesia to the area. The physician may place a penile block by injecting 1% lidocaine (without epinephrine) around the base of the penis. This will effectively reduce the child's pain. Ice packs can then be placed for 5 to 10 min, after which manual reduction should be attempted (Fig. 58-2*A* to *C*). The physician's index fingers are placed on the leading edge of the edematous foreskin, and the thumbs are placed on the glans. Thumb pressure is directed inward toward the body as the prepuce is pushed back over the glans. Once reduction is complete, the prepuce should lie over the end of the glans and the urethral opening should not be visible (Fig. 58-2*C*). If retraction

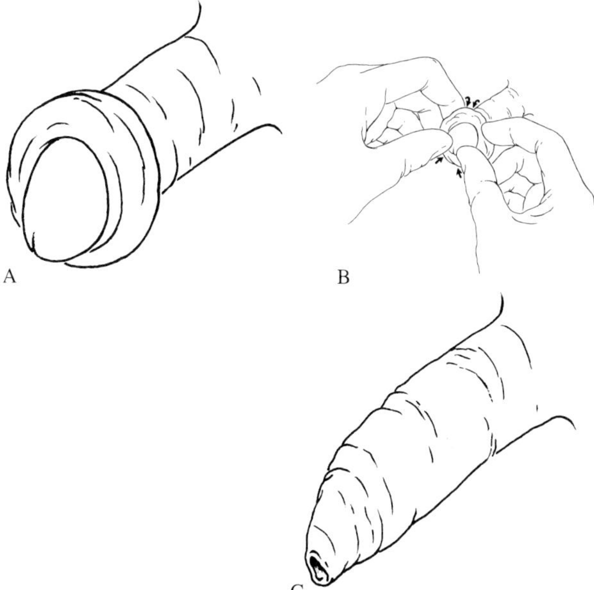

FIG. 58-2 *A*. Paraphimosis. *B*. Manual retraction of the prepuce over the glans. *C*. Normal position of the prepuce.

of the prepuce is successful and the child is able to urinate spontaneously, then the child can be discharged with urologic follow-up. If the prepuce cannot be retracted, then emergent urologic consultation is needed for circumcision.

Balanitis/Balanoposthitis

Balanitis and balanoposthitis are infections of the glans and foreskin. Both are relatively more common in the uncircumcised male (6 percent) but may also be found in circumcised children (3 percent). Balanitis may be caused by entrapment of organisms under a poorly retractable foreskin. Monilial infections are also associated with balanoposthitis in infants (Fig. 58-3). In the adolescent, syphilis must also be considered as a cause.

Signs and Symptoms

Signs and symptoms include swelling, erythema, penile discharge, dysuria, bleeding, and, rarely, ulceration of the glans. Phimosis can occur but is uncommon. A careful examination of the base of the penis should be performed to look for a strand of hair, which may cause strangulation and edema.

Management

Local care with soaks and topical antibiotic ointment is recommended. The addition of oral antibiotics, such as cephalexin or amoxicillin for 10 days, may be reserved for the more severe

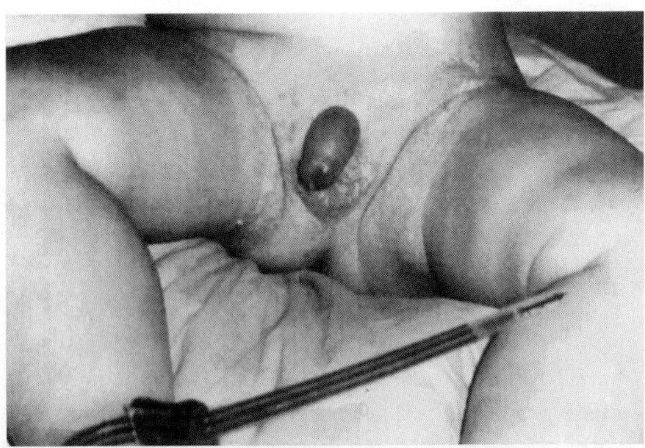

FIG. 58-3 Balanoposthitis in an infant with monilial diaper rash.

cases. The patient should be followed within 2 days to assure that symptoms have resolved. Children with repeated episodes may be referred to a urologist for elective circumcision.

Priapism

Priapism is a prolonged painful erection unaccompanied by continued sexual stimulation. It is relatively uncommon in childhood except in patients with sickle cell disease. In this group, priapism occurs in about 3 to 10 percent of patients.

Signs and Symptoms

Patients often have a delayed presentation, possibly as a result of embarrassment. The patient is noted on physical examination to have an erect penis, which is firm on the dorsal surface (corpora cavernosum) and soft on the ventral surface (corpora spongiosum) and the glans. The patient should be asked about placement of urethral/penile foreign bodies and the bladder palpated for enlargement. Urinary retention may be associated with priapism and can easily be relieved by placement of a urinary catheter.

Diagnostic Evaluation

Priapism is a clinical diagnosis based on physical examination; however, the physician may wish to send for a complete blood count, looking for evidence of leukemia or anemia; a hemoglobin electrophoresis, looking for possible sickle cell disease; renal function tests, if there has been significant urinary retention; and, if the patient has suffered perineal trauma, a retrograde cystourethrogram. Color Doppler US may be used to determine if the priapism is secondary to a low-flow or a high-flow state.

Management

Treatment is based on the presumed etiology of the priapism. Providing oxygen, hydration, and analgesics to the patient with sickle cell disease may alleviate the priapism; if not, an exchange transfusion of the patient's blood with 30 mL/kg of packed cells is performed in an effort to get the patient's hemoglobin to above 10 g/dL. Patients with leukemia may receive hydration and analgesics and appropriate treatment for their cancer. A urinary catheter should be inserted to relieve bladder distension. Once medical management is initiated, the patient should be admitted for observation. Urologic consultation is recommended in all cases. The timing of surgical management of priapism is controversial. Some authors recommend waiting no longer than 24 h of medical management, followed by intracavernous injection of a vasoconstrictor (epinephrine, ephedrine, phenylephrine) and, if unsuccessful, followed by surgical shunting of blood from the cavernosum to the spongiosum or the glans. Intravenous ketamine hydrochloride has been used to treat priapism in the newborn.

For a more detailed discussion, see Gausche M: Genitourinary problems, chap. 58, p. 355, in *Pediatric Emergency Medicine: A Comprehensive Study Guide*.

59 Urinary Tract Diseases

Marianne Gausche

URINARY TRACT INFECTION

Urinary tract infection (UTI) is a frequent cause of fever in the infant and child. In a recent metaanalysis of children from 0 to 36 months of age with fever, 7 percent of male infants less than 6 months of age and 8 percent of female infants less than 1 year of age had UTI. Other studies have shown an overall incidence of 3 to 5 percent in girls and 1 percent in boys.

Signs and Symptoms

Signs and symptoms vary with the age of the patient. They may be nonspecific in the infant, including fever, vomiting, and irritability. In the older child, they may be more localized, including frequency, urgency, dysuria, and hematuria.

Patients with abdominal or flank pain, high fever, vomiting, or other systemic signs must be evaluated for pyelonephritis.

Diagnostic Evaluation

Obtaining an adequate urine for culture is the most important step in establishing the diagnosis of UTI. Approximately 20 percent of young children with a documented UTI have a normal urinalysis or reagent strip for leukocytes and nitrites. There are a number of methods of obtaining a urine sample; these include (1) bagging the perineum, (2) taking a clean catch, (3) catheterizing the urinary tract, and (4) suprapubic aspiration. Although bagging the perineum is easy and noninvasive, it is the least reliable method. Older children with adequate instruction and/or supervision may be able to provide a clean catch specimen.

Suprapubic aspiration is a simple but invasive procedure that relies on the fact that the bladder is an intraabdominal organ in the infant and child less than 2 years of age. It is best to perform the procedure when the bladder is full. Landmarks for aspiration are one fingerbreadth above the symphysis pubis and in the midline. The infraumbilical abdomen is prepped with povidone solution, and a small wheal of 1% lidocaine is injected subcutaneously with a 27-gauge needle. A 22-gauge, 1½-in needle with a 10-mL syringe is then placed at a 60 to 90° angle cephalad, in the midline, above the symphysis pubis. The physician exerts negative pressure on the syringe as the needle is inserted and continues until urine is obtained. The needle is withdrawn and the abdomen cleaned of the povidone solution, after which a bandage is placed over the aspiration site. Complications of the procedure are uncommon; they include hematuria, bowel perforation, cystitis, and abdominal wall hematoma or infection.

Other studies, such as electrolytes and renal function tests, should be obtained on all patients with signs of dehydration or toxicity and on all infants, all males, and patients with signs of upper tract infection.

Management/Radiologic Evaluation of the Urinary Tract

Neonates, females with recurrent UTI or pyelonephritis, and males of any age should undergo radiologic evaluation for urinary tract abnormalities. As many as 50 percent of these patients will show congenital anatomic abnormalities on radiologic evaluation.

The radiologic evaluation of the urinary tract has become more sophisticated in recent years. Table 59-1 summarizes the types of diagnostic tests and their indications.

The most common anatomic abnormality of the urinary tract is vesicoureteral reflux (VUR). It is usually diagnosed in the first decade of life and resolves spontaneously in most cases. Voiding cystourethrogram (VCUG) is the diagnostic test of choice for boys and girls with suspected urethral pathology. Otherwise girls can be evaluated for VUR with isotope cystography (IC).

Renal cortical scintigraphy (RCS) is displacing intravenous urography (IVU) as the diagnostic test of choice in the diagnosis of upper tract infections. With RCS, dimercaptosuccinic acid (DMSA labeled with technetium 99m) is injected intravenously, and the patient is scanned with a gamma camera approximately 2 h later.

TABLE 59-1 Diagnostic Tests and Their Indications

Diagnostic test	Indication(s)
Renal cortical scan	Pyelonephritis; UTI and fever
Voiding cystourethrogram	Vesicoureteral reflux; initial evaluation of boys with UTI; initial evaluation of girls with UTI (in some centers)
Isotope cystography	Vesicoureteral reflux; initial evaluation of girls with UTI without suspected urethral pathology
Renal ultrasonography	Hydronephrosis; nephrolithiasis
Diuretic renography	Obstructive uropathies
Intravenous pyelogram	Nephrolithiasis; isolated renal trauma
Computed tomography	Renal and abdominal trauma

This procedure has many advantages over IVU, including the facts that

1. Visualization is not obscured by bowel contents, as with IVU.
2. The use of highly osmotic agents is not required.
3. Allergic reactions are rare.
4. It is more sensitive in patients with poor renal function.
5. It delivers a lower dose of radiation to the gonads.

Renal cortical scintigraphy should be performed on patients with fever and UTI to determine upper tract involvement. Clinical signs and symptoms, laboratory evaluation, or sonography are not reliable in determining pyelonephritis. An algorithm for the radiologic evaluation of the child with its first UTI is summarized in Fig. 59-1.

Antibiotic therapy is directed at the presumed infecting organism until results of the urine culture are obtained. Almost 80 percent of community-acquired organisms causing UTI are resistant to ampicillin; therefore amoxicillin or trimethoprim/sulfamethoxazole (TMP/SMZ) are first-line therapies. Other antibiotic regimens include sulfisoxazole (Gantrisin), 120 to 150 mg/kg/24 h orally every 6 h, or cephalexin (Keflex), 25 to 50 mg/kg/24 h orally every 6 h. Older children (above 6 years of age) may benefit from the addition of phenazopyridine (Pyridium) to the treatment regimen. Pyridium can be given 10 mg/kg/day in three divided doses for 2 to 3 days or until the patient is less symptomatic.

Criteria for admission are listed in Table 59-2. All neonates and infants below 3 months of age, patients with pyelonephritis,

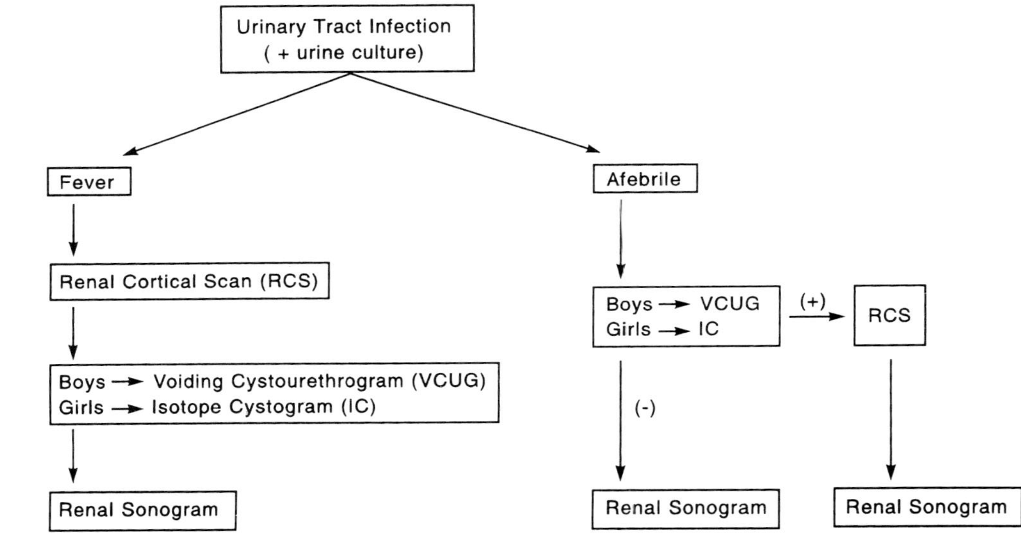

FIG. 59-1 Algorithm for the radiographic evaluation of the child with its first UTI. (Adapted from Andrich MP, Majd M: Diagnostic imaging in the evaluation of the first urinary tract infection in infants and young children. *Pediatrics* 90:436, 1992.)

TABLE 59-2 Admission Criteria for Children with Urinary Tract Infection

Neonate
Pyelonephritis
Known urinary tract abnormality
Urinary tract obstruction (stone)
Ureteral stents or other urinary tract foreign bodies
Immunocompromised
Vomiting and dehydration
Renal insufficiency

immunocompromised patients, and those with known urinary tract obstruction should be admitted for intravenous antibiotics. Intravenous antibiotic therapy, which includes an aminoglycoside such as gentamicin 7.5 mg/kg/24 h every 8 to 12 h, should continue until the sensitivity of the organism is known and the patient's clinical status is improved. Once stable, patients may be discharged on the appropriate oral antibiotic and treated for a total of 14 days.

UROLITHIASIS

Urolithiasis is stone formation in the bladder, ureter, or kidney. It is less common in children than in adults but nevertheless occurs in approximately one case per 7500 pediatric hospital admissions (Table 59-3). The incidence of urolithiasis varies by geographic

TABLE 59-3 Causes of Urolithiasis in North American Children

Cause	Number, %
Metabolic	162 (32.9)
Idiopathic hypercalcuria	
Cystinuria	
Myeloproliferative disorders	
Hyperoxaluria	
Renal tubular acidosis	
Primary hyperparathyroidism	
Hypercortisolism	
Other	
Endemic (urate)	10 (2.2)
Developmental anomalies of the genitourinary tract	160 (32.5)
Infection	21 (4.3)
Idiopathic	139 (28.3)

location. It is highest in the southeastern and western United States (1 per 1380 hospital admissions). In the United States, most urinary calculi (58 percent) are calcium oxalate or calcium phosphate. Urolithiasis is rare in blacks but affects girls and boys equally, with a mean age of 9 years at presentation.

Signs and Symptoms

Patients may present with abdominal or flank pain (44 percent), hematuria (38 percent), fever (15 percent), and other urinary tract complaints (18 percent). Flank pain is not as common in children, especially those below 5 years of age, as in adults. The emergency physician should assess for history of recurrent UTI, frequent bouts of abdominal pain, family history of stones, history of microscopic or gross hematuria, passage of stones or gravel in the urine, intake of vitamins C and D, hydration status, recent trauma, and genitourinary surgery. A routine physical examination should be performed, including evaluation of the blood pressure and normal growth parameters.

Diagnostic Evaluation

A urinalysis, urine culture, and renal function studies should be obtained on all children with possible urinary tract stones. Urinalysis may reveal hematuria (gross or microscopic), or it may be entirely normal. Once the diagnosis is suspected from history, physical examination findings, and laboratory analysis, a renal ultrasound or an intravenous pyelogram (IVP) is performed to confirm the diagnosis. The IVP is the diagnostic test of choice for locating and outlining the size of renal stones and identifying obstruction. Renal ultrasound may be useful in those patients who are pregnant, have renal insufficiency, or are allergic to contrast media. Ultrasound cannot distinguish obstructive from nonobstructive causes of hydronephrosis.

Management

In the emergency department, patients are evaluated for signs of infection and given adequate hydration. Morphine sulfate 0.1 mg/kg IV or IM or other narcotic agents are given to control pain. Further diagnostic studies will need to be initiated but are not emergent and should be done in consultation with a pediatric urologist.

Patients with complete urinary obstruction, intractable pain, dehydration, a solitary kidney, renal insufficiency, or inability to keep fluids down may have to be admitted. Today, with extracorporeal shock wave lithotripsy, medical management for urolithiasis may predominate. Some 16 percent of pediatric patients with urinary stones will have a recurrence, so close follow-up and outpatient dietary management are critical.

For a more detailed discussion, see Gausche M: Urinary tract diseases, chap. 59, p. 364, in *Pediatric Emergency Medicine: A Comprehensive Study Guide.*

---

60 Specific Renal Syndromes

Roger Barkin

ACUTE GLOMERULONEPHRITIS

Glomerulonephritis is a histopathologic diagnosis, acutely associated with clinical findings of hematuria, edema, and hypertension. Patients under 2 years of age are rarely affected.

Glomerulonephritis probably results from the deposition of circulating immune complexes in the kidney. These immune complexes are deposited on the basement membrane, reducing glomerular filtration.

Diagnostic Findings

There is usually a preceding streptococcal infection or exposure 1 to 2 weeks before the onset of glomerulonephritis. An interval of less than 4 days may imply that the illness is an exacerbation of preexisting disease rather than an initial attack. Fever, malaise, abdominal pain, and decreased urine output are often noted.

The physical findings reflect the duration of illness. Initial findings may be only mild facial or extremity edema with a minimal rise in blood pressure. Patients uniformly develop fluid retention and edema and commonly have hematuria (90 percent), hypertension (60 to 70 percent), and oliguria (80 percent). Fever, malaise, and abdominal pain are frequently reported. Anuria and renal failure occur in 2 percent of children. Circulatory congestion as well as hypertensive encephalopathy may be noted.

Ancillary Data

An abnormal urinalysis with microscopic or gross hematuria is noted. Erythrocyte casts are present in 60 to 85 percent of hospitalized children. Proteinuria is generally under 2 $g/m^2/24$ h. Hematuria (Fig. 60-1) and proteinuria (Fig. 60-2) may present independently and require a specific evaluation. Leukocyturia and hyaline and granular casts are common.

The fractional excretion of sodium as a reflection of renal function may be reduced. The blood urea nitrogen (BUN) is elevated disproportionately to the creatinine.

Total serum complement and specifically C3 is reduced in 90 to 100 percent of children during the first 2 weeks of illness, returning to normal within 3 to 4 weeks. Ongoing low levels suggest the presence of chronic renal disease. The antistreptolysin (ASO) is elevated, consistent with a previous streptococcal infection. Anemia, hyponatremia, and hyperkalemia may be present.

Management

Fluid and salt restriction is essential to normalize intravascular volume. Diuretics are often required. Elevated blood pressure may require specific pharmacologic management. Specific complications such as congestive heart failure, renal failure, and hyperkalemia must be anticipated and treated.

Recovery is usually complete. Over 80 percent of patients recover without residual renal damage. A nephrologist generally should be consulted.

NEPHROTIC SYNDROME

Nephrotic syndrome is associated with increased glomerular permeability, producing massive proteinuria. Hypoalbuminemia results, producing a decrease in the plasma osmotic pressure. The shift of fluids from the vascular to the interstitial spaces shrinks the plasma volume, thereby activating the renin-angiotensin system and enhancing sodium reabsorption. Edema develops.

The etiology is generally idiopathic but has been associated with glomerular lesions. Intoxications, allergic reactions, infection, and other entities have also been associated with the syndrome (Table 60-1). Males have a higher incidence of primary nephrotic syndrome than females.

The renin-angiotensin-aldosterone system produces an increased reabsorption of sodium chloride and worsens the edema state. Serum cholesterol levels rise and remain high even after resolution of urinary protein loss.

Diagnostic Findings

Patients frequently present with edema, often with a history of a preceding flulike syndrome. Edema initially is present periorbitally

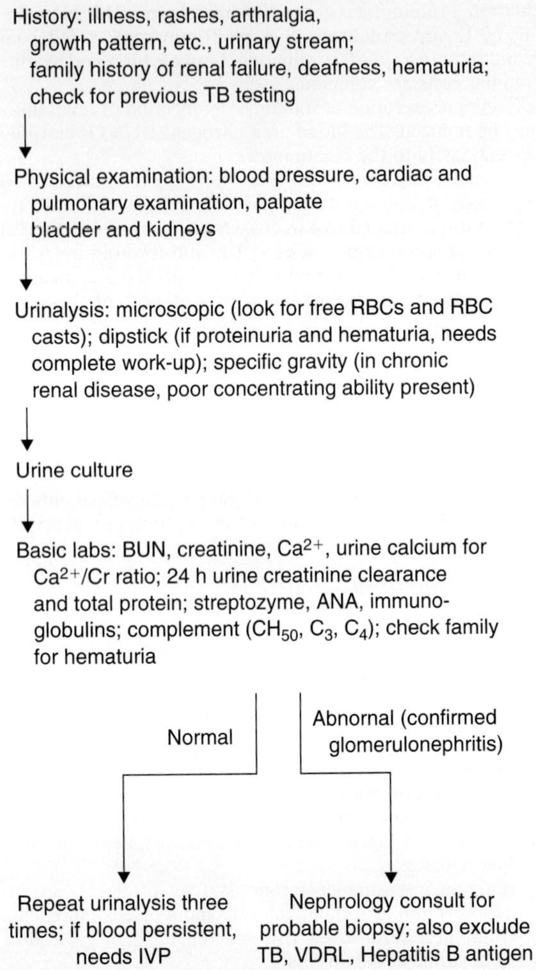

History: illness, rashes, arthralgia, growth pattern, etc., urinary stream; family history of renal failure, deafness, hematuria; check for previous TB testing

↓

Physical examination: blood pressure, cardiac and pulmonary examination, palpate bladder and kidneys

↓

Urinalysis: microscopic (look for free RBCs and RBC casts); dipstick (if proteinuria and hematuria, needs complete work-up); specific gravity (in chronic renal disease, poor concentrating ability present)

↓

Urine culture

↓

Basic labs: BUN, creatinine, Ca^{2+}, urine calcium for Ca^{2+}/Cr ratio; 24 h urine creatinine clearance and total protein; streptozyme, ANA, immunoglobulins; complement (CH_{50}, C_3, C_4); check family for hematuria

Normal → Repeat urinalysis three times; if blood persistent, needs IVP

Abnornal (confirmed glomerulonephritis) → Nephrology consult for probable biopsy; also exclude TB, VDRL, Hepatitis B antigen

Fig. 60-1. Evaluation for hematuria. [From Barkin RM, Rosen P (eds): *Emergency Pediatrics: A Guide to Ambulatory Care,* 4th ed. St. Louis: Mosby-Year Book, p 246, 1994, with permission.]

and may become generalized, associated with weight gain. Ascites may be caused by edema of the intestinal wall, often associated with abdominal pain, nausea, and vomiting. Pleural effusion or pulmonary edema may occur. Malnutrition may be noted secondary to protein loss.

Blood pressure may be decreased if the intravascular volume is depleted or increased in the presence of significant renal disease. Blood pressure is elevated in approximately 5 to 10 percent of these patients. Renal failure may develop.

Infection is probably the most common complication, related to the increased risk of peritonitis and concomitant immunosuppression due to the glucocorticoid therapy. Immune protein levels, including IgG, are low due to urinary losses. The blood of children is hypercoagulable, leading to an increased risk of thromboembolism. Renal vein thrombosis may be underrecognized but should be suspected if hematuria, flank pain, and decreased renal function occur.

Hypoalbuminemia is common, as well as proteinuria and hyperlipidemia. A 24-h urine collection reveals a protein excretion of >3.5 g protein/1.73 m^2/24 h. A spot protein/creatinine ratio >3.0 is noted. Blood urea nitrogen and creatinine are elevated in 25 percent of children. Serum complement is decreased. Plasma cholesterol carriers (low-density lipoprotein and very low density lipoprotein) are increased. Elevated lipids result from increased synthesis as well as catabolism of phospholipid. Imaging studies, especially ultrasound, should document normal renal structure.

A renal biopsy should be considered if the following poor prognostic signs are present:

- Age over 6 years
- Azotemia
- Decreased complement
- Hematuria
- Persistent hypertension
- No response to glucocorticoids

Management

Management should focus on assuring hemodynamic stability and a balanced intake and output. Subsequent evaluation is noted in Fig. 60-3. The majority of patients should be hospitalized initially, usually in consultation with a nephrologist. Hypovolemia is treated with albumin and fluids. Hypertension is carefully watched for and treated if it occurs.

After diagnosis and stabilization, the patient without complications (<16 years, normal complement, no gross hematuria, no

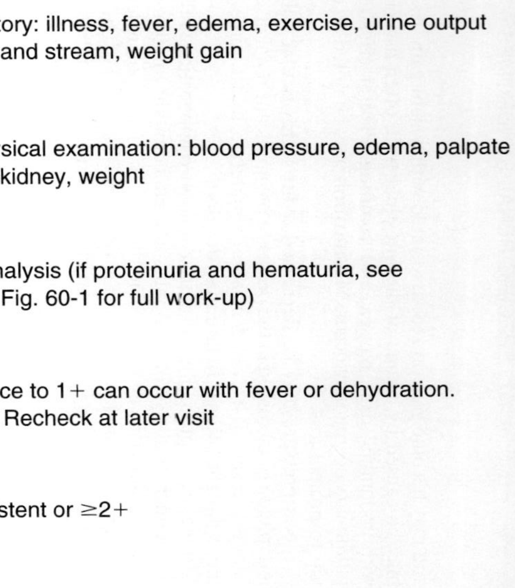
History: illness, fever, edema, exercise, urine output and stream, weight gain
Physical examination: blood pressure, edema, palpate kidney, weight
Urinalysis (if proteinuria and hematuria, see Fig. 60-1 for full work-up)
Trace to 1+ can occur with fever or dehydration. Recheck at later visit
Persistent or ≥2+

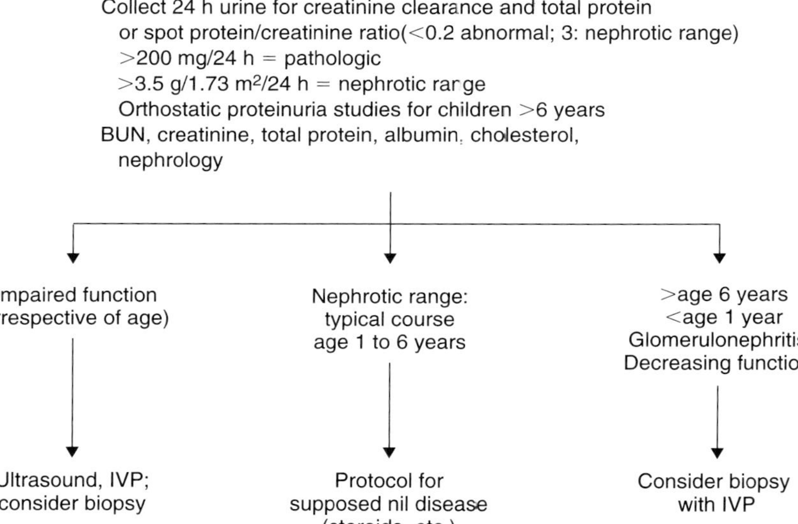

Fig. 60-2. Evaluation for proteinuria. [From Barkin RM, Rosen P (eds): *Emergency Pediatrics: A Guide to Ambulatory Care,* 4th ed. St. Louis, MO: Mosby-Year Book, p 247, 1994, with permission.]

TABLE 60-1 Evaluation of Renal Failure

Prerenal	Intrarenal	Postrenal
Ultrasound: normal	Ultrasound: can have increased renal density or slight swelling	Ultrasound: dilated bladder or kidney
Serum BUN to creatinine ration >15 : 1		History and exam may be diagnostic
Urine Na^+ <15 meq/L	Urine Na^+ >20 meq/L	Indexes not helpful
Urine osmolality >500 mOsm/kgH_2O	Urine osmolality <350 mOsm/kgH_2O	
Urine to plasma creatinine ratio >40 : 1	Urine to plasma creatinine ratio <20 : 1 (often <5 : 1)	
Fractional excretion of Na^+ <1 (<2.5 in neonates)	Fractional excretion of Na^+ >2 (>2.5 in neonates)	

$$\text{Fractional excretion of Na}^+ = \frac{\text{Urine Na}^+\ (\text{meq/L})}{\text{Plasma Na}^+\ (\text{meq/L})} \times \frac{\text{Plasma creatinine (mg/dL)}}{\text{Urine creatinine (mg/dL)}}$$

Source: From Barkin RM, Rosen P (eds): *Emergency Pediatrics: A Guide to Ambulatory Care*, 4th ed. St. Louis, MO: Mosby-Year Book, p 738, 1994, with permission.

large protein loss) is started on prednisone at a dose of 2 mg/kg/24 h up to 80 mg/24 h and tapered once a response is noted. Nearly three-quarters of patients will respond within 14 days. Treatment continues for about 2 months but is reinstituted if relapse is noted. Other pharmacologic agents may ultimately be needed. Salt and water restriction should be initiated.

Diuretics may be needed if there is pulmonary edema or respiratory distress. However, they must be used judiciously to avoid vascular volume depletion and electrolyte abnormality. Salt restriction is required.

Signs of infection must be watched for, since these patients are considered immune-compromised. Deep vein punctures are avoided if possible so as not to trigger a deep vein thrombosis.

HEMOLYTIC-UREMIC SYNDROME

Nephropathy, microangiopathic hemolytic anemia, and thrombocytopenia are noted in patients with hemolytic uremic syndrome (HUS), which commonly occurs in children under 5 years of age, following an episode of gastroenteritis or respiratory infection. Siblings may also develop the disease due to a familial genetic component. The illness has an acute onset with rapid progression to renal failure and thrombocytopenia.

Etiology

Associated infections can be found with HUS. *Escherichia coli* serotype 0157:H7 is the most commonly found organism, producing a cytotoxin that inhibits protein synthesis, leading to cell death in gastrointestinal organs.

Shigella, Salmonella, and group A streptococci may be associated with HUS, as well as coxsackievirus, influenza, and respiratory syncytial virus (RSV).

Diagnostic Findings

Patients usually have a recent history of gastroenteritis with vomiting, bloody diarrhea, and crampy abdominal pain up to 2 weeks before the onset of HUS. Children who develop HUS without a prodrome of gastroenteritis have a poor prognosis. Low-grade fever, pallor, hematuria, oliguria, and gastrointestinal bleeding occur. Central nervous system (CNS) deterioration can occur, with a spectrum of symptoms ranging from irritability to seizures or coma.

There is a tremendous spectrum of severity of clinical disease, ranging from mild elevation of BUN with anemia to total anuria

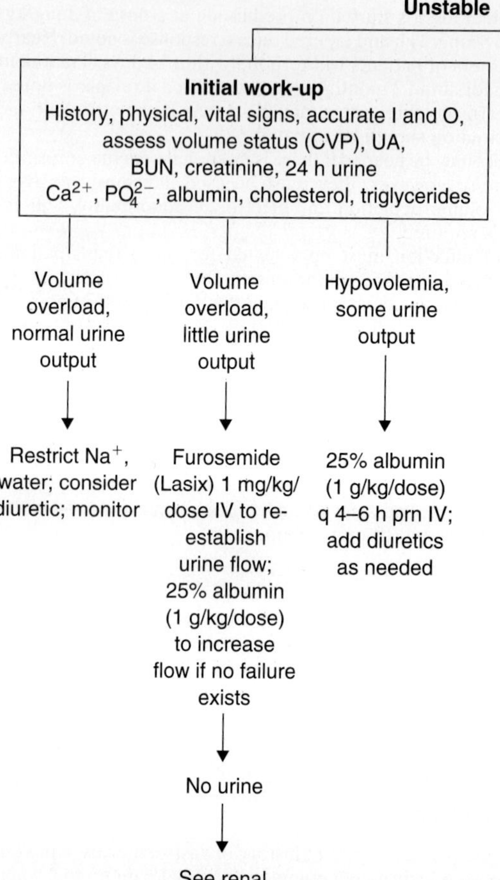

Fig. 60-3. Management of nephrotic syndrome. [From Barkin RM, Rosen P (eds): *Emergency Pediatrics: A Guide to Ambulatory Care,* 4th ed. St. Louis, MO: Mosby-Year Book, p 735, 1994, with permission.]

syndrome (proteinuria >3.5 g/1.73 m²/24 h)

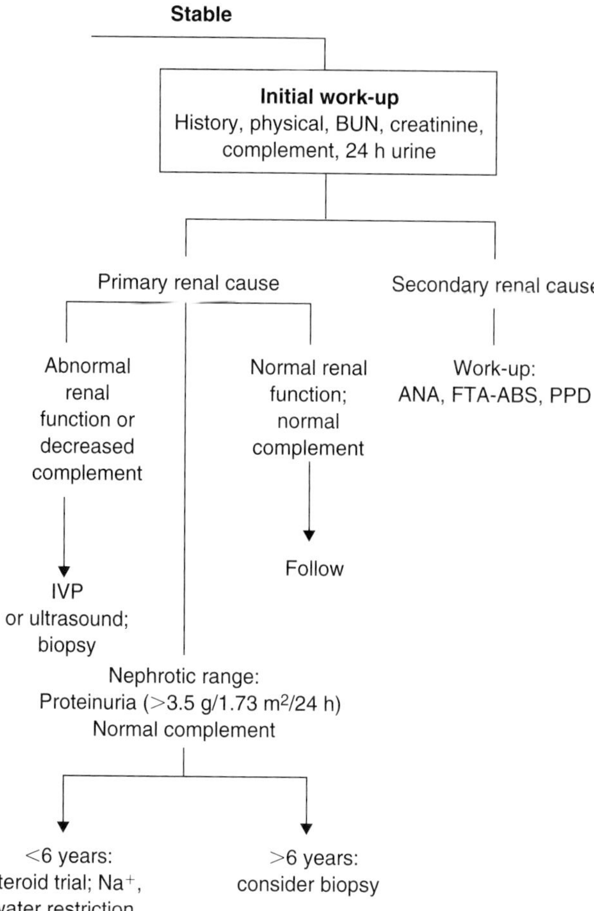

due to acute nephropathy with severe anemia and thrombocytopenia.

Ultimately, patients may develop hypertension; evidence of anemia, such as pallor, petechiae, and easy bruising; hepatosplenomegaly; and edema. Hypertension occurs in up to 50 percent of patients. Irritability or lethargy may develop. Seizures occur in 40 percent of the cases. Hyponatremia and hypocalcemia are common. Acute abdominal conditions, including intussusception, bowel perforation, and toxic megacolon, can occur. Hepatic and pancreatic injury can also occur in HUS. Cardiac involvement includes the possibility of cardiomyopathy, myocarditis, and high-output failure.

There may be recurrences, often without a prodrome; these are associated with a high mortality rate.

Laboratory evaluation should include assessment of renal function, including electrolytes, BUN, creatinine, and urinalysis. Hematologic studies reveal low hemoglobin with a microangiopathic, hemolytic anemia. Burr cells are common. Platelets are usually decreased below 50,000/mm^3. Coagulation studies are usually normal.

Management

Initial stabilization is obviously mandatory. All of these patients need admission to an appropriate medical center. Volume overload may occur secondary to anemia. Hypertension may occur and appears to be caused by increased renin levels. Renal failure requires meticulous balancing of intake and output with specific treatment of hyperkalemia, acidosis, hypocalcemia, hyperphosphatemia, and other metabolic abnormalities. Peritoneal dialysis may be required, especially when the BUN is over 100 and when congestive heart failure, encephalopathy, or hyperkalemia is present or anuria has been present for 24 h.

A hemoglobin under 5 g/dL or hematocrit less than 15 percent generally requires treatment with packed red blood cells, infused slowly. Platelet survival is shortened, and platelet infusions may be required in children with active bleeding. Seizures require specific management and are usually caused by hypertension or uremia. Acute treatment includes support, stabilization, and anticonvulsants as well as a consideration of emergency dialysis.

ACUTE RENAL FAILURE

Impairment of the kidney's ability to regulate urine volume and composition produces problems with hemostasis. This is usually associated with a decreased glomerular filtration rate (GFR).

The etiology of acute renal failure may be categorized on the basis of the type of renal injury. It may be prerenal (decreased perfusion of the kidney), intrarenal (damage to the actual nephron), or postrenal (downstream obstruction of the urinary tract) (Table 60-1).

Prerenal patients have decreased perfusion of the kidney. Dehydration is usually causative, secondary to vomiting, diarrhea, diabetic ketoacidosis, or decreased intravascular volumes associated with nephrotic syndrome, burns, or shock.

Intrarenal failure results from direct, intrinsic damage to the nephrons caused by glomerulonephritis (hematuria, proteinuria, edema, and hypertension), hemolytic uremic syndrome, nephrotoxic exposures, crush injuries, sepsis, or disseminated intravascular coagulation.

Obstruction leads to postrenal failure and may be accompanied by symptoms, although blockage may be insidious and without symptoms. Causes of postrenal obstruction include posterior urethral valves, ureteropelvic junction abnormalities, renal stones, and trauma.

Diagnostic Findings

The history may reflect the underlying disease and the category of renal failure encountered. The physical examination will help determine the mechanism. It is essential to evaluate for hypovolemia, volume overload, hypertension, or obstruction.

Patients may have oliguria with urine output under 1 mL/kg/h or be nonoliguric with an output excessive for the volume status. Azotemia may be noted.

Laboratory evaluation should include electrolytes, studies of renal function, and a search for the underlying pathology. The creatinine clearance is a good measure of GFR and is useful in initial assessment and ongoing monitoring. A 24-h urine is normally needed.

$$\text{Creatinine clearance (mL/min/1.73 m}^2) = \frac{UV}{P} \times \frac{1.73}{SA}$$

where U = urinary concentration of creatinine (mg/dL); V = volume of urine divided by the number of minutes in collection period (24 h = 1440 min) (mL/min); P = plasma concentration of creatinine (mg/dL); and SA = surface area (m^2).

A rapid approximation can be made using the formula

$$\text{Creatinine clearance (mL/min/1.73 m}^2) = \frac{0.55 \times \text{ht (cm)}}{P}$$

where ht = height in centimeters and P = plasma concentration of creatinine (mg/dL). Normal values are as follows:

Newborn and premature: 40 to 65 mL/min/1.73 m^2
Normal child: 109 mL (female) or 124 mL (male)/min/1.73 m^2
Adult: 95 mL (female) or 105 mL (male)/min/1.73 m^2

A single voided urine in adults has been of some use in assessing renal function. In patients with stable renal function, a spot protein/creatinine ratio of >3.0 represents nephrotic-range proteinuria; a ratio of <0.2 is normal (see Table 60-1). Ultrasonography is also important in the evaluation of these patients. Combining data from serum, urine, and ultrasonography helps differentiate among prerenal, intrarenal, and postrenal failure.

Management

Initial management must focus on stabilization with correction of fluid imbalance (Fig. 60-4). If the intravascular volume is adequate or overloaded, urine output may be enhanced by furosemide (Lasix), usually in an initial dose of 1 mg/kg/dose, increased up to 6 mg/kg/dose. Mannitol may be administered if there is no response to furosemide. The dose is 0.5 to 0.75 g/kg/dose IV. These agents should not be used if obstruction is present.

In oliguric or anuric patients with decreased intravascular volume, fluid may be administered slowly, often in conjunction with monitoring of the central venous pressure. Low-dose dopamine may occasionally be utilized to increase renal blood flow and glomerular filtration rate. Those with high urine output must receive a significant amount of fluid to avoid hypovolemia.

Hypertension may be caused by fluid overload or high renin secretion. Children having acute hypertension with a diastolic pressure over 100 mmHg should be treated parenterally because of the risk of seizures, encephalopathy, and other sequelae. Only a mild reduction is needed, usually to the diastolic range of about 100 mmHg. Nitroprusside is useful for reduction of pressure.

Hyperkalemia causes membrane excitability with possible cardiac dysrhythmias. A potassium over 6.5 meq/L can cause elevation of the T wave. Specific and immediate treatment for a potassium over 7.0 meq/L is required, including calcium chloride 20 to 30 mg/kg slowly, sodium bicarbonate 1 to 2 meq/kg/dose, and glucose/insulin infusion of 1 mL/kg of $D_{50}W$ followed by 1 mL/kg of $D_{25}W$ and 0.5 U/kg of regular insulin per hour to keep serum glucose between 120 and 300 mg/dL. Kayexalate at 1 g/kg/dose every 4 to 6 h mixed with 70% sorbitol, PO or rectally, may be useful after initial stabilization.

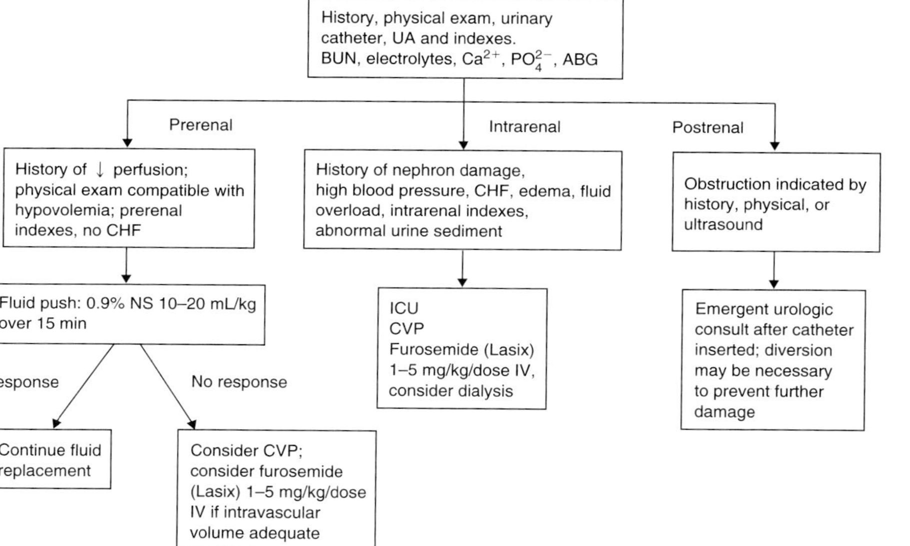

Fig. 60-4. Acute renal failure: initial assessment and treatment. [From Barkin RM, Rosen P (eds): *Emergency Pediatrics: A Guide to Ambulatory Care,* 4th ed. St. Louis, MO: Mosby-Year Book, p 740, 1994, with permission.]

Other abnormalities that may need specific treatment include anemia, metabolic acidosis, hyponatremia, and hyperphosphatemia.

Dialysis may be required for unresponsive fluid overload, severe hyperkalemia, severe hyponatremia or hypernatremia, unresponsive metabolic acidosis, a BUN over 100 mg/dL, and altered level of consciousness secondary to uremia. Such patients obviously require hospitalization.

For a more detailed discussion, see Barkin R: Specific renal syndromes, chap. 60, p. 368, in *Pediatric Emergency Medicine: A Comprehensive Study Guide.*

SECTION X
DERMATOLOGIC EMERGENCIES

61 Petechiae and Purpura

Julia A. Rosekrans

Petechial rashes are the most serious dermatologic problem seen in the acute care setting because they may be symptomatic of significant life-threatening illnesses that require rapid intervention. They can occur because of increased capillary fragility, because of decreased ability to clot, or because of traumatic injury (Table 61-1).

PETECHIAE DUE TO SEPSIS

Septic illness causes petechiae *both* by local vasculitis and through consumption of coagulation factors. Petechial rashes in acute infections can range from a few scattered small petechiae to the pattern of widespread purpura and shock seen in purpura fulminans.

Etiology

The major cause of purpura fulminans is meningococcemia caused by the gram-negative bacteria *Neisseria meningitidis.* Other bacteria—including gonococcus, *Salmonella typhi,* and *Escherichia coli*—may also cause bacterial sepsis with petechiae. Rocky Mountain spotted fever is a rickettsial disease spread by tick bites in endemic regions.

Many children with viral illnesses develop petechiae even though they are not severely ill.

Clinical Findings

Most children and adolescents with septic illnesses appear toxic, with high fever, delirium, and occasionally hypotension. Not all children "look sick," however, and occasionally a bacteremic patient with a significant pathogen is not recognized until a blood culture is reported as positive.

Petechiae and purpura are hemorrhages in the skin that do not

TABLE 61-1 Differential Diagnosis of Purpura

Infectious
Acute
Meningococcemia
Rocky Mountain spotted fever
E. coli sepsis
Gonococcemia
Subacute bacterial endocarditis
Atypical measles
Echovirus 9, 4, 7
Epstein-Barr virus
Coxsackie A9
Neonatal
Rubella
Toxoplasma
Cytomegalovirus
Syphilis
Thrombocytopenic
Idiopathic thrombocytopenic purpura
Leukemia
Systemic lupus erythematosus
Hemangioma with platelet trapping
Nonseptic normal platelet count
Henoch-Schönlein purpura (anaphylactoid purpura)
Coagulation disorders
Trauma, including child abuse

disappear when capillary blood is pressed out of the skin—they do not blanch. The rash may be identified before the child is brought in for evaluation or may develop during the examination. Small, fresh lesions are red, while large lesions are blue to purple in appearance. Lesions darken and change color over several days as hemoglobin degrades and the hemorrhage resolves.

Petechiae above the nipple line suggest increased intravenous pressure in the superior vena cava and may result from vomiting or coughing. Petechiae seen in an acral distribution, on the hands and feet, suggest infectious vasculitis.

Diagnosis

Laboratory evaluation is essential to identify the organism causing the infection. A complete blood count to evaluate both total white cells and total platelet count is helpful in estimating severity of illness. Blood cultures are mandatory because some children with a normal clinical examination will be bacteremic. A lumbar puncture may be needed to diagnose meningitis.

Complications

A child with purpura fulminans runs a risk of vascular compromise that can lead to loss of digits and sloughing of affected areas of skin if the child survives the underlying infection. Meningitis frequently complicates septic illnesses.

HENOCH-SCHÖNLEIN PURPURA

Anaphylactoid purpura is a systemic vasculitis. Although the striking pattern of distribution of purpura may be the most obvious manifestation of the illness, most children also have visceral and joint involvement.

Etiology

Infectious illnesses such as mild viral respiratory infections and streptococcal pharyngitis have been implicated as agents that initiate an immune complex response. The immune complex reacts with blood vessel walls, causing capillary leaking.

Clinical Findings

The presentation of this illness is quite variable. Children may present with abdominal pain, joint pain, or even seizures as a first symptom of Henoch-Schönlein purpura (HSP). On the other hand, the typical rash may develop before any systemic symptoms. Some children have no difficulty beyond the rash.

Abdominal pain may resemble appendicitis. In addition, some children develop intussusception. In most children, abdominal pain lasts for only 24 h, but it can be severe enough that a child will refuse to eat or drink. Many children have microscopic intestinal bleeding and guaiac-positive stools.

Arthralgia or arthritis, especially of feet and hands, is seen in about 80 percent of children. This is usually mild and transient. Sometimes a complaint that the child will not walk will not be recognized as HSP for several days if the rash is not present initially.

Renal involvement is very common, and most children will have microscopic hematuria at some point during the illness. A few children develop nephrotic syndrome, which can progress to chronic renal failure.

Central nervous system involvement is a rare manifestation of

HSP. Children with vasculitis of cerebral vessels may present with seizures, coma, or paralysis.

The rash may begin with urticaria, which progresses to palpable purpura over 24 h. Frequently, the initial skin lesions are palpable purpura 1 or 2 mm in diameter. The acral distribution of the rash is its most characteristic finding. It is symmetrical and most prominent on the buttocks and thighs, although it can also be seen on the hands and arms; the genitalia are often involved. Most skin changes last for about 4 to 6 weeks and then resolve permanently.

Management

Most children can receive care at home with outpatient follow-up and no active treatment other than mild analgesics for pain control.

Inpatient treatment should be considered for children with significant joint pain, especially if they are too large for parents to carry them. Children with abdominal pain may need intravenous fluids if they refuse to eat. Prednisone, 2 mg/kg/day, has been used to treat abdominal pain, although studies of its efficacy remain controversial.

IDIOPATHIC THROMBOCYTOPENIC PURPURA

The sudden appearance of petechiae and ecchymoses in no particular distribution over the body may signal a decrease in the number of platelets. Idiopathic thrombocytopenic purpura is a common cause of an acute low platelet count in children. Easy bruising is usually preceded, by about 2 weeks, by a viral respiratory infection.

Clinical Findings

Many children have very mild, self-limited illnesses. Bruises appear spontaneously on areas of the body, such as the abdomen and chest, where bruises from mild trauma do not usually appear. In severe cases, the skin findings may be accompanied by bleeding from the oral cavity or the gastrointestinal and genitourinary systems. The physical examination is otherwise normal, with no significant lymphadenopathy and no enlargement of the spleen.

Diagnosis

A complete blood count is needed both to identify the low platelet count and to assess the total white cell count and hemoglobin. Antibody titers are not a necessary part of the initial evaluation.

Differential Diagnosis

Other illnesses in which platelets are destroyed rapidly include autoimmune collagen vascular disease, especially lupus. Some drugs, including thiazides, quinidine, and sulfa antibiotics, can produce immunologic toxicity to platelets.

Diseases such as leukemia, lymphoma, and myeloma may cause thrombocytopenia by decreasing megakaryocytes in bone marrow, so that fewer platelets are produced.

Complications

In severe cases, bleeding into vital organs can occur. Intracerebral hemorrhage is the most serious potential complication.

Management

Most cases are mild and self-limited and require only close follow-up. When the illness is more severe, prednisone has been used to decrease abnormal antibodies. Intravenous gamma globulin is also given to interrupt the process of platelet destruction. Splenectomy is a rare management strategy for patients whose illness does not remit spontaneously. A child with a platelet count below 50,000 requires inpatient management.

CHILD ABUSE

Bruises that are caused by nonaccidental injury are important to recognize so that appropriate supervision can be instituted. The child must be protected from further injury. Normal traumatic bruises occur over bony prominences. Toddlers commonly fall and bruise elbows, knees, and foreheads. It is unusual to bruise the abdomen or trunk during normal play. When an adult slaps a child, the slap will typically hit a cheek or the buttocks. Some bruises occur in obvious patterns, such as bite marks, cord marks from being tied up, or belt shapes from a beating.

One should consider abuse if there is a discrepancy between the appearance of bruises and the reported cause. A complete blood count is important to identify platelet abnormalities. In selected cases, further clotting studies may be needed. A skeletal bone survey may be helpful for infants under 18 months with clear nonaccidental bruises to identify subtle unsuspected fractures. A complete discussion of child abuse is provided in Chap. 119.

For a more detailed discussion, see Rosekrans JA: Petechiae and purpura, chap. 61, p. 377, in *Pediatric Emergency Medicine: A Comprehensive Study Guide.*

62 Pruritic Rashes

Julia A. Rosekrans

Parents frequently decide to consult a physician if their child has a rash that causes itching and discomfort. Some rashes that present with itching as a primary symptom are acute problems that can be diagnosed and rapidly treated. Others are chronic problems for which control measures other than cure can be emphasized (Table 62-1).

ATOPIC DERMATITIS

This chronic relapsing condition appears in children who have a tendency to produce specific IgE when exposed to environmental antigens. It is associated with other atopic conditions, including allergic rhinitis and asthma, that may be seen in the affected child or in family members.

Clinical Findings

In infancy, cheeks and extensor surfaces of the legs are most commonly affected. Later in childhood, the antecubital and popliteal fossae are most affected. Children with extensive atopic dermatitis are most likely to have problems as adults when there is a diffuse pattern of skin involvement.

The rash may range in severity from dry, itchy skin to weeping, open fissures. The most important and consistent symptom is itchiness, which may be severe enough to interfere with sleep.

Associated physical findings include signs of scratching, rubbing, and other atopic problems. Some children show very shiny, buffed fingernails from constant rubbing. Denny's lines on the lower eyelid and allergic shiners are commonly seen and may relate to rubbing the eyes or to venous stasis due to nasal congestion. Hypopigmented patches on the face may be quite pronounced in children with dark or tanned skin.

Differential Diagnosis

The most commonly confused conditions are scaly or papulovesicular disorders such as seborrheic dermatitis, scabies, contact dermatitis, or tinea corporis. Some metabolic problems such as Hurler syndrome and phenylketonuria may include eczematous rashes. Histiocytosis X may present with a rash that resembles atopic dermatitis but does not respond to appropriate treatment.

TABLE 62-1 Pruritic Rashes

Chronic
Atopic dermatitis
Seborrhea
Acute
Urticaria
Scabies
Insect bites
Head lice
Contact dermatitis

Complications

The most common acute complication is bacterial superinfection. The skin of children with atopic dermatitis is colonized with *Staphylococcus aureus,* which can cause abscesses, cellulitis, and lymphangitis.

Cataract formation is a possible chronic complication. Keratoconus (an abnormally shaped cornea) may develop in adolescents.

Management

Since there is no cure for atopic dermatitis, education of the family must be aimed toward relief of dryness, inflammation, and itching.

Baths should be limited, and soap should be mild and nonperfumed. Bath oils may be helpful in maintaining skin hydration. Topical moisturizers such as Eucerin and skin lotions are very soothing after a bath.

Inflammation is treated with topical glucocorticoid ointments. Care must be taken to avoid powerful fluorinated preparations that are systemically absorbed and can cause permanent thinning of the skin. High-potency glucocorticoids may be used to briefly quell a severe flare; however, a rapid change to less powerful ointments is very important.

Antihistamines of the H_1 type such as diphenhydramine hydrochloride (4 to 6 mg/kg/24 h, not to exceed 300 mg divided into 3 or 4 doses daily) and hydroxyzine hydrochloride (2 to 4 mg/kg/24 h, divided into 2 or 3 doses) are commonly used to relieve the itch.

CONTACT DERMATITIS

Contact between the skin and irritating substances can cause a vesicular itchy rash. Some material will cause a contact dermatitis reaction in nearly all people. Other substances will cause reactions only in people who are sensitized to a specific chemical.

Clinical Findings

Erythema and a papulovesicular eruption develop on the skin that has been in contact with sensitizing material. When the reaction is to a contact with a plant, the rash may appear to be in lines like the edge of a leaf or a stem. An eruption in a discrete area such as ear lobes or the back of the wrist could indicate contact with a metal such as nickel found in earrings or a wristwatch.

Diagnosis

The diagnosis of contact dermatitis is made by recognizing the sudden development of a vesicular weeping eruption in a pattern suggestive of contact with a suspicious allergen. If it is necessary to identify the particular allergen, patch testing to elicit reactions in a controlled fashion may be useful.

Differential Diagnosis

Other pruritic vesicular rashes include atopic dermatitis, ichthyoses, and scabies.

Management

The first step in treating contact dermatitis is removing the sensitizing material. In the case of Rhus dermatitis, this includes washing the skin and any clothing that may carry Rhus oleoresin. Once the reaction has begun, fluid from the blisters does not spread the reaction either to other parts of the patient's skin or to other people. There may be some delay in the appearance of the rash on thicker areas of skin. If new lesions appear over several days, the child is probably being reexposed.

Topical glucocorticoids may help to relieve some of the inflammation. However, the rash can last for several weeks. In severe cases, systemic steroids such as prednisone (1 to 2 mg/kg/24 h over 7 to 10 days) can be helpful. The medication must be tapered gradually because the inflammation often rebounds.

Systemic H_1 antihistamines such as hydroxyzine can help relieve itching. Cool compresses with tap water or Burow's solution are important in relieving discomfort.

PEDICULOSIS

Head lice are frequently discovered by school nurses or day-care workers. This infestation can cause such anxiety that medical attention may be requested at any time of the day.

Clinical Findings

Scratching the scalp may be the first sign of head lice. Nits are commonly found close to the scalp, especially behind the ears and at the nape of the neck. Nits may be confused with dandruff and can be identified because the egg cases are firmly stuck to the hair shaft.

Head lice spread from child to child by direct contact. Combs and hats can act as fomites that spread the infestation.

Differential Diagnosis

Dandruff, seborrhea, and neurotic excoriation of the scalp can all be confused with head lice.

Complications

Bacterial superinfection of the scalp may develop as a result of scratching. While it is recognized that body lice can spread typhus and relapsing fever, there are no reports that head lice are implicated in spreading blood-borne diseases.

Management

Treatment requires education to prevent reinfection as well as eradication of the infestation.

There are several insecticides available as shampoos or cream rinses that are very effective at killing adult lice and nits. Permethrin 1% cream rinse (Nix) is available without prescription and has an excellent safety record.

All members of a household should be treated at the same time. A second treatment should be done after 7 days. Insecticides will usually kill the larva inside the egg cases; however, the nits may be very difficult to dislodge. Diluted vinegar seems to soften nit cement and can be used with a fine-tooth comb to remove the nits. Because lice are very heat-sensitive, clothing and bedding that are washed and dried in a hot-air dryer will be effectively cleaned. Clothing or hats that cannot be heat-treated can be disinfected by sealing them in a plastic bag for 4 weeks. Any lice that hatch out will starve in this time. Parents must be warned that pruritus can last for several weeks after successful treatment. Multiple treatments with insecticides can lead to contact dermatitis. Antihistamines by mouth and topical hydrocortisone cream may help alleviate itching.

SCABIES

This very pruritic skin infestation is caused by a mite, *Sarcoptes scabiei.* It is quite contagious and spreads readily from one person to the next.

Clinical Findings

The earliest symptom is itching, which may be present before any burrow or papule can be seen. In adults and older children, papules develop on the hands and wrists, especially in the interdigital webs, elbows, belt line, and gluteal cleft. Infants, however, may develop papules and vesicles all over their bodies, including the palms and soles. Infants often have scabies on the face and scalp, while this area is rarely affected in older children.

Because of intense scratching, burrows are frequently a site for bacterial superinfection, and impetigo may be the presenting chief complaint.

Diagnosis

Scraping papules and fresh vesicles may yield the mite itself or, more often, its stool pellets. However, the sudden onset of very pruritic papules in a child with other affected family members is very suggestive of scabies even if the mite cannot be found.

Differential Diagnosis

Atopic dermatitis, papular urticaria, and simple insect bites are often confused with scabies. Because it is so contagious, it is uncommon to find scabies in a child without other affected family members. A family history of pruritic papules is an important diagnostic feature.

Complications

Secondary infection with *Streptococcus* or *Staphylococcus* is the most common complication of this dermatitis. Acute glomerulonephritis secondary to streptococcal skin infection related to scabies has been described.

Management

All close personal contacts as well as the affected child must be treated with an insecticide. Permethrin cream (Elimite) can be applied to the body overnight and then rinsed off. A second treatment after 7 days is suggested.

Clothing and bed linen should be washed with ordinary soap at usual temperatures to eliminate any mites that are present. Infestations can usually be controlled without insecticide sprays.

Antihistamines by mouth may be necessary to control itching for several weeks after treatment is initiated.

PAPULAR URTICARIA

Young children frequently develop an intense hypersensitivity reaction to insect bites. The initial reaction to an insect bite or sting may begin as a typical wheal and flare but then progress to a hard papule that persists for several days.

Papular urticaria is seen in preschool children, especially infants in the second summer season, when they are exposed to insect bites. Usually only one member of a family is affected.

Clinical Findings

Dome-shaped papules in crops on areas of the body that are exposed to insect bites develop acutely. The reaction may be severe enough to cause vesicles and bullae. In most cases, no discrete puncture wound can be seen. The papules last for up to 2 weeks.

Complications

Scratching can lead to bacterial superinfection from impetiginization to cellulitis.

Management

To be protected from further insect bites, the child should wear pants and long sleeves, with an insect repellent such as DEET applied to the clothes. If the bites are coming from fleas, treating infested pets is extremely important. Topical hydrocortisone cream applied to the papules may be helpful. Oral antihistamines may be necessary to control itching.

URTICARIA

Hives are a benign, self-limited problem; they cause alarm because they appear suddenly and cause itchy discomfort. They are the most common pediatric dermatologic problem seen in emergency departments.

Medications, seafoods, strawberries, peanuts, and tomatoes are among the commonly recognizable causes of hives. Insect stings may cause local urticaria or progress to a systemic anaphylactic reaction.

Many respiratory infections, including viruses and group A beta-hemolytic strep, are responsible for hives. If a child develops hives while taking antibiotics for a respiratory infection, it may be difficult to decide whether the child is actually allergic to the medication. It has been reported that with follow-up skin testing, more than 90 percent of children who develop hives while taking ampicillin have no evidence of ampicillin allergy.

Clinical Findings

Urticaria occurs on all parts of the body. It is very pruritic and transient, lasting from a few minutes to several hours. It typically appears on areas of skin that are warm or that are under pressure, such as under waist bands. It is accentuated by heat and often develops after a bath or when the child is wrapped in warm clothing.

Differential Diagnosis

Urticaria and erythema multiforme are frequently confused. Two clinical points can help to differentiate these conditions. Erythema multiforme is a fixed skin reaction. Individual lesions last for several days. Subcutaneous epinephrine can be given to clear urticaria, but it does not change erythema multiforme.

Management

If urticaria is severe, subcutaneous epinephrine (1 : 1,000) at a dose of 0.01 mL/kg (maximum 0.3 mL) will give some short-term relief, and H_1 antihistamines can be used for long-term control.

Topical antihistamines and glucocorticoids do not help to control urticaria. Systemic glucocorticoids have been used for chronic severe urticaria but are not needed for most cases.

ERYTHEMA MULTIFORME

The definition of this hypersensitivity reaction is controversial and includes a variety of skin problems, from minor itching and urticarialike lesions to severe blistering and desquamation.

The agents most commonly responsible for erythema multiforme are infections and drug exposure. Sulfa products and phenytoin are medications commonly recognized as causing severe reactions. Penicillin and cephalosporins can also cause erythema multiforme.

Recurrent herpes simplex and *Mycoplasma pneumoniae* are infectious agents that can lead to erythema multiforme reactions.

No specific inciting agent is identified for about 50 percent of cases.

Clinical Findings

There are several clinical syndromes within the erythema multiforme group. All have similar pathophysiologic findings.

Erythema multiforme minor is a condition of urticarialike lesions with little systemic reaction. The lesions are different from common urticaria because they are fixed in the skin and fade slowly over a week's time. They do not blister, but they are usually pruritic. They can be differentiated from urticaria because they do not clear when subcutaneous epinephrine is given. The lesions may develop a characteristic target shape, or they may remain as round-topped papules. They last for about a week, becoming darker as they start to resolve.

Stevens-Johnson syndrome is more severe, with fever, general malaise, and blistering of mucous membranes. The epidermal lesions may blister, and when the blisters are small, they may look like varicella. The mucous membranes of the mouth can become deeply eroded and crusted. Conjunctivae and urogenital mucous membranes also become inflamed.

Toxic epidermal necrolysis (TEN) is the most severe variant of erythema multiforme. Dramatic blisters develop rapidly over all areas of the body. High fever and severe mucous membrane involvement are common.

Complications

Mild cases resolve completely. Problems with maintaining fluid balance and adequate nutrition may develop in cases with oral blistering. Lesions that are severely blistered may be deep enough to produce scarring. There is a serious risk of mortality in patients with TEN who have significant disruption of the normal skin's protective barrier.

Management

Mild cases need only symptomatic care with oral antihistamines. When mucous membranes become involved, intravenous fluids and hyperalimentation may be needed. The use of systemic glucocorticoids is controversial. Mildly affected patients do well without them. For patients with TEN, the increased risk of complications, such as gastrointestinal hemorrhage and sepsis, outweighs the potential value of decreasing blistering, and glucocorticoids should not be used. There is some suggestion that in moderate cases, blistering may be diminished if glucocorticoids are initiated within the first 2 weeks of an eruption.

For a more detailed discussion, see Rosekrans JA: Pruritic rashes, chap. 62, p. 381, in *Pediatric Emergency Medicine: A Comprehensive Study Guide.*

63 Superficial Skin Infections

Julia A. Rosekrans

Children are brought to the emergency department for treatment when their parents recognize that there is a condition that they cannot treat at home. They often have questions about the contagiousness of the rash, especially when a child attends day care.

IMPETIGO AND ECTHYMA

The most common skin infection in children is impetigo. It develops as a secondary problem when the normal protective barrier of the skin is broken. Impetigo often complicates pruritic skin problems. Impetigo is superficial, involving the papillary epidermis, whereas ecthyma involves the entire thickness of the epidermis.

Etiology

There are two clinically distinguishable types of impetigo. Bullous impetigo is caused by *Staphylococcus aureus.* Both *S. aureus* and group A beta-hemolytic streptococci (GABHS) are involved in nonbullous impetigo and ecthyma.

Clinical Findings

Bullous impetigo begins as small papules, which develop into 1- to 2-cm bullae. These thin-walled bullae rupture easily, and the shiny, wet, red base of the blister is usually all that is seen. The lesions are found most often on the buttocks and perineum or on the face, but they can also occur anywhere on the body.

Nonbullous impetigo forms a pustular reaction with a serous honey-colored crust. The lesions may be described as pruritic if the infection is a complication of an insect bite or other pruritic dermatitis. Sometimes the lesions spread, leaving a central clear healed area. Regional lymph nodes may be enlarged if the infection is deep or has been present for a long period of time. Ecthyma, because it is deeper, is often painful and may involve lymphangitis or surrounding cellulitis.

Differential Diagnosis

Herpes simplex lesions often resemble impetigo, and a viral culture may be needed if identification is required. Varicella and contact dermatitis may resemble the vesicle stage of impetigo.

Tinea capitis that has progressed to kerion formation looks as if it were impetiginized; however, the reaction is a response to the fungal infection.

Complications

Impetigo, because it is so superficial, rarely causes any scarring; however, ecthyma does tend to leave scars. Poststreptococcal glomerulonephritis has been seen when nephrogenic strains of streptococci cause the skin infection. There have not been any reports of rheumatic fever or carditis due to impetigo.

Management

Treatment of impetigo depends on antibiotic therapy. In widespread cases, oral antibiotics active against staphylococci are needed. Dicloxacillin, 20 to 50 mg/kg/24 h divided into four doses, or cefadroxil, 30 mg/kg/24 h in two doses, works well. Two-percent mupirocin (Bactroban) ointment is also effective in many situations, especially when the infection is localized.

STAPHYLOCOCCAL SCALDED-SKIN SYNDROME

This superficial skin infection is characterized by erythema and generalized blistering and peeling of skin over the whole body. It is a serious systemic illness that carries a risk of mortality.

Etiology

The illness is caused by an infection with a strain of *S. aureus* that produces an epidermolytic toxin. The infecting bacteria may be located in the nose, conjunctivae, or even an infected umbilical stump.

Clinical Findings

This syndrome is most often seen in children below 5 years of age. Children with this illness are usually febrile and often complain of painful skin. The rash begins with generalized erythema and quickly progresses to formation of large bullae, with desquamation of large sheets of skin. Serous crusts may be seen around the nose and mouth.

Differential Diagnosis

In the initial erythematous phase, scarlet fever, toxic shock syndrome, severe erythema multiforme, and even sunburn may be considered.

Management

Fluid loss, electrolyte imbalance, heat loss, and pain control are problems that must be managed along with antibiotics to eradicate staphylococci. Most children are treated with intravenous antibiotics such as cefazolin or nafcillin. Analgesics such as acetaminophen are needed for pain. Mild lubricant creams may be helpful in the healing stages to reduce skin discomfort.

FUNGAL INFECTIONS

Fungi are simple plants that lack chlorophyll and obtain nourishment from other living or dead organic material. Superficial fungal infections of the epidermis, hair, or nails are caused by dermatophytes.

Tinea Capitis

Fungal infections of the scalp are most commonly seen in children between 2 and 10 years of age.

Etiology

Most cases in the United States are caused by *Trichophyton tonsurans. Microsporum audouinii* is seen in less than 10 percent of cases. *Microsporum canis* can also cause infection but is usually transmitted from an infected cat rather than a dog.

Clinical Findings

Typical patches of tinea capitis are round or oval areas of alopecia about 1 to 5 cm in diameter. Stubby hair shafts that have broken off at the level of the scalp cause a "black dot" appearance.

Occasionally, tinea capitis can resemble flaky dandruff without any clear patches of alopecia. Close examination will still show black dots. If kerion formation occurs, occipital and cervical lymphadenopathy will sometimes be accompanied by low-grade fever.

Diagnosis

Hairs that are infected by *Microsporum* species will fluoresce yellow-green in the presence of long-wave ultraviolet light produced by a Woods lamp. Unfortunately, this organism causes the minority of infections.

Potassium hydroxide (KOH) preparation of hair and scalp scrapings will show spores and hyphae either alongside or within the hair shaft.

Fungal cultures should be obtained routinely because the course of therapy can be quite long.

Differential Diagnosis

Circumscribed areas of alopecia can result from noninfectious conditions such as alopecia areata and trichotillomania. Traction alopecia from tight braiding can cause hairs to break off close to the scalp. Seborrhea, dandruff, and psoriasis can be confused with the diffuse scaly form of tinea capitis. Kerion formation is most often confused with bacterial skin infections; however, the exudate of the kerion is sterile.

Complications

Complete destruction of the hair follicle with scarring and permanent baldness can result if the condition is untreated.

Treatment

Initial therapy for tinea capitis is oral griseofulvin at a dose of 15 mg/kg/day. This must continue for at least 6 weeks. Oral prednisone may be helpful in reducing the inflammatory kerion response.

Fungal spores remain viable for a long period of time. Barrettes, combs, and brushes must be washed frequently. All family members should be checked for infection, since this is quite contagious. A child can be permitted to return to school after 1 week of griseofulvin therapy.

TINEA CORPORIS

Dermatophyte infections of the epidermis are superficial and less problematic than tinea capitis. They can be found on any part of the body.

Etiology

Microsporum canis and *Trichophyton mentagrophytes* are responsible for tinea corporis. Any organism that can cause tinea capitis can also cause tinea corporis.

Clinical Findings

Lesions may appear as papules, vesicles, or eczematous plaques. However, the most recognizable pattern is the classic oval ringworm shape of an expanding inflammatory border with a clear central area.

The rash is often pruritic. Regional lymph nodes are usually not involved unless the lesion becomes impetiginized.

Diagnosis

A KOH preparation of material from the scaly inflammatory border should be used to confirm the presence of hyphae. Cultures are not usually needed because topical treatment is generally very effective.

Differential Diagnosis

Pityriasis rosea, granuloma annulare, and atopic dermatitis are sometimes confused with tinea corporis.

Complications

With treatment, infections usually clear completely without any scarring.

Management

Topical therapy may result in relief of itching within a week; however, therapy should continue for a minimum of 2 to 3 weeks after initial clearing.

Several effective topical antifungal medications are available without prescription, including tolnaftate (Tinactin), miconazole (Micatin), haloprogin (Halotex), and clotrimazole (Lotrimin). All are used by rubbing cream into the affected area twice a day. Failure to improve after 3 weeks of treatment is reason for further evaluation.

For a more detailed discussion, see Rosekrans JA: Superficial skin infections, chap. 63, p. 388, in *Pediatric Emergency Medicine: A Comprehensive Study Guide.*

64 Exanthems

Julia A. Rosekrans

Viral illnesses often produce characteristic skin rashes and clinical symptoms that help to categorize the illness. Besides recognizing the rash, the physician should be prepared to discuss the course of the illness, risk to others, incubation period, and potential complications (see Table 64-1).

RUBEOLA (MEASLES)

The number of cases of measles has dropped precipitously since live attenuated virus vaccine was introduced in 1963. Today most cases occur as community epidemics when there are high rates of inadequately immunized children. Measles virus is a single-stranded RNA paramyxovirus. The virus is transmitted by droplet spread and is highly contagious. There is an incubation period of about 9 to 12 days between exposure and the onset of symptoms. A patient with the illness is most contagious during the prodromal period, starting about 3 days before the onset of the rash, and is considered contagious for about 4 days thereafter.

Clinical Findings

Typical measles begin with a prodrome of respiratory symptoms. Cough, conjunctivitis, and coryza (nasal congestion) are usually present. Koplik's spots, tiny white spots on erythematous buccal mucosa opposite the lower molars, appear during the prodrome and last for about 24 h. They are usually still present when the rash begins.

The exanthem appears about 14 days after exposure. It begins at the hairline behind the ears and then spreads from the head to the feet over about 3 days. It is erythematous and maculopapular. Although individual spots may be seen initially, these become confluent over time. The patient looks most ill on the second or third day, with high fever, brassy cough, and photophobia. In a healthy child, the illness lasts for about 7 days.

Complications

Otitis media is the most common complication of measles. Respiratory complications include croup and laryngitis. The most common problem for which children with measles require hospitalization is pneumonia. Encephalitis with neurologic sequelae can occur.

TABLE 64-1 Differential Diagnosis of Morbilliform Rashes

Viral	Drug-induced reaction
Measles	Ampicillin
Rubella	Nonsteroidal anti-inflammatories
Roseola	Barbituates
Fifth disease	Phenytoin
Infectious mononucleosis	Sulfa antibiotics
Pityriasis rosea	Thiazides
Bacterial	Reactive erythema
Scarlet fever	Urticaria
Toxic shock syndrome	Erythema multiforme
Kawasaki syndrome	Rocky Mountain spotted fever

Management

There is no treatment for measles other than symptomatic support with bed rest and analgesics.

Live attenuated measles vaccine given within 72 h of exposure can provide some protection by stimulating active antibody production. Immune serum globulin 0.25 mL/kg IM, to a maximum of 15 mL, will prevent or modify the disease if given within 6 days of exposure.

Documented cases of measles should be reported to local public health authorities to reduce the possibility of an epidemic.

RUBELLA (GERMAN MEASLES)

This mild viral illness is significant because of its teratogenic effects. Rubella is a single-stranded RNA virus.

Droplet spread through the respiratory route results in a high rate of transmission among susceptible people. The incubation period is 14 to 23 days, with a period of infectiousness from 1 week before to about 5 days after the rash appears. Infants with congenital rubella syndrome can spread infection because they shed virus for months after birth. There is a high rate of subclinical infection, and many adults are immune without a history of having the illness.

Pathophysiology

The cause of the rash is not fully understood. In a research setting, virus can be recovered from papules on the skin as well as from skin that appears normal. The skin rash is probably due to an antigen-antibody reaction.

Clinical Findings

Rubella in children is a very mild disease, although parents sometimes describe children as being unusually fussy. Slight fever and marked lymphadenopathy with prominent postauricular and suboccipital lymph nodes usually occur at the same time that the rash is present. The rash itself is a nonspecific, diffuse, erythematous, maculopapular eruption. Older children often complain of transient joint pain.

Serologic tests can be done if it is necessary to reach a definitive diagnosis. This is not useful acutely.

Complications

Arthritis or arthralgia may begin during the prodrome or can follow the rash. This does not appear to predispose to arthritis later in life. Rare complications include thrombocytopenia or encephalitis.

The most significant complication is fetal malformation following a maternal rubella infection during the first or second trimester of pregnancy. The infection affects the organ system that is undergoing most rapid development at the time of the viremia. Since there is no treatment for the infection, maternal infection should be prevented by maintaining a high rate of herd immunity among young children and by immunization of adults before pregnancy occurs.

Management

This self-limited disease requires only symptomatic treatment. Nonsteroidal anti-inflammatory medication may be needed to control symptoms of arthritis.

ROSEOLA (EXANTHEM SUBITUM)

Human herpesvirus C has recently been identified as the cause of roseola. This common illness rarely occurs before about 6 months of age or after 2 years.

Most cases appear in spring and early fall. The illness is spread by respiratory droplets and has an incubation period of about 5 to 15 days.

Clinical Findings

The most characteristic feature of this illness is a well-looking child despite high fever. There does not appear to be a prodrome. The fever comes on suddenly and persists for 3 to 4 days. The rash appears as the fever vanishes and resolves within 48 h.

Febrile seizures may occur with this illness. Some infants have a bulging fontanelle without other meningeal symptoms, and results of lumbar punctures are unremarkable.

Complications

There are no known complications of this illness.

Management

Symptomatic care is all that is needed.

FIFTH DISEASE (ERYTHEMA INFECTIOSUM)

This mild disease is usually recognized in school-age children.

Etiology

Parvovirus B19, a single-stranded DNA virus, was identified as the cause of fifth disease in 1975.

Clinical Findings

The rash develops abruptly, with bright red cheeks giving the "slapped cheek" appearance. A maculopapular, faintly pink rash develops on the trunk and extremities, then clears in a lacy pattern. The rash fades over several days but can reappear intermittently for several weeks, especially when skin is exposed to sun or a warm bath. The child occasionally has a low-grade fever but generally seems quite well.

Complications

In a healthy person, there are no apparent complications. Adults may develop transient arthritis, although this is rare in children.

Parvovirus has been associated with bone marrow suppression and aplastic crisis in children with sickle cell anemia. Infection during pregnancy can result in fetal death or red cell aplasia with fetal hydrops.

Management

The disease is self-limited in children and requires no therapy. Serologic testing is suggested for pregnant women who develop the disease or are in close contact with children who have the illness.

SCARLET FEVER

This exanthem results from a reaction to erythrogenic toxin produced by several strains of group A beta-hemolytic streptococci

(GABHS). It can develop in association with strep pharyngitis and can also be seen with impetigo or cellulitis.

Clinical Findings

A sandpaper rash begins in skin folds such as the groin, axillae, and antecubital areas. The area around the mouth and nose is not erythematous, giving an appearance of circumoral pallor. Generalized lymphadenopathy is common. The exanthem usually develops within 12 to 48 h after onset of fever and chills. Desquamation progresses in the same pattern as the rash.

Complications

Scarlet fever carries the same risks as a GABHS infection without a rash. It is no more serious, although its name sounds worse to many parents. The risks of rheumatic fever and glomerulonephritis exist, but at the same rate as for streptococcal infections without rash.

Management

Oral penicillin VK, 15 to 50 mg/kg/24 h divided into three doses, or erythromycin, 20 to 50 mg/kg/24 h in three to four divided doses, is adequate to control disease spread. Children should not return to school until 24 h after starting antibiotics.

CHICKENPOX

This common childhood illness is a primary viral infection with a typical clinical course and rash. Varicella zoster is a herpes-type virus.

The incubation period for chickenpox is 14 to 21 days. Most cases occur in children under 14 years of age because the virus is so common. The method of viral spread is not clear, and both direct contact and airborne spread have been documented.

Clinical Findings

The illness begins with a mild 1- or 2-day prodrome of respiratory symptoms and low-grade fever. The rash appears on the trunk as small red papules that progress to tiny vesicles, giving the appearance of a "dew drop on a rose petal." Crops of vesicles develop for 3 to 5 days, so that all stages of the lesions can be found at the same time on any part of the body. When the vesicles dry and crust, they are thought not to be infectious.

Subclinical infections are common, so many adults who are not known to have had the disease are actually immune. Although varicella usually gives lifelong immunity with the first infection, second attacks can occur.

Complications

The most common complications are bacterial superinfections of the skin lesions and otitis media. Since varicella is a systemic illness, all body systems have been described with effects of the infection. Adolescents are more at risk for complications than young children. Inpatient care may be needed for children with cellulitis, pneumonia, hepatitis, or encephalitis.

Most adults have some shallow varicella scars. These occur most often in lesions that have become superinfected.

Management

For children with uncomplicated illnesses, treatment is symptomatic and supportive. Antihistamines such as diphenhydramine may help control itching. Oatmeal baths are also quite soothing.

Acyclovir inhibits herpesvirus DNA polymerase. It can be given in intravenous form to immune-compromised children or children with significant complications of chickenpox. Oral acyclovir will decrease the duration of development of skin lesions in healthy children if it is given within the first 24 h of rash appearance. It should be considered for therapy in household contacts and in adolescents, whose illness is often more problematic.

Children who are at high risk for severe or complicated infections should be given varicella zoster immune globulin (VZIG) if it can be given within 48 h of varicella exposure. The dose is 125 U/10 kg of body weight, with a maximum dose of 625 U.

HERPES ZOSTER

After a primary varicella infection, the varicella zoster virus persists in a latent condition in spinal sensory nerve root ganglia. The virus can erupt years later. Tingling pain usually precedes the appearance of vesicles, which occur in two or three crops within one dermatome. The most common area of involvement is the thoracic area, where several adjacent dermatomes may be involved. The lumbosacral area is also commonly involved. The least commonly involved areas in children are the cranial nerves;

however, since eruption here can involve the cornea, this pattern is the most medically worrisome.

Complications

Serious complications usually occur only in immunosuppressed patients. For most people, the eruption is troublesome and painful but self-limited. Postherpetic pain without any reappearance of skin lesions is more common in adults than in children.

Acyclovir and VZIG are useful in managing this type of herpes-virus eruption.

HERPES SIMPLEX

The clinical manifestations of infection with herpes simplex virus range from recurrent cold sores to encephalitis.

Two types of herpes simplex virus are known to cause infection in humans, type 1 (HSV-1) and type 2 (HSV-2). Both types can cause similar clinical patterns; however, HSV-1 is more common and tends to be found in oral infections, whereas HSV-2 is usually associated with genital infections. Both viruses can cause subclinical infection, and both remain latent within the body after initial infection.

This virus is species-specific and affects only humans. It is passed by direct contact, either with another person who has an active infection or with droplets on fomites. Lesions that are clinically inapparent can shed the virus. The incubation period is variable and ranges from 1 day to 4 weeks.

Clinical Findings

Herpes gingivostomatitis is a primary infection usually caused by HSV-1. The peak incidence of this infection is seen in children less than 5 years of age. Children appear quite ill, with high fever, painful vesicles on the tongue and mucous membranes, and regional lymphadenopathy. They frequently drool and refuse to eat. The fever may last for a week, with sores persisting for up to 2 weeks.

Herpetic whitlow is a painful inoculation of herpes virus onto a finger. This often happens in children who suck their fingers. A primary infection with fever, local pain, regional lymphadenopathy, and general malaise may develop.

Genital herpes usually results from sexual contact with an infected partner; however, it can also develop from self-inoculation from an oral infection, with virus spread on the patient's hands or from contact with fomites. A primary reaction will include painful local vesicles, regional lymphadenopathy, and fever.

Not all patients develop recurrent local herpes after a primary infection. In addition, many primary infections are subclinical, so patients with recurrent local eruptions may not have had a severe primary illness. When a local reaction begins, most people describe itching and burning in the region for a day before vesicles appear. Pain can last for a brief time or up to a week. There is no lymphadenopathy, and viral shedding rapidly decreases. While some people know that their local reactions are triggered by exposure to sun, spicy foods, stress, or trauma, many patients cannot determine a specific trigger mechanism.

Neonatal herpes simplex infection carries a serious risk of mortality or long-term morbidity. It is usually caused by HSV-2 and results from either intrauterine or intrapartum exposure; however, infants with postpartum infection can be infected by exposure to any adult with an active herpes infection, including cold sores. Infants may develop disseminated systemic illness, infection limited to the skin, or encephalitis without any skin lesions. Symptoms may develop as late as 6 weeks after birth.

Diagnosis

Herpes simplex infections can be identified by performing a Tzanck smear. Material from the base of a fresh vesicle is stained with Giemsa stain. Multinucleated giant cells can be identified easily.

Confirmation of infection with viral culture may be necessary, especially for genital lesions.

Differential Diagnosis

Other vesicular rashes can be confused with primary herpes infections. Hand-foot-and-mouth disease and herpangina resemble gingivostomatitis. Impetigo and herpes labialis are often confused, since both produce a yellow serous crust with surrounding erythema. Gram stain or Tzanck smear may help to distinguish them. Herpetic whitlow is often confused with bacterial cellulitis, since the involved finger is usually swollen and erythematous.

Complications

Most herpes infections resolve without scarring. Problems are related only to the pain of the eruption. Neonatal herpes can disseminate and cause an encephalitis or death.

Management

Acyclovir inhibits DNA synthesis and will shorten the course of a primary infection if started early in the illness. This drug has not been approved for use in children with gingivostomatitis, and the long-term effects of acyclovir in children are not known. It has been used in genital herpes infections at a dose of 200 mg every 4 h for 5 doses a day for 10 days.

Local acyclovir 5% ointment applied in a small amount six times a day may provide some relief of symptoms and shorten viral shedding for localized perioral or genital infections.

Intravenous acyclovir is recommended for neonatal herpes infections when systemic illness or encephalitis is present. Because infants with skin lesions may develop encephalitis as a late complication, some authorities recommend oral acyclovir during the first few months after birth.

If no treatment is given, as many as 70 percent of affected infants will develop disseminated infection. There is a 50 percent chance of mortality with systemic illness. Infants with herpes encephalitis usually develop permanent long-term neurologic sequelae.

Local symptomatic care includes analgesics, cool compresses, ice packs, and forcing of fluids. Children with oral primary herpes infections may have so much pain that they refuse to drink and require intravenous fluids.

ENTEROVIRUSES

Many viral exanthems occur that are not clinically significant enough for an exact etiology to have been sought. Nonspecific viral rashes may be maculopapular, scarlatiniform, vesicular, or urticarial. A few clinical syndromes can be differentiated. Most of these rashes come to our attention because a child has fever, is fussy, or demonstrates other systemic symptoms.

Clinical Findings

Hand-foot-and-mouth syndrome is caused by coxsackievirus A16 and occasionally A5 and A10. It is seen most commonly in summer and fall. The incubation period is variable, usually a few days. A prodrome of low fever, malaise, and abdominal pain may precede the rash. A child may complain of a sore mouth or painful hands and feet. Vesicles about 5 mm in diameter are found on the palms, the soles of the feet, the buttocks, and sometimes the trunk. Oral lesions usually appear later on the soft palate, gingivae, and tongue. The illness lasts about 3 to 6 days and resolves without problems. Occasional cases of myocarditis, pneumonia, and meningoencephalitis have been reported.

Herpangina is an exanthem of tiny vesicles on the soft palate, uvula, and tonsils. It can be produced by several enteroviruses as well as by herpes simplex. Sore throat and pain with eating are the most common complaints. Fever, headache, myalgia, and vomiting may be present.

Management

Analgesics for pain, a soft diet, and bed rest, if needed, are used for symptomatic care. Good hand-washing may help to reduce viral spread. Many infections are subclinical, and isolation from day care is impractical.

PITYRIASIS ROSEA

This self-limited disorder is usually seen in adolescents and young adults who seek medical care because the rash is spreading.

Clinical Findings

The distribution of the rash is diagnostic. Most cases begin with a single large, oval, scaly patch about 2 to 5 cm in diameter. This "herald patch" may not be noticed until the secondary eruption develops. Crops of small, oval, scaly patches appear on the trunk parallel to skin cleavage lines, creating a "Christmas tree" pattern. The herald patch fades quickly, while the secondary patches may take several weeks to fade. Some patients report mild itching. Occasionally, a patient may have pharyngitis and malaise.

Differential Diagnosis

Other scaly lesions may be confused with pityriasis rosea. Tinea corporis is often mistaken for the herald patch. The most important differential consideration is secondary syphilis, and a serologic test should be ordered in all sexually active teenagers.

Management

Most patients require only reassurance and education. Exposure to sunlight may hasten disappearance of the rash. Topical glucocorticoids do not seem to shorten the course, although moisturizers may stop the itching. Whether treated with them or not, the rash resolves without sequelae.

For a more detailed discussion, see Rosekrans JA: Exanthems, chap. 64, p. 392, in *Pediatric Emergency Medicine: A Comprehensive Study Guide.*

65 Infant Rashes

Julia A. Rosekrans

SEBORRHEIC DERMATITIS

This chronic condition with greasy, scaly skin may also be seen in adolescents; however, it is most commonly a parental concern when it develops in a young infant.

Minor problems such as dandruff and significant problems such as Letterer-Siwe disease may be confused with seborrhea. Psoriasis, yeast infections, and atopic dermatitis all share similarities in appearance.

Management

Low-potency topical glucocorticoids are used to treat inflamed, weeping areas. Scales on the scalp can be softened with mineral oil and washed off with mild shampoo. Diaper rash often requires treatment with antifungal medication to eradicate superinfection with *Candida*.

The process is chronic and follows a relapsing course until it resolves spontaneously, usually before 1 year of age. Infants with seborrhea do not have increased problems with seborrhea or acne as adolescents.

DIAPER DERMATITIS

Many different skin problems occur in the diaper area. Almost every diapered infant will develop some diaper rash, but only about 10 percent of infants will have serious problems.

Clinical Findings

Diaper rash due to chafing occurs mainly on the thighs and around the waist, where skin folds rub together. Skin is mildly reddened and dry and may be lichenified. This type of rash tends to appear quickly and resolve quickly.

Irritant diaper rash occurs on exposed skin surfaces and tends to spare intertriginous folds. Skin is reddened, with papules, vesicles, and scaly lesions on the lower abdomen, buttocks, and inner thighs.

Candida diaper dermatitis appears as reddened skin with sharply demarcated margins. Pustules and vesicles may be present at the edges of the affected area.

A painful, bright, glistening red eruption around the anus is characteristic of group A beta-hemolytic strep infection.

Management

The mainstay of treatment of diaper dermatitis is keeping the skin as dry as possible. Frequent diaper changes and the use of cornstarch powder to reduce friction may help to reduce the development of diaper rash.

When an inflamed rash is present, it is important to avoid rubbing the skin, and it may be necessary to rinse the baby in warm water in a sink rather than cleaning with a washcloth or premoistened wipe. Emollients containing zinc oxide provide good barrier protection and decrease friction.

If a rash has started, hydrocortisone cream (1%) applied in a thin coat two or three times a day may help to reduce inflammation.

Candida diaper rash can be treated with topical imidazole or nystatin in combination with 1% hydrocortisone cream. It is important to avoid fluorinated glucocorticoids, since they are absorbed excessively from occluded skin such as the diaper area.

Perianal streptococcal infection should be treated with oral antibiotics, either penicillin or erythromycin.

Diaper dermatitis usually responds well to outpatient care. Follow-up evaluation should be suggested for infants who have not improved within 7 days.

For a more detailed discussion, see Rosekrans SA: Infant rashes, chap. 65, p. 399, in *Pediatric Emergency Medicine: A Comprehensive Study Guide.*

SECTION XI
ORAL, EAR, NOSE, AND THROAT EMERGNECIES

66 Ear and Nose Emergencies

John P. Santamaria / Thomas J. Abrunzo

ACUTE OTITIS EXTERNA

Acute otitis externa refers to any inflammatory condition of the external ear. It is important to determine the severity of the infection, recognize unusual presentations, prevent complications, and avoid pitfalls in management.

Pseudomonas species are the most common cause of acute otitis externa. Other bacteria, including *Staphylococcus* species, *Streptococcus* species, gram-negative organisms, and diphtheroids, are less frequently isolated. *Aspergillus,* which causes approximately 90 percent of fungal cases, is more common in patients who are immunosuppressed or have uncontrolled hyperglycemia.

Diagnostic Findings

Local itching and mild pain are common early symptoms. Edema and increased tissue tension develop as bacterial invasion progresses. Pain is exacerbated by traction to the pinna, pressure on the tragus, or movement of the jaw from side to side.

If the condition is untreated, swelling of the ear canal will occur and an exudate may develop. In patients with a fungal etiology, white, yellow-green, or dark pigmented masses composed of hyphae are seen.

Acute otitis externa is characterized by local symptoms; systemic toxicity suggests another diagnosis.

Differential Considerations

A retained foreign body can exactly mimic the presentation of acute otitis externa of infectious etiology, becoming apparent only after thorough cleansing of the ear canal.

A furuncle, or localized pyogenic infection, is most frequently caused by *Staphylococcus aureus.* If this is not fluctuant, treatment should be begun with warm compresses and systemic antibiotics such as a first-generation cephalosporin, amoxicillin with clavulanic acid, dicloxacillin, or erythromycin, depending on local sensitivities.

Eczematous changes of the pinna and ear canal include atopic dermatitis, seborrheic dermatitis, dyshidrosis, and contact dermatitis. When edema of the ear canal prevents adequate visualization of the tympanic membrane and exudate is present in the canal, it may be impossible to distinguish otitis externa from otitis media with perforation.

Management

Cleansing of the ear canal has several advantages. Examination is improved, the exudate removed from the canal can no longer cause an inflammatory response, and topical medications can better contact the diseased area. Suction, dry mopping, curetting, and irrigation have all been used with success.

When topical medication is instilled directly, enough should be used to completely fill the canal. The use of a wick is particularly advantageous when significant edema is present so that medication is maintained in direct contact with the epithelial surface. Topical agents may be directly instilled into the external acoustic canal or applied to a wick. Wicks are removed within 2 days of placement to avoid a foreign-body reaction.

Commonly used antibiotic glucocorticoid topical preparations are effective against *Pseudomonas,* other gram-negative bacteria, and staphylococci. They also have anti-inflammatory and antipruritic effects. Based on efficacy, cost, risk of allergic reaction, and development of bacterial resistance, antiseptic drops—such as boric acid or aluminum acetate—are recommended in early cases.

Fungal otitis externa should be followed by an otolaryngologist. Topical tolnaftate therapy for several weeks is usually effective.

Malignant otitis externa, almost always caused by *Pseudomonas aeroginosa,* is refractory to conventional treatment. It has a high mortality and typically occurs in adults with diabetes mellitus. Malignant otitis externa in children is rare, primarily affecting diabetic adolescents and others who are immunosuppressed. Deeper tissue invasion explains the necrosis, local thrombosis, and vasculitis that can occur. Similar involvement of contiguous structures such as cartilage, bone, the mastoid air spaces, lymph glands, and parotid gland is possible. Sequelae are generally limited to facial nerve paresis, stenosis of the external canal, and hearing loss. Malignant otitis externa requires prolonged intravenous antibiotic therapy and possible surgical debridement. It should be managed by the otolaryngologist.

OTITIS MEDIA AND MASTOIDITIS

Otitis media includes the clinical syndromes of acute suppurative otitis media and otitis media with effusion. Significant overlap exists in their pathology, pathophysiology, microbiology, clinical findings, and treatment. The incidence peaks between the ages of 6 and 13 months, when examination is most difficult. It is necessary to appreciate the wide range of normal tympanic and middle ear findings so that otitis media is not overdiagnosed and other, more dangerous processes overlooked.

Mastoiditis is an important and treatable albeit uncommon complication of acute suppurative otitis media.

Anatomy and Pathophysiology

Eustachian tube dysfunction is most important in the pathogenesis of otitis media. In health, the eustachian tube has three major functions: equilibration of middle ear and atmospheric air pressures, protection from secretions of the nasopharynx, and clearance of middle ear secretions into the nasopharynx. The eustachian tube becomes congested as a result of allergy, infection, or anatomic predisposition. Accumulated secretions serve as a culture medium. Suppuration and rupture of the tympanic membrane may result. Supine positioning and shorter eustachian tube length in young children enhances reflux of nasopharyngeal pathogens into the middle ear, thus predisposing to otitis media. Hematogenous spread of bacteria into the middle ear is possible in newborns, but uncommon.

The posterior wall of the middle ear communicates with the mastoid antrum and air cells via the aditus. The mucous membrane lining the tympanic cavity and mastoid structures is continuous.

Etiology

Otitis media and mastoiditis have similar microbiologic origins. *Streptococcus pneumoniae* is the most common bacterial isolate in otitis media at all ages. *Haemophilus influenzae* also remains an important pathogen throughout childhood and adulthood. *Branhamella catarrhalis* has increased in importance since the early 1980s. Group A streptococci and *S. aureus* are isolated much less frequently. *Chlamydia trachomatis* is difficult to isolate but is known to cause otitis media in infants below 6 months of age.

Mycoplasma pneumoniae should be considered in cases unresponsive to initial therapy or when tympanic bullae are present. The role of viruses is poorly understood. The role of anaerobes is somewhat controversial. During the first 2 weeks of life, there is significant risk of infection with *S. aureus,* Group B streptococci, and gram-negative enteric bacteria.

Diagnostic Findings

Historical findings include local symptoms of ear pain, discharge, and hearing loss. Systemic symptoms such as fever, headache, malaise, gastrointestinal irritation, altered behavior, and anorexia may also be present.

Pneumatic otoscopy is an essential component of the ear examination, especially in the crying child. After inspection of the pinna, postauricular area, and external auditory canal for inflammation, a pneumatic otoscope with a well-fitting speculum should be used to evaluate the color, lucency, light reflex, bony landmarks, and mobility of the tympanic membrane.

Classic tympanic membrane findings in acute otitis media are redness, opacity, absence of landmarks, alteration of the light reflex, and lack of mobility. Tympanic membrane immobility is the only reliable sign of otitis media in the crying child, since abnormalities in the color, lucency, light reflex, and landmarks can be false-positive findings.

The uncooperative child must be adequately immobilized before otoscopy is attempted. Any foreign bodies and cerumen must be removed. Curettage, suction, and irrigation are most commonly used for cerumen removal and should be mastered by the emergency physician.

Redness and swelling over the mastoid area may be seen in more advanced cases of mastoiditis. Outward, downward protrusion of the pinna is suggestive of subperiosteal abscess. Computed tomography or magnetic resonance imaging may be helpful in the diagnosis of mastoiditis, brain abscess, or lateral sinus thrombosis.

Differential Considerations

Care must be taken not to overdiagnose otitis media, especially in the young child, who is at greater risk of having an unrecognized, more serious bacterial disease. A crying, otherwise normal child can have physical findings almost identical to those in a child with acute otitis media. Partially treated meningitis, for example, can smolder and present later in a fulminant state. Even when the diagnosis of otitis media is certain, other coexistent illnesses must be considered.

Otitis externa and otitis media with perforation may be impossible to differentiate unless the ear canal is thoroughly cleansed.

Complications

Complications of acute otitis media include tympanic perforation, mastoiditis, cholesteatoma, facial paralysis, labyrinthitis, and infectious eczemoid dermatitis. Intracranial suppurative complications such as meningitis, brain abscess, encephalitis, and lateral sinus thrombosis may be heralded by symptoms as vague as worsening ear pain on antibiotics, persistent headache, intractable emesis, or behavior change. More specific symptoms, such as meningismus, visual changes, papilledema, seizure, and focal neurologic findings, may not be present, especially when the patient is "partially treated" with oral antibiotics.

Management

Amoxicillin or trimethoprim/sulfamethoxazole is recommended as a first-line agent for acute otitis media. If these are not effective, amoxicillin/clavulanate or erythromycin/sulfisoxazole will provide broad coverage. Some beta-lactamase-producing strains of *B. catarrhalis* are resistant to cefaclor and cefprozil. Cefixime may not cure infections caused by *S. aureus* but may be desirable for its once-a-day dosing schedule. Single-dose intramuscular ceftriaxone (50 mg/kg) has been shown to be as effective as 10 days of oral amoxicillin. Antibiotic recommendations should be continually reevaluated based on current patterns of microbiologic resistance and availability of new drugs.

In neonates, the possibility of hematogenously spread disease, including that from gram-negative bacilli or *S. aureus,* requires a complete septic work-up, admission, and intravenous broad-spectrum antibiotics pending culture results. The rarity of this occurrence has prompted some authorities to recommend that in the otherwise well neonate over 2 weeks old, otitis media without systemic toxicity can be treated on an outpatient basis with oral antibiotics. A cautious approach is recommended, especially if fever is present.

There is to date no conclusive evidence supporting the efficacy of topical or systemic glucocorticoids, decongestants, or antihistamines in the treatment of otitis media. Their use is not recommended. In particular, glucocorticoids should not be used when the risk of concurrent varicella infection exists.

Mastoiditis should be managed by an otolaryngologist. Before microbiologic confirmation, a broad-spectrum intravenous cephalosporin, such as ceftriaxone, can be used. Alternatively, a penicillinase-resistant penicillin, such as oxacillin, in combination with an aminoglycoside, such as gentamicin, can be used.

The patient with otitis media should be rechecked if symptoms worsen or if no improvement occurs within 3 days. Otherwise, reevaluation in 2 weeks is appropriate. Worsening on antibiotics may be a sign of suppurative complication. At least partial improvement is expected after 3 days of treatment. Follow-up is necessary after treatment to assess for persistent middle ear effusion.

The child with concomitant systemic bacterial infection or toxic appearance may require hospitalization and intravenous antibiotics.

FOREIGN BODY OF THE NOSE AND EAR

The removal of nasal and aural foreign bodies can be very difficult. Optimally, physical examination confirms the history, and removal is uneventful. Often, however, the history is vague, the examination difficult, and the foreign body not easily grasped. Removal attempts under suboptimal conditions may precipitate bleeding, edema, and movement of the foreign body to a less accessible location.

The size and shape of nasal and aural foreign bodies are limited only by the volumes to which the normal structures of the nose and ear can expand. This is evidenced by innumerable case reports of large retained foreign bodies. Some go unnoticed for long periods of time.

Diagnostic Findings

In the absence of a clear history, helpful clues include epistaxis, pain, fever, discharge, and alteration of sense of smell or hearing. Bleeding and purulent discharge can impede the physical examination.

Both sides of the nose and both ears must be examined. Children who have one foreign body are at greater risk for several. Foreign bodies have masqueraded as chronic infections, tumors, recurrent epistaxis, and generalized body odor (bromidrosis).

Plain radiographs will miss the many nonradiopaque objects. A rhinolith is a mineralized nasal foreign body. Gradually increasing in size, it is usually discovered as an incidental finding on plain radiograph. Although rarely indicated, more sensitive radiographic techniques can demonstrate the presence of a foreign body in the posterior portion of the nose, which is not readily visualized on examination. In difficult cases, radiographic studies can be used prior to removal to demonstrate the size and position of a retained foreign body.

Complications

Complications occur as a result of the foreign body, examination, or removal. Blockage of the external auditory canal or nares can interfere with normal function. Infection can closely follow the presence of a foreign body in both the ear and the nose. Occlusion of the sinus ostia in the anterior part of the nasal cavity and the eustachian tube posteriorly can predispose to sinusitis and otitis media. Undiscovered nasal foreign bodies may present with recurrent epistaxis due to mucosal erosion and local irritation. An expanding rhinolith may impinge on contiguous structures, complicating removal or predisposing to infection. A case of meningitis and death secondary to a foreign body is reported in the literature.

Adequate restraint of the child and careful use of conscious sedation before instrumentation will minimize potential complications. Overzealous restraint can cause vascular compromise or ecchymosis. Inadequate restraint can increase the risk of tympanic membrane trauma and perforation.

Foreign bodies that are pushed into the nasopharynx can be swallowed or aspirated.

Management

The first priority is to do no harm. Any case with a low probability of successful removal in the emergency department should be referred to an otolaryngologist. It is true that the first attempt at removal is the most likely to be successful, since removal attempts may stimulate bleeding, mucosal edema, and movement of the object to a less accessible area.

Although many cases will not require elaborate supplies, it is prudent to be prepared for complications before attempting removal (Table 66-1).

After the procedure has been explained to the child and family, adequate immobilization should be ensured. Optimally this is achieved with the child's cooperation; more often, assisted immobilization with or without sedation is required. The availability of sufficient personnel will reduce the chance of injury to the child and emergency department staff. One person assigned to each limb and a fifth to control the head may be necessary with larger, stronger children. Use of an immobilization device fashioned from sheets or a papoose board may reduce the number of holders required.

TABLE 66-1 Equipment for Examination and Removal of a Nasal or Aural Foreign Body

Immobilization device (sheet or papoose board)
Sedative medications (Chap. 8)
Otoscope for instrumentation under direct visualization
Nasal speculum
Headlight (optional)
Topical vasoconstrictor (phenylephrine 0.125%–0.5%, cocaine 4%, or epinephrine 1 : 1000)
Alligator or Hartman forceps
Wire loop or curette
Suction apparatus, including catheters of various sizes
No. 8 Foley or Fogarty catheter (optional)

No attempts at removal should be made without a good light source. For most foreign bodies of the nose and ear, direct visualization and instrumentation through an otoscope is adequate. A nasal speculum and headlight are preferable for nasal foreign bodies. Vertical opening of the nasal speculum will avoid septal damage. Topical vasoconstriction may reduce intranasal tissue edema and aid foreign-body removal.

The shape, location, and composition of the foreign body, along with physician preference, influence the removal technique and instrument employed. Insects are usually easier to remove and cause less trauma when they are not wiggling their bodies or flapping their wings. It is generally recommended that they be killed with alcohol before removal is attempted. Wood and other vegetable matter tends to swell when wet and is best removed before irrigating the ear canal. Mineral-based foreign bodies, such as round plastic beads, are difficult to grasp. When possible, forceps are used to grasp the foreign body. Round, fragile objects may be more successfully removed by placing a wire loop curette behind the foreign body or by using an adhesive of the Super Glue type on a cotton-tipped applicator.

Familiarity with the use of a curette is particularly helpful in removal of excess cerumen deposits. A curette with a small loop with rounded, smooth edges that is slightly bent at the juncture of the shaft and the curette ring is best to facilitate cerumen removal. Otic drops can soften hard cerumen prior to removal attempts. After cerumen removal, the canal should be checked for trauma, which could predispose to infection. If the canal is traumatized, prophylactic therapy for acute otitis externa should be considered.

To avoid damage to the ear canal or tympanic membrane while using an otoscope, curette, or other instrument near the ear canal, part of that hand should be anchored against the child's head. If the child's head moves suddenly, the examining hand and instrument will then move with it.

Small aural foreign bodies close to the tympanic membrane may be removed by irrigation with tap water at body temperature. A 30- to 60-mL syringe attached to a plastic infusion catheter or, preferably, a butterfly needle tubing cut off about 3 cm from the hub will deliver adequate volumes for irrigation at adequate pressures. The soft, flexible butterfly tubing is inserted atraumatically into the external acoustic meatus, directing the water inflow around a partial obstruction and allowing the foreign body to be removed with lateral water outflow. The myriad of methods advocated for the removal of aural and nasal foreign bodies attests to the fact that no single technique is universally successful. Some practitioners remove foreign bodies with suction apparatus or small-size Foley catheters.

Since children may pack a nose or ear with several objects at once, a thorough check for other objects is advisable after a foreign body is removed.

The successful management of foreign bodies in the ear and nose requires careful patient selection, proper equipment, and a planned, coordinated approach to the child. If emergency department removal is not possible and immediate removal is not necessary, the child can be started on oral antibiotics to cover normal upper respiratory flora and referred to an otolaryngologist as an outpatient.

EPISTAXIS

Nosebleeds tend to occur in the preteenage population and are almost exclusively anterior in location, at either the nasal vestibule or the plexus of vessels on the anterior, inferior portion of the nasal septum (Little's area, Kiesselbach's plexus). Much less commonly, occult bleeding from the respiratory and gastrointestinal tracts can present as epistaxis.

Diagnostic Findings

History of recent trauma, upper respiratory illness, allergy, or exposure to dry air may be obtained. Prolonged bleeding or easy bruisability in the patient or family members are important clues to systemic disorders. In bilateral epistaxis, the history of which side bled first usually reveals the bleeding site. The physician must ask how much bleeding occurred, but should expect an overestimation.

A history of behavior change, pallor, or orthostatic dizziness suggests significant blood loss. Altered mental status and delayed capillary refill may be the only physical findings to suggest hypovolemia. Sustained tachycardia and tachypnea may be noted. Hypotension is a late finding.

Supplies, including suction apparatus, should be readied before attempting evaluation of the child with epistaxis, so that treatment can accompany examination. The head-down position will lessen the risk of aspiration from swallowed blood. Careful physical examination usually will reveal the bleeding point. Positioning a small child in a parent's lap with manual restraint is often helpful. Optimal examination is facilitated by the use of a headlamp and nasal speculum. The speculum should be opened in a rostrocaudal direction to avoid damage to the nasal septum. Removal of blood with a Fraser suction tip can aid in localization of the bleeding point.

Demonstration of blood under the nails may be evidence of nose picking. Associated lymphadenopathy or evidence of other bleeding suggests systemic disease.

Stat hemoglobin and typing/crossmatching of blood are indicated if there is clinical evidence of hypovolemia. Epistaxis alone is usually self-limiting and does not warrant evaluation for a coagulation defect.

Management

No treatment is required for patients whose bleeding resolves spontaneously or with direct pressure. The number of recurrences, general health of the patient, and hydration status should be considered in deciding whether or not to treat a nosebleed.

All equipment should be readied before immobilizing the child. Yankaur suction tips for suction of particulate matter (emesis) and Fraser tips for removal of blood are especially important. The use of a headlamp leaves both of the physician's hands free to use the nasal speculum, suction apparatus, and other equipment.

Packing the nose with topical thrombin followed by 10 min of firm, constant pressure is safe, effective, and technically simpler and better tolerated than silver nitrate cautery. It is helpful to remove as much fresh blood and clot as possible before attempting this procedure.

Cautery of the bleeding site and the immediately surrounding area may be helpful if packing with thrombin is ineffective. The child's thin nasal septum must be considered at risk for perforation when cautery is done. A cotton pledget can be soaked in phenylephrine hydrochloride (0.125 to 0.5%), epinephrine (1:1000), or cocaine (4%) and placed in the nose for 10 min. Injection of the site with 1 to 2 mL of lidocaine with epinephrine (1:100,000) has both tamponading and vasoconstrictive effects. Systemic effects should be anticipated.

It is uncommon for childhood epistaxis to require nasal packing. Packing should be done in consultation with an otolaryngologist. Nasal sponges are easily inserted when dry, can be cut to size, and expand when moistened. Packing with petrolatum gauze is much more uncomfortable and is poorly tolerated by small children. Complications include syncope during packing, sinusitis, bacteremia, local infection, toxic shock syndrome, and iatrogenic sleep apnea if bilateral sponges or packs are placed. Packing should be removed within 2 days and antibiotic coverage provided while the packing is in place. Recommended antibiotics cover normal nasal flora. Amoxicillin is usually adequate, but better staphylococcal coverage (cefaclor, erythromycin ethylsuccinate, and amoxicillin with clavulanate potassium) is prudent. Erythromycin is a good choice for the older child.

Posterior bleeds are suspected when a bleeding site cannot be visualized and anterior packs are not effective. In-hospital management by an otolaryngologist is indicated. Foley catheters and pneumatic nasal catheters are better tolerated by patients than petrolatum gauze nasal packs. Eustachian tube obstruction and subsequent iatrogenic otitis media can occur. A posteriorly placed pack, arterial ligation, pterygopalatine fossa block, and embolization are rarely needed in a child.

Pediatric epistaxis, usually a result of local trauma and dry nasal mucosa, is likely to recur. Humidifiers and petroleum jelly rubbed onto the anterior nasal septum and the skin at the nasal orifice may be helpful. Fingernails should be kept short. Habitual nose-pickers may benefit from having their hands covered with socks during sleep.

RHINITIS

Rhinitis is the single most frequent cause of nasal discharge. It is a major cause of school absenteeism and missed parental workdays. Its incidence reflects the child's age, contact with other children, and general state of health. Estimates have ranged between 6 and 21 episodes per year.

TABLE 66-2 Response to Treatment of Infectious and Allergic Rhinitis

	Infectious	Allergic
Decongestants	Fair	Fair
Antihistamines	Poor	Good
Glucocorticoids	None	Excellent
Immunotherapy	None	Variable
Cromolyn	None	Fair
Antibiotics/antivirals	Disease-specific	None

Diagnostic Findings

The examiner should ask about known precipitants; discharge quality, quantity, and timing; factors that improve or worsen the discharge; and associated symptoms. Previous episodes, known sensitivities, medications, and prior therapy are potentially important. History of topical decongestant use should be sought.

The nasal mucous membrane is best examined with a good light source and nasal speculum. A large-caliber otoscope speculum can also be used.

Immobilization of the uncooperative child is necessary. Swelling, erythema, and secretions are evidence of inflammation. Laboratory and radiographic evaluation are not needed in the acute management of infectious or allergic rhinitis.

Therapeutic Trial

Therapy is disease-specific. Therapeutic options for patients with allergic and infectious rhinitis are outlined in Table 66-2.

Decongestants (vasoconstrictors) may be used orally or topically. Therapy with topical decongestants must be limited to 5 days to minimize rebound phenomena. A single injection of dexamethasone and oral decongestants for a few days may facilitate removal of topical therapy. Others advocate use of nasal decongestant spray on one side only. The unsprayed side improves in approximately 3 days.

Evidence of bacterial infection should prompt antibiotic use. Antibiotics effective against *Streptococcus pneumoniae* and *Haemophilus influenzae* (amoxicillin, trimethoprim/sulfamethoxazole, cefaclor) are first-line agents.

When avoidance, decongestants, and antihistamines fail, glucocorticoids, cromolyn sodium, and immunotherapy may be used by the continuing care physician. Inhaled glucocorticoids cause less adrenal suppression and are preferred to oral preparations.

SINUSITIS

Sinusitis is a bacterial inflammation of the paranasal sinuses associated with nasal mucosal inflammation and obstruction of the sinus ostia. The condition is most often manifested as a prolongation or complication of viral upper respiratory tract infection. Children average six to eight upper respiratory infections per year, and it is estimated that 0.5 to 5 percent develop sinusitis.

Symptoms may vary from the more common persistent, purulent rhinorrhea and cough to the less common symptoms of fever, headache, facial pain, and swelling.

Predisposing clinical problems include allergies, rhinitis, foreign bodies, choanal atresia, cleft palate, neoplasm, septal deviation, adenoidal hypertrophy, polyps (allergic, cystic fibrosis), dental infection, immunodeficiency, and immotile cilia syndromes (such as Kartagener syndrome). Swimming, trauma, and rhinitis medicamentosa may also cause mucosal swelling and obstruction of the sinusal ostia.

Common bacteria isolated from patients with acute sinusitis include

Streptococcus pneumoniae—25 to 30 percent
Moraxella (Branhamella) catarrhalis—15 to 20 percent
Haemophilus influenzae—15 to 20 percent
Group A streptococci—2 to 5 percent

Staphylococci and anaerobes are more important pathogens in chronic sinusitis.

Diagnostic Findings

The key to differentiating an uncomplicated upper respiratory infection from sinusitis is the unusual severity or protraction of symptoms found in the latter. Measures of severity may include fever above 39.0°C, purulent nasal discharge, and periorbital swelling. Protracted (>10 days) findings are common, including nasal discharge (clear or purulent), cough that is frequently worse at night, bad breath, and facial pain and periorbital edema that are worse in the morning. Fatigue, malaise, decreased appetite, and weight loss are sometimes noted. Headache, dental pain, and facial tenderness are less common complaints in children than in adults.

Sphenoidal sinusitis is uniquely associated with frontal, temporal, or retroorbital pain, which may be the only symptom. It is rare in children. Since isolated sphenoidal sinusitis can result in severe intracranial complications (extension to the brain) in the absence of the typical respiratory prodrome, it is an important consideration in the differential diagnosis of headache.

On physical examination, one may find purulent drainage from the middle meatus, boggy nasal mucosa, postnasal drip, and cobblestoning of the posterior pharynx. Transillumination is of limited value in children because of the variable development of sinuses before the age of 8 to 10 years. In older children, it is useful to note whether light transmission is normal or absent.

The white blood cell count may help in assessing patient response to infection. Blood cultures may occasionally be useful in the toxic patient. If a sinus puncture is done, the material should be sent for Gram stain and culture for aerobes and anaerobes.

Radiologic plain film examination of children has variable reliability. Normal sinus films are helpful. Abnormal sinus films are difficult to interpret, although after 6 years of age the interpretation can be more definitive. Sinusitis appears as clouding, mucoperiosteal thickening greater than 4 mm, or air fluid levels within the sinuses, with the last being most helpful in defining acute infection. Preferred plain views include the following:

Occipitomental (Waters) views for maxillary sinuses
Anteroposterior (Caldwell) views for frontal and ethmoidal sinuses
Submentovertex views for sphenoidal sinus
Lateral views for sphenoidal sinuses

For most small children, where maxillary sinusitis is suspected, a single Waters view may suffice. With equivocal plain radiographs, computed tomography is indicated as the definitive evaluation of acute or chronic infection. It is usually indicated if the child is seriously ill, has had recurrent episodes, or has chronic disease or suspected suppurative complications.

Differential Considerations

In evaluating the patient with suspected sinusitis, other entities that cause comparable presentations must be excluded. An acute upper respiratory tract infection or allergy may initially have similar symptoms, while a foreign body, neoplasm, or polyp commonly causes unilateral drainage and obstruction, possibly as predisposing factors in the development of sinusitis. Functional and organic causes of headache should also be excluded.

Complications

Sinusitis can seed the systemic circulation, resulting in septicemia. Local extension can result in facial cellulitis, facial abscess, periorbital and orbital cellulitis, osteomyelitis of the skull (Pott's puffy tumor), cavernous sinus thrombosis, epidural abscess, subdural empyema, meningitis, and brain abscess.

Management

Though sinusitis resolves spontaneously in 40 percent of cases, antibiotic therapy is indicated to hasten resolution of symptoms and prevent complications. For the nontoxic patient, a 2- to 3-week course of one of several agents is appropriate: amoxicillin (50 mg/kg/24 h) q8h PO, amoxicillin with clavulanic acid (50 mg/kg/24 h) q8h PO, cefaclor (40 mg/kg/24 h) q8h PO, or trimethoprim/sulfamethoxazole (10 mg TMP/50 mg SMX/kg/24 h) q12h PO. Failure to respond justifies the addition of specific coverage for *S. aureus* (dicloxacillin 50 mg/kg/24 h q6h PO) and anaerobic organisms. In toxic children and those with evidence of sphenoidal sinusitis, inpatient admission and parenteral antibiotics are indicated initially.

The use of standard doses of antihistamines, decongestants, glucocorticoids, and cromolyn sodium is controversial regarding efficacy in the treatment of sinusitis. Input from the consultant pediatrician or otolaryngologist is useful in developing a specific, personalized therapeutic regimen.

Needle or surgical drainage is necessary in those patients who are unresponsive to antibiotics. Antral puncture by an otolaryngologist is indicated if there is severe pain that is unresponsive to medical management; sinusitis in a seriously ill, toxic child; an unsatisfactory response; or suppurative complications; or if the patient is immunocompromised.

Recurrent or refractory sinusitis is sometimes further evaluated by antral lavage to establish a definitive bacteriologic diagnosis. Persistent infection that is unresponsive to multiple antibiotics is treated surgically by the creation of an antral window or by endoscopic enlargement of the osteomeatal unit.

Degree of toxicity, ability to tolerate oral fluids, complicated or serious disease, age of the patient, and reliability of follow-up will dictate whether inpatient management is necessary. Immunocompromised hosts will frequently require inpatient therapy.

For a more detailed discussion, see Santamaria JP, Abrunzo TJ: Ear and nose emergencies, chap. 66, p. 401, in *Pediatric Emergency Medicine: A Comprehensive Study Guide.*

67 Emergencies of the Oral Cavity and Neck

Thomas J. Abrunzo / John P. Santamaria

DENTOALVEOLAR INFECTIONS

Infections originating from dental structures begin in the periodontium or in the dental pulp. Periodontal infections tend to localize to intraoral soft tissue and seldom extend to deeper structures of the face and neck. Periodontitis is a chronic inflammation and infection of the dental-gingival interface. Pericoronitis is an acute, localized infection caused by food particles and microorganisms that have become trapped under the gum flaps (opercula) of partially erupted or impacted teeth. Dental infections can extend locally to involve deep fascial spaces of the mandible, causing Ludwig's angina. *Bacteroides, Peptostreptococcus, Actinomyces,* and *Streptococcus* are common pathogens of orofacial infections arising from odontogenic sources.

Diagnostic Findings

A history of recent restoration or extraction; tactile (lingual) sensation of a change in restoration surface; and thermal, percussion, or chemical sensitivity suggest failed dental therapy, dental fracture, or new caries as a cause of pain. Pain, fever, gingival swelling, and purulent gingival discharge suggest periodontal abscess, periapical abscess, pulpitis, pericoronitis, or gingivitis.

Dental examination includes a search for discoloration, fractures, swelling, fluctuance, and percussion tenderness. Gentle probing of the suspicious area may disclose tenderness or purulent discharge. Anterior cervical adenopathy may be present.

A panoramic radiograph of the dentition and mandible may reveal evidence of primary dental disease or secondary involvement of the maxilla or mandible. Computed tomography (CT) of the orofacial area may be necessary to diagnose infection of the deep fascial space.

Management

Caries require analgesics and dental referral. Pulpitis and periapical abscess also require analgesia, with warm compresses, and systemic antibiotics, usually penicillin or erythromycin. Incision and drainage may be necessary. Pericoronitis and periodontitis

TABLE 67-1 Oral Ulcers: Diagnostic Considerations

Aphthous stomatitis
Acute necrotizing gingivostomatitis (trench mouth: Vincent's angina)
Autoimmune
Candidiasis (oral thrush)
Chemical (antineoplastic)
Drugs (phenytoin)
Epstein-Barr virus
Erythema multiforme/Stevens-Johnson syndrome
Hand-foot-and-mouth disease
Herpangina
Herpes simplex
Herpetic gingivostomatitis
Malignancy (leukemia)
Radiation-induced
Syphilis (primary and secondary)
Traumatic
Varicella zoster
Vitamin deficiency (scurvy)

are treated similarly; irrigation and gentle debridement of opercula, with removal of retained debris, may obviate the need for incision and drainage.

Uncomplicated dental infection is usually treated on an outpatient basis; deep fascial space infections require hospitalization.

GINGIVOSTOMATITIS

Gingivitis presents as tender, swollen, edematous, sometimes friable gum tissue with or without vesiculation or ulceration. Gingivitis may be accompanied by stomatitis, which presents as either diffuse erythema or vesicoulceration. Ulcers appear as circumscribed loss of epithelium or local tissue necrosis (Table 67-1).

Diagnostic Findings

History of specific exposures frequently assists in diagnosis: chemotherapy causes mucositis; phenytoin causes gingival hyperplasia;

nutritional deprivation causes scurvy; physical disability may predispose to poor hygiene. Fever is a common symptom in most infections except those due to *Candida.*

The presence of posterior pharyngeal ulcers is likely to represent Coxsackie virus. Buccal and lingual vesicles and maculovesicles on the hands and feet (hand-foot-and-mouth disease) are also caused by an enterovirus (Coxsackie A-5, 10, and 16). Primary herpes simplex infection usually manifests itself by high fever and swollen, red, friable gums with diffuse oropharyngeal mucosal lesions that may become confluent. It can be differentiated from trench mouth (Vincent's angina) by the latter's isolated gingival involvement. Syphilis may present in its primary stage as oral, lingual, and tonsillar chancres and, in its secondary stage, as mucous patches, which are superficial, excoriated, weeping, exudative lesions found anywhere in the oropharynx. Erythema multiforme is an exanthem of erythematous macules or papules with superimposed vesicles, primarily of the upper extremity and trunk, that evolve into annular or target lesions. An enanthem of mucosal blistering occurs in the Stevens-Johnson form of erythema multiforme. The stomatitis of *Candida* appears as white, flocculent, confluent patches found diffusely over the tongue and oropharyngeal mucosa.

Laboratory evaluation is not helpful in most cases of gingivostomatitis. A complete blood count (CBC) may be useful in the diagnosis of leukemia and Epstein-Barr virus (EBV) infection. The Monospot test is also helpful to detect EBV titers. The diagnosis of syphilis can be made by serologic studies and dark-field exam.

Management

Gingivitis is significantly improved with good oral hygiene (toothbrushing and use of a mouthwash). Children with stomatitis, ulcers, or severe sore throat may benefit symptomatically from gargling or careful oral administration of a combination of kaopectate, diphenhydramine, and viscous lidocaine. Overuse of lidocaine may, however, cause seizures. Systemic analgesics are sometimes necessary.

Candida usually responds to nystatin swabbing. Trench mouth is thought to respond to penicillin. Syphilitic ulcers require benzathine penicillin, tetracycline, or erythromycin, with serologic follow-up at specified intervals. Stevens-Johnson syndrome can be life-threatening, and the patient should receive prompt consultation and admission.

PHARYNGITIS

Diagnostic Findings

Infants and toddlers with pharyngitis may manifest nonspecific irritability, poor feeding, anorexia, drooling, or oral lesions. Older children can verbalize and localize pain to the throat. Epiglottitis in the older child may present as the "worst" sore throat.

Respiratory symptoms, such as clear rhinorrhea, cough, hoarseness, or mucosal ulcers, suggest a viral etiology. Epstein-Barr virus and cytomegalovirus (CMV) infection often have associated pharyngeal inflammation, diffuse lymphadenopathy, and hepatosplenomegaly. Herpangina causes small vesicular lesions and punched-out ulcers in the posterior pharynx. Hand-foot-and-mouth disease causes vesicles and ulcers in the areas noted. Pharyngoconjunctival fever is characterized by low-grade fever, follicular conjunctivitis, sore throat, and cervical lymphadenopathy.

Headache, vomiting, abdominal pain, and scarlatiniform (fine, erythematous, sandpaper) rash are noted with streptococcal pharyngitis. Onset is typically acute, with fever, throat pain, and dysphagia. It most often occurs in late winter and early spring. Diphtheria presents as an adherent, grayish pharyngeal membrane with bull neck and toxic appearance. History of exposure to the tissue or secretions of infected small animals may suggest tularemia. Pharyngitis accompanied by rash, joint pain, and urethral or vaginal discharge may indicate gonorrhea. Asymptomatic carriage of gonorrhea is not unusual. Urticaria, wheezing, or stridor may indicate an allergic etiology.

Rapid detection of streptococci by latex agglutination or enzyme immunoassay is useful when positive. False positives with latex agglutination are uncommon (specificity, 88 to 100 percent), but false negatives occur frequently (sensitivity, 72 to 95 percent). A negative rapid screening test should be confirmed by a routine streptococcal culture using aerobic culture technique and sheep-blood medium with a bacitracin disk. Specific swabbing of tonsillar tissue yields the most success in detection of streptococci.

Local suppurative complications (severe dysphagia, stridor, dysphonia, and odynophagia) may require more aggressive diagnostic testing, such as soft tissue radiographs of the lateral neck and a CT scan of the neck. Surgical incision and drainage may be necessary.

A complete blood count, Epstein-Barr virus (EBV) titers (Monospot), syphilis screening tests, and cultures for *Neisseria gonorrhoeae* are indicated for atypical presentations. The presence of a positive gonococcal culture in a young child is a marker for sexual abuse and must be reported to the appropriate social service investigators. Additional studies may be useful in the seriously ill or immune-compromised patient in order to exclude nonsuppurative complications of streptococcal infection. These tests may include urinalysis, assessment of immunologic response to infection {anti-streptolysine-O (ASO), Streptozyme}, renal function tests, and electrocardiogram.

Complications

Suppuration can spread to contiguous tissue, causing peritonsillar abscess (quinsy), life-threatening Lemierre's "postanginal sepsis" (aerobic or anaerobic bacteremia from septic thrombophlebitis of the tonsillar vein), and Ludwig's angina (submandibular abscess). Hematologic spread may result in mesenteric adenitis, meningitis, brain abscess, cavernous sinus thrombosis, suppurative arthritis, endocarditis, osteomyelitis, sepsis, and septic embolization to the lung.

Nonsuppurative syndromes due to streptococcal infection include scarlet fever, rheumatic fever, and glomerulonephritis. Unrecognized gonococcal or syphilis infections can disseminate systemically. Untreated diphtheria may progress to seizures or respiratory failure.

Management

Antibiotics for streptococcal pharyngitis should generally be administered for a total of 10 days. Optimal initial management in areas of low rheumatic fever prevalence include oral penicillin, 250 mg twice a day for children under age 12 and 500 mg twice a day for children over age 12. Where poor compliance and follow-up are issues, intramuscular benzathine penicillin is given, 600,000 U for children under 60 lb and 1,200,000 U for children over 60 lb. Penicillin-allergic patients can be treated with erythromycin ethylsuccinate, 40 mg/kg/day in two to four doses daily for 10 days. Sulfa and tetracycline are not effective.

Indications for tonsillectomy for recurrent sore throats are controversial.

Other bacterial diseases require specific and supportive management. If diphtheria is suspected, diphtheria antitoxin is given along with penicillin or erythromycin. Tularemia requires streptomycin or gentamicin.

Allergic entities frequently require epinephrine, 1:1000, 0.01 mL/kg/dose, SQ. Antihistamines, such as diphenhydramine, 1.25 mg/kg/dose IM or PO and glucocorticoids such as prednisone, 2 mg/kg/dose PO, are also used.

PERITONSILLAR ABCESS

Peritonsillar abscess (quinsy) is the most common deep infection of the head and neck. Usually a complication of bacterial tonsillitis, it can also occur with EBV infection. Peritonsillar abscess is rare in children under 12 years of age.

Diagnostic Findings

The history is usually of gradually increasing pharyngeal discomfort and ipsilateral otalgia, followed by trismus, dysarthria and, less commonly, dysphagia and odynophagia. Drooling is not unusual. The voice has a muffled, "hot potato" quality. Patients are often toxic.

Examination of the oropharynx may sufficiently distinguish peritonsillar cellulitis from an abscess. Cellulitis is commonly associated with diffuse swelling and edema in the peritonsillar region. An abscess causes varying degrees of trismus due to a peritonsillar mass effect with displacement of the soft palate medially and the uvula contralaterally. Fluctuance can frequently be palpated. There is usually ipsilateral cervical adenopathy.

The white blood cell count may be elevated. The throat culture will often document a streptococcal infection. Blood and tonsillar aspirate cultures are useful for directing antibiotic therapy. A CT of the head and neck is vital for delineating the extent of involvement if extension from the peritonsillar space is suspected and the patient is not responding to standard antibiotic therapy.

Differential Considerations

Peritonsillar abscess is sometimes difficult to distinguish from uncomplicated tonsillitis or peritonsillar cellulitis. Peritonsillar abscess may be confused with peripharyngeal space infections, cervical adenitis and abscess, foreign bodies, dental infections, tetanus, salivary gland infections, and tumors.

Complications

Extension beyond the peritonsillar space produces complications. Peripharyngeal extension may be heralded by spiking fevers, chills, neck stiffness and pain, torticollis toward the opposite side (from sternocleidomastoid spasm), and swelling around the parotid gland. Necrotizing fasciitis has been reported as a lethal complication. Airway obstruction, aspiration pneumonia, mediastinitis, lung abscess, thrombophlebitis, and sepsis have also been reported.

Management

Generally, patients will require hospitalization for hydration, intravenous antibiotics, analgesia, and surgical drainage, if indicated. Antibiotics usually include a third-generation cephalosporin, such as ceftriaxone (100 mg/kg/24 h q12h IV) or cefotaxime (150 mg/kg/24 h q8h IV). Many clinicians add penicillin G (25 to 50 mg/kg/24 h or 40,000 to 80,000 U/kg/24 h q4h IV) initially if the child is toxic. If resolution is slow, nafcillin 100 to 150 mg/kg/24h q4h IV (or equivalent) is started.

Needle aspiration is sometimes used diagnostically to differentiate between cellulitis and abscess. Some otolaryngologists employ needle aspiration therapeutically instead of incision and drainage in cooperative patients. Tonsillectomy, after the acute episode, is advocated by many but appears necessary only infrequently in children for recurrent problems or slow resolution of symptoms.

RETROPHARYNGEAL ABSCESS

Retropharyngeal abscess is a local accumulation of pus in the prevertebral soft tissue of the upper airway.

Complications

The most serious acute complications are airway obstruction and aspiration. The abscess may rupture into the esophagus, mediastinum, or lungs. Empyema and pneumonia can result. Blood vessels may be eroded, and hemorrhage can occur. Inadequate drainage can allow reformation of the abscess.

Management

The standard approach to airway maintenance is vital, since airway obstruction and aspiration can occur at any time. Patients will require hospitalization for hydration, intravenous antibiotics, analgesia, and surgical drainage. Antibiotics usually include penicillin G 25 to 50 mg (40,000 to 80,000 U)/kg/24 h q4h IV or nafcillin (or equivalent) 100 to 150 mg/kg/24 h q4h IV. A third-generation cephalosporin such as ceftriaxone (100 mg/kg/24 h q12h IV) or cefotaxime (150 mg/kg/24 h q8h IV) may also be added. Emergent surgical intervention and drainage are necessary, with particular attention to the airway and ventilation.

CERVICAL LYMPHADENOPATHY

Lymphadenopathy is enlargement of one or more lymph nodes. Benign lymph node enlargement and lymphadenitis account for most childhood neck masses.

Staphylococcus aureus and group A streptococci account for 60 to 85 percent of primary lymphadenitis in children. Less common etiologic agents include *Mycobacterium tuberculosis,* nontuberculous mycobacteria, and anaerobic bacteria. Rare causes include *Francisella tularensis* (tularemia), *Yersinia pestis* (plague), *Brucella melitensis* (brucellosis), *Chlamydia* species, *Mycoplasma* species, *Treponema pallidum* (syphilis), *Actinomyces israelii, Streptococcus pyogenes, Haemophilus influenzae, Pseudomonas aeroginosa,* and *Toxoplasma gondii* (toxoplasmosis).

Mucocutaneous lymph node syndrome (Kawasaki disease) is associated with aneurysmal dilatation of the coronary vessels. Early recognition and treatment can reduce mortality from this complication. The presence of cervical adenitis and fever for several days should prompt examination for other clinical findings of this syndrome: stomatitis, conjunctivitis, polymorphous exanthem, peripheral edema, and desquamation of the hands and feet.

Noninfectious causes of lymphadenopathy include traumatic soft tissue swelling, malignancy, congenital muscular torticollis, branchial cleft cyst, thyroglossal duct cyst, cystic hygroma, lymphangioma, and vascular abnormalities. Some developmental abnormalities are detected only after secondary infection occurs.

Diagnostic Findings

Time of symptom onset and clinical course should be clearly defined. History should include information about upper respiratory infection, concurrent sore throat, duration of symptoms, skin lesions of the scalp or face, fever, dental problems, pets, and exposure to tuberculosis or other infections.

The most useful differentiating finding in examination of an enlarged lymph node is the presence or absence of inflammation. A "hot" node presents with erythema, warmth, tenderness, and sometimes fluctuance. Examination of the scalp, teeth, neck, and tonsils often reveals a primary infection. "Cold" or apparently uninflamed nodes require a thorough search for associated disease such as cat-scratch disease, tuberculosis, nontuberculous mycobacterial infections, and malignancy. A painless, firm neck mass should be considered malignant until proven otherwise. A thorough otolaryngologic and systemic examination with detailed notation of all lymph nodes, including the axillae and groin, should be noted. If malignancy is suspected, a complete blood count with differential may reveal anemia, thrombocytopenia, or abnormal white blood count with immature cells.

If tuberculosis is suspected, a 5-TU PPD skin test should be placed intradermally on the volar aspect of the forearm. If anergy is suspected, a control skin test should be placed on the contralateral volar forearm. Nontuberculous mycobacteria may weakly react to PPD.

Spontaneously draining nodes provide an excellent opportunity for culture. In the immunocompromised patient in the neonate, or when antibiotic therapy has failed, the abscess material should be cultured for aerobic and anaerobic bacteria, mycobacteria, and fungi.

Differential Diagnosis

Regional lymph node enlargement can be a response to tonsillitis, peritonsillar abscess, dental pathology, scalp trauma or infection, ear disease, or other antigenic stimulation in the head and neck. Second, cervical lymphadenopathy may be a manifestation of systemic disease. Mononucleosis (frequently); sarcoidosis, tuberculosis, or Kawasaki's disease (less commonly); and toxoplasmosis, syphilis, and other systemic diseases (rarely) can cause inflammatory changes in the cervical lymph nodes. If neither a site of inflammation in the head and neck nor evidence of systemic disease can be detected, primary lymph node enlargement should be suspected.

Management

As always, life-threatening respiratory and cardiovascular compromise should be treated first.

If primary lymph node infection is suspected and the child has been in an endemic area or has been exposed to tuberculosis, a 5-TU PPD skin test and a suitable control to exclude anergy should be placed. Historical or clinical clues may suggest an unusual microbiotic etiology. Specific antigenic skin tests are available for some of the nontuberculous mycobacteria, but culture is the only reliable means of confirming the diagnosis. Tuberculosis is treated by medical means, but nontuberculous mycobacterial infections usually require complete node excision.

"Hot" or suppurative nodes are most commonly caused by group A beta-hemolytic streptococci (*S. pyogenes*) and penicillin-resistant *S. aureus.* A majority of the staphylococcal species are resistant to penicillin. A semisynthetic penicillin such as dicloxacillin is the drug of choice, but the greater palatability of cephalexin and amoxicillin-clavulanic acid make them superior choices. Erythromycin should be considered when cost is a concern.

Toxic appearance, advanced disease, young age, unreliable follow-up, unresponsiveness to oral therapy, immunocompromised host, or inability to tolerate oral medications may make outpatient therapy impractical. Inpatient management should include a semisynthetic penicillin, such as intravenous oxacillin. A short course of intravenous antibiotics may bring enough improvement to allow completion of therapy on an outpatient basis.

The therapy of "cold" lymphadenopathy is determined by the disease process.

Follow-up in 2 to 3 days is helpful to assess the progress of therapy, read skin tests if placed, and observe for fluctuance. If fluctuance occurs or if the patient is unresponsive to optimal medical management, surgical consultation should be requested. Incision and drainage of the nodes by the emergency physician should be avoided, since a persistent draining sinus can result, especially when the infection is caused by nontuberculous mycobacteria. Distinction between bacterial and mycobacterial disease by physical examination is not reliable. Total surgical excision of the node is curative, prevents a draining sinus, and allows a clear etiologic diagnosis. Suspected embryonic remnants should be evaluated by a surgeon for possible excision.

Children with suspected malignancy should be followed very closely by an otolaryngologist. In a review of 178 pediatric cases of malignant head and neck tumors, one of six malignant neck masses had an associated nasopharyngeal tumor. If questions about follow-up exist or if the patient appears toxic, further evaluation and treatment should be completed on an inpatient basis.

For a more detailed discussion, see Abrunzo TJ, Santamaria JP: Emergencies of the oral cavity and neck, chap. 67, p. 411, in *Pediatric Emergency Medicine: A Comprehensive Study Guide.*

Section XII
Eye Emergencies

68 | Eye Emergencies

Katherine M. Konzen

Children with eye problems present in many ways and may appear impressively disfigured. The physician must remember certain important guidelines when facing the patient with ocular disease.

1. The cardinal rules of resuscitation—airway, breathing, circulation—must be remembered. In a patient with multiple trauma or severe systemic disease, the life-threatening conditions must be evaluated and managed first. The eye must be protected from further damage.
2. A thorough and complete history is taken. Has the child had previous eye problems or surgeries? Does he or she have underlying health problems? Does he or she wear glasses or contact lenses? If the injury was caused by trauma, when and where did it occur? Who saw it? What type of instrument was involved? Who else was involved? What was done for the patient prior to arrival in the emergency department? In the absence of trauma, is eye pain present? Has there been eye discharge or exposure to others with similar conditions? Has there been use of systemic or topical medications?
3. The visual acuity in both eyes must always be checked. Information about the unaffected eye can help guide the assessment of the affected eye.
4. The emergency physician should begin with a general physical examination and build rapport with the child while looking for other underlying injuries or signs of systemic illness. The eye examination is performed in a logical, methodical manner. Toys or other objects that hold the child's interest are useful and allow proper evaluation of the visual fields. The eye is touched and dilated only after a thorough systemic examination, and only if indicated.
5. All of the possibilities must be considered before the eye is manipulated. If the possibility of a globe perforation exists, the eye must not be touched. If there is concomitant head trauma, the pupils must not be dilated.

6. The emergency physician must know when to stop and consult an ophthalmologist.

PHYSICAL EXAMINATION OF THE EYE AND DIFFERENTIAL CONSIDERATIONS

A thorough and systematic eye examination is divided into six major categories: vision, lids and orbit, anterior segment, pupils and extraocular movements, posterior segment, and intraocular pressure.

Vision

Some method of testing visual acuity must be available for both the preverbal and the verbal child. For the very young child, the ability to focus on an object such as a toy may give a rough assessment of visual acuity. For the older child, Snellen letters or Allen figures are useful to check visual acuity in both eyes. Vision can be impaired from any obstruction of the visual pathway.

Lids and Orbit

The lids are examined by noting the ability to raise and lower them and noting any erythema, edema, lacerations, or ecchymosis. Children with periorbital cellulitis will often have significant edema and erythema of both the upper and lower eyelids. The upper lid must be everted to rule out the presence of a foreign body by firmly grasping the lashes at the lid margin and everting the lid against countertraction at the superior tarsal margin, using a cotton-tipped applicator.

Examination of the orbit includes palpation for defects in the orbital bony structure or for subcutaneous emphysema. Orbital fractures are often accompanied by ecchymosis, lid swelling, proptosis, and limitation in extraocular movements. Sinus fractures may be associated with subcutaneous emphysema. The presence of exophthalmos or enophthalmos is noted.

Anterior Segment

The sclera and conjunctiva are inspected for swelling, erythema, foreign bodies, hemorrhage, or discharge. Diseases of the cornea and conjunctiva are divided into two main categories, infection and trauma. In North America, the most common corneal infection causing permanent visual impairment is herpes simplex. Throughout the rest of the world, the most common agent is trachoma. Traumatic injuries to the cornea should be considered in even the youngest of children. Fluorescein examination for a corneal abrasion may be appropriate during the initial examination. The corneal light reflex is evaluated for both briskness and adequacy of response. Self-inflicted thermal wounds from curling irons, microwave popcorn bags, or other mechanisms should be thoroughly evaluated.

Acute iritis (anterior uveitis) is rare in children and may be associated with juvenile rheumatoid arthritis or sarcoidosis. The possibility of iritis should be considered in a child who presents with sudden unilateral onset of pain, photophobia, and redness. Infections of the uvea can be caused by bacteria, fungi, viruses, or helminths. Measles, mumps, and pertussis may be associated with a uveitis; however, this is not due to direct invasion of the infectious agent, but rather to some other mechanism.

Trauma can cause damage to the anterior chamber. A hyphema occurs when there is hemorrhage into the anterior chamber. Hyphemas can cause considerable damage to the eye and must be managed by an ophthalmologist. The iris should be evaluated for shape and contour. Under penlight or direct ophthalmoscopic examination, the lens should be clear. If opacification is present, cataracts should be considered. Depending on the type of trauma, cataract formation can occur within days or years of injury. Either infection or injury to the anterior chamber can lead to increased intraocular pressure. Glaucoma can manifest itself any time after an insult to the eye. Pain and blurred vision should suggest the possibility of glaucoma. Tonometry can help to make the diagnosis.

Pupils and Extraocular Movements

Pupils should be black, round, symmetrical, and equally reactive to light. Changes in the anterior chamber, lens, or vitreous may result in a pupil that is not black. A ruptured globe or intracranial process can lead to pupil asymmetry. Pupillary assessment includes evaluation for an afferent pupillary defect known as a Marcus Gunn pupil, in which pupillary constriction is delayed and diminished in both eyes when light is shone into the affected eye as compared to the normal eye. A Marcus Gunn pupil is evidence of injury to the anterior visual system and is a poor prognostic sign. Extraocular movements in all visual fields are assessed and deficits clearly noted.

Posterior Segment

The posterior segment comprises the vitreous, retina, and optic nerve. The direct ophthalmoscope can be used to examine for papilledema, hemorrhages, retinal detachment, and intraocular foreign bodies. Chronic conditions including uveitis can cause deposits in the vitreous. Endophthalmitis (infections inside the eye) may result from a penetrating injury, worsening superficial infection, or surgery. Children will present with unilateral severe pain in or around the eye and compromised vision. Purulent exudate in the vitreous will show up as a greenish color on the ophthalmoscopic examination. Often a hypopyon (pus in the anterior chamber) is seen.

Blunt or penetrating trauma to the eye can lead to a vitreous hemorrhage. Other causes of hemorrhage include diabetes mellitus, hypertension, sickle cell disease, leukemia, retinal tears, central retinal vein occlusion, and tumor. Presentation of these patients is usually due to sudden loss of vision or diminished vision.

Retinal artery and retinal vein obstruction are relatively uncommon in the pediatric population. Etiologies include trauma and other systemic entities. Retinal artery occlusion can be due to emboli in patients with endocarditis or systemic lupus erythematosus or can result from hypercoagulability in patients with sickle cell disease. When central retinal artery occlusion occurs, there is sudden, painless loss of vision in one eye. Ophthalmoscopic examination reveals the cherry-red spot of the fovea, a pale optic nerve, and markedly narrowed arteries. A Marcus Gunn pupil may be present. Ophthalmologic consultation must be immediate.

Retinal vein obstruction also leads to sudden, painless loss of vision, which varies depending on the extent of the obstruction. Retinal hemorrhages and a blurred, reddened optic disk may be seen. Arteries are often narrowed, veins are distended, and there may be white exudates. Retinal vein obstruction can occur in trauma as well as leukemia, cystic fibrosis, and retinal phlebitis.

Retinal tears can lead to vitreous hemorrhage, causing diminished vision in the affected eye. Retinal detachment may take years to develop after a tear. As the detachment progresses, patients may have a visual field deficit or may complain of lightning flashes in the affected eye. Ophthalmoscopic examination will reveal a lighter-appearing retina in the area of detachment.

The optic nerve is responsible for the transmission of visual information to the cortex. Disruptions in this transmission can lead to visual loss. Optic neuritis is usually due to inflammation or demyelination. It is characterized by an abrupt, rapid, unilateral loss of vision, while pain is variable. Rarely does optic neuritis present as a separate entity in children. Most often it is caused by meningitis, viral infections, encephalomyelitis, and demyelinating diseases. Lead poisoning and long-term chloramphenicol therapy are other known culprits.

Various toxins have been associated with impaired vision. Most act on the ganglion cells of the retina or optic nerve, causing visual defects. Methyl alcohol can cause sudden, permanent blindness. Other recognized toxins include sulfanilamide, quinine, quinidine, and halogenated hydrocarbons.

Finally, one must consider that visual loss can result from faulty conductance to the visual cortex of the brain. Head trauma, hypoglycemia, leukemia, cerebrovascular accidents, and anesthetic accidents can all be associated with cortical blindness.

Intraocular Pressure

If acute glaucoma is of concern, intraocular pressure is measured. This should not be undertaken, however, if the possibility of a ruptured globe exists. Accurate measurement is accomplished by slit-lamp tonometry or a hand-held tonometer. In a patient with acute glaucoma, rough tactile measurement of intraocular pressure can be made by gentle palpation of the globes with the fingers through the eyelids. An extremely firm eye can easily be detected.

ERRORS TO AVOID

In managing eye emergencies, some common mistakes to be avoided include forgetting to examine the unaffected eye, not thoroughly examining the injured eye, failing to consider and recognize globe perforation, overprescribing topical anesthetics and steroids, using eyedrops or ointment when a perforation exists, and failing to ensure proper follow-up for the patient.

COMMON EYE COMPLAINTS

The Red Eye

History is extremely important in differentiating the etiology of the red eye. Although conjunctivitis is very common in childhood, other etiologies must be thoroughly considered prior to arriving at the diagnosis. Time of onset, exposure to chemicals or noxious stimuli, exposure to other children with similar problems, presence of systemic illness, history of trauma, photophobia, and excessive tearing are all important in the consideration of the differential diagnosis.

Eye Pain

Eye pain often can be difficult to characterize in the younger child. Superficial eye pain is frequently associated with epithelial abnormalities such as a corneal abrasion, whereas deep eye pain is more often associated with increased intraocular pressure or uveitis. Eye pain associated with burning makes one consider dry eyes, allergies, or irritation secondary to chemicals or noxious stimuli. Pain caused by bright light is associated with iritis, uveitis, and glaucoma.

Eye pain in children results from a variety of causes, including corneal abrasions, conjunctivitis, episcleritis, acute dacrocystitis, congenital glaucoma, uveitis, optic neuritis, hordeolum, herpes zoster, and a wide array of trauma. One must attempt to characterize the pain and then thoroughly search for the underlying etiology.

Excessive Tearing

Usually noted in infants, excessive tearing can be due to nasolacrimal obstruction or be secondary to bacterial, viral, or allergic conjunctivitis. Sometimes an infant with a corneal abrasion or glaucoma will present with tearing.

Eye Discharge

Purulent eye discharge is most often associated with bacterial conjunctivitis. Viral and allergic conjunctivitis are more often associated with mucoid discharge. Patients with blepharitis have crusting in addition to the discharge.

NONTRAUMATIC EYE DISORDERS

Eyelid Infections

Eyelid infections are frequent throughout childhood. The glands of Zeis are sebaceous glands that are attached directly to the hair follicles; the meibomian glands are sebaceous glands that extend through the tarsal plate. Eyelid infections (blepharitis) often involve one of these glands. The most common infections of the eyelid include chalazion, hordeolum, impetigo contagiosa, and herpes simplex.

Clinical Findings

A chalazion is a lipogranuloma of the meibomian gland. It presents as a painless, hard nodule and is often located in the midportion of the tarsus, away from the lid border; it is caused by obstruction of the gland's duct. Chalazions are uncommon during infancy but frequently occur during childhood. A hordeolum or style is a purulent staphylococcal infection in the glands of Zeis. Initially, the swelling may be diffuse, but it usually becomes a localized swelling of the lid margin. Impetigo contagiosa is a pyoderma that usually presents with vesicles, then develops a yellowish crust, which occurs due to local invasion by staphylococci or streptococci.

In patients with impetigo, there can often be an underlying seborrheic dermatitis. Herpes simplex can present on the eyelids of children and can lead to latent infection, which may persist throughout life and be reactivated. Recurrent infection often involves the cornea. Herpetic blepharitis is characterized by the formation of vesicles, which break down and form a yellowish crusted surface.

Differential Diagnosis

The differential diagnosis of a chalazion includes rhabdomyosarcoma, capillary hemangiomas, dermoids, orbital cysts, molluscum contagiousum, sarcoidosis, fungal infections, foreign bodies, and juvenile xanthogranuloma. Differentiation is made by lack of response to local therapy and/or biopsy.

The differential diagnosis of a hordeolum includes contact dermatitis and allergic conjunctivitis. Itching is a more prominent feature in the latter two entities and is not usually associated with a hordeolum.

Impetigo contagiosa and herpes simplex can be easily confused. Cultures should be obtained to ascertain etiology.

Management

Chalazions are usually treated with warm compresses and antistaphylococcal antibiotic ointment (erythromycin ophthalmic ointment or polymixin B sulfate) or ophthalmic drops. Antibiotic treatment should continue for several days after rupture of the chalazion to prevent recurrence. If there is a lack of response to medical treatment, surgical incision and drainage under general anesthesia is recommended for younger children.

Treatment of hordeolums is similar to that for chalazions. Recurrence commonly results from autoinoculation and inattention to good hygiene.

Impetigo contagiosa should be treated with removal of crusts and local antistaphylococcal/antistreptococcal antibiotics. A cotton-tipped applicator soaked in baby shampoo can be used to clean the lid margins. Bacitracin ophthalmic ointment is often effective; however, topical erythromycin and gentamicin can be used. If systemic impetigo is present, oral antibiotics should be initiated.

Herpes simplex blepharitis should be treated with vidarabine ophthalmic ointment and trifluorothymidine topical drops. Topical and oral acyclovir should be considered but may be of limited value. Treatment of herpes simplex will be discussed in further detail in the sections that follow.

Cellulitis of the Periorbital and Orbital Region

Periorbital infections are common in childhood and usually resolve with appropriate therapy and without sequelae.

Periorbital infections, particularly sinusitis, may cause infection or severe inflammation in the orbital tissues, leading to a preseptal or orbital cellulitis. The proximity of the paranasal sinuses to the orbital walls and the interconnection between the venous system of the orbit and the face allow infection to spread from the sinuses to the orbit, either directly or via the bloodstream. The orbital venous system is devoid of valves, so that two-way communication with the venous system of the nose, face, and pterygoid fossa is allowed. The superior and inferior ophthalmic veins drain directly from the orbit and empty into the cavernous sinus. Orbital and facial infections can lead to cavernous venous thrombosis. The orbital periosteum and septum are important anatomic structures that help to limit direct spread of infection. The orbital periosteum acts as a barrier to the spread of infection from the sinuses; however, it may become eroded if a periorbital abscess develops. The orbital septum may also limit the spread of infection from the preseptal space to the orbit.

The following classification for orbital infections has been described:

Class 1. Periorbital or Preseptal Cellulitis

Cellulitis is confined to the anterior lamella tissue due to a lack of flow through the ethmoid drainage vessels. Lid edema and erythema may be mild or severe. The globe ordinarily is not involved, so that vision and function remain normal.

Class 2. Orbital Cellulitis

Orbital tissue is infiltrated with bacteria and cells that extend through the septum into the orbital fat and other tissues. Manifestations usually include proptosis, impaired or painful movement, and periocular pain. Visual acuity may be impaired, and septicemia may be present.

Class 3. Subperiosteal Abscess

Purulent material collects between the periosteum and the orbital wall. Medial wall involvement causes the globe to be displaced inferiorly or laterally. Symptoms include edema, chemosis, and tenderness with ocular movement; vision loss and proptosis vary in severity.

Class 4. Orbital Abscess

When pus accumulates within the orbital fat inside or outside the muscle cone, an orbital abscess has developed. The infectious process becomes localized and encapsulated, unlike orbital cellulitis, which tends to be more diffuse. Exophthalmos, chemosis, ophthalmoplegia, and visual impairment are generally severe; systemic toxicity may be impressive.

Class 5. Cavernous Sinus Thrombosis

This results from extension of an orbital infection into the cavernous sinus. Nausea, vomiting, headache, fever, pupillary dilation, and other systemic signs may be present. There is marked lid edema and early onset of third, fourth, and sixth cranial nerve palsies.

Clinical Findings

Most of the clinical findings are described with each class of infection. Preseptal or periorbital cellulitis is marked by periorbital edema, erythema, and tenderness but is not accompanied by proptosis, ophthalmoplegia, or loss of visual acuity. Chemosis and conjunctivitis may be present, as well as fever and leukocytosis. In young children who present with fever and other systemic signs, a lumbar puncture and intravenous antibiotics should be considered because of the possibility of underlying meningitis. In younger children, *Haemophilus influenzae* type B can produce a distinctive type of bluish-purple hue in the eyelid. It is often accompanied by fever, irritability, otitis media, and bacteremia.

Patients with orbital cellulitis present similarly but have further development of ophthalmoplegia, proptosis, pain on eye movement, worsening chemosis, and changes in vision. Fever and leukocytosis are often seen. If the orbital cellulitis is secondary to sinusitis, then headache, rhinorrhea, and swelling of the nasal mucosa may also be present.

At times, swelling of the eyelid may be so severe that further evaluation is necessary. Computed tomography (CT) has been useful in distinguishing periorbital cellulitis from orbital cellulitis but has its limitations in making a definitive diagnosis of a subperiosteal abscess from reactive subperiosteal edema.

Management

In patients with very mild periorbital cellulitis and no history of fever or other systemic illness, a thorough physical examination is recommended, but laboratory investigation may be unnecessary. Mild cases of preseptal cellulitis due to local trauma or a conjunctivitis can be treated with oral antibiotics covering activity against *Staphylococcus aureus.* For cellulitis secondary to bug bites, oral antihistamines and warm compresses may also be helpful. Close follow-up is mandatory.

For patients requiring hospitalization, a complete blood count, blood cultures, lumbar puncture, and CT of the head may be warranted.

The following management scheme has been recommended by several authors:

1. All patients hospitalized for orbital inflammation should receive opthalmologic and otolaryngologic consultation.
2. Broad-spectrum antimicrobial therapy should be instituted at once while blood or intraoperative culture results are awaited.
3. Attempts must be made to determine whether the cellulitis is of preseptal or postseptal origin. Computed tomography of the head is a helpful diagnostic aid but cannot make the definitive diagnosis.
4. Surgical indications include diminishing visual acuity, lack of improvement despite adequate antibiotics, or spiking fevers suggesting possible development of orbital abscess or cavernous venous thrombosis.

Posttraumatic suppurative cellulitis is treated by early incision and drainage of the infected space, coupled with parenteral antibiotics. Tetanus prophylaxis should be considered. Sufficient coverage for *S. aureus* and *Streptococcus pyogenes* is necessary. Anaerobic coverage should be instituted following animal and human bites. Intravenous antibiotics are recommended for a minimum of 48 to 72 h, after which consideration of oral therapy may be appropriate.

Children below 5 years of age without a history of trauma should be placed on appropriate coverage against *H. influenzae* type B, *Streptococcus pneumonia,* and group A beta-hemolytic streptococci. A third-generation cephalosporin is ideal for this particular situation. Children above age 5 do not generally require coverage for *Haemophilus*; antimicrobials should be similar to those used for the treatment of severe sinusitis.

Orbital cellulitis secondary to sinusitis should be managed with the consultation of ophthalmology and otolaryngology. Intravenous antibiotics should consist of a third-generation cephalosporin and a penicillinase-resistant penicillin. If the potential for an anaerobic infection exists, clindamycin may be substituted for the penicillinase-resistant penicillin. Frequent ophthalmologic examination with thorough clinical reassessment is warranted to determine response to treatment and need for surgical intervention.

Complications

In addition to the previously mentioned complications of cavernous venous thrombosis and meningitis, blindness has been associated with postseptal cellulitis. In the preantibiotic era, up to 20 percent of patients with postseptal inflammation developed blindness. Alarmingly, recent studies report a 10 percent incidence of blindness resulting from orbital complications of sinusitis. Clearly, broad-spectrum antibiotics and modern surgical techniques have not totally alleviated this devastating complication. In fact, negative or equivocal CT findings have often contributed to an inappropriate delay in surgical intervention. Computed tomography of the head alone cannot determine patient management; clinical judgment must prevail.

Scleritis and Episcleritis

Scleritis is uncommon but can be associated with juvenile rheumatoid arthritis or various infectious processes, including herpes simplex, varicella zoster, mumps, syphilis, and tuberculosis. Most patients present with severe eye pain.

The thin vascular membrane between the sclera and the conjunctiva is called the episclera. Inflammation of this area produces some irritation, but not the severe pain associated with scleritis. Episcleritis is also associated with a variety of diseases, including varicella zoster, syphilis, Henoch-Schönlein purpura, erythema multiforme, and penicillin sensitivity. Episcleritis often presents as a distinct area of injected conjunctiva with dilated vessels in the involved layer of tissue. Differentiation may be helped by the administration of topical phenylephrine, as it constricts vessels dilated by conjunctivitis but not those vessels involved in scleritis or episcleritis. Management consists of treating the underlying disease and some combination of oral nonsteroidal anti-inflammatory agents, topical glucocorticoids, and cycloplegics.

Ophthalmia Neonatorum

Conjunctivitis in the newborn period (first 28 days of life) is not uncommon. Because of the potential complications from ocular infections in infancy, neonates presenting with symptoms mandate a thorough evaluation. Important guidelines for evaluation include the following:

1. A detailed maternal history must be obtained, including prenatal care, history of or exposure to venereal disease, duration of rupture of membranes, type of delivery, agent used for ocular prophylaxis at birth, recent exposures to someone with conjunc-

tivitis, and timing of onset of symptoms. History should also include a description of excessive tearing, type and amount of exudate, and elucidation of systemic signs of illness in the baby, such as fever, vomiting, irritability, or lethargy.
2. Physical examination must be thorough, including a comprehensive eye examination searching for evidence of eyelid erythema, edema, discharge, corneal ulceration, globe perforation, or foreign body. In addition, the general physical examination must be complete; special attention must focus on the skin and the respiratory and genitourinary systems for evidence of concomitant systemic involvement.
3. Conjunctival scrapings should be obtained for Gram stain, Giemsa stain, and viral and bacterial cultures, including *Neisseria.* A rapid antigen test is sensitive and specific for *Chlamydia* and can be obtained easily from the conjunctiva. Culture is usually not necessary.

Differential Diagnosis

Chemical Conjunctivitis Chemical conjunctivitis caused by silver nitrate drops in the immediate newborn period occurs in almost 10 percent of newborns. Signs of this type of conjunctivitis include bilateral conjunctival hyperemia and mild discharge, which begin in the first 24 h of life and usually subside within 48 h. Gram stain reveals no organisms and only a few white blood cells. The inflammation is typically quite mild and does not require intervention.

Chlamydial Infection Chlamydia infections (*Chlamydia trachomatis*) have a typical incubation period of 1 to 2 weeks but can occur earlier if there was premature rupture of membranes. The overall incidence of chlamydial ophthalmia is approximately 20 to 40 cases per 1000 births annually. The prevalence of chlamydial infections in pregnant women ranges from 2 to 23 percent; transmission rates from infected mothers range from 23 to 70 percent. Typically, the conjunctiva becomes hyperemic and edematous, with the palpebral conjunctiva more involved than the bulbar conjunctiva. Unilateral purulent involvement is characteristic. Neonates may also have evidence of a concomitant otitis media or pneumonia. Samples are obtained by scraping the palpebral conjunctiva of the lower lid. The diagnosis is confirmed by identification of chlamydial antigen, detection of intracellular inclusions from the Giemsa stain, or isolation of the organism. Antigen detection tests are rapid, sensitive, and specific and are the most efficient means of confirming the diagnosis. Gram stain is not helpful.

Management

Systemic therapy is absolutely essential in the treatment of this condition. The treatment of choice is oral erythromycin (40 to 50 mg/kg/day) for a 2- to 3-week course to eliminate both conjunctival and nasopharyngeal colonization. Administration of a topical agent is unnecessary. Since *Chlamydia* is the most frequent sexually transmitted disease, prevention by detection in the mother prior to delivery is essential. Early studies suggested that the administration of erythromycin ointment prophylaxis in newborns was effective in preventing chlamydial conjunctivitis but not in altering the rate of development of pneumonia or nasopharyngeal infection. Recent studies have revealed that neonatal ocular prophylaxis with erythromycin does not reduce the incidence of chlamydial conjunctivitis. Chlamydial conjunctivitis can lead to chronic changes of conjunctival scarring and micropannus formation. Fortunately, these long-term ocular sequelae are quite rare.

Bacterial conjunctivitis The role of other bacteria in the newborn period is not quite as clear. Conjunctivitis can be caused by *S. aureus, Haemophilus* spp, *S. pneumoniae,* and enterococci. Many studies have also shown that these bacteria, in addition to *Corynebacterium, Proprionibacterium, Lactobacillus,* and *Bacteroides,* can be normal flora. Typically, the conjunctiva is red and edematous, with some amount of exudate. Diagnosis is made by Gram stain and culture. Broad-spectrum topical antimicrobial therapy is initiated, although there are no good studies in this population to document the necessity or efficacy of topical therapy. If cultures have been obtained, antimicrobial therapy can be tailored to treat the offending organism. Untreated cases of bacterial conjunctivitis could potentially progress to corneal ulceration, perforation, endophthalmitis, and septicemia.

Gonococcal ophthalmia neonatorum With the appearance of antibiotics and postnatal prophylaxis, the current incidence in the United States is thought to be 2 to 3 cases per 10,000 live births. The mean incubation period is 6.5 days, with a range of 1 to 31 days. Gonococcal ophthalmia neonatorum classically presents as a purulent, bilateral conjunctivitis. Conjunctival hyperemia, chemosis, eyelid edema, and erythema may also be seen. This entity is diagnosed by Gram stain, revealing gram-negative intracellular diplococci. Cultures should be sent immediately on blood and chocolate agar because the organisms die rapidly at room temperature. Cultural growth usually occurs within 2 days. Infants with conjunctivitis may have other manifestations of localized disease, including rhinitis, anorectal infection, arthritis, and meningitis. Neonates with suspected gonococcal conjunctivitis or any neonate with fever and conjunctivitis should have a sepsis evaluation, including a lumbar puncture.

Management

Treatment must be systemic; there is no role for oral or topical antibiotics. Neonates without meningitis should be treated for 7 days with either ceftriaxone or cefotaxime. If meningitis is present, treatment continues for 10 to 14 days. If the organism is sensitive to penicillin, penicillin G can be substituted. Treatment must also include frequent saline irrigation of the eyes. Parents should be screened for gonococcal disease. An infant born to a mother with known active gonococcal infection should receive one dose of ceftriaxone immediately after delivery.

Herpes Simplex Most neonates with herpes simplex become colonized during the birth process. Neonatal herpes simplex may occasionally present first as conjunctivitis. The onset is generally 2 to 14 days after birth. Characteristics are not clinically distinctive; however, unilateral or bilateral epithelial dendrites are virtually diagnostic. Fluorescein staining reveals these defects. It is important to obtain a parental history of herpes. Often conjunctivitis leads to further disseminated infections, which carry a high morbidity and mortality rate. The conjunctivitis can be diagnosed with conjunctival scrapings, looking for multinucleated giant cells and intranuclear inclusions. A fluorescent antibody test should be obtained, followed by a viral culture.

Management

Treatment should consist of intravenous acylovir for 10 days and topical trifluorothymidine. Parents must be aware of the high risk of recurrence of keratitis later in life; an ophthalmologist ought to follow these children closely. Recurrences are treated with topical therapy alone. Neonatal herpes simplex can lead to the development of keratitis, cataracts, chorioretinitis, and optic neuritis, in addition to numerous other ocular problems. Long-term follow-up studies have shown that more than 90 percent of neonates with neurologic sequelae from herpes simplex infection also have some type of ocular abnormality.

Viral Etiologies (Nonherpetic)

Other viral causes of conjunctivitis in neonates are infrequent. Conjunctivitis in a sibling or parent is the most likely source of infection. Hands or other fomites are the modes of transmission. Diagnosis is made by history of recent exposure and clinical findings. Usually infections are self-limited; often topical antimicrobials are prescribed to avoid secondary infection, but they are probably of limited value. Education regarding hand-washing and nonsharing of washcloths and towels is necessary.

Obstructed Nasolacrimal Duct Congenital nasolacrimal duct obstruction is often recognized only when the infant presents with a history of recurrent ocular infections. The blockage is frequently caused by failure to canalize a membrane called the valve of Hasner, which is located at the lower end of the nasolacrimal duct. Affected infants often present with pooling of tears onto the lower lid and cheeks and maceration of the eyelids. When these infants cry, their tears fail to arrive at the external nares. It is important to differentiate nasolacrimal obstruction from congenital glaucoma. Congenital glaucoma presents with tearing, photophobia, and a cloudy, enlarged cornea. Redness is not a major feature of glaucoma. Conservative treatment consists of massaging the lacrimal sac, suppressive topical antimicrobials, and warm compresses. Probing of the nasolacrimal system is not recommended until after 1 year of age, because 95 percent of children younger than 13 months will experience spontaneous opening of the lacrimal duct.

Noninfectious Etiologies The differential diagnosis of the red eye in the neonate should also include noninfectious etiologies. Corneal abrasions can be detected in infants and may often be secondary to a scratch from the infant's fingernail. Conjunctival hyperemia may be present; fluorescein staining is diagnostic. Trauma to the eye during delivery can also cause a corneal abrasion or laceration. Foreign bodies are rare in the neonatal period but should be considered in the evaluation.

Conjunctivitis Beyond the Neonatal Period

Conjunctivitis is a frequently encountered entity in children. Considerations in management include the child's age, onset of conjunctivitis (acute being less than 2 weeks, chronic lasting longer than 2 weeks), previous history of conjunctivitis, trauma, type of eye discharge, unilateral or bilateral symptoms, photophobia, lacrimation, pain, change in visual acuity, previous history of herpes simplex, exposure to a contact with conjunctivitis, and associated systemic symptoms of fever, sore throat, or rash. It is crucial to differentiate conjunctivitis from more serious conditions. Conjunctivitis in older children is characterized by normal vision, a gritty sensation in the eye, diffuse injection, and exudate. Photophobia and lacrimation are not usually associated with conjunctivitis. Keratitis and iritis typically are associated with impaired vision, true pain, photophobia, and lacrimation. Clinically, viral conjunctivitis is difficult to distinguish from bacterial conjunctivitis. Marked exudate, severe injection, and lid matting are more typical of bacterial or chlamydial infections. Preauricular adenopathy is often associated with viral infections. Follicles on the palpebral conjunctivae are more indicative of viral or chlamydial infections.

Viral Conjunctivitis

Adenoviruses are the most common cause of viral conjunctivitis in children. There are a few clinical syndromes associated with this group of viruses, including pharyngoconjunctival fever, epidemic keratoconjunctivitis, and nonspecific follicular conjunctivitis. Pharyngoconjunctival fever is most common in children and is associated with an upper respiratory tract infection, regional lymphadenopathy, and fever. The illness is usually self-limited, lasting 1 to 2 weeks, and is due to serotypes 3, 4, and 7. Spread can occur by droplet transmission, although numerous epidemics have been linked to swimming pools. Epidemic keratoconjunctivitis is more common in the second to fourth decades of life and causes preauricular lymphadenopathy with diffuse superficial keratitis. Serotypes 3, 8, and 19 are associated. Instruments in eye clinics have been linked to its transmission.

Enteroviral infections from particular Coxsackie and echoviruses may cause conjunctivitis but are often associated with other clinical signs, including rash or aseptic meningitis. Acute hemorrhagic conjunctivitis is caused by enterovirus 70 or Coxsackie A 24 and also occurs in epidemics. Transmission is by direct contact, with an incubation of less than 2 days. Clinically, patients present with sudden onset of unilateral ocular redness, excessive tearing (epiphora), photophobia, pain, purulent discharge, and eyelid swelling, which develop in a span of 6 to 12 hours. The eye pain is typically a burning, foreign-body sensation, which is thought to be due to discrete patches of epithelial keratitis (diagnosed with fluorescein staining). In 80 percent of cases, the other eye becomes involved within 24 h. Most impressive are the subconjunctival hemorrhages associated with these viruses. They are usually located beneath the superior bulbar conjunctivae. Malaise, myalgias, fever, headache, and upper respiratory tract symptoms may also accompany the conjunctivitis. Conjunctival scrapings for a viral culture yield identification of the virus. Ophthalmologic sequelae are rare; less than 5 percent of cases develop a secondary bacterial conjunctivitis.

Management Treatment is symptomatic with cool compresses. Many physicians prescribe a topical antimicrobial to prevent secondary bacterial infection, but this practice has not been proven to be effective.

Herpes Simplex and Varicella Zoster

Vesicular lesions on the eyelid can be due to herpes simplex, varicella zoster, impetigo, or contact dermatitis. History and a general physical examination should aid in the diagnosis. Of all herpes simplex infections, less than 1 percent involve the eye. Infections are characterized by unilateral follicular conjunctivitis with vesicles localized to the eyelids. Preauricular lymphadenopathy is commonly present. Some 50 percent of the patients develop keratitis within 2 weeks. The virus remains latent in the sensory ganglion and lacrimal glands. Approximately 25 percent of all children will have recurrences; these usually begin with corneal involvement. Long-term complications include necrotizing stromal disease, diffuse retinitis, and scarring. In children, herpes simplex is the most common cause of severe corneal ulceration and is second only to trauma as a cause of corneal blindness.

Ocular involvement with varicella is relatively uncommon, occurring in less than 5 percent of cases. In chickenpox, the conjunctiva can become involved through two mechanisms. Eyelid vesicles can slough virus into the conjunctival cul-de-sac, or vesicle formation can take place on the conjunctival surface. Occasionally, the cornea is involved. Fluorescein staining of the cornea and conjunctiva is necessary.

Zoster is uncommon in children, with only 5 percent of all zoster occurring in children younger than 5 years of age. Zoster infections of the eye notably follow the distribution of the first division of the trigeminal nerve. Lesions are usually located on the forehead and upper eyelid.

Trifluorothymidine is the preferred agent for treatment of herpes simplex because of its increased solubility, diminished toxicity, and lack of viral resistance. Approximately 95 percent of the corneal ulcers treated with it are cured within 2 weeks; however, treatment should be extended for 1 additional week after resolution of the lesions. For herpetic eye lesions, systemic acyclovir is not recommended because the drug does not penetrate the avascular cornea.

Gonococcal Conjunctivitis

Gonococcal eye infections can occur in prepubertal children. A nonvenereal mode of transmission has been suggested. Certain patients have presented with a negative history and physical examination suggestive of abuse. Some of these patients have occasionally shared a bed with a parent. Interestingly, isolates collected from selected patients have identical sensitivities to that obtained from a parent. Intravenous antibiotics are still recommended for this age group.

Gonococcal conjunctivitis can occur in sexually active children and adolescents; the mode of transmission is similar to that in adults. Treatment may consist of either 1 g of ceftriaxone IM once plus saline irrigation or, alternatively, 1 g IM/IV for 5 days plus saline irrigation.

Allergic Conjunctivitis

Seasonal and Perennial Allergic Conjunctivitis Itching is frequently the hallmark of allergic conjunctivitis. Seasonal allergic conjunctivitis has its onset of symptoms in either the fall or the spring. Patients with sensitivity to grass have more symptoms in the spring, while individuals sensitive to ragweed have more symptoms in the fall. Patients often complain of bilateral itchy, watery eyes with a burning sensation. The conjunctivae are mildly inflamed, with varying degrees of edema. Perennial allergic conjunctivitis is a variant with symptoms on a year-round basis, and often allergens such as dust, mites, animal dander, and feathers are responsible for it. This conjunctivitis represents a type I hypersensitivity reaction.

Management

Treatment consists of a combination of topical vasoconstrictors, antihistamines, and glucocorticoids. Systemic antihistamines may be of some benefit. Cromolyn sodium has also been shown to be effective when used as a prophylactic agent.

Vernal Conjunctivitis Vernal keratoconjunctivitis is a rare condition mainly affecting children under the age of 10. It is common in warm, dry climates, and males have a 2:1 ratio of being affected. Often there is a significant history of atopy. The peak incidence is between April and August. Patients usually have a history of bilateral itching, foreign-body sensation, clear mucoid discharge, photophobia, and injection. The giant papillae involve the upper tarsal conjunctiva and consist of large "cobblestone" papillae. The pathophysiology is not entirely clear; IgE and IgG are thought to play a role. Treatment is the same as for seasonal allergic conjunctivitis.

Special Forms of Conjunctivitis

Patients with Stevens-Johnson syndrome may have severe conjunctival involvement. In the acute phase of the disease, the palpebral and ocular conjunctivae can scar together. Often goblet cells are lost in the conjunctival epithelium, and the mucous layer of tear film is lost. Since the mucous layer allows tear film to stick to the surface of the eye, the dry-eye state of Stevens-Johnson syndrome is characterized by abundant tears that do not cover the surface of the eye because they are unable to adhere to it. Treatment consists of a combination of topical lubricants and antibiotics.

A chronic blepharoconjunctivitis can be caused by *Pthirus pubis* when the eyelashes are infected by the nits or the bug itself. The only recognized lice to infect the eyelashes are pubic lice. Family members should be screened. The type of conjunctivitis seen with lice results from a hypersensitivity reaction. Systemic treatment of the organism is necessary for successful eradication. Eye ointments have been used for treatment because they are thought to paralyze and smother the lice. A cotton-tipped applicator should be used for debridement prior to the placement of the ointment.

Molluscum contagiosum can cause a conjunctivitis when the virus is shed into the eye. Typically, it causes a chronic conjunctivitis that does not respond to topical antimicrobials. The problem results from the virus protein, which is toxic to the eye. One may see lesions on the eyelids that are often buried between the eyelashes. Eradication of the virus requires that the lesions be opened with a needle and the central core of the umbilicated region removed. Bleeding into the core is considered definitive treatment.

Contact lenses can cause a conjunctivitis; this is particularly common in teenagers. Lens wear should be discontinued, and storage and cleaning solutions must be replaced to prevent further contamination. Corneal ulcers should always be considered in the patient who wears contact lenses and presents with a red eye. The patient should see an ophthalmologist.

Other systemic diseases presenting with eye findings that mimic a conjunctivitis include ataxia-telangiectasia, where large, tortuous vessels are noted on the bulbar conjunctivae. Conjunctival injection is also noted in Kawasaki syndrome, but exudate is absent. Patients with Lyme disease may develop an nonspecific conjunctivitis with or without eye pain.

Keratoconus

Keratoconus is a condition of unknown etiology characterized by thinning of the central cornea. It has been associated with conditions including atopy, aniridia, trisomy 21, Marfan syndrome, retinal dystrophies, Ehlers-Danlos syndrome, and congenital rubella. Thinning is usually manifested in adolescence and becomes progressive, sometimes leading to disruption of the deep layers of the cornea and rupture of Descemet's membrane. Presenting symptoms are corneal edema, blurry vision, and pain. Treatment consists of conservative management with hard contact lenses. Occasionally, corneal transplant must be considered.

Glaucoma

Childhood glaucoma is extremely rare but should be mentioned. Children can present with a red, teary, photophobic eye. The differential diagnosis includes uveitis and conjunctivitis. One should consider glaucoma in the diagnosis if there is a past history of eye trauma, retinopathy of prematurity, Marfan syndrome, or any systemic condition associated with eye inflammation. Secondary glaucoma can also occur in patients with neurofibromatosis, aniridia, Sturge-Weber syndrome, Lowe syndrome, chronic uveitis, and iridocorneal dysgenesis. Diagnosis is dependent on measuring the intraocular pressure, which can be difficult in children. Normal eye pressure in children ranges from 10 to 22 mmHg. An ophthalmologist must immediately be involved in the care and treatment of children with suspected glaucoma. Immediate medical management includes a combination of miotics, adrenergic agents, and carbonic anhydrase agents. Diamox is most often used at an oral dose of 15 mg/kg/day.

Leukocoria

A white spot on the pupil can be due to a congenital cataract, coloboma, retinopathy of prematurity, retinal dysplasia, congenital toxoplasmosis, old vitreous hemorrhage, retinoblastoma, or retinal detachment, in addition to a wide variety of other hereditary, developmental, inflammatory, and miscellaneous conditions. It is essential for a patient presenting with leukocoria to have a thorough fundoscopic examination by an ophthalmologist.

Aniridia

Aniridia presents as an apparent absence of the iris but has many variations. The pupil appears as large as the cornea, while the iris remains as a small residual structure. The patient's visual acuity is extremely poor due to macular hypoplasia; nystagmus and photophobia are often present. Two-thirds of patients have a hereditary autosomal dominant condition, while one-third of cases are sporadic. Approximately 20 percent of infants with sporadic aniridia develop a Wilms' tumor, other genitourinary defects, or mental retardation. Other ocular defects associated with aniridia include a displaced lens, cataracts, corneal epithelial dystrophy, and glaucoma.

For a more detailed discussion, see Konzen KM: Eye emergencies, chap. 68, p. 419, in *Pediatric Emergency Medicine: A Comprehensive Study Guide.*

Section XIII
Gynecologic and Obstetric Emergencies

69 Pediatric and Adolescent Gynecology

Michael Van Rooyen

Gynecologic problems are not uncommon in childhood and adolescence. The emergency physician must be familiar with the examination of the prepubertal patient as well as the sexually active adolescent.

THE GYNECOLOGIC EXAMINATION

Evaluation of Premenarchal Patients

The evaluation of prepubescent patients requires particular sensitivity to the emotional concerns of the patient and the family. Continuous reassurance during the examination is necessary, particularly in cases where sexual abuse is an issue. Children are best examined by placing them in either the frog-leg position or the prone knee-chest position. The child may be positioned on the mother's lap. In the frog-leg position, an assistant may help the examiner by supporting the buttocks from underneath to facilitate abdominal relaxation.

Inspection of the vagina focuses on identifying the normal perineal landmarks and evidence of congenital abnormalities, as well as signs of trauma, foreign bodies, lacerations, excoriation, skin lesions, or vaginal discharge. An otoscope may be used to check for vaginal lacerations or foreign bodies. If abdominal pain or an abdominal mass is suspected, a rectal examination may be helpful. A speculum examination is usually indicated in prepubertal children only when there is a question of trauma, and is best performed under anesthesia. A bimanual examination in prepubescent girls is not routinely indicated.

Vaginal cultures are obtained by gently swabbing the vaginal introitus or by lavaging the introitus with a small amount of saline. In suspected sexual misconduct, cultures for *Neisseria gonorrhoeae* and *Chlamydia trachomatis* are obtained, and slide preparations for *Trichomonas* may be indicated. Children with vaginal discharge may require a sample for wet mount and Gram stain to screen for candidal infections or bacterial vaginosis.

GYNECOLOGIC DISORDERS OF INFANCY AND CHILDHOOD

Congenital Vaginal Obstruction

Congenital obstruction of the vagina affects up to 0.1 percent of all full-term female infants. The most common etiology is imperforate hymen. Less common are vaginal atresia and transverse vaginal septum. In neonates with imperforate hymen, the hymenal ring occludes the vaginal opening and impairs the normal flow of mucoid secretions from the uterus. If the disorder is not detected, vaginal obstruction and uterine distension, termed *hydrocolpos,* may develop.

The patient with hydrocolpos may present with abdominal distension and bulging of the membrane that occludes the vaginal introitus. Another common complaint is abdominal pain associated with urinary retention. The child may develop constipation, detrusor spasm, and hydronephrosis. If congenital vaginal obstruction remains undiagnosed until puberty, the patient may present with noncyclic lower abdominal pain and amenorrhea. The obstructed flow of menstrual blood, termed *hematocolpos,* often presents with abdominal distension, urinary complaints, and a dark-blue, bulging introitus. The treatment of imperforate hymen is surgical.

Patients with transverse vaginal septum or vaginal atresia may present in a similar fashion. The evaluation of the complaint of vaginal outlet obstruction includes a search for associated congenital renal anomalies.

Labial Adhesions

Etiology

Labial adhesions, also called labial agglutination, represent a condition in which the epithelial tissue around the labia minora becomes fused to form labial syncytia. It is characterized by a thin midline film of tissue that connects both sides of the labia minora. The etiology of this disorder is unknown. The child is usually brought to the physician by the parents with the concern that the vagina is "closing." Adhesions are characterized by a vertical connecting line that forms a central seam or raphe.

Management

The treatment in asymptomatic girls is expectant, since the condition is usually self-limiting. In children with local recurrent irritation and adhesions, estrogen cream applied to the adhesions at bedtime for 3 to 4 weeks will usually facilitate labial opening. The cream is used only until separation has occurred, as prolonged use can lead to breast growth. Surgical separation is not effective, as adhesions will recur.

Prepubertal Vaginal Bleeding Due to Trauma

The most common cause of genital trauma in childhood is accidental injury due to a fall. Straddle-type injuries may lead to blunt or penetrating trauma to the vulvar region, depending on the mechanism of injury. Vaginal hematomas are common in blunt injuries to the perineum and are usually apparent on physical examination. Penetrating trauma to the perineum from falling on a sharp object requires careful evaluation to exclude injury to the urethra, rectum, and peritoneum. Significant abdominal pain may or may not be present.

Vaginal hematomas are treated conservatively with cool packs and sitz baths. Early gynecologic or surgical consultation should be considered in cases of vaginal laceration. Urinalysis and rectal examination are done to exclude the possibility of urethral or rectal involvement. General anesthesia may be required to fully explore the extent of a vaginal laceration.

Urethral Prolapse

Urethral prolapse is the protrusion of the urethral mucosa through the urethral meatus, producing red, edematous mucosa at the meatus. Most cases occur in African American children. Patients may present with painless vaginal spotting, dysuria, or hematuria. If left untreated, urethral prolapse may progress to mucosal thrombosis and necrosis.

Warm compresses or sitz baths are used to shrink the swelling of urethral tissue. Subsequent application of estrogen cream may encourage healing. Surgical management to excise redundant tissue may be required if the condition persists or the urethral tissue has become gangrenous.

TABLE 69-1 Tanner Stages

Stage	Breast	Pubic Hair
Stage 1 (prepubertal)	Elevation of papilla	No pubic hair
Stage 2	Age 9.8 to 10.5 years: Elevation of papilla and areolar diameter enlarged	Sparse hair on labia majora
Stage 3	Age 11.2 to 11.4 years: Enlargement without separation of breast and areola	Dark, coarse, curled hair over mons
Stage 4	Age 12.0 to 12.1 years: Secondary mound of areola and papilla above the breast	Adult-type hair, abundant, limited to mons
Stage 5	Age 13.7 to 14.6 years: Recession of areola to contour of the breast	Adult-type hair in quality and distribution

Precocious Puberty

Normal puberty occurs over a wide range of ages. Precocious puberty is defined as *the appearance of secondary sex characteristics before the age of 8, or the appearance of menarche before the age of 9.* The most common form of precocious puberty is idiopathic and simply represents early sexual development. True precocious puberty is secondary to premature maturation of the pituitary and results in both menstruation and ovulation. Pseudo-precocious puberty is not secondary to pituitary control, and menses may occur without ovulation.

Increased growth is often the first change in precocious puberty, followed by breast development and the appearance of pubic hair. Menarche may occur before the appearance of secondary sex characteristics. Precocious puberty can result in diminished stature due to early closure of epiphyseal plates. Familiarity with the Tanner staging criteria may be helpful to the emergency physician (Table 69-1).

Patients with suspected precocious puberty are referred to a pediatric endocrinologist to rule out McCune-Albright syndrome, ovarian tumors, and central nervous system disorders.

Genital Tract Infections in Children

Vulvovaginitis

Vulvovaginitis is the most common gynecologic problem in childhood and adolescence. Vaginitis can be produced by a variety of infections and irritants. The differential diagnosis in vaginitis varies with age. Childhood vaginitis may be manifested by vaginal discharge or minimal vaginal bleeding. Adolescents may have normal vaginal discharge, and the presence of vaginitis may be heralded by a change in discharge or pruritus and vulvar irritation.

Historical considerations include an overview of hygienic practices, the use of irritating soaps or constrictive clothing, underlying medical disorders, and the possibility of sexual abuse. The presence of pruritus and odor, the character and amount of discharge, and the patient's menstrual and sexual history should be assessed.

Most childhood vulvovaginitis is due to irritation of the vulva and secondary involvement of the lower third of the vaginal canal. Inadequate local hygiene in the young child is the most common predisposing factor in nonspecific vulvovaginitis. Vaginal cultures will yield mixed nongonorrheal bacteria. Treatment includes antimicrobial therapy when indicated and encouraging proper hygiene and preventative measures (Table 69-2).

Vaginal foreign bodies may cause vaginal infection and present with purulent, bloody discharge. Common offenders include small toys, tissue paper, or crayons. The infection usually subsides after removal of the foreign body. In children this may need to be done under general anesthesia.

TABLE 69-2 Nonspecific Vulvovaginitis in Children

Causes
Poor toilet hygiene following bowel evacuation
Tight-fitting underclothing
Lack of proper bathing
Irritative agents: bubble baths, harsh soaps
Vaginal foreign bodies
Upper respiratory infections
Treatment
Elimination of the irritative agents
Improved local hygiene
Sitz baths (2 tbsp baking soda and lukewarm bathwater)
Aveeno oatmeal baths
Loose-fitting underclothing
Antibiotics directed by culture and sensitivity

On occasion, bacterial upper respiratory infections may precede a vaginal infection by 3 to 5 days. Symptoms include severe vulvar irritation. Cultures may confirm the presence of respiratory flora, including Group A beta-hemolytic streptococci or *Staphylococcus aureus.* Specific bacterial infections should be confirmed by culture before antimicrobial treatment is instituted.

Specific Vulvovaginal Infections

Candidal Vaginitis

Vulvovaginitis due to *Candida albicans* is uncommon during infancy and childhood. The most common presenting symptom is intense pruritus and a thick, whitish, nonodorous discharge. Diagnosis may be made by preparing a wet mount with potassium hydroxide (KOH) preparation. Treatment is with antifungal agents.

Shigella Vaginitis

Vulvovaginitis can be caused by organisms from the intestinal tract. *Shigella* vaginitis presents with persistent vaginal irritation unresponsive to antifungal agents. It can be treated with a 10-day course of ampicillin.

Parasitic Vulvovaginitis

Parasites that can cause vulvar pruritus, irritation, and discharge include pinworms (*Enterobius vermicularis*), roundworms (*Ascaris lumbricoides*), and whipworms (*Trichuris trichiura*). Diagnosis is best made by performing a "tape test" by pressing a piece of cellophane adhesive tape against the perianal area in the early morning to recover the parasitic ova, which can be identified by microscopic examination. The treatment for pinworms is mebendazole, given as a single dose of 100 mg and repeated in 2 weeks. Roundworms and whipworms may be treated with mebendazole 100 mg twice daily for 3 days.

GYNECOLOGIC DISORDERS OF ADOLESCENCE

The Gynecologic Examination

Adolescents who are sexually active require a complete sexual history and a full speculum and bimanual examination to evaluate for sexually transmitted illnesses and disorders related to pregnancy. A complete and candid history may be difficult to obtain in the presence of a parent, and it is important to reassure the patient that the history will remain confidential. The male physician examining a patient should be accompanied by a female chaperone.

Dysmenorrhea

Primary dysmenorrhea is pain with menstruation that is not associated with recognized pelvic pathology. It most commonly occurs during normal menstruation. Secondary dysmenorrhea is pain that occurs during menses that is caused by an underlying abnormality, such as endometriosis, chronic pelvic inflammatory disease, uterine pathology such as myomas or polyps, and genitourinary anomalies such as bicornuate uterus or cervical stenosis. Primary dysmenorrhea is much more common than secondary dysmenorrhea, particularly in adolescents.

Patients most commonly complain of crampy lower abdominal pain prior to or at the start of menses. Symptoms typically last for the first 24 to 48 h of the menstrual period. Associated symptoms may include headaches, including migraines, low back pain, nausea, and vomiting.

Patients are examined to rule out causes of secondary dysmenorrhea. Initial treatment of mild dysmenorrhea includes the use of aspirin, ibuprofen, or naproxen, which is effective in 80 to 90 percent of cases. Patients with refractory or incapacitating pain may be treated with oral contraceptives.

Dysfunctional Uterine Bleeding

Etiology

Dysfunctional uterine bleeding (DUB) is defined as vaginal bleeding that may be irregular (metrorrhagia), excessive in duration and amount (menorrhagia), or both (menometrorrhagia). Dysfunctional uterine bleeding most commonly occurs within the anovulatory phase but may occur during ovulation. While DUB can occur in adolescence, it is most commonly seen in older women at the end of their reproductive years.

Patients present with excessive vaginal bleeding, which should be quantified by the examiner. Physical examination is directed at ruling out potential life threats, such as hemorrhagic shock and coagulopathy. Vital signs should include measurement of orthostatic blood pressure. The patient is evaluated for signs of blood loss, including pallor and decreased capillary refill. The evaluation of the patient must include a pelvic examination to exclude vulvar and cervical pathology or uterine masses. Laboratory testing should include pregnancy testing, hemoglobin, and coagulation profile if the suspicion of a coagulopathy exists.

Management

The management of patients with dysfunctional uterine bleeding is directed initially toward stabilization and subsequently toward searching for underlying pathology. Patients may be categorized into three groups to simplify the management of DUB. Those with minimal bleeding may be reassured and observed. Patients with moderate bleeding may be treated with medroxyprogesterone 10 mg/day orally for 5 days. If bleeding persists, this regimen may be repeated for a total of three cycles, after which normal menses should occur.

Patients with severe vaginal bleeding and unstable vital signs are treated aggressively. Management of shock must begin with immediate stabilization and circulatory resuscitation, followed by laboratory evaluations to determine the etiology and degree of bleeding. After the patient is stabilized, treatment with high-dose estrogens such as Premarin 40 mg every 4 h for up to 24 h may be used, followed by treatment with oral preparations. Subsequent evaluation is important to rule out underlying pathology, and supplemental iron may be prescribed to prevent iron-deficiency anemia.

Mittelschmerz

Mittelschmerz is pain upon ovulation caused by peritoneal irritation from minor ovarian bleeding. This disorder, which presents with lower abdominal pain in midcycle, is benign and resolves spontaneously. It must be distinguished from ectopic pregnancy, ovarian torsion, and appendicitis.

Premenstrual Syndrome

Premenstrual syndrome is a constellation of symptoms attributable to the ovulatory cycle. It is characterized by vague pelvic pain, weight gain, headaches, and variations in mood. Premenstrual edema, also related to the ovulatory cycle, is most appropriately managed conservatively but may require salt restriction or a short course of a mild diuretic 3 days before the onset of menses.

Ovarian Cysts

Ovarian cysts are most commonly painless and are usually discovered on routine pelvic examination. Ovarian cysts may be associated with menstrual irregularities and are normally less than 6 cm in diameter. Cysts may rupture and cause lower abdominal pain and hemoperitoneum; they may therefore be confused with appendicitis or ectopic pregnancy.

Ovarian Torsion

Ovarian torsion, or twisting of the ovary and adnexa, is an uncommon but important cause of abdominal pain. Torsion may present with intermittent unilateral abdominal pain, low-grade fever, and a tender mass on pelvic examination. Predisposing factors include ovarian enlargement from pregnancy, ovarian cysts, and polycystic ovary disease. Although ultrasound may be helpful, laparoscopy is the most reliable diagnostic procedure.

Genital Tract Infections

Vulvovaginitis in Adolescents

Various factors affecting the vaginal physiology in adolescents and adults determine the types of infections that occur in this age group. Protective factors include an acidic vaginal pH, thick protective epithelium, commensal bacterial flora, and physiologic mucus secretion.

Candidal Vaginitis

Vulvovaginitis due to *C. albicans* is relatively common in adolescence and adulthood. Patients present with thick vulvovaginal discharge associated with intense pruritus and inflammation. A KOH preparation will reveal pseudohyphae and branching spores. Treatment is with antifungal agents.

Trichomonas Vaginitis

Vaginitis caused by *Trichomonas* is typically sexually transmitted. Patients complain of frothy yellowish or greenish discharge, which is foul-smelling. The vaginal mucosa and the cervix may have a spotted "strawberry" appearance. The diagnosis is confirmed by a wet mount demonstrating motile, flagellated trichomonads. Treatment is with metronidazole, which may be given as a single dose of 2 g or as 250 mg three times daily for 7 days in adolescents. The presence of *Trichomonas* in children indicates the possibility of sexual abuse.

Gardnerella Vaginitis

Gardnerella vaginitis results from overgrowth of an organism that may be found in the normal vaginal flora. Patients often complain of white or greyish discharge with a "fishy" odor. A KOH prep may reveal characteristic "clue" cells, which are epithelial cells that have been invaded by bacteria. Effective treatments include metronidazole 250 mg three times daily for 7 days or clindamycin 300 mg twice daily for 7 days.

Herpetic Vulvovaginitis

Herpetic vulvovaginitis is a sexually transmitted disease usually caused by the herpes simplex II virus. However, in up to 10 percent of cases, it is caused by herpes simplex I virus. Genital herpes most commonly presents with labial or perianal vesicles, which rupture and progress to painful ulcerations. Inguinal lymphadenopathy may be present. Genital herpes infections are self-limiting but recurrent. The course of the disease may be shortened by administration of acyclovir 200 mg every 4 h for 10 days.

Bartholin's Abscess

A Bartholin cyst is an enlargement of the Bartholin gland, located on the lateral border of the labia majora. Presenting symptoms include a red, tender mass on the lateral introitus and progressive pain. Treatment requires incision and drainage.

For a more detailed description, see Van Rooyen M: Pediatric and adolescent gynecology, chap. 69, p. 435, in *Pediatric Emergency Medicine: A Comprehensive Study Guide.*

Section XIV
Hematologic Emergencies

70 Anemias

David F. Soglin / Jane E. Kramer

Anemia is defined as a hemoglobin concentration more than two standard deviations below the mean. The normal hemoglobin concentration varies by age and, in the postpubertal population, by sex. Infants reach a nadir in hemoglobin concentration at 2 to 3 months of life, at which time the mean hemoglobin is only 11.5 g/dL. This nadir is deeper and occurs at a younger age in premature infants. In general, 11 g/dL defines the lower limit of normal for the prepubertal patient population.

Patients with mild anemia are usually asymptomatic. Even children with moderate to severe anemia may be asymptomatic if the problem develops slowly. Symptomatic patients may present with fatigue, irritability, or shortness of breath on exertion. Physical examination may reveal pallor, tachycardia, and a systolic ejection murmur from increased cardiac output. When hemoglobin drops rapidly, the child may develop dizziness, orthostatic hypotension, or high-output cardiac failure.

The history and physical examination play important roles in determining the etiology of anemia. A thorough diet history may suggest nutritionally induced anemia. A family history of hemoglobinopathy or a hereditary membrane disorder would guide a diagnostic workup. Physical examination may reveal findings that aid in the evaluation of the anemia.

Anemias are most easily classified by red blood cell (RBC) size and evidence of bone marrow activity. The size of RBCs is measured as mean corpuscular volume (MCV), the normal values of which vary with age. Bone marrow activity is reflected by the reticulocyte count. Correcting the measured reticulocyte count for the degree of anemia allows an accurate determination of marrow activity. An estimate of the corrected reticulocyte count is obtained by multiplying the measured reticulocyte percent by the ratio of measured hematocrit to normal hematocrit [Retic (HCT measured/HCT normal)].

The appearance of the RBCs on the peripheral smear, total number of RBCs, and red cell distribution width (a measure of anisocytosis, the variability in RBC size) are also helpful in determining the etiology of anemia.

MICROCYTIC ANEMIA

Microcytic anemia is defined by an MCV lower than two standard deviations below the mean. The vast majority of microcytic anemia in young patients is caused by iron deficiency.

Iron Deficiency

Risk factors for iron-deficiency anemia include age between 6 months and 2 years, decreased prevalence or duration of breast-feeding, lack of use of iron-fortified formulas, early introduction of whole cow's milk into the diet, and low socioeconomic status. Premature infants are at greater risk for iron-deficiency anemia than full-term infants.

Iron-deficiency anemia develops slowly, and patients rarely present with acute symptoms. The diagnosis is usually made on the basis of the history and complete blood count (CBC) results showing anemia, microcytosis, and a high red cell distribution width (RDW). The reticulocyte count is not elevated. Thrombocytosis is common in iron-deficiency anemia. In the usual setting, a trial of iron therapy is both diagnostic and therapeutic. Ferrous sulfate is administered in an amount sufficient to provide 5 to 6 mg/kg of elemental iron per day in three divided doses for approximately 3 months. An increase in the reticulocyte count is typically seen in a matter of days, and the hemoglobin level increases in 1 to 2 weeks. Diagnostic tests useful in the evaluation of iron-deficiency anemia include an elevated free erythrocyte protoporphyrin level, reduced serum iron, elevated total iron binding capacity (TIBC), and reduced ferritin level. Ferritin, however, is an acute-phase reactant, and in the face of infection may be elevated despite the presence of iron-deficiency anemia.

Thalassemia

Thalassemias are inherited defects resulting in the inability to synthesize sufficient quantities of various globin chains of the hemoglobin molecule. The production of beta chains is most commonly affected. The defect is most common in people of Mediterranean ancestry and is present in a very small percentage of American blacks. In general, the disease is classified as thalassemia minor or major, which correspond to heterzygous and homozygous states, respectively. The heterozygous form of thalassemia is often referred to as thalassemia trait.

Thalassemia trait produces marked microcytosis out of proportion to the degree of anemia. There is typically a high total RBC count and narrow RDW, which helps differentiate thalassemia trait from iron-deficiency anemia. In beta-thalassemia trait, the hemoglobin concentration is often 2 to 3 g/dL below normal values. A hemoglobin electrophoresis will demonstrate an elevated A_2 component and in some cases an elevated level of fetal hemoglobin (Hgb F). Patients with alpha-thalassemia trait have normal hemoglobin electrophoreses.

Beta-thalassemia major produces severe hemolytic anemia with marked microcytosis. It usually presents within the first year of life. Pallor, jaundice, and hepatosplenomegaly are often present. Because patients require lifelong transfusion therapy, the use of uncrossmatched blood is avoided except in the most dire circumstances. The major side effect of long-term transfusion therapy is iron overload, which adversely affects multiple organs, especially the pancreas, liver, and heart.

Lead Poisoning

Lead poisoning must be considered in the child with microcytic anemia. High levels of lead can interfere with hemoglobin production, but much of the anemia seen with lead poisoning is actually due to concomitant iron deficiency. It is reasonable to screen all children with microcytic anemia for lead toxicity, even if iron deficiency is present.

NORMOCYTIC ANEMIA

Though less common than microcytic anemias, the differential diagnosis of normocytic anemia in childhood is vast (Table 70-1). The first determination is whether the anemia is due to decreased production or increased loss or destruction of RBCs. A corrected reticulocyte count will allow the practitioner to make this initial decision.

NORMOCYTIC ANEMIA WITH ELEVATED RETICULOCYTE COUNT

If the corrected reticulocyte count is high and there is no evidence of blood loss, a hemolytic anemia is likely. The workup for a patient with hemolytic anemia includes a Coombs test to determine if hemolytic anemia is immunologic in nature. Immune hemolytic anemia may be the result of a drug reaction, infection, collagen

TABLE 70-1 Normocytic Anemia

Blood loss (high reticulocyte count)
Hemolytic anemia (high reticulocyte count)
Immune
Autoimmune hemolytic anemia
Neonatal-maternal blood group incompatibility
Nonimmune
Microangiopathic
Disseminated intravascular coagulation (DIC)
Hemolytic uremic syndrome (HUS)
Macroangiopathic
Artificial cardiac valve
Membrane abnormalities
Spherocytosis
Elliptocytosis
Stomacytosis
Metabolic abnormalities
G6PD deficiency
Pyruvate kinase deficiency
Hemoglobinopathies
Nonhemolytic anemia (low or normal reticulocyte count)
Abnormality isolated to red cell line
Chronic hemolytic anemia with concurrent aplastic crisis
Transient erythroblastopenia of childhood (TEC)
Chronic disease
Renal insufficiency
Diamond-Blackfan anemia
Abnormality affecting other cell lines
Bone marrow infiltration
Leukemia
Lymphoma
Tumor metastasis
Acquired aplastic anemia

vascular disorder, or malignancy, but most commonly no etiology is determined.

Patients often present acutely with severe anemia, pallor, jaundice, and hemoglobinuria. Transfusions may be necessary with severe symptomatic anemia, but this can be difficult because the circulating antibody causes "incompatibility" in vitro and rapid destruction of transfused RBCs in vivo. Immunosuppression with prednisone is frequently adequate to diminish RBC destruction, so that the patient's brisk reticulocytosis can repair the anemia. Intravenous gamma globulin is also useful. In severe cases, plasmapheresis may be necessary.

The differential diagnosis for nonimmune hemolytic anemia

include micro- and macroangiopathic destruction, membrane disorders, metabolic abnormalities, and hemoglobinopathies, which are discussed in detail in Chap. 71.

Microangiopathic RBC destruction can occur with disseminated intravascular coagulation and hemolytic uremic syndrome. The peripheral smear will demonstrate schistocytes, burr cells, and other RBC fragments.

Membrane disorders such as spherocytosis and elliptocytosis are hereditary in nature. Hereditary spherocytosis results in a hemolytic anemia due to splenic destruction of red blood cells. The disease is often apparent in infancy, and while the degree of anemia varies widely, it rarely results in a hematologic emergency. Laboratory studies reveal anemia, reticulocytosis, and hyperbilirubinemia. Many patients develop pigmentary gallstones. The diagnosis is confirmed by osmotic fragility studies. Splenectomy is curative. The major hematologic crisis is aplastic anemia, which is usually secondary to a parvovirus infection.

Hereditary elliptocytosis is another inherited defect that can occasionally result in significant hemolytic anemia. The peripheral smear reveals the characteristic elliptocytes. As in hereditary spherocytosis, splenectomy is curative. Aplastic crisis can occur.

Inherited metabolic disorders such as pyruvate kinase and glucose-6-phosphate dehydrogenase (G6PD) deficiencies also cause chronic hemolysis. Pyruvate kinase deficiency may present because of an increase in hemolysis or due to an aplastic crisis. There are multiple variants of G6PD, some of which cause severe hemolysis with relatively minor exposure to oxidant challenges. The A variant is seen in approximately 10 percent of African American males and becomes symptomatic only after a significant challenge from a drug or infection. Typically, aspirin in therapeutic doses does not pose a problem for these patients. Sulfonamides, antimalarials, and naphthalene can precipitate hemolysis.

NORMOCYTIC ANEMIA WITH LOW RETICULOCYTE COUNTS

A low reticulocyte count in the face of significant anemia indicates bone marrow underproduction. If the abnormality is isolated to the RBC line, the primary considerations are transient erythroblastopenia of childhood (TEC) and an aplastic crisis complicating an underlying hemolytic anemia (see the discussion of sickle cell disease in Chap. 71).

An acquired red cell aplasia, TEC spares the white blood cells and platelets and resolves after a number of weeks. It typically affects children between 1 and 4 years of age. Supportive therapy is usually sufficient because patients are typically hemodynamically stable and recover spontaneously. Transfusions may be necessary in symptomatic patients. Glucocorticoids have not been shown to speed recovery.

Other entities in the differential of normocytic anemia with low to normal reticulocyte counts and no abnormalities of other cell lines include anemia of chronic disease, inflammatory processes, and decreased erythropoietin from renal insufficiency. Diamond-Blackfan anemia is a congenital RBC aplasia that usually presents in the first year of life with severe anemia. Occasionally other congenital abnormalities are associated, such as cleft palate, skeletal anomalies, and congenital heart disease.

Thrombocytopenia or white blood cell abnormalities associated with normocytic anemia and poor reticulocyte response suggests marrow infiltration or acquired aplastic anemia.

Acquired aplastic anemia in the absence of an underlying hemolytic anemia has been associated with drugs and infections. Often no etiology is determined. The prognosis is quite poor, and bone marrow transplantation is often required. Blood transfusion is performed judiciously in patients who are candidates for bone marrow transplantation because of the dangers of sensitization.

MACROCYTIC ANEMIA

Macrocytic anemia is uncommon in pediatric patients. Folate and vitamin B_{12} deficiencies can result in megaloblastic anemia. These are rare in otherwise healthy children. Chemotherapy and malabsorption can lead to folate depletion, as can rapid turnover of RBCs. Many patients with sickle cell anemia are treated with folate supplementation for that reason.

For a more detailed discussion, see Soglin DF, Kramer JE: Anemias, chap. 70, p. 447, in *Pediatric Emergency Medicine: A Comprehensive Study Guide.*

---

71 Sickle Cell Disease

David F. Soglin / Jane E. Kramer

Sickle cell anemia (SCA) is a chronic hemolytic anemia that is most common among African Americans. It is also seen in people of Mediterranean, Indian, and Middle Eastern descent. It is secondary to a hemoglobinopathy that occurs when valine is substituted for glutamic acid in the 6 position of the beta chain. In addition to patients with hemoglobin SS (Hb SS), the diagnosis of SCA is applied to patients with hemoglobins SC, S beta-thalassemia, and SD. Patients with double heterozygous states are typically less seriously affected than those with Hb SS.

Patients with a single abnormal gene for Hb S have sickle cell trait. The concentration of Hb S is typically 40 percent, and the large percentage of normal hemoglobin allows the patients to remain asymptomatic except under the most severe hypoxic stress. However, the hypoxic environment of the renal medulla can cause localized sickling even in patients with sickle cell trait, leading to hematuria and isosthenuria.

Patients with SCA experience a number of complications that are likely to bring them to the emergency department.

VASOOCCLUSIVE CRISIS

The most common of the sickle cell crises, vasoocclusive pain, presumably occurs when sickled red blood cells (RBCs) obstruct blood flow and cause tissue ischemia. Dactylitis, or hand-foot syndrome, is vasoocclusion in the metacarpal or metatarsal bones. This is often the earliest presentation of SCA. It is common in young infants, who present with hand and foot swelling and tenderness, refusal to walk, and irritability. The swelling is most marked on the dorsal surface, and there may be radiologic evidence of avascular bony necrosis.

Older patients typically experience vasoocclusive pain crises in the long bones, back, joints, and abdomen. There is a great deal of individual variation in number and severity of painful crises. Fetal Hb seems to have a mitigating effect.

As there is no diagnostic test or clinical finding that will identify patients in vasoocclusive crisis, the diagnosis is made on the basis of history alone. A complete blood count and reticulocyte count is indicated. Typically, patients remain at baseline levels of Hb and hematocrit during a painful event. Therapy consists of hydration at 1½ to 2 times maintenance and analgesia. Oxygen has not been shown to be beneficial in the management of pain crises unless hypoxemia is a complicating factor.

Pain relief is achieved with a variety of analgesics, depending on the severity of the crisis. Oral agents such as acetaminophen, nonsteroidal anti-inflammatory drugs (NSAIDs), and codeine used separately or in combination are the mainstays of treatment for mild to moderate pain. Such management frequently allows the child with a painful vasoocclusive crisis to remain at home. Parenteral agents such as morphine and mixed agonist-antagonist agents such as nalbuphine are frequently used in the emergency department setting. Although meperidine has been commonly used in the past, the availability of other potent analgesics has reduced its use for SCA vasoocclusive pain. Ketorolac tromethathine is a relatively new NSAID that can be given orally or intramuscularly for acute pain. There is limited experience with ketorolac in children.

ACUTE CHEST SYNDROME

Patients with SCA presenting with chest pain, hypoxemia, and infiltrates on chest radiograph are termed to have "acute chest syndrome" (ACS). Fever may be present. Acute chest syndrome can result from pneumonia or pulmonary infarction due to vasoocclusion. It is difficult to differentiate vasoocclusion from pneumonia in patients with ACS. Lung scans are not useful in establishing a diagnosis. In the majority of patients with ACS, no infectious etiology is isolated. When the etiology is bacterial pneumonia, *Pneumococcus* is the most common organism. *Mycoplasma* causes approximately 15 percent of events. Most adults and many children probably have pulmonary infarcts secondary to vasoocclusion.

The mainstay of therapy for pulmonary infarction in patients with SCA is early blood transfusion, with consideration of exchange transfusion. Patients are often treated with antibiotics because of the difficulty in eliminating an infectious etiology. All patients receive hydration, oxygen, and analgesics.

INFECTION

Patients with SCA are at high risk for infection with encapsulated bacteria, especially *Pneumococcus.* Overwhelming pneumococcal sepsis is a common cause of mortality. Although prophylactic penicillin and vaccines for pneumococci and *Haemophilus influenzae* type B have reduced the incidence of sepsis in this vulnerable population, it remains the major cause of death in the young patient with SCA. Children below 3 years of age are particularly susceptible to bacteremia.

Children below 5 years of age with SCA who present to the emergency department with fever are at high risk for bacteremia. Complete blood counts and blood cultures are obtained, and most of these children are promptly treated with parenteral antibiotics effective against *Streptococcus pneumoniae* and *H. influenzae.* Although hospital admission is generally recommended, some institutions use a long-acting cephalosporin such as ceftriaxone along with close outpatient follow-up. Older children, who are less susceptible to overwhelming sepsis, can be managed on an individual basis depending on the height of the fever, the appearance of the child, findings on physical examination, and results of laboratory tests.

In addition to overwhelming sepsis, children with SCA are susceptible to other infections such as pneumonia, meningitis, and osteomyelitis. The etiology is most frequently encapsulated organisms. The most common organism identified as the cause of osteomyelitis in patients with SCA is *Staphylococcus*; however, these patients are at increased risk for *Salmonella* osteomyelitis.

CEREBROVASCULAR ACCIDENTS

Cerebrovascular accidents (CVAs) are common in children with SCA and are thought to be due to intimal damage and RBC sickling. Because simple blood transfusions increase the viscosity of the blood, exchange transfusion is the management of choice. These patients are at high risk for subsequent CVAs and are usually managed with long-term blood transfusions to maintain their percentage of Hb S below 30 percent. Exchange transfusion is unnecessary in the chronic phase of transfusion therapy. Iron overload may develop with chronic transfusions.

SPLENIC SEQUESTRATION

Splenic sequestration crisis occurs when RBCs become entrapped in the spleen, resulting in a sudden drop in the Hb and hematocrit. Affected patients present with a history of decreased exersize tolerance. The physical examination reveals pallor, splenomegaly, and often signs of high-output heart failure. Laboratory studies demonstrate marked anemia and a high reticulocyte count. In patients with SS hemoglobinopathy, splenic sequestration occurs almost exclusively in young children, because as the SCA patients age, they undergo "autosplenectomy." Patients with Hb SC or Hb SB thalassemia often have persistent splenomegaly and thus remain at risk for sequestration crises into adulthood.

The mainstay of therapy is rapid blood transfusion. Fluid expansion can be used in the initial stages of resuscitation if blood is not immediately available, but it must be used carefully because volume overload and congestive heart failure can result. Exchange transfusions can be used instead of simple blood transfusions if fluid overload is a concern. Occasionally splenectomy is necessary.

APLASTIC CRISIS

Viral infections, especially with parvovirus, can result in marrow suppression. Children with SCA are susceptible to even brief bone marrow suppression because of the extremely short half-life of the sickle cell. Patients may present in a decompensated state, complaining of fatigue and shortness of breath. There will be a significant drop in Hb from baseline and little or no reticulocytosis. Some patients can be managed with supportive care and close observation, because the marrow often rebounds in a matter of days. Many patients, however, will require a transfusion of packed RBCs. Folate deficiency is common in patients with SCA and may be responsible for a small percentage of aplastic crises. Folate supplementation is provided for these patients.

For a more detailed discussion, see Soglin DF, Kramer JE: Sickle cell disease, chap. 71, p. 451, in *Pediatric Emergency Medicine: A Comprehensive Study Guide.*

72 Bleeding Disorders

David F. Soglin / Jane E. Kramer

HEMOPHILIA

Hemophilia is an X-linked recessive disorder of coagulation caused by deficiency of factor VIII (hemophilia A) or factor IX (hemophilia B or Christmas disease). The percentage of factor present determines the severity of the disease: 5 to 25 percent denotes mild disease with no tendency for spontaneous hemorrhage; 1 to 4 percent, moderate disease; and <1 percent, severe disease with proclivity to spontaneous hemorrhage. Two-thirds of American hemophiliacs have severe disease. In both hemophilia A and B, prothrombin time (PT) and bleeding time are normal and partial thromboplastin time (PTT) is prolonged. The same types of bleeding occur in both diseases. Bruising, hemarthroses, and intramuscular hematomas predominate. Intracranial hemorrhage is less common but can be devastating when it occurs.

TYPES OF BLEEDING

Acute Hemarthrosis

Knees, elbows, and ankles are the most commonly affected joints. It is generally agreed that even if joint bleeding cannot be confirmed, treatment is indicated. This philosophy is based on the potentially crippling sequelae of hemarthrosis.

Symptomatic treatment of hemarthroses consists of splinting, ice, immobilization, elastic bandages, and analgesia with acetaminophen with or without codeine. A single factor infusion to raise levels to 25 to 30 percent is usually sufficient to terminate bleeding. A joint that has bled repeatedly may require several doses of factor. Range of motion and physical therapy are instituted as soon as possible. Hip bleeds are especially worrisome, because pressure within the joint can lead to aseptic necrosis of the femoral head. Factor replacement to 50 to 75 percent levels with subsequent daily replacement to 30 percent may be necessary.

Intramuscular Bleeds

Such hemorrhage is usually identifiable by pain, tenderness, and swelling in the muscle, and is treated with factor replacement to 30 percent levels. Forearm, calf, and hand bleeding can result in a compartment syndrome. Vascular compromise or nerve paralysis from compartment syndrome requires fasciotomy. Iliopsoas hemorrhage, which can be massive, presents with flexion of the thigh, groin and abdominal pain, and paresthesias below the inguinal ligament from femoral nerve compression. Ultrasound or computed tomography (CT) can confirm the diagnosis. Compartment syndromes and psoas hemorrhages are treated with correction to achieve factor levels of 50 to 60 percent and require admission for observation and continued factor replacement.

Intracranial Hemorrhage

A potentially devastating complication, intracranial bleeding may be traumatic or spontaneous. Presenting symptoms include headache, vomiting, and seizures. Forceful blows to the head, regardless of symptoms, are empirically treated with factor replacement. Symptomatic children need factor replacement to 100 percent levels.

Other Bleeding Manifestations

Subcutaneous hemorrhage, abrasions, and lacerations that do not require sutures do not require factor replacement.

Painless gross hematuria can occur. An anatomical source for the bleeding is usually not found. Treatment with factor may not be necessary if the bleeding is spontaneous. Use of epsilon aminocaproic acid (EACA) is probably contraindicated because of the risk of ureteral clot formation. Prednisone is advocated by some to decrease the duration and degree of hematuria. Factor replacement is necessary before laceration repair, lumbar puncture, surgery, and dental extractions.

MANAGEMENT ISSUES

Intramuscular injections, aspirin, and jugular and femoral venipuncture are avoided. Simple peripheral venipuncture is followed by at least 5 min of pressure to the site.

Factor replacement for hemophilia A is accomplished by transfusion with cryoprecipitate or a variety of factor VIII concentrates, which are preferred for convenience and safety. Hemophilia B is treated with factor IX complex concentrates, which also contain factors II, VII, and X, or more recently licensed pure factor IX. The former carry the risk of disseminated intravascular coagulation and thromboembolism, especially in patients with crush injuries.

As indicated above, the amount of factor to be delivered will depend on the nature and severity of the bleeding episode. For significant bleeds, treatment with factor replacement is generally required every 12 h until healing occurs.

The following formulas may be used to calculate factor replacement:

1. Factor VIII (units) = weight (kg) × 0.5 × desired increment (%) of factor VIII level (i.e., 1 U/kg of factor VIII raises the level by 2 percent).
2. Factor IX (units) = weight (kg) × 1.0 × desired increment (%) of factor IX level (i.e., 1 U/kg of factor IX raises the level by 1 to 1.5 percent).

Patients with hemophilia A who have developed inhibitors (IgG antibodies to the missing factor) present special problems. Some 10 to 20 percent of severe hemophiliacs form factor inhibitors. Treatment of bleeding episodes in these children depends on inhibitor titer and the severity of the bleeding. Children with low titers and minor hemorrhage may respond to factor VIII therapy. Some children with inhibitors demonstrate an anamnestic response, with high titers of antibody appearing rapidly after factor VIII administration. Alternatives for treating patients with high titers of inhibitor include factor IX concentrates (50 to 100 U/kg); activated factor IX concentrate (Feiba or Autoplex), which has a higher degree of success; porcine factor VIII; plasmapheresis and factor replacement; or high-dose factor VIII (>100 U/kg).

Today's concentrates, through a combination of improved donor screening and viral attenuation techniques (pasteurization and steam/vapor or solvent-detergent treatment), appear safe in terms of disease transmission.

Some investigators recommend the use of glucocorticoids for the management of hematuria or recurrent joint bleeds. Epsilon aminocaproic acid (Amicar) is a clot stabilizer for use in intraoral bleeds, and desmopressin (DDAVP) increases factor VIII levels in patients with mild hemophilia. Useful for minor bleeds, DDAVP is administered intravenously over 30 min (0.3 μg/kg). Von Willebrand's patients are treated with DDAVP as well.

VON WILLEBRAND DISEASE

Von Willebrand disease exists when there is decreased or defective von Willebrand Factor (vWF), which is necessary for platelet adhesion to blood vessel walls. Classification systems separate quantitative deficiencies of vWF and Factor VIII coagulant protein (factor VIII:C) (Type I, classic) from qualitative abnormalities [Types II (variant) and III (severe)].

Clinical manifestations include epistaxis, easy bruising, menorrhagia, and bleeding after dental extraction. Posttraumatic and postsurgical hemorrhage can occur, but hemarthroses are uncommon. Many people exhibit no clinical problems with bleeding in spite of biochemical abnormalities. Typical laboratory findings include a normal PT and platelet count, with a prolonged bleeding time and an aPTT that may be normal or prolonged. Measurement of antigenic vWF (vWF:ag) and ristocetin cofactor activity can usually confirm the diagnosis.

The treatment for hemorrhage in these patients is the administration of cryoprecipitate, which contains intact vWF, or intermediate-purity fractionated factor VIII concentrate (Humate P). Most other factor VIII concentrates do not contain vWF. Type I von Willebrand disease is often amenable to desmopressin therapy, which corrects the bleeding time for 3 to 4 h and avoids the infectious risks of cryoprecipitate.

ACQUIRED COAGULOPATHIES

Acquired abnormalities of coagulation include vitamin K deficiency, liver disease, disseminated intravascular coagulation (DIC), thrombocytopenia, and platelet dysfunctions.

Vitamin K deficiency leads to decreases in the vitamin K-dependent factors (II, VII, IX, and X) and prolongation of the

PT. It can be seen in malabsorption syndromes, biliary obstruction, and prolonged diarrhea, and it can be caused by drugs such as diphenylhydantoin, phenobarbital, isoniazid, and coumarin. Vitamin K deficiency can also lead to hemorrhagic disease of the newborn unless supplementation is provided routinely at delivery. The liver is the site of production of the clotting factors, although factor VIII is produced elsewhere as well, and severe liver disease causes coagulation defects that can mimic DIC.

DISSEMINATED INTRAVASCULAR COAGULATION

In DIC there is simultaneous activation of coagulation and fibrinolysis. Microthrombi form in small blood vessels, leading to occlusion and tissue ischemia. Excessive bleeding occurs due to thrombocytopenia, consumption of clotting factors, and fibrinolysis. In pediatric patients, the leading cause of DIC is overwhelming infection. While bleeding is the predominant symptom, thrombotic damage can occur in most organ systems. Common ischemic complications include hemorrhagic necrosis of the skin, renal failure, seizures and coma, hypoxemia, and pulmonary infarcts. Laboratory findings in DIC usually include hemolytic anemia with schistocytes, thrombocytopenia, prolonged PT and PTT, and decreased fibrinogen with increased fibrin split products.

Management depends on the underlying disorder. The patient is stabilized and transfused if significant bleeding has occurred. Therapeutic options include factor replacement, anticoagulants, and antifibrinolytics. Factor replacement is accomplished with fresh frozen plasma (10 to 15 U/kg) to keep the PT <115 s. For severe hypofibrinogenemia, cryoprecipitate, which contains 10 times more fibrinogen than plasma, can be used. The dose of cryoprecipitate is 1 bag/3 kg in infants and 1 bag/5 kg in children. Platelet transfusion is considered when platelet counts are <120,000/μL.

Heparin therapy may be helpful in the presence of widespread thrombosis, but it remains controversial. It does not replace the use of fresh frozen plasma or platelets. Repeated measurements of the coagulation profile and blood and platelet counts are essential.

PLATELET DISORDERS

Normally functioning platelets are a necessary component of the clotting process. A deficit in platelet number or function can lead to excessive bleeding following injury (Table 72-1). Platelet dysfunction can be congenital, resulting from defects in receptors, platelet–vessel wall adhesion (von Willebrand disease, Bernard Soulier syndrome), platelet-platelet interaction (Glanzmann's

TABLE 72-1 Platelet Abnormalities

Thrombocytopenia
Immune disorders
Immune thrombocytopenic disorders
Autoimmune disease (systemic lupus erythrematosus)
Infectious-related (Epstein-Barr viruses, hepatitis B)
Infection
Sepsis with or without DIC
Bone marrow failure
Infiltration (leukemia, lymphoma)
Aplastic anemia
Drug-related
Congenital
Wiskott-Aldrich syndrome
Thrombocytopenia-absent radius syndrome
Hemolytic-uremic syndrome
Platelet dysfunction
Congenital defects
Receptor defects
Platelet–vessel wall adhesion defects
Von Willebrand's disease
Bernard Soulier syndrome
Platelet-platelet interaction defects
Glanzmann's thrombasthenia
Platelet secretion defects
Acquired defects
Drug interactions

thrombasthenia), platelet secretion, and other miscellaneous syndromes. Acquired platelet dysfunction is caused most commonly by aspirin. Even minor platelet dysfunction can result in easy bruisability and significant bleeding from mucosal membranes or after minor procedures.

Deficits in platelet number are much more common in pediatric patients. Thrombocytopenia is defined as a platelet count less than 150,000/μL. Platelet counts below 20,000/μL indicate severe thrombocytopenia, and in that range, particularly when counts drop below 10,000/μL, there is significant risk for life-threatening hemorrhage and intracranial bleeding.

Symptomatic patients may present as well-appearing children with a petechial or purpuric rash. At times the extensive ecchymoses in the absence of a history of significant trauma can wrongly suggest child abuse. With lower counts, patients may develop significant bleeding and bruising from minor trauma, mucosal bleeding, hematuria, or hematochezia. In addition to the skin findings, the physical examination should focus on lymphadenopathy and liver and spleen enlargement. Involvement of other bone marrow elements also help guide the workup.

The differential diagnosis of thrombocytopenia is extensive, but the single most common cause in the well-appearing child is immune (idiopathic) thrombocytopenic purpura (ITP). Other causes include autoimmune diseases such as systemic lupus erythematosus and secondary immune destruction of platelets from infectious agents such as hepatitis B and Epstein-Barr viruses. Sepsis can cause destruction of platelets.

Bone marrow infiltration from leukemia, lymphoma, and other malignancies may initially present with thrombocytopenia but will often have associated hepatosplenomegaly, anemia, and abnormalities of the white blood cells. Decreased production of platelets can also occur in aplastic anemia or from drug effects. Cancer chemotherapy agents typically depress production of all cell lines, and idiosyncratic immune reactions leading to thrombocytopenia may be seen following administration of various agents. In the pediatric population, this is particularly seen with valproic acid, phenytoin, and trimethoprim/sulfamethoxazole.

Wiskott-Aldrich syndrome is an X-linked disorder with thrombocytopenia, immunodeficiency, and eczema. Typically these patients are identified as newborns because of bleeding and petechiae. The immunodeficiency presents later in infancy, and the eczema is frequently not severe until later. Thrombocytopenia-absent radius syndrome (TAR) is autosomal recessive and presents in the neonatal period with petechiae and typical upper limb anomalies.

HEMOLYTIC UREMIC SYNDROME

Hemolytic uremic syndrome presents with a triad of acute renal failure, microangiopathic hemolytic anemia, and thrombocytopenia. The thrombocytopenia is usually mild to moderate. The typical presentation is that of a pale, somewhat lethargic young child with a prodromal history of a gastrointestinal infection. Abdominal pain, vomiting, and bloody diarrhea are common, as are acute renal failure and neurologic manifestations. Laboratory examination typically reveals anemia with red blood cell fragmentation, thrombocytopenia, electrolyte and acid-base disturbances, and elevated blood urea nitrogen and serum creatinine. Dialysis may be necessary.

IMMUNE THROMBOCYTOPENIC PURPURA

Immune thrombocytopenic purpura is the most common cause of thrombocytopenia in a well-appearing young child. Children typically have a history of a preceding viral illness. The platelet surface is covered with increased amounts of IgG, and the spleen removes the affected platelets from the circulation.

Patients present with the acute onset of bruising, petechiae, and purpura. The children have normal physical examination other than the skin findings. Mucosal or gastrointestinal bleeding can occur. The most serious complication, intracranial hemorrhage, occurs in less than 1 percent of patients and almost exclusively with platelet counts under 10,000/μL.

The diagnosis of ITP is likely when the complete blood count (CBC) reveals thrombocytopenia in association with normal red and white blood cell numbers and morphology. Definitive diagnosis is made by bone marrow examination. Although bone marrow aspiration may be necessary to conclusively rule out aplastic or infiltrative disease, with mild to moderate thrombocytopenia and the absence of signs, symptoms, or CBC results suggesting another diagnosis, and no plans for treatment, careful observation without bone marrow aspiration may be appropriate in some cases.

Treatment of patients with ITP is controversial. Most patients demonstrate a return to normal platelet counts within 3 months. Glucocorticoids can hasten recovery but are not necessary in most patients who have only skin manifestations and platelet counts above 30,000/μL. Intravenous gamma globulin has been shown to increase counts in patients with profound thrombocytopenia and may be useful during active bleeding or intracranial hemorrhage. Transfused platelets will be rapidly destroyed due to the immune response and have no role in management except in cases of life-threatening hemorrhage. In that circumstance, massive platelet transfusions along with intravenous gamma globulin are administered.

For a more detailed discussion, see Soglin DF, Kramer JE: Bleeding disorders, chap. 72, p. 454, in *Pediatric Emergency Medicine: A Comprehensive Study Guide.*

73 Blood Components

David F. Soglin / Jane E. Kromer

Transfusion of blood and blood components is often necessary in the emergency department. Whole blood, packed red blood cells

(PRBCs), platelets, granulocytes, fresh frozen plasma, cryoprecipitate, specific clotting factors, albumin, and immunoglobulins each have specific indications and risks associated with their use.

Whole Blood

Transfusion of whole blood is rarely needed but may be indicated for prompt restoration of red cells and volume after trauma or surgery. After 24 h of storage, whole blood has lost platelet and granulocyte function. Activity of labile clotting factors V and VIII is also diminished greatly within 3 to 5 days. Further, the risk of transfusion reactions is doubled because of the volume of foreign proteins and antibodies that are transferred in whole blood.

Packed Red Blood Cells

Packed red blood cell units contain approximately 50 mL of plasma and have a hematocrit ranging from 70 to 80 percent. There are no functional platelets or granulocytes in this preparation. For patients with a previous history of febrile reactions to transfusions or if the risk of cytomegalovirus (CMV) transmission is to be particularly avoided, filtered, leukocyte-poor red cells are recommended. Patients with recurrent or severe allergic reactions to transfusions should receive PRBCs that have been saline-washed.

Platelet Concentrate

These preparations contain approximately 5.5×10^{10} platelets in 50 to 70 mL of plasma. They should be ABO- and Rh-compatible, but crossmatching is not necessary. In children, the dose is estimated at 0.2 to 0.4 U/kg. Platelets transfusions are indicated for patients with thrombocytopenia or platelet dysfunction who are actively bleeding. They should be used in consultation with the patient's hematologist.

Granulocyte Concentrates

Transfusion of white cells is not an emergency department procedure. The severely neutropenic ($<1500/mm^3$) patient, if febrile, must be cultured, treated with antibiotics, and admitted, since the risk of sepsis is high.

Fresh Frozen Plasma

This product is plasma frozen within 6 h of collection. It contains all clotting factors, including labile factors V and VIII. ABO compatibility is important, but crossmatching is not necessary. Fresh frozen plasma (FFP) is used at a dose of 10 to 20 mL/kg to treat coagulopathies secondary to unknown factor deficiencies, disseminated intravascular coagulation, and chronic liver disease, and to compensate for excessive warfarin or dicumarol treatment. The risk of disease transmission is similar to that of whole blood transfusion, and allergic reactions are possible. Fresh frozen plasma is not indicated for volume expansion.

Cryoprecipitate

Cryoprecipitate is prepared by slow thawing of FFP at 4°C and subsequent refreezing of the protein precipitate, which is rich in fibrinogen, factor VIII, and von Willebrand factor. Cryoprecipitate does not require crossmatching. It is used to treat Von Willebrand disease and congenital hypofibrinogenemia. It can be used for patients with hemophilia A, although factor VIII concentrate is preferred.

Antihemophilic Factor (VIII)

This is a freeze-dried preparation of factor VIII:C (the procoagulant activation or antihemophilic factor) that gives a higher dose of Factor VIII per volume than cryoprecipitate. It is used to treat classic hemophilia (hemophilia A). Current heat and chemical treatment greatly diminish the infectious transmission risks. Recombinant factor VIII with no risk of infectious transmission is also available.

Factor IX Complex

This product contains vitamin K–dependent factors II, VII, IX, and X. It is made from large pools of human plasma and therefore carries the risk of transmission of infections. A heat-treated form of factor IX is also available to treat hemophilia B (Christmas disease).

Albumin

Available in both 5% and 25% solutions, albumin is most frequently used for blood volume expansion. Heat and chemical treatment eliminates the infectious transmission risk, and it contains no blood group antibodies. Only the 5% solution is isosmotic with plasma, and the 25% solution is never used to treat shock without other fluids.

Immune Globulins

These antibody-rich preparations are occasionally used in the emergency department (ED) to treat conditions such as rabies, tetanus, or varicella as postexposure disease prophylaxis.

Indications for Transfusion

Transfusion of blood in the ED is usually performed because of shock secondary to acute blood loss.

Blood typing (for ABO and Rh) takes about 5 min, and screening for antibodies and crossmatching takes 30 min or more. The use of O-negative (universal donor) blood is reserved for life-threatening hemorrhage. The accompanying risks of minor blood group incompatibility are overshadowed in this situation. The use of group- and Rh type–specific blood is preferred over O-negative transfusions when time precludes complete crossmatching. The formula for calculating the volume (V) of packed red blood cells (in milliliters) to infuse is as follows:

$$V = (\text{desired hemoglobin in g/dL} - \text{observed hemoglobin in g/dL}) \times \text{weight in kilograms} \times 3$$

Thus, 3 mL of PRBC per kilogram will raise the hemoglobin by 1 g/dL.

COMPLICATIONS

Acute Hemolytic Transfusion Reactions

Acute hemolytic transfusion reactions (AHTR) occur immediately and are almost always due to ABO incompatibility. The transfused cells are lysed by complement and IgM antibodies. Symptoms include fever, chills, back or chest pain, nausea and vomiting, dyspnea, flushing, tachycardia, and hypotension. Disseminated intravascular coagulation, hyperkalemia, shock, renal failure, and death may ensue. Hemoglobinemia and hemoglobinuria are present.

Delayed Hemolytic Transfusion Reactions

Delayed hemolytic transfusion reactions (DHTR) are directed at non-ABO antigens on transfused cells. They are delayed because an anamnestic immune response must develop to increase antibody production. Signs and symptoms include fever, anemia, jaundice, and, rarely, hemoglobinuria. No treatment is usually required.

Febrile Nonhemolytic Transfusion Reactions

Febrile nonhemolytic transfusion reactions (FNHTR) are benign and self-limiting; they account for the great majority of transfusion reactions, and occur most commonly in the multiply transfused patient. This condition is caused by recipient antibodies to donor leukocytes and platelets. It may be difficult to distinguish from AHTR, and so the transfusion must be stopped and tests for hemolysis performed. Once an AHTR is ruled out, antipyretics may be given.

Allergic Transfusion Reaction

Allergic transfusion reactions are of two types, which have different etiologies: urticarial and anaphylactic. Urticarial reactions are produced by IgE antibodies to plasma proteins, leading to histamine release, hives, and pruritus. The transfusion must be interrupted and the patient watched closely for signs and symptoms of anaphylaxis. An antihistamine such as diphenhydramine, 1 mg/kg/dose, should be administered. When the urticaria fades, the transfusion can be resumed.

Anaphylactic reactions occur in patients with congenital IgA deficiency who have high-titer IgG anti-IgA antibodies. Activation of a complement and chemical mediator cascade precipitates increased vascular permeability, resulting in angioedema, respiratory distress, urticaria, and shock. The transfusion is stopped, epinephrine administered, and blood pressure stabilized with crystalloid and vasopressive agents if necessary.

Massive Transfusion

This generally refers to the transfusion of one or more blood volumes within 24 h. Risks involved include hypothermia if a blood warmer is not used, hyperkalemia, hypocalcemia, and coagulation disorders from the dilution of platelets and clotting factors.

INFECTIOUS COMPLICATIONS

Viral Hepatitis

Approximately 3 to 10 percent of transfusion recipients will develop hepatitis, as defined by elevated transaminases. Most of this is caused by non-A, non-B hepatitis virus (usually hepatitis C virus). Current screening tests greatly diminish the chances of transmitting posttransfusion hepatitis.

Human Immunodeficiency Virus

The risk of human immunodeficiency virus (HIV) transmission has been greatly reduced through routine screening of donor blood for anti-HIV antibodies and screening for high-risk behaviors.

Cytomegalovirus

Neonates and immunocompromised children should receive leukocyte-poor, CMV antibody–negative blood to avoid risk of systemic CMV infection.

For a more detailed discussion, see Soglin DF, Kramer JE: Blood components, chap. 73, p. 459, in *Pediatric Emergency Medicine: A Comprehensive Study Guide.*

SECTION XV
ONCOLOGIC EMERGENCIES

74 Oncologic Emergencies

Brenda N. Hayakawa

Approximately 10 percent of childhood deaths are related to cancer. Patients frequently present to the emergency department with complications related to tumors and their treatment.

COMMON PEDIATRIC MALIGNANCIES

Acute Leukemias

Acute leukemia is the most common childhood malignancy (Table 74-1); 75 percent of these are of the acute lymphoblastic type (ALL). Acute myelogenous leukemia (AML) is much less common than ALL, accounting for 25 percent of acute leukemia.

The peak incidence of ALL occurs between the ages of 3 and 5 years. Overall, about 60 to 70 percent of patients survive more than 5 years beyond diagnosis, with many patients considered cured. The prognosis for AML is much poorer.

The signs and symptoms of acute leukemia reflect involvement of bone marrow by leukemic cells. Common presentations include pallor, fatigue, petechiae, purpura, bleeding, and fever. Lymphadenopathy, hepatomegaly, and splenomegaly reflect extramedullary involvement. Bone pain results from leukemic involvement of the periosteum and bone, causing the patient to limp or even refuse to walk. Joint pain may mimic nonmalignant disease, such as juvenile rheumatoid arthritis. Other nonspecific symptoms include anorexia, lassitude, low-grade fever, and irritability.

The leukocyte count is greater than $10{,}000/mm^3$ in approximately half of patients with ALL. However, neutropenia may be encountered and may predispose to serious infections. Most patients will be anemic and thrombocytopenic.

Despite hematologic abnormalities in the peripheral blood

TABLE 74-1 Distribution of Cancer in Children Aged 0 to 14 Years: New Cases, 1973–1982

Cancer	Percent
Leukemia	30
CNS	19
Lymphoma	13
Neuroblastoma	8
Soft tissue sarcoma (including rhabdomyosarcoma)	7
Wilms' tumor	6
Bone	5
Retinoblastoma	3
Liver	1
Other	8

Source: Adapted from National Cancer Institute. Ries LA, Hankey BF, Miller BA, et al (eds): *Cancer Statistics Review 1973–88*, NIH Publication No. 91-2789. Bethesda, MD: National Cancer Institute, 1991, p II-11.

count, the diagnosis of leukemia is confirmed only by bone marrow aspiration and biopsy. Further characterization of the leukemic blasts determines the particular treatment regimen. Treatment consists of combination chemotherapy for induction of remission, central nervous system (CNS) preventative therapy, consolidation, and maintenance therapy.

Complications of Leukemia

Complications of leukemia include CNS involvement, which may be present at the time of initial diagnosis or can occur in patients who relapse. Patients may present with headache, nausea, vomiting, irritability, papilledema, or other signs of raised intracranial pressure. Diagnosis is confirmed through the demonstration of leukemic blasts in the cerebrospinal fluid.

Leukemia may relapse in the testes, where it causes painless, usually unilateral testicular enlargement. Testicular biopsy confirms leukemic infiltrate. Testicular leukemia is often indicative of bone marrow relapse.

Hematologic complications include anemia, hemorrhage, and hyperleukocytosis. In the absence of hemorrhage, the anemia most often develops gradually. Patients with a hemoglobin greater than 10 g/dL usually do not require immediate therapy. Blood products administered to leukemia patients are usually irradiated to minimize the occurrence of posttransfusion graft-versus-host disease.

Hemorrhage is most often due to thrombocytopenia. Petechiae, bruising, and mucosal bleeding may be seen with platelet counts below 20,000/mm^3, but significant spontaneous internal hemorrhage is more likely with platelet counts below 10,000/mm^3. Most cases of spontaneous intracranial hemorrhage are associated with a platelet count below 5000/mm^3. Platelet transfusions are warranted for patients with a platelet count in the range of 20,000 to 50,000/mm^3 who have significant bleeding, such as epistaxis, gingival bleeding, or gross gastrointestinal hemorrhage. Platelets are administered at a dose of 0.2 U/kg or 6 U/m^2. Prophylactic use of platelet transfusions for the nonbleeding patient with a platelet count below 20,000/mm^3 is controversial and should be done in consultation with a hematologist.

Hemorrhage can also occur secondary to disseminated intravascular coagulation (DIC). Disseminated intravascular coagulation may occur in the setting of sepsis, newly diagnosed or relapsing acute nonlymphocytic leukemia, hyperleukocytosis, and disseminated neuroblastoma. Initial management includes treatment of the underlying condition and replacement of coagulation factors with fresh frozen plasma (10 mL/kg). Platelet and packed red blood cell (PRBC) transfusions may be necessary, as well as vitamin K (5 mg IV for infants and young children; 10 mg IV for older children).

Hyperleukocytosis, with an initial white blood cell (WBC) count $>$100,000/mm^3, may be seen with acute leukemias and chronic myelocytic leukemia. Unlike red blood cells (RBC) and platelets, WBC are large and not easily deformed, and they contribute significantly to blood viscosity. Patients may be asymptomatic but more often are dyspneic, are confused or agitated, or experience blurred vision. Physical examination may reveal plethora, cyanosis, signs of right ventricular failure, papilledema, or priapism. Arterial blood gas may show an acidemia. The chest radiograph may show a diffuse interstitial infiltrate. Patients with hyperleukocytosis are at risk for tumor lysis syndrome and are treated with intravenous hydration, alkalinization measures, and allopurinol and admitted for antileukemic therapy. Thrombocytopenia is corrected to a platelet count of at least 20,000/mm^3, as there is a significant risk of intracranial hemorrhage with hyperleukocytosis. Leukapheresis is an option prior to initiation of chemotherapy.

Neutropenia may occur at time of diagnosis as well as after chemotherapy. The febrile neutropenic patient is at significant risk of serious infection (see "Common Complications of Childhood Cancer," below).

Although hypercalcemia, with a serum calcium > 10.5 mg/dL, is more commonly associated with adult malignancies, it may occur with ALL, non-Hodgkin's lymphoma, neuroblastoma, and Ewing sarcoma. Disruptions in calcium homeostasis, excessive bone resorption by tumor, and, rarely, ectopic parathyroid hormone production are the usual causes. Clinically, patients may experience nausea, vomiting, constipation, polyuria, lethargy, and subsequent dehydration. Treatment begins with intravenous hydration with normal saline, followed by furosemide to promote calcium excretion.

Other metabolic complications include hyperuricemia and syndrome of inappropriate antidiuretic hormone, which are discussed further below.

Hodgkin's Disease

Hodgkin's disease is a malignancy arising in the lymph nodes that may spread to other local nodes and lymphatic channels. The malignant cell is the Reed-Sternberg cell. The first peak in incidence occurs from ages 13 to 35 years, with a late peak at 50 to 75 years.

The majority of pediatric patients present with painless supraclavicular or cervical lymphadenopathy. Nodes are rubbery and matted and, unlike reactive nodes, do not decrease in size. A lymph node is considered enlarged if it is greater than 10 mm at its greatest diameter, with the exceptions of an epitrochlear node, which is considered enlarged at 5 mm, and an inguinal node, at 15 mm. The abdominal examination may reveal hepatomegaly or splenomegaly, which indicates more advanced disease. Systemic symptoms occur in a third of the patients and include unexplained fever, weight loss, and night sweats.

The differential diagnosis of Hodgkin's disease includes other causes of lymphadenopathy, such as infectious mononucleosis, mycobacterial infections, toxoplasmosis, or other metastatic malignancies. A screening complete blood count (CBC) and chest radiograph are indicated, as well as a tuberculin skin test. Patients are referred for lymph node biopsy if the node is enlarging after 2 to 3 weeks, remains enlarged and has not returned to normal size by 5 to 6 weeks, or is associated with an abnormal chest radiograph finding such as mediastinal enlargement.

Once the diagnosis of Hodgkin's disease is confirmed and histologically classified, patients undergo further workup for staging, which may include exploratory laparotomy and splenectomy. Treatment regimens include multidrug chemotherapy and/or radiation.

TABLE 74-2 Mediastinal Tumors in Children

	Malignant	Benign
Anterior	Non-Hodgkin's lymphoma Hodgkin's disease Teratocarcinoma Thymoma Sarcoma	Teratoma Cystic hygroma Thymic cyst Hemangioma Bronchogenic cyst Lipoma
Middle	Non-Hodgkin's lymphoma Hodgkin's disease Rhabdomyosarcoma Teratocarcinoma Other sarcoma	Bronchogenic cyst Granuloma Teratoma Esophageal cyst Diaphragmatic hernia
Posterior	Neuroblastoma Ganglioneuroblastoma Ewing's sarcoma Pheochromocytoma Lymphoma	Ganglioneuroma Neurolemmoma Neurofibroma Enterogenous cyst

Source: Adapted from King RM, Telander RL, Smithson WA, et al: Primary mediastinal tumors in children. *J Pediatr Surg* 17:512, 1982.

Non-Hodgkin's Lymphomas

Non-Hodgkin's lymphomas (NHL) are a heterogeneous group of malignancies of lymphatic tissue. They usually present in children over 5 years of age. Childhood NHL are rapidly proliferating and are often disseminated in extranodal tissues at the time of presentation. Epstein-Barr virus and immunodeficiency diseases have been linked to this malignancy.

Clinically, NHL may rarely present as an isolated, painless adenopathy in the cervical, supraclavicular, or inguinal areas. Intrathoracic tumors may present with supraclavicular adenopathy, cough, wheezing, chest pain, or signs and symptoms of superior vena cava obstruction. Mediastinal lymphomas are more commonly of the lymphoblastic (T-cell) type. Burkitt or non-Burkitt undifferentiated types can present with abdominal involvement causing pain, nausea, vomiting, distension, ascites, or bowel obstruction. Right-lower-quadrant pain reflects distal ileal, appendiceal, or cecal involvement and may mimic appendicitis. Abdominal lymphoma may be the lead point of an intussusception. Bone, bone marrow, and the CNS are common sites of metastasis.

Initial laboratory studies include a CBC to assess for leukemia. Chest radiograph may reveal a mediastinal mass. Other mediastinal tumors in children are listed in Table 74-2. Patients with isolated nodal enlargement suspicious of lymphoma are referred to an appropriate facility for biopsy. Patients presenting with an abdominal mass may be evaluated by abdominal ultrasound or computed tomography or (CT). Multiagent chemotherapy is the mainstay of treatment, with up to 80 percent long-term disease-free survival.

Central Nervous System Tumors

The second most common group of pediatric malignancies is those of the CNS. Associations of CNS tumors with genetic diseases occur, such as neurofibromatosis with optic gliomas and tuberous sclerosis with giant-cell astrocytomas.

Tumors arising in the supratentorial region include cerebral astrocytoma, optic glioma, and craniopharyngioma. These more commonly occur in the neonatal and infancy period. Infratentorial tumors such as cerebellar astrocytoma, medulloblastoma, ependymoma, and brainstem glioma are more commonly seen after 2 years of age.

Supratentorial tumors may cause headache, seizures, or visual impairment. Truncal ataxia or incoordination is typical of infratentorial tumors. Impingement of the brainstem may lead to cranial nerve palsies or Horner syndrome. Raised intracranial pressure (ICP) in infants and toddlers may manifest as vomiting, anorexia, irritability, developmental regression, or impaired upward gaze ("sunsetting" sign). There may be excessive enlargement of the head circumference and persistently palpable cranial sutures. Parents may note a change in behavior or personality in their child. Older children may complain of headache, fatigue, or vomiting. Headaches that are recurrent, intense, incapacitating, or changing in character or that awaken the patient from sleep raise the suspicion of a malignancy. In addition, patients may have back pain, bladder or bowel dysfunction, or focal neurologic deficits that suggest spinal cord or cauda equina involvement.

Tumors of the CNS may be diagnosed by CT which can detect up to 95 percent of CNS lesions. Magnetic resonance imaging (MRI) is more sensitive than CT in detecting tumors. Treatment is multimodal, utilizing surgical resection, chemotherapy, and radiation therapy.

Wilms' Tumor

Wilms' tumor (nephroblastoma) is the most common pediatric abdominal malignancy. Most Wilms' tumors occur under the age of 6 years and present with a nontender or tender abdominal mass. If present, hematuria is usually microscopic. Systemic symptoms such as fever, anorexia, vomiting, or weight loss are infrequent, and the child may appear well. Hypertension may result from increased renin activity. Rarely, associated congenital abnormalities such as aniridia, hemihypertrophy, and genitourinary tract defects may be present.

The differential diagnosis includes other conditions presenting with an abdominal or pelvic mass. Initial workup includes a CBC, urinalysis, blood urea nitrogen (BUN), and creatinine, and also plain radiographs of the chest and abdomen. Ultrasound is a noninvasive means of evaluating a renal mass. Patients suspected of a Wilms' tumor are referred for further evaluation and management, which includes surgical resection and chemotherapy.

Neuroblastoma

Neuroblastoma is a malignant tumor arising from sympathetic neuroblasts in the adrenal medulla and sympathetic chain. It is the most common extracranial solid tumor in childhood, usually presenting within the first 4 years of life. Presenting signs and symptoms are most often related to the local effects of the primary or metastatic tumor. Two-thirds of neuroblastomas arise in the abdomen and pelvis and may present as an abdominal mass, bowel obstruction, or edema of the lower extremities and scrotum due to compression of venous and lymphatic drainage. Impingement of renal vasculature may lead to renin-mediated hypertension. Other sites of origin include the posterior mediastinum and neck. Horner syndrome, with unilateral ptosis, miosis, and anhydrosis, may occur with cervical or high thoracic involvement. Tumors of the paraspinal ganglia may grow around and through the intervertebral foramina, causing spinal cord or nerve root compression. This may cause radicular pain, motor and sensory deficits, bladder or bowel incontinence, or paraplegia. At the time of diagnosis, more than half of the patients with neuroblastoma will have metastases involving the lymph nodes, bone marrow, cortical bone, liver, or skin. Lung or brain involvement is rare and usually represents end-stage or relapsing disease. Retrobulbar involvement can cause proptosis or periorbital ecchymosis. Bone pain and limping may be related to bone and bone marrow disease. Massive hepatomegaly due to liver involvement, more common in infants, can cause respiratory compromise or liver failure. Skin manifestations appear as bluish, nontender subcutaneous nodules. They occur rarely outside of infancy. Paraneoplastic syndromes seen with neuroblastoma include opsoclonus, myoclonus, and cerebellar ataxia. Tumor secretion of vasoactive intestinal peptide may cause an intractable secretory diarrhea that results in hypokalemia and dehydration.

A CBC may reveal neutropenia or pancytopenia due to marrow involvement. Chest radiography may show a posterior mediastinal mass, which may cause impingement on the upper airway. Abdominal radiographs may reveal a mass displacing normal tissues. Abdominal ultrasound or CT scan may reveal a suprarenal mass. Lytic lesions and periosteal reaction may be seen on radiographs of painful areas of bone.

Primary Bone Tumors

Common primary pediatric malignancies of the bone include osteosarcoma and Ewing's sarcoma. Osteosarcoma has a predilection for the metaphysis of long bones, particularly around the knee. Ewing's sarcoma may also arise in extraosseous tissues.

Local pain, the most common symptom, may be exacerbated with activity and cause a limp. The pain may be intermittent, remitting for several weeks and later returning with increasing severity. Other presentations include a palpable mass, fever, or pathologic fracture. Back pain may be an early symptom of spinal cord compression.

Plain radiographs of the affected bone reveal bony destruction and soft tissue swelling. Later, the tumor may extend through the periosteum, causing new malignant bone deposition, which results in the characteristic radiographic sunburst sign, or it may cause a multilaminar periosteal reaction that results in an "onion peel" appearance on a radiograph. Osteosarcoma may metastasize to the lung, causing pulmonary hemorrhage, pneumothorax, or, rarely, superior vena cava obstruction.

Patients with radiographic changes suggestive of a bone tumor are referred to an orthopedist for confirmational biopsy and further management.

Rhabdomyosarcoma

Rhabdomyosarcoma is a malignant solid tumor arising from mesenchymal tissue that normally forms striated muscle. It most often presents as a painless mass. The most common site of origin is the head and neck region. Orbital tumors may present with periorbital swelling, proptosis, or ophthalmoplegia. Parameningeal tumors arising around the nasopharynx and paranasal sinuses may cause nasal obstruction, pain, sinusitis, or epistaxis. Tumor extension toward the meninges may cause cranial nerve palsies, meningeal irritation, headache, and vomiting. Chronic otitis media and otalgia may be due to middle ear involvement. Genitourinary tract involvement may manifest with hematuria or urinary obstruction. Vaginal tumors may present with vaginal hemorrhagic discharge and may mimic a vaginal foreign body. Rhabdomyosarcoma of the extremities or trunk usually presents as an enlargening soft tissue mass. Common sites of metastasis include lymph nodes, lungs, bones, bone marrow, brain, spinal cord, and heart.

Head or neck lesions may be evaluated by CT scan. Ultrasound is a useful initial tool to define a pelvic mass. Plain radiographs of the affected area of the limb or trunk should be obtained. Patients with a soft tissue mass must be referred for diagnostic biopsy. Treatment of rhabdomyosarcoma is multimodal, utilizing surgery, chemotherapy, and radiation.

Retinoblastoma

Retinoblastoma is the most common intraocular tumor of childhood. In 30 percent of cases, the disease is bilateral. Infants and young children are most commonly affected. Retinoblastoma most commonly presents with leukokoria, or a white pupil. Other presentations include strabismus and intraocular hemorrhage. The disease may be localized to the orbit, or it may metastasize to the brain, liver, kidneys, and adrenals. Plain radiographs of the orbits may reveal deposition of calcium. Unilateral disease is predominantly treated with enucleation. In bilateral disease, vision in at least one eye may be preserved by the use of radiation therapy.

COMMON COMPLICATIONS OF CHILDHOOD CANCER

The emergencies encountered in the cancer patient result from tumor or therapy-induced infectious or hematologic complications, metabolic derangement, or structural consequences of tumor compression.

Infectious Complications

Infection is the leading cause of death in children with cancer. The single most important factor is the development of neutropenia due to replacement of healthy bone marrow by malignant cells or from myelosuppressive chemotherapy. The best estimate of production of neutrophils is the absolute neutrophil count (ANC), calculated as the total white blood cell count multiplied by the percentage of band cells plus polymorphonuclear neutrophils (PMN). Patients are defined as being neutropenic if their ANC is less than 500/mm^3. These patients are at significant risk of bacteremia or fungemia. The risk decreases and plateaus as the ANC approaches 1000/mm^3. There are also qualitative abnormalities of granulocyte function that result from chemotherapy or radiation therapy. Impairment in cell-mediated immunity is more commonly encountered with Hodgkin's disease, with lymphomas, and in patients treated with chemotherapy and glucocorticoids. Impaired cell-mediated immunity results in a greater risk for fungal, mycobacterial, and viral infections. Impairment of humoral immunity more commonly occurs with chronic lymphocytic leukemia or chemotherapy and after splenectomy. Splenectomized patients are at greatly increased risk for sepsis with encapsulated bacteria such as *Pneumococcus* and *Haemophilus influenzae.* In addition, mechanical barriers such as the skin and mucous membranes may be broken down by infection, by chemotherapy, or iatrogenically from intravenous catheters and other long-term indwelling venous access devices. Patients are at risk of infection from their own endogenous flora as well as nosocomial pathogens from previous recent hospitalizations. The virulence of the infection depends on the extent of the host's immune defect. About 75 percent of neutropenic cancer patients with fever have an infection, most commonly bacterial. Of the nonneutropenic cancer patients with fever, approximately 17 percent have associated infection. The common pathogens are listed in Table 74-3.

Evaluation of the child with cancer and fever includes a careful history and physical examination. Particular attention is paid to occult sites of potential infection, such as the oropharynx, axillae, groin, perineum, sites of previous invasive procedures, and along the tract of any indwelling venous access device. It is important to note that fever may be the only positive sign and that other findings, such as exudates, adenopathy, fluctuance, warmth, and swelling, may be absent. A child with early pneumonia may not have cough or sputum production. Rales are frequently absent on chest auscultation.

Initial investigations include a chest radiograph, urinalysis and urine culture, CBC, and two sets of blood cultures obtained from different sites. If an indwelling catheter is present, one blood specimen is obtained from the line and one from a peripheral vein. An aspirate for Gram stain and culture is sent from any area suggestive of focal infection. An arterial blood gas is obtained from patients suspected of having pneumonia or sepsis.

Prompt initiation of empiric antibiotic therapy in the febrile neutropenic child has been associated with a reduction in morbidity and mortality. Combination therapy has been the usual approach to provide broad-spectrum antibiotic coverage (Table 74-4). An aminoglycoside and beta-lactam or two beta-lactam drugs are used to provide gram-negative bacterial coverage. Addition of a penicillinase-resistant penicillin provides gram-positive bacterial coverage. The development of broad-spectrum antibiotics has made monotherapy a growing option for initial empiric therapy. Ceftazi-

TABLE 74-3 Common Pathogens in Children with Cancer

Bacteria
- Gram-positive aerobes
  - *Staphylococcus aureus*
  - Coagulase-negative staphylococci
  - Alpha-hemolytic streptococci
  - Enterococci
- Gram-negative aerobes
  - Enterobacteriaceae (*Escherichia coli, Klebsiella pneumoniae*)
  - *Pseudomonas aeruginosa*
  - *Enterobacter, Citrobacter, Serratia*
  - Anaerobes

Fungi
- *Candida* species
- *Aspergillus* species
- *Cryptococcus*

Parasites
- *Pneumocystis carinii*
- *Cryptosporidium* species
- *Strongyloides stercoralis*

Viruses
- Herpes simplex virus
- Varicella zoster virus
- Cytomegalovirus

Source: Adapted from Pizzo PA, Rubin M, Freifeld A, Walsh TJ. The child with cancer and infection: I. Empiric therapy for fever and neutropenia, and preventive strategies. *J Pediatr* 119:679, 1991.

dime, a third-generation cephalosporin with good activity against *Pseudomonas aeruginosa,* has been efficacious when used in patients with fever and neutropenia. Some institutions will extend the gram-positive coverage using a penicillinase-resistant penicillin or vancomycin along with ceftazidime.

Modifications to Therapy

Patients with a focus of infection may require modifications in therapy. Signs or symptoms suggestive of an infection along the gastrointestinal tract warrant extended anaerobic coverage with either metronidazole or clindamycin. The presence of a pulmonary infiltrate may represent a bacterial, viral, fungal, or parasitic infection. Patients with diffuse or interstitial infiltrates receive trimethoprim/sulfamethoxazole (TMP/SMX) for possible *Pneumocystis carinii* infection, as well as erythromycin for *Legionella* and *Mycoplasma* coverage. In the face of neutropenia, these antibiotics are

TABLE 74-4 Empiric Antibiotic Therapy for the Febrile Neutropenic Patient

Rationale	Drug	Dose
Gram negative coverage	Gentamicin	5–7.5 mg/kg/day IV divided q8h
	or	
	tobramycin	(as for gentamicin)
PLUS antipseudomonal penicillin	Ticarcillin	200–300 mg/kg/day IV divided q4–6h
	or	
	mezlocillin	(as for ticarcillin)
	or	
	piperacillin	(as for ticarcillin)
	OR	
Third-generation cephalosporin alone	Ceftazidime	100–150 mg/kg/day IV divided q8h
or		
with antipseudomonal penicillin	As above	As above
If immediate-type penicillin allergy	Aztreonam	75–150 mg/kg/day IV divided q6h
	plus aminoglycoside	as above
Gram-positive coverage: Penicillinase-resistant penicillin	Oxacillin	100–200 mg/kg/day IV divided q4–6h
	or	
	nafcillin	(as for oxacillin)
If indwelling central venous catheter	Vancomycin	40 mg/kg/day IV divided q6h
Pulmonary infiltrates,		
interstitial	Broad-spectrum antibiotics	As above
or	plus	
diffuse	trimethoprim/sulfamethoxazole	15–20 mg/kg/day IV divided q6h (based on TMP component)
	plus	
	erythromycin	30–50 mg/kg/day IV divided q6h
Patchy or localized	Broad-spectrum antibiotics	As above

Source: Adapted from Pizzo PA, Rubin M, Freifeld A, et al: The child with cancer and infection: I. Empiric therapy for fever and neutropenia, and preventative strategies. *J Pediatr* 119:679, 1991.

added to the baseline broad-spectrum therapy. In the neutropenic patient with a patchy or localized infiltrate, broad-spectrum antibiotic therapy should suffice.

Fungal Infections

Cancer patients who are febrile and neutropenic are at risk for fungal infections, particularly *Candida* species. In the pediatric patient, the oral cavity is the most common site of fungal infection. It may present asymptomatically as punctate foci or diffuse erythematous mucosal plaques and ulcerations. Any patient with difficulty breathing, hoarseness, or stridor should be considered to have epiglottic or laryngeal candidiasis. A KOH preparation of a scraping reveals hyphae. A scraping from the base of a lesion is sent for fungal and viral culture. Neutropenic patients who are afebrile and able to tolerate oral medication may be treated with topical antifungal agents such as clotrimazole. If there has been minimal response with clotrimazole, ketaconazole (5 to 10 mg/kg/day divided qid or bid) or fluconazole (2 to 8 mg/kg once daily) may be tried. Patients with oral or esophageal candidiasis who have not responded to or are unable to tolerate topical therapy are candidates for intravenous antifungal agents such as amphotericin B. Those with suspected epiglottic or laryngeal involvement may require airway support and close observation.

Viral Infections

Herpes simplex virus (HSV) infections tend to be localized, even in the immunocompromised patient, and commonly involve the mouth, nares, esophagus, genitals, and perianal region. Pain is the predominant presenting symptom. Disruption of the mucosa may promote secondary bacterial infection. Laboratory diagnosis is confirmed through viral culture or direct immunofluorescence studies on the inoculated tissue culture. Immunocompromised patients with mild mucocutaneous disease may be started on oral acyclovir (200 mg PO five times a day). Patients with moderate or severe HSV infection are admitted for intravenous acyclovir therapy (250 mg/m^2 IV q8h).

Varicella zoster virus (VZV) infections in an immunocompromised patient are associated with significant morbidity and mortality. Patients with Hodgkin's disease, non-Hodgkin's lymphoma, solid tumors, and bone marrow transplant are particularly at risk. Diagnosis of VZV infection is usually based on the characteristic vesicular lesions. Laboratory confirmation is by positive culture of the virus from scraping of the base of the lesions. Direct immunofluorescence staining of the vesicular fluid smear or tissue specimen is also rapid and accurate. A chest radiograph is obtained to assess for pneumonia. Liver transaminases may be elevated in varicella hepatitis. Cancer patients with VZV infection are usually admitted for intravenous acyclovir. Varicella zoster seronegative patients who are seen within 96 h of virus exposure receive varicella zoster immune globulin at a dose of 125 U/10 kg IM with a maximum dose of 625 U.

Parasitic Infections

Pneumocystis carinii (PC) is the most common parasitic infection in the immunocompromised patient. Children with hematological malignancies are most at risk. Typically, the patient will present with fever, dry cough, tachypnea, and intercostal retractions, without detectable rales. The chest radiograph may be normal in early disease but later progresses to bilateral alveolar infiltrates. Atypical radiographic findings include lobar consolidation and effusion. Arterial blood gas analysis reveals a decrease in P_{CO_2}, normal or decreased P_{CO_2}, and increased pH. Diagnosis is confirmed by bronchoalveolar lavage or open lung biopsy. Immunocompromised patients are started on empiric therapy with TMP/SMX pending definitive diagnosis, as well as erythromycin for empiric *Legionella* coverage.

Tumor Lysis Syndrome

Tumor lysis syndrome (TLS) results from the rapid degradation of tumor cells and release of the intracellular metabolites uric acid, phosphate, and potassium in excess of their renal clearance. The result is hyperuricemia, hyperphosphatemia, and in some cases hyperkalemia.

The syndrome occurs prior to or within several days after the initiation of cancer therapy. It is more commonly seen in patients with a large tumor cell load or rapidly growing tumors such as Burkitt's lymphoma and T cell lymphoma-leukemia. The syndrome is generally not seen with nonlymphomatous solid tumors.

Uric acid, a product of purine catabolism from nucleic acids, usually exists as a soluble form. However, with excessive amounts, it may precipitate in the renal collecting ducts, leading to obstruction, oliguria, azotemia, and renal failure. The phosphate concentration in lymphoblasts is four times higher than in normal lymphocytes. Calcium phosphate crystals start to form when the calcium phosphate product exceeds 60 mg/dL, and the crystals become trapped in the renal microvasculature. The result is renal failure and hypocalcemia. Potassium is a major intracellular electrolyte which, with TLS, can cause hyperkalemia as well as exacerbate existing hyperkalemia due to renal failure. Cardiac complications include ventricular arrhythmias and asystole.

Signs and symptoms of TLS include nausea, vomiting, lethargy, abdominal or back pain, and change in urine color and amount. Hypocalcemia may manifest as muscle weakness, spasms, tetany, convulsions, altered level of consciousness, photophobia, or abdominal pain.

All patients with possible TLS require a CBC, electrolytes, BUN, creatinine, glucose, calcium, phosphate, uric acid, urinalysis, and electrocardiogram (ECG).

Therapy is directed at treatment of hyperuricemia and hyperphosphatemia and prevention of renal failure. Hydration is important in facilitating uric acid and phosphate excretion. Intravenous fluid is administered at a minimum of twice the patient's maintenance rate, aiming at a urine specific gravity of less than 1.010. Uric acid production may be reduced with allopurinol. Alkalinization of the urine increases uric acid solubility and excretion. This is achieved by adding one ampule (44 meq) of sodium bicarbonate to each liter of D_5W 0.2*N*/S to keep the urine pH around 7 or 7.5. Urine pH greater than 7.5 may promote precipitation of hypoxanthine and calcium phosphate, while uric acid crystals tend to form at a pH less than 7. Calcium supplementation for hypocalcemia is indicated only in patients who are severely symptomatic with a normal serum phosphate. Hyperkalemia may be reduced by calcium gluconate (100 to 200 mg/kg/dose, slowly by IV), sodium bicarbonate, and insulin along with dextrose (see Chap. 56). Sodium polystyrene sulfonate (Kayexalate) per rectum in the neutropenic patient may create a perirectal infection and is therefore to be avoided. Dialysis is indicated for persistent hyperkalemia, uric acid concentrations exceeding 10 mg/dL, creatinine >10 mg/dL, phosphate >10 mg/dL, and symptomatic hypocalcemia.

Syndrome of Inappropriate Antidiuretic Hormone

The syndrome of inappropriate antidiuretic hormone (SIADH) results in excessive free water retention and subsequent fall in serum sodium concentration. In pediatric cancer patients, SIADH is often related to chemotherapeutic agents such as vincristine or cyclophosphamide.

Clinically, patients may present with weight gain, fatigue, lethargy, confusion, seizures, or coma. Typical laboratory studies reveal hyponatremia, hypoosmolality (often less than 260 mosm/L), and an increase in urine osmolality and urine sodium concentration.

Asymptomatic patients may be treated with fluid restriction to about two-thirds of their usual maintenance needs. Those symptomatic patients with hyponatremia and seizures or coma require prompt correction of the serum sodium concentration to approximately 125 meq/L with 3% saline.

Superior Vena Cava Syndrome

Superior vena cava (SVC) syndrome refers to the signs and symptoms resulting from obstruction of the SVC. Although usually due to extrinsic compression of the SVC and its branches, up to half of the cases may have concomitant intravascular thrombosis. In children, compression of the narrow, more compliant trachea poses an additional complication.

Superior vena cava syndrome occurs most commonly in non-Hodgkin's lymphoma and Hodgkin's disease. The presence of central venous catheters predisposes to vascular thrombosis and SVC syndrome. When structures surrounding the SVC and trachea enlarge, they cause compression and result in clotting and edema formation, impeding airflow and blood return from the head, neck, and upper thorax. Collateral vessels become enlarged but provide inadequate compensation. In children and adolescents, symptoms of SVC syndrome may progress rapidly over several days, unlike in adults, where the onset is more insidious.

Patients present with edema and plethora of the face, conjunctivae, neck, and upper torso. Tortuous collateral veins appear on the chest and upper abdomen. Headache, papilledema, seizures, coma, cerebral hemorrhage, and engorgement of retinal veins are a result of cerebral venous hypertension. Compression of the tracheobronchial tree may cause tachypnea, wheezing, stridor, orthopnea, or cyanosis. Other presentations include vocal cord paralysis, Horner's syndrome, and, in extreme cases, lower cervical or upper thoracic spinal cord compression. Fatalities from SVC syndrome are related to airway obstruction, cerebral edema, or cardiac compromise.

Chest radiography reveals superior mediastinal widening and occasionally a pleural or pericardial effusion. The trachea may appear deviated or narrowed. A complete blood count with differential may show evidence of leukemia or lymphoma.

The first priority in management is to protect and secure the airway. If SVC syndrome is due to central venous catheter thrombosis, a thrombolytic agent such as urokinase may avert the need to remove the catheter. Radiation has been the traditional mode of therapy for tumor-induced SVC syndrome; however, chemotherapy is an effective alternative. Some patients will require empiric therapy prior to tissue diagnosis to reduce the compressive effects of the tumor.

Supportive therapy includes minimizing cerebral hypertension by elevation of the head of the bed. Intravenous hydration may be more efficient through a low-pressure lower extremity vein. Upper extremity phlebotomy is avoided, as these veins are under high pressure and may bleed excessively. Correction of electrolyte abnormalities and treatment of hyperuricemia should be initiated.

Spinal Cord Compression

Spinal cord compression due to a tumor occurs in approximately 4 percent of pediatric cancer patients. Extradural metastatic tumors such as soft tissue sarcomas, neuroblastoma, and lymphoma account for the majority of cases. About two-thirds of patients may complain of muscle weakness, limp, or increased fatigue. Other common findings include back pain, which may be localized or radicular, sensory deficits, or change in bladder and bowel function. Hydrocephalus may result from physical obstruction from a high cervical tumor or elevated cerebrospinal fluid protein levels. Most patients will usually have objective neurologic deficits at the time of presentation.

Plain spine radiographs will show an abnormality in less than 50 percent of these patients. Contrast myelography or MRI provides a more definitive study.

Spinal cord compression is a true neurologic emergency. Treatment begins with dexamethasone to reduce tumor-related edema. Myelography or MRI is done immediately in those patients with progressive neurologic deficit or within 24 in stable symptomatic patients without loss of function. Epidural masses require immediate decompression with glucocorticoids, radiation therapy, or laminectomy.

Central Nervous System Emergencies

Children with cancer may present with CNS abnormalities such as altered mental status, intracranial hemorrhage, and seizures. Metabolic or structural insults to the reticular activating system or cerebral hemispheres may alter the patient's level of consciousness and may or may not be accompanied by raised intracranial pressure (ICP). Electrolyte abnormalities, hypoxia, renal or hepatic failure, DIC, and sepsis are some common metabolic derangements. Primary CNS tumors and metastatic lesions may present with acute mental status changes; CNS infections may be diffuse or localized. Cerebrovascular accidents (CVA) may complicate acute leukemia as a result of cerebral arterial or venous thrombosis or intracranial hemorrhage. Seizures may arise from a metabolic abnormality, infection, or metastatic disease, or as a complication of CNS therapy.

The initial evaluation includes a CBC, electrolytes, glucose, creatinine, BUN, phosphate, calcium, uric acid, magnesium, and coagulation studies. Arterial blood gas or oxygen saturation is obtained to evaluate for hypoxia. A CT scan of the head without contrast can assess for tumor or intracranial bleed.

Treatment for patients with altered mental status begins with support and protection of the airway and breathing. If raised ICP is suspected, hyperventilation to a P_{CO_2} of 25 to 30 mmHg will help reduce cerebral blood flow. Dexamethasone is given to patients with an intracranial tumor in order to decrease cerebral edema. Prompt surgical consultation is recommended if a mass lesion or hemorrhage is demonstrated on CT scan. If meningitis is suspected, defer lumbar puncture but initiate antibiotics prior to the CT scan. Thrombocytopenia and coagulopathy are corrected, especially in the presence of an intracranial hemorrhage.

Gastrointestinal Emergencies

In addition to the more common causes of acute abdominal pain, pediatric cancer patients are at risk for unique conditions, such as esophagitis, gastric ulcers, typhlitis (a severe necrotizing cecitis occurring in neutropenic patients), perirectal abscess, pancreatitis, and cholecystitis. Leukemic infiltrates can accumulate in the stomach and small bowel, predisposing to intussusception and bowel obstruction. Hemorrhagic necrosis of the mucosal layer can occur, and may be related to vascular insufficiency, coagulation abnormalities, or chemotherapeutic agents. Agranulocytic necrosis is a result of bacterial invasion of the bowel wall and is complicated by perforation. Fungal lesions can invade the gastrointestinal tract or solid organs. Perirectal cellulitis and abscess result from anaerobic and gram-negative bacteria invading the perirectal area. Gastrointestinal hemorrhage can result from thrombocytopenia, coagulopathy, mucosal ulceration, or abnormal tumor vessels.

Evaluation of the cancer patient with acute abdominal pain includes characterization of the pain and associated symptoms. The abdominal examination begins with careful observation, gentle palpation, and serial reexamination. Rectal examination is key in detecting pelvic and perirectal disease, and neutropenia is not a contraindication to this maneuver.

Laboratory workup includes a CBC, blood and urine cultures, urinalysis, electrolytes, glucose, and amylase. A chest radiograph is done to assess for pneumonia, and abdominal films may reveal bowel obstruction, perforation, or pneumatosis intestinalis.

Patients with an acute abdomen are admitted and started on intravenous hydration. Nonneutropenic patients with esophagitis and presumptive gastric stress ulcers may benefit from H_2 antagonists. Thrombocytopenia and coagulopathies are corrected in the presence of hemorrhage. Patients with typhlitis must be started on broad-spectrum antibiotics. Early surgical consultation is recommended. Indications for laparotomy include evidence of perforation, persistent gastrointestinal hemorrhage despite correction of existing coagulopathies, and clinical deterioration.

For a more detailed discussion, see Hayakawa BN: Oncologic emergencies, chap. 74, p. 463, in *Pediatric Emergency Medicine: A Comprehensive Study Guide.*

SECTION XVI
NONTRAUMATIC BONE AND JOINT DISORDERS

75 Infectious Musculoskeletal Diseases

Diana Mayer

SEPTIC ARTHRITIS

Septic arthritis is an infection occurring within a joint space. In the vast majority of cases, it is of bacterial etiology. Septic arthritis occurs more commonly in children than in adults. Males are more frequently affected than females. In 80 percent of cases, the infection involves a joint of the lower extremity.

Seeding of the joint with bacteria occurs either by hematogenous spread, by direct inoculation, or by spread from an adjacent site of infection. Direct inoculation most commonly affects the knee. In the pediatric population, septic arthritis resulting from a spread from a contiguous focus is uncommon. However, in infants, metaphyseal osteomyelitis can spread to the joint via blood vessels that bridge the epiphysis.

In the first 2 months of life, *Staphylococcus aureus* and group B streptococci are the most common pathogens. However, infection with gram-negative organisms such as *Escherichia coli* can occur. From 3 months to about 3 years, *S. aureus* is a common pathogen. After approximately 3 years of age, *S. aureus* predominates until adolescence, when *Neisseria gonorrhoeae* becomes a frequent pathogen. Other bacteria commonly implicated in septic arthritis, especially in younger patients, include pneumococcus and group A streptococci. *Haemophilus influenzae* type B was a common pathogen in children less than 3 years of age until the advent of a highly effective vaccine.

Immunosuppressed patients are particularly vulnerable to infection with gram-negative organisms, including *Pseudomonas*. Patients with sickle cell disease are susceptible to infection with *Salmonella* species.

A majority of cases of septic arthritis involve one joint. Neonates and young infants are prone to infection of the hip. The first manifestation of disease may be nonspecific irritability. Parents may note that the baby appears to be in pain when the diaper is changed. As the disease progresses, the baby holds the hip flexed and abducted, which allows for maximum opening of the joint capsule and helps relieve pressure. The presence of lethargy may indicate concomitant meningitis. In older infants and children, the knee is more commonly affected. Patients old enough to ambulate may begin to walk with a limp or may refuse to walk. Septic arthritis of the knee and most other joints is characterized by warmth, the presence of an effusion, and, in the majority of cases, significant limitation of range of motion. Most patients are febrile.

Gonococcal arthritis is likely in any postpubertal patient with joint pain and fever. It usually accompanies asymptomatic disease of the genitourinary tract. In the early stages, patients may complain of fever, chills, and polyarthralgia. The knee, ankle, and especially the joints of the wrist, hand, and fingers are affected. Some patients develop tenosynovitis. A rash may develop that can consist of petechiae, papules, and pustular lesions with erythematous halos. Monoarticular arthritis can eventually occur.

Laboratory Evaluation

The laboratory evaluation of suspected septic arthritis includes a complete blood count, erythrocyte sedimentation rate, and blood cultures. In most patients, the white blood count and the erythrocyte sedimentation rate will be elevated. Many patients, especially neonates and young infants, will have positive blood cultures.

The mainstay in the diagnosis of septic arthritis is analysis of joint fluid. The fluid from a septic joint is often turbid. While there is considerable overlap in the cell count between bacterially mediated arthritis and other causes of joint inflammation, the white blood cell count in a septic joint is generally greater than 50,000 to 75,000/mL and is associated with more than 75 percent neutrophils. The percentage of glucose in an infected joint is often less than 50 percent of that in the serum. Table 75-1 contrasts the characteristics of joint fluid under various conditions. Up to 70 percent of patients may have a positive joint culture except in the case of gonococcal arthritis, where the culture is usually negative. Up to 50 percent of patients have a positive Gram stain. In infants, if clinical findings are indicative of or cannot exclude meningitis, a lumbar puncture is indicated. Radiographic studies may be useful in demonstrating the presence of a joint effusion.

TABLE 75-1 Differential Diagnosis of Joint Fluid

	Normal	*Bacterial*	*Inflammatory*
Appearance	Clear	Turbid, purulent	Clear or turbid
Leukocytes	<100 cells/mm^3	$>50{,}000$ cells/mm^3	500–75,000 cells/mm^3
Neutrophils, %	25	>75	50
Glucose Synovial/Blood	$>50\%$	$<50\%$	$>50\%$

TABLE 75-2 Treatment of Septic Arthritis

	Organisms	Initial antibiotics
Neonates	Group B *Streptococcus* *Staphylococcus aureus* Gram-negative enteric bacilli[a] *Candida*[a] *Neisseria gonorrhoea*[a]	Nafcillin and gentamicin
Infants	*Staphylococcus aureus* *Haemophilus influenzae*	Ceftriaxone
Children	*S. aureus* Group A *Streptococcus* *Streptococcus pneumoniae* *H. influenzae*	Nafcillin or cefuroxime if hemophilus influenzae type B (HIB) vaccination is not up to date
Teens	*N. gonorrhoea* *S. aureus*	Ceftriaxone
Immunosuppressed	Gram-negative enteric bacilli	Cetriaxone
Sickle cell anemia	*Salmonella* spp.	Cetriaxone
Puncture wounds	*Pseudomonas aeruginosa*	Ceftazidime plus gentamicin and carbenicillin plus gentamicin

[a] Rare.

The differential diagnosis of septic arthritis includes transient synovitis, traumatic hemarthrosis, and osteomyelitis.

Treatment of septic arthritis consists of antibiotic therapy directed at the likely bacterial organisms and drainage of the involved joint. In neonates, antibiotic treatment usually consists of nafcillin and an aminoglycoside. Older infants and children under 10 years of age can be treated with nafcillin or a second- or third-generation cephalosporin. If *N. gonorrhoeaea* is a possibility, ceftriaxone is the drug of choice. Table 75-2 summarizes treatment.

The procedure used for drainage depends to some degree on the joint involved. In the case of the hip, urgent arthrotomy is indicated to avoid permanent damage to the vulnerable femoral head. Arthrotomy should also be strongly considered in septic arthritis of the shoulder. In the case of a septic knee, serial aspiration is preferred, although in some instances arthrotomy may be required.

OSTEOMYELITIS

Osteomyelitis is an infection of the bone. In the pediatric age group, it is most common between the ages of 3 and 12. Boys are more commonly affected than girls.

Seeding of the bone with bacteria occurs either by hematogenous spread, by direct inoculation, or by extension from an adjacent septic joint. The anatomy of the growth plate may contribute to the development of osteomyelitis.

The most common etiology of osteomyelitis is *S. aureus.* In neonates, group B streptococci and enteric gram-negative organisms are possible causes, and in unvaccinated infants older than 4 to 6 weeks of age, *h influenzae* type B can occur. In patients sustaining puncture wounds to the foot, *Pseudomonas aeruginosa* is a potential pathogen. *Salmonella* is a consideration in patients with sickle cell disease.

Neonates may demonstrate few clinical findings other than irritability, fever, and some resistance to movement of a limb. Older infants and children may be able to localize discomfort over the affected site. Limp is a common finding in ambulatory patients. Most patients are febrile. In some cases, the physical examination reveals erythema, warmth, and swelling over the area of bone involvement.

Laboratory assessment includes a complete blood count, erythrocyte sedimentation rate, blood culture, and radiograph of the affected area. The white blood count may be normal or elevated, but the erythrocyte sedimentation rate is usually increased. Blood cultures are positive about 50 percent of the time. Radiographs are usually unremarkable during the first week of the illness. Around day 7, mottling and demineralization of bone are seen. New periosteal bone formation becomes evident around day 10.

Radionuclear scanning with technetium 99m is more sensitive than radiography early in the course of disease. Increased uptake is often observed within 1 to 2 days after the onset of infection. In some cases, a gallium 67 citrate bone scan or magnetic resonance imaging may be helpful. In suspected *Pseudomonas* osteomyelitis of the foot following a puncture wound, a bone biopsy and culture of the lesion may be desirable.

Treatment for osteomyelitis is directed at eradicating the infection. Antibiotic coverage for *S. aureus* is always indicated. Other antibiotic coverage depends on the age of the patient and the clinical situation. In general, hospitalization is warranted.

TABLE 75-3 Treatment of Osteomyelitis

	Organisms	Initial treatment
Neonates	Group B *Streptococcus* *Staphylococcus aureus* Gram-negative enterics	Nafcillin and gentamicin May add penicillin if cultures indicate group B *Streptococcus*
Infants	*S. aureus* *Haemophilus influenzae*	Nafcillin and cefotaxime
Older children	*S. aureus*	Nafcillin
Teens	*N. gonorrhoea*	Ceftriaxone
Sickle cell anemia patients	*Salmonella* *S. aureus*	Nafcillin/cefotaxime or ceftriaxone
Puncture wounds/ IV drug abusers	*Pseudomonas aeruginosa*	Ceftazidime plus gentamicin or carbenicillin plus gentamicin

Table 75-3 lists antibiotic coverage for osteomyelitis under various circumstances.

INTERVERTEBRAL DISKITIS

Intervertebral diskitis is an acute infection of the vertebral disk occasionally seen in children. Affected patients are usually below 5 years of age. Most commonly, the lumbar area is involved. The common pathogen is *S. aureus*; less commonly, pneumococcus and gram-negative organisms are involved. Rarely, the infection results from tuberculosis.

Most cases are preceded by an upper respiratory infection. Infants may become irritable and refuse to sit. Toddlers may refuse to walk. Older children may complain of back or leg pain and may develop a limp. If the lesion occurs at the lower thoracic or upper lumbar area, the child may have gastrointestinal symptoms.

The physical examination may show a loss of lordosis. Tenderness along the vertebrae, mild fullness of the paraspinal muscles secondary to irritation, and occasionally hip pain and stiffness can occur.

Radiographs of the involved area may demonstrate a narrowing of the disk space and, eventually, erosion of the vertebral end plates. The erythrocyte sedimentation rate is usually elevated. In about 40 percent of cases, blood cultures are positive. In some patients, computed tomography (CT) may be helpful.

Affected children can usually be managed as outpatients, with antibiotic therapy directed against *S. aureus.* Despite treatment, older children commonly develop spontaneous spinal fusion.

LYME DISEASE

Lyme disease is caused by the spirochete *Borrelia burgdorferi* and is transmitted by the *Ixodes* tick species. In the United States, it is clustered mainly along the East Coast, the northern Midwest, and the West Coast.

The disease occurs in three stages. The first stage begins around 1 week after inoculation by the tick and is marked by a characteristic rash known as erythema chronicum migrans. The lesion starts as an erythematous papule or macule that spreads outward to form an enlarging circle with a red rim and central clearing. It often disappears within 4 weeks of the initial tick bite. Many patients develop secondary skin lesions. Many patients experience fever, malaise, lethargy, and headache. Some patients complain of myalgias and suffer meningismus.

The second stage of the illness begins around 4 weeks after the onset. Patients commonly develop aseptic meningitis, but they can suffer other neurologic complaints, including encephalitis, multiple radiculopathies, chorea, and ataxia. In this stage some patients also develop cardiac conduction abnormalities.

The third stage of the illness is also characterized by the development of arthritis, which may be the presenting complaint. Large joints are most commonly affected, especially the knee, although virtually any joint can be involved. In some cases, the arthritis is migratory. Although the affected joints are swollen and painful, they are rarely red. Many patients suffer multiple attacks of arthritis, which can occur years after the initial infection, despite treatment with antibiotics.

The differential diagnosis of Lyme arthritis includes acute rheumatic fever, juvenile rheumatoid arthritis, and postinfectious virally induced arthritis. Laboratory studies include a complete blood count, antinuclear antibody, rheumatoid factor, urinalysis, electrocardiogram, throat culture and streptococcal screen, and Lyme disease titers. Joint fluid in patients with active arthritis may contain up to 100,000 white blood cells per milliliter, with a preponderance of polymorphonuclear leukocytes.

Antibiotic treatment of Lyme disease shortens the course of disease and can prevent the development of chronic illness. In some cases it effectively treats established chronic arthritis and neurologic symptoms. Oral treatment with penicillin or tetracycline is indicated in early disease. Treatment with tetracycline may be more effective than penicillin in preventing late complications. Children under 9 years of age should not receive tetracycline. Penicillin-allergic patients can receive erythromycin. Patients with evidence of neurologic involvement or chronic arthritis are treated with high-dose intravenous penicillin. Ceftriaxone is also effective. Symptomatic arthritis may respond to therapy with high-dose aspirin.

ACUTE SUPPURATIVE TENOSYNOVITIS

The palmar surface of the hand is vulnerable to suppurative tenosynovitis, which usually occurs as an extension of a localized infection.

Physical examination of the hand reveals erythema and tenderness along the tendon sheath. Patients hold the affected finger in a flexed position, and active or passive extension provokes intense pain. The affected finger is diffusely swollen.

The most common bacterial etiologies are *S. aureus* and group A streptococci. In adolescents and sexually abused children, *N. gonorrhoeae* is a likely possibility.

Management consists of therapy with antibiotics and surgical drainage. Therefore, orthopedic consultation is indicated.

For a more detailed discussion, see Mayer D: Infectious musculoskeletal diseases, chap. 75, p. 475, in *Pediatric Emergency Medicine: A Comprehensive Study Guide.*

---

76 Inflammatory Musculoskeletal Disorders

Diana Mayer

REACTIVE AND POSTINFECTIOUS ARTHRITIS

In many inflammatory and infectious disorders, arthritis is an associated finding. Both ulcerative colitis and Crohn disease can result in arthritis in children. Gastroenteritis caused by *Shigella, Salmo-*

nella, and *Campylobacter* can also produce arthritis. Multiple viral infections, including hepatitis, Epstein-Barr virus, rubella, and adenovirus, are also associated with arthritis. Infection with *Mycoplasma pneumoniae* is occasionally associated with arthritis. Reiter syndrome consists of urethritis, conjunctivitis, and arthritis. It can follow infections caused by *Shigella* and, in sexually active individuals, sexually transmitted disease. The treatment of reactive arthritis usually consists of therapy with anti-inflammatory agents. Definitive therapy is predicated upon accurate diagnosis of the primary disease process.

TRANSIENT SYNOVITIS

A common cause of nontraumatic hip pain is transient synovitis, which is also referred to as toxic synovitis. It is presumed to be an inflammatory process and often follows an upper respiratory infection. The disorder is usually seen in children between the ages of 18 months and 7 years and is most common during the second year of life.

The presenting complaint in a toddler may be refusal to walk. Older patients may complain of hip or knee pain. Patients may be afebrile or have a low-grade fever. Physical examination reveals pain localized to the hip. Some resistance to range of motion is present.

Laboratory studies are useful in distinguishing transient synovitis from a septic hip. In transient synovitis, the white blood cell count and erythrocyte sedimentation rate are usually normal or only slightly elevated. Radiographic findings are usually not helpful. However, in older children with hip pain, Legg-Calvé-Perthes disease is a diagnostic possibility, and follow-up films are indicated.

The treatment of transient synovitis is bed rest and therapy with anti-inflammatory agents. The prognosis is excellent.

JUVENILE RHEUMATOID ARTHRITIS

Juvenile rheumatoid arthritis (JRA) encompasses a spectrum of clinically distinct inflammatory diseases that have their onset in childhood. Juvenile rheumatoid arthritis is classified as polyarticular, which involves about 50 percent of patients; pauciarticular, which affects about 35 percent; and systemic-onset, affecting the remaining 15 percent.

Polyarticular disease involves more than four joints and is further categorized as rheumatoid factor–positive or rheumatoid factor–negative. Both types of disease are more common in girls, but rheumatoid factor–positive disease is more likely to result in severe arthritis. The onset of illness may be insidious or fulminant. Arthritis often begins in large joints and is symmetrical. Symptoms are worse in the morning. Affected joints are swollen and warm, although erythema is unusual. While discomfort on range of motion exists, joint pain is generally not severe. Many patients have significant involvement of the joints of the hand, and up to half have involvement of the cervical spine, which in severe cases can result in atlantoaxial instability. Some patients have involvement of the temporomandibular joint. Occasionally arthritis occurs in the cricoarytenoid joint, where it can result in hoarseness of the voice.

Systemic involvement in polyarticular disease includes fever, irritability, and occasional hepatomegaly. In severe cases, significant growth disturbances can occur.

Pauciarticular disease involves four or fewer joints. It is categorized as type I or type II. Type I has its onset in early childhood and is associated with the presence of antinuclear antibodies. Large joints are most commonly affected, although hip involvement is unusual. Severe joint destruction is uncommon. However, up to 30 percent of patients with pauciarticular disease develop chronic iridocyclitis. Other systemic manifestations of disease are generally mild.

Type II pauciarticular disease is more common in boys, has an onset in later childhood, and is not associated with antinuclear antibodies. As is the case with pauciarticular disease type I, large joints are most commonly involved. Hip involvement and sacroiliitis can occur, as can Achilles tendinitis. Unlike patients with type I disease, these patients may develop chronic spondyloarthropathies, especially of the lumbar area. Patients with type II disease are also at risk for acute iridocyclitis.

Systemic-onset disease occurs throughout childhood. Unlike with the other forms of JRA, systemic manifestations predominate. Intermittent spiking fever is often the initial manifestation of disease. The fever is often accompanied by a characteristic rash, which appears as pink, often coalescent, macules that commonly develop on the trunk and extremities. The rash is transient and recurrent. Hepatosplenomegaly and lymphadenopathy are common. Eventually, patients develop joint involvement, which tends to be polyarticular. The onset of joint disease may be significantly delayed, which can obscure the diagnosis of JRA.

Systemic-onset JRA is often associated with chronic, debilitating arthritis. Other complications include the development of pericarditis, and in some cases pericardial effusion. Myocarditis and pleuritis can also occur. Some patients develop anemia. Episodes of severe disease can be accompanied by abdominal pain.

The differential diagnosis of JRA includes acute rheumatic fever, systemic lupus erythematosus, bacterial arthritis, reactive arthritis, and neoplastic diseases, especially leukemia. The workup of suspected JRA includes a complete blood count, renal function studies, and an erythrocyte sedimentation rate. Patients with myocarditis or pericarditis require an electrocardiogram and echocardiogram.

The treatment of JRA consists of aggressive therapy with anti-inflammatory agents. The initial treatment is usually aspirin, although other nonsteroidal agents are also commonly utilized. In severe cases, cytotoxic drugs or gold salts may be effective. Patients with severe pericarditis or myocarditis may respond to prednisone.

SYSTEMIC LUPUS ERYTHEMATOSUS

Systemic lupus erythematosus (SLE) is an inflammatory disease of probable autoimmune etiology that affects multiple organ systems. About 20 percent of cases of SLE begin in childhood and adolescence. After puberty, the disease is far more common in females.

Complaints in patients with SLE include fever, malaise, weight loss, and fatigue. Skin manifestations include the characteristic erythematous rash extending from the malar regions across the bridge of the nose. Some patients develop alopecia. About half of pediatric patients will complain of joint pain, and most will eventually develop joint disease. Aside from pain, symptoms include morning stiffness and swelling. Clinically, the patient's pain may be disproportionately greater than the degree of swelling would suggest. Joint involvement is usually symmetrical. Other musculoskeletal complaints include tenosynovitis and periostitis. Myalgia and diffuse muscle weakness can also occur. In approximately 15 percent of patients, avascular necrosis occurs, most commonly in the femoral head. Involvement of serosal membranes, including the pleura, peritoneum, and pericardium, is a prominent aspect of SLE and leads to complications that include pleuritis with or without pleural effusion, peritonitis, and pericarditis. Pericarditis can occasionally result in a clinically significant pericardial effusion. Cardiac complications include myocarditis and myocardial infarction.

Pulmonary disease includes pneumonitis and, on occasion, pulmonary hemorrhage. Involvement of the central nervous system can result in alterations of mental status, seizures, or cerebrovascular accidents. Most patients develop renal disease, which can ultimately result in renal failure. Hematologic abnormalities include anemia, thrombocytopenia, and leukopenia.

In all patients with suspected SLE, a complete blood count, prothrombin time (PT), partial thromboplastin time (PTT), and erythrocyte sedimentation rate are indicated, as are serum electrolytes, blood urea nitrogen, and creatinine. A urinalysis will often reveal microscopic hematuria and proteinuria. Antinuclear antibody, rheumatoid factor, complement studies, and quantitative immunoglobulins are indicated but are not clinically useful in the emergency department. If there is evidence of a coagulopathy, lupus anticoagulant and antiphospholipid antibody tests are indicated.

Therapy is directed primarily at ameliorating the underlying inflammatory process. In mild disease, nonsteroidal anti-inflammatory agents may suffice. Ibuprofen is not recommended because of a possible link with aseptic meningitis. More severe manifestations or flareups of quiescent disease may respond to therapy with glucocorticoids. In patients with acute, severe symptoms, high-dose pulse therapy with intravenous glucocorticoids may be necessary. In extremely severe cases, such as rapidly progressive renal disease, immunosuppressive agents such as cyclophosphamide (Cytoxan) or azathioprine (Imuran) are added to glucocorticoid therapy. The use of both glucocorticoids and immunosuppressive agents in patients with severe disease results in an increased risk of opportunistic infection.

RHEUMATIC FEVER

Acute rheumatic fever (ARF) is an systemic inflammatory condition that is a complication of group A beta-hemolytic streptococcal pharyngitis. It does not occur after cutaneous infection. The disorder is thought to be autoimmune. Acute rheumatic fever generally develops about 2 to 3 weeks following the pharyngitis.

The initial manifestations of ARF include fever, anorexia, and fatigue. Joint complaints are common and range from arthralgias to frank arthritis. The arthritis tends to move from joint to joint and is therefore termed *migratory*. It generally affects the large joints of the extremities. The arthralgia associated with ARF is especially intense at night. A predominant characteristic of the arthritis of ARF is the disproportionate severity of the pain when compared to the clinical findings. The joint symptoms tend to resolve within a month and leave no permanent damage.

Cardiac disease can affect all layers of the heart, including the pericardium, and is responsible for most of the morbidity associated with ARF. The carditis can be clinically silent or severe enough to result in congestive heart failure. Involvement of the valves, especially the mitral and aortic, results in significant long-term morbidity. A common manifestation of rheumatic carditis is the development of a new murmur, which most commonly reflects mitral regurgitation.

Chorea occurs in up to 10 percent of patients and can be the only manifestation of disease. It consists of random, purposeless movements, most commonly involving the muscles of the extremities and face, that in some cases are preceded by behavioral changes. The duration of chorea varies, but it is a self-limited process.

The dermatologic manifestations of ARF include erythema marginatum, which is an intermittent, red, slightly raised rash that occurs most commonly on the trunk and extremities. Subcutaneous nodules are painless, movable lesions that may develop late during the course of illness. They are rare.

The differential diagnosis of ARF includes JRA, septic arthritis, bacterial endocarditis, leukemia, and SLE. In addition, postinfectious arthritis can mimic ARF.

The diagnosis of rheumatic fever is usually made by utilizing a combination of clinical and laboratory findings. These are summarized in the modified Jones criteria. The presence of two major and one minor or one major and two minor criteria is highly correlated with ARF. In addition to the criteria, virtually all children have serologic evidence of an antecedent streptococcal infection. A negative throat culture, however, does not rule out ARF. An electrocardiogram is indicated, as is an echocardiogram to assess heart size as well as the structural and functional integrity of the valves.

Patients with suspected ARF are admitted to the hospital. Penicillin is indicated to eradicate any residual carriage of group A *Streptococcus.* Patients with arthritis but without carditis are managed with high-dose aspirin. Patients with evidence of significant carditis are treated with prednisone. It is important that, especially in patients with isolated arthralgia, therapy with anti-inflammatory agents be withheld until a definitive diagnosis is ruled out. Chorea may respond to haloperidol.

Recurrent attacks can be prevented by prophylactic administration of antibiotics, most commonly by monthly injections of benzathine penicillin. First attacks can be prevented by aggressive diagnosis and treatment of streptococcal pharyngitis.

ENTHESOPATHIES

Enthesopathy, also known as enthesitis, is an inflammation of tendons, ligaments, and fascia at their sites of attachment. Enthesopathies are found in a variety of rheumatologic disorders, including juvenile ankylosing spondylitis, psoriasis, inflammatory bowel disease, and seronegative enthesopathy and arthropathy (SEA) syndrome.

Tenderness from enthesopathy may be noted in the chest wall, iliac crest, ischial tuberosity, posterior or plantar surface of the heel, metatarsophalangeal area, and anterior tibial tuberosity.

Pain resulting from enthesopathies is treated with nonsteroidal anti-inflammatory agents.

ANKYLOSING SPONDYLITIS

Ankylosing spondylitis is a rheumatic disorder that can present in later childhood or adolescence. It is most common in males. Some 90 percent of patients are HLA B27–positive.

The disorder is predominantly characterized by involvement of the sacroiliac joints and the lumbar spine. Many patients have associated peripheral arthritis. Affected patients often complain of hip, back, and thigh pain that is worse at night and improves with movement. Systemic symptoms including fatigue and low-grade fever may be present. A significant percentage of patients develop acute iridocyclitis.

The physical examination may reveal tenderness over the sacroiliac joints and loss of range of motion of the lumbar spine. Ultimately, there is radiographic evidence of destruction of the sacroiliac joints. A complication of ankylosing spondylitis is vertebral fusion.

The primary treatment of ankylosing spondylitis is nonsteroidal anti-inflammatory agents. Physical therapy is an important adjunct to medical management.

For a more detailed discussion, see Mayer D: Inflammatory musculoskeletal disorders, chap. 76, p. 480, in *Pediatric Emergency Medicine: A Comprehensive Study Guide.*

---

77 Structural Musculoskeletal Disorders

Diana Mayer

LEGG-CALVÉ-PERTHES DISEASE

Legg-Calvé-Perthes disease results from avascular necrosis of the femoral head. The cause is unknown. It is most common in boys, and occurs most often in patients between 5 and 9 years of age.

Children may complain of pain in the hip, thigh, or groin. Some patients may refuse to walk. Passive movement of the hip may be limited by spasm of the adductor and iliopsoas muscles. Restriction of medial rotation and abduction may also be noted.

Early in the disease there may not be radiographic changes, although some widening of the joint space may be observed. This is followed sequentially by the appearance of a microfracture of a portion of the proximal femur's secondary ossification center, enhanced radiodensity, and then collapse of the infarcted lesion. Radionuclear scanning may be helpful. Initially, decreased uptake is noted, correlating with a diminished blood supply. As healing begins, increased uptake is observed.

The treatment of Legg-Calvé-Perthes disease includes bed rest and traction, and in some cases bracing.

SLIPPED CAPITAL FEMORAL EPIPHYSIS

Slipped capital femoral epiphysis is characterized by posterior displacement of the proximal femoral epiphysis on the femoral neck. It is most often seen in obese adolescent males. In up to 25 percent of cases, patients have bilateral disease.

Patients usually complain of hip or knee pain. Most patients walk with a noticeable limp. Physical examination of the hip reveals limited medial rotation, inability to fully flex and extend, and limited abduction and lateral rotation.

Early findings include growth plate widening and irregularity. As the lesion progresses, slippage of the epiphysis posteriorly on the femoral neck occurs.

Depending on the degree of slippage, treatment varies from in situ stabilization and pinning to osteotomy. In the emergency department, orthopedic consultation is indicated.

OSGOOD-SCHLATTER DISEASE

Osgood-Schlatter disease results from inflammation and possibly avulsion of the tibial tuberosity. It is thought to be secondary to forceful use of the quadriceps. It is usually seen in physically active teenagers.

Patients complain of pain below the knee exacerbated by physical activity and kneeling. The physical examination reveals tenderness and possibly swelling over the tibial tubercle. A radiograph may reveal irregularity or prominence of the tibial tubercle.

Management consists of temporary restriction of activity and relief of pain with nonsteroidal anti-inflammatory drugs (NSAIDs). The problem is self-limited. Rarely, a retained ossicle

TABLE 77-1 Generalized Joint Hypermobility Criteria[a]

1. Passive hypertension of the fingers so that they lie parallel with the extensor aspect of the forearm
2. Passive opposition of the thumbs to the flexor aspect of the forearm
3. Hyperextension of the elbows >10°
4. Hyperextension of the knees >10°
5. Flexion of the trunk with knees extended so that palms rest on the floor

[a] Generalized joint hypermobility = 3 or more of the above criteria.

within the patellar tendon can cause discomfort in adulthood and require surgical excision.

HYPERMOBILITY SYNDROME

Hypermobility of the joints occurs in approximately 5 to 12 percent of school-age children, most commonly in girls. Joint pain is a common complaint and may be worse at night. The knees and hands are most frequently affected. More than one joint is usually involved.

The physical examination is the key to the diagnosis. Hypermobility syndrome is established if patients have three or more of the criteria listed in Table 77-1.

Treatment includes NSAIDs for relief of pain and physical therapy, especially muscle-strengthening exercises.

NON-MALIGNANT TUMORS

Osteoid Osteomas

Osteoid osteoma is a relatively common benign tumor. It frequently causes pain, especially at night. The most common areas affected are the femur and tibia. Radiographs demonstrate a radiolucent center of osteoid tissue encircled by sclerotic bone. Surgical removal of the lesion is curative.

Nonossifying Fibromas

Nonossifying fibromas are most commonly seen in preadolescents and adolescents. They can also cause chronic pain. Occasionally, pathologic fractures can occur. Radiographs reveal a characteristic scalloped lesion. Treatment is not required.

Osteochondromas

Osteochondromas, also called cartilaginous exostoses, are occasionally seen in children and adolescents. The most commonly affected areas are the proximal tibia and distal femur. The lesion may result in a noticeable mass or a pathologic fracture. Radiographs demonstrate sessile or pedunculated lesions. These lesions should be biopsied and usually require removal.

Enchondromas

Patients with enchondromas may present with a mass or pathologic fracture. The metacarpals, metatarsals, and phalanges are most commonly involved. Lesions in these areas are typically benign. Diaphyseal tumors may have malignant potential. Radiographs show thinning bone with cortical bulging and stippled calcification. Orthopedic consultation is indicated.

Solitary Bone Cysts

Solitary bone cysts start near the epiphyseal plate and extend toward the diaphysis during growth. Most often they are found incidentally. Especially in the lower extremity, these lesions are prone to associated fracture and require excision. Therefore, orthopedic consultation is indicated.

For a more detailed discussion, see Mayer D: Structural musculoskeletal disorders, chap. 77, p. 484, in *Pediatric Emergency Medicine: A Comprehensive Study Guide.*

SECTION XVII
TOXICOLOGIC EMERGENCIES

78

General Principles of Poisoning: Diagnosis and Management

Timothy Erickson

There has been a 96 percent decline in the number of pediatric poisoning deaths over the past few decades. Over 60 percent of poisonings reported to the American Association of Poison Control Centers (AAPCC) occur in children under the age of 17 years. Most exposures in this age group are accidental and result in minimal toxicity. Thus, the pediatric population accounts for only 10 percent of hospital admissions due to poisonings. The majority of these poisonings result from ingestions. They may also result from inhalation and from intravenous, dermal, ocular, and environmental exposure. Nonaccidental causes of drug toxicity include recreational drug abuse, suicide attempts, and Munchausen syndrome by proxy.

Iron supplements are the single most common cause of pediatric unintentional ingestion fatalities. Antidepressants, cardiovascular medications, salicylates, hydrocarbons, and pesticides follow in order of decreasing mortality.

HISTORY

The essential history of the poisoned patient includes the toxin or medication to which the child was exposed, the time of the exposure or ingestion, what other medications were available to the child, and how much was taken. The emergency physician should always assume the worst-case scenario.

PHYSICAL EXAMINATION

A comprehensive physical examination may provide valuable clues regarding the ingestion or exposure. Since many drugs and toxic

TABLE 78-1 Toxic Vital Signs

Bradycardia
P Propranolol (beta blockers)
A Anticholinesterase drugs
C Clonidine, calcium channel blockers
E Ethanol/alcohols
D Digoxin, Darvon (opiates)
Tachycardia
F Free base (cocaine)
A Anticholinergics, antihistamines, amphetamines
S Sympathomimetics
T Theophylline
Hypothermia
C Carbon monoxide
O Opiates
O Oral hypoglycemics, insulin
L Liquor
S Sedative hypnotics
Hyperthermia
N Neuroleptic malignant syndrome, nicotine
A Antihistamines
S Salicylates, sympathomimetics
A Anticholinergics, antidepressants
Hypotension
C Clonidine
R Reserpine (antihypertensive agents)
A Antidepressants
S Sedative hypnotics
H Heroin (opiates)
Hypertension
C Cocaine
T Theophylline
S Sympathomimetics
C Caffeine
A Anticholinergics, amphetamines
N Nicotine

agents have specific effects on the heart rate, temperature, blood pressure, and respiratory rate, monitoring the vital signs may direct the clinician toward the proper diagnosis (Table 78-1). Additionally, the patient's level of consciousness, pupillary size, and potential for seizures may be directly affected by the poison in a dose-dependent fashion. Other diagnostic clues are obtained from the

TABLE 78-2 Toxic Physical Findings

Miosis
C Cholinergic, clonidine
O Opiates, organophosphates
P Phenothiazines, pilocarpine, pontine bleed
S Sedative hypnotics

Mydriasis
A Antihistamines
A Antidepressants
A Anticholinergics, atropine
S Sympathomimetics (cocaine, amphetamines)

Seizures
O Organophosphates
T Tricyclic antidepressants
I Isoniazid, insulin
S Sympathomimetics
C Camphor, cocaine
A Amphetamines
M Methylxanthines
P PCP
B Beta blockers
E Ethanol withdrawal
L Lithium
L Lead

Diaphoretic skin
S Sympathomimetics
O Organophosphates
A ASA (salicylates)
P PCP

Red skin: Carbon monoxide, boric acid
Blue skin: Cyanosis, methemoglobinemia

Breath odors

Bitter almonds	Cyanide
Fruity	DKA, isopropanol
Oil of wintergreen	Methylsalicylates
Rotten eggs	Sulfur dioxide, hydrogen sulfide
Pears	Chloral hydrate
Garlic	Organophosphates, arsenic, DMSO
Mothballs	Camphor

skin and breath odor (Table 78-2). Several groups of toxins consistently present with recognizable patterns or signs. Recognizing these toxic syndromes or "toxidromes" may expedite not only the diagnosis of the toxic agent but its management as well (Table 78-3).

DIAGNOSTIC AIDS/LABORATORY

In a child with a significant or unknown ingestion, baseline laboratory studies include a complete blood count, electrolytes, blood urea nitrogen and creatinine, glucose, and arterial blood gas. If

TABLE 78-3 Toxic Syndromes

Anticholinergics [tricyclic antidepressants (TCAs) antihistamines]
HOT as a hare
DRY as a bone
RED as a beet
BLIND as a bat
MAD as a hatter

Cholinergics (organophosphates)
D Diarrhea, diaphoresis
U Urination
M Miosis, muscle fasciculations
B Bradycardia, bronchosecretions
E Emesis
L Lacrimation
S Salivation

Sympathomimetics (cocaine, amphetamines)
Mydriasis
Tachycardia
Hypertension
Hyperthermia
Seizures

Narcotics
Miosis
Bradycardia
Hypotension
Hypoventilation
Coma

Withdrawal
Alcohol
Benzodiazepines
Barbiturates
Antihypertensives
Opioids

the arterial blood gas reveals a metabolic acidosis, calculating the anion gap can assist in formulating a differential diagnosis. A metabolic acidosis with an increased anion gap results from the presence of organically active acids and is characteristic of several toxins and various other disease states (Table 78-4). Normal anion gap acidosis results from loss of bicarbonate (diarrhea, renal tubular acidosis) or from addition of chloride-containing compounds (NH_4Cl, $CaCl_2$). The anion gap can be calculated from serum electrolytes as follows:

$$\text{Anion gap calculation} = \text{Na} - (\text{Cl} + \text{HCO}_3) \quad (\text{normal} = 8 \text{ to } 12)$$

TABLE 78-4 Toxic GAPS

Metabolic acidosis/elevated anion gap	
A Alcoholic ketoacidosis	**P** Paraldehyde, phenformin
C Carbon monoxide, cyanide	**I** Iron, isoniazid
A ASA (salicylates)	**L** Lactic acidosis
T Toluene	**E** Ethyelene glycol
M Methanol	
U Uremia	
D DKA	
Elevated osmolar gap	
M Methanol	
E Ethylene glycol	
D Diuretics (mannitol)	
I Isopropyl alcohol	
E Ethanol	

Source: Adapted from Bryson.

If ingestion of a toxic alcohol, such as methanol or ethylene glycol, is suspected, calculation of the osmolal gap is critical. The osmolal gap is the difference between the measured osmolality and that calculated from major osmotically active molecules in the serum.

$$\begin{aligned}\text{Calculated osmolality} &= 2(\text{Na}) + \text{glucose}/18\\ &\quad + \text{BUN}/2.8 + \text{ETOH}/4.6\\ \text{Osmolality gap} &= \text{measured osmolality}\\ &\quad - \text{calculated osmolality (normal } <10)\end{aligned}$$

When a particular drug or toxin is known or highly suspected, blood or serum can be tested for specific drug levels. These levels confirm the ingestion and often guide medical management. Commonly available tests are listed in Table 78-5.

TABLE 78-5 Serum Drug Levels

Acetaminophen	Lithium
Carbon monoxide	Methanol
Cholinesterase	Methemoglobin
Digitalis	Phenobarbital
Ethanol	Phenytoin
Ethylene glycol	Salicylate
Iron	Theophylline
Lead	

TABLE 78-6 Toxicology and Radiology

Noncardiogenic pulmonary edema
M Meprobamate, mountain sickness
O Opiates
P Phenobarbital
S Salicylates

Toxins radiopaque on radiographs
C Chloral hydrate
H Heavy metals
I Iron
P Phenothiazines
E Enteric-coated preps (salicylates)
S Sustained-release products (theophylline)

Toxicology screening can be helpful in the diagnosis of the unknown ingestion, but it has limitations. Blood toxicology screens may be negative if the drug has a short half-life and the specimen is not obtained immediately after the exposure. The urine toxicology screen may be of greater value, since the drug's metabolites continue to be excreted in the urine for 48 to 72 h following the ingestion. Toxicology panels typically screen for drugs of abuse, such as narcotics, amphetamines, canabinoids, phencyclidine (PCP), and cocaine. However, since most of these screens are qualitative, the mere detection of a drug does not necessarily entail toxicity. A grave error can also occur if the physician assumes the child ingested nothing simply because the toxicology screen is reported as negative, and the actual drug ingested has not been included in the screen.

Radiologic testing can prove valuable with certain ingestions, particularly those that are radiopaque or those that may induce a noncardiogenic pulmonary edema or chemical pneumonitis (Table 78-6).

MANAGEMENT

Stabilization

The cornerstone of management of the patient with a suspected overdose is supportive care, with particular attention to the airway, breathing, and circulation. Resuscitative measures are instituted prior to antidotal therapy or gastric decontamination.

In the child with an altered level of consciousness or in whom a bedside glucose oxidase test documents hypoglycemia, intravenous dextrose is administered at 0.5 to 1.0 g/kg, given as 2 to 4 mL/kg of $D_{25}W$ for the child or 50 mL (one ampule) of $D_{50}W$ for the adolescent. If intravenous access is difficult or unobtainable, 1 mg of glucagon is administered intramuscularly.

In addition to dextrose, naloxone is given to the child or adolescent with lethargy or coma. Naloxone is a specific opiate antagonist with minimal side effects. The initial dose is 0.1 mg/kg intravenously or 2 mg for children weighing over 20 kg. Often, additional doses of naloxone are required for certain opiates such as codeine, methadone, and propoxyphene, which have high potency and a prolonged half-life. If an intravenous line cannot be established, naloxone may be administered via the endotracheal tube, intramuscularly, or intralingually.

Gastric Decontamination

Whether a patient is managed with syrup of ipecac, gastric lavage, cathartics, or activated charcoal depends on the toxicity of the particular drug, the quantity and time of ingestion, and the patient's condition. If the child ingests a nontoxic agent or a very small amount of a poison unlikely to cause toxicity, no gastric decontamination measures are indicated. However, if the child is symptomatic or the toxin ingested may cause delayed toxicity, aggressive gastric evacuation is necessary. Several clinical trials have been conducted to determine which of the gastric decontamination modalities are most efficacious. However, these studies must be critically interpreted prior to their definitive application in the clinical setting.

Gastric Evacuation

Induction of Emesis

Syrup of ipecac is the most commonly used emetic agent. The American Academy of Pediatrics recommends that parents keep syrup of ipecac at home in the event that the child suffers a potentially toxic ingestion. See Table 78-7 for dosage.

Ipecac can be expected to induce vomiting within 20 to 60 min. The recovery of ingested material in the vomitus is approximately 30 percent if ipecac is administered 1 to 2 h postingestion. Unfortunately, most children experience three or more episodes of vomiting, which delays the administration of activated charcoal. Ipecac is contraindicated in children less than 6 months of age, in patients with evidence of a diminished gag reflex and potential for coma or seizures, and in the ingestion of most hydrocarbons, acids, alkalis, and sharp objects.

TABLE 78-7 Doses for Gastric Decontamination

Syrup of ipecac: For patients 6–12 months of age: 5–10 mL with 15 mL/kg clear fluids; patients 12 months–12 years: 15 mL ipecac plus 8 oz of clear fluids; patients over 12 years: 30 mL ipecac plus 16 oz water.
Activated charcoal: Dose of 1–2 g/kg prepared as a slurry in water or sorbitol to achieve a 25% concentration. For repetitive dosing: 1 g/kg every 2–4 h without sorbitol or cathartic.
Cathartics: Sorbitol (35% solution): 4 mL/kg of commercial solution diluted 1 : 1
Magnesium sulfate (10% solution): 1–2 mL/kg
Magnesium sulfate (10% solution): 1–2 mL/kg

Gastric Lavage

Gastric lavage mechanically removes toxins from the stomach using a large-bore orogastric tube irrigated with aliquots of normal saline. This mode of gastric decontamination is preferred in the intoxicated child with a depressed level of consciousness. In most cases, airway protection by endotracheal intubation prior to the lavage is recommended. Gastric lavage is contraindicated in ingestions of most hydrocarbons, acids, alkalis, and sharp objects. Although gastric lavage is relatively safe when performed properly, complications of aspiration, esophageal perforation, electrolyte imbalance, and hypothermia have been described. Gastric lavage is most effective if performed within 1 to 2 h postingestion; at best, it removes up to 40 percent of the ingested toxin.

Chemical Decontamination

Activated charcoal Activated charcoal is an odorless, tasteless, fine black powder that is effective in adsorbing many toxins. It has now become the most frequently used and most effective gastric decontamination agent. It is most beneficial when administered soon after the ingestion. The recommended initial dose of activated charcoal is summarized in Table 78-7.

For many drugs, such as theophylline, aspirin, phenobarbital, digitoxin, and carbamazepine, multiple dosing of activated charcoal may enhance elimination due to enterohepatic or enteroenteric circulation of the drug. Repetitive use of charcoal preparations premixed with cathartics like sorbitol is avoided, since dehydration and electrolyte imbalance may result. Although charcoal is probably the safest method of decontamination, rare cases of constipation, obstruction, and aspiration have been reported.

Activated charcoal is neither effective nor indicated in heavy metal poisonings, as with iron or lithium, or following ingestion of acids or alkalis where endoscopy may be required.

Cathartics Cathartics are osmotically active agents that eliminate toxins from the gastrointestinal tract by inducing diarrhea. The most common agents are sorbitol, magnesium citrate, and magnesium sulfate. No studies exist evaluating cathartics as the sole decontamination modality in the overdose setting. However, studies investigating the use of sorbitol in combination with activated charcoal have found that it enhances charcoal's palatability. In the pediatric population, cathartic agents can result in hypermagnesemia, dehydration, and severe electrolyte imbalances if used excessively or repeatedly.

Whole bowel irrigation Originally used as a preoperative bowel preparation, whole bowel irrigation is now used in the overdose setting to "flush" the toxin down the gastrointestinal tract. In theory, it may also produce a concentration gradient that allows previously absorbed toxins to diffuse back into the gastrointestinal tract. The solution used is a polyethylene glycol electrolyte solution that does not appear to create fluid or electrolyte disturbances. The dose is 0.5 L/h for smaller children and 1 to 2 L/h for adolescents. The irrigation process is continued until the rectal effluent is clear, which is usually in 2 to 6 h. Whole bowel irrigation has been used in the pediatric population with minimal to no side effects and has been effective in ingestions of iron, button batteries, and cocaine packets.

Antidotes

Although a majority of poisonings in pediatrics respond to supportive care and gastric decontamination alone, there are a few toxins that require antidotes (Table 78-8). The purpose of antidotal therapy is to reduce the agent's toxicity by inhibiting the toxin at the effector site or target organ, reduce the toxin's concentration, or enhance the excretion of the toxin.

Hemodialysis/Hemoperfusion

Although hemodialysis is recommended for a wide variety of toxins, it is necessary in only a few severely poisoned patients. Drugs that may be adequately dialyzed include those with a low molecular weight, low volume of distribution, low protein binding, and high water solubility. Examples include salicylates, theophylline, uremia-causing agents, methanol, barbiturates, lithium, and ethylene glycol. Theophylline is also responsive to charcoal hemoperfusion.

TABLE 78-8 Antidotes

Toxin	Antidote
Acetaminophen	*N*-acetylcysteine
Benzodiazepines	Flumazenil
Beta-blockers	Glucagon
Calcium channel blockers	Calcium
Carbon monoxide	Oxygen
Cyanide	Amyl nitrate, sodium nitrate, sodium thiosulfate
Digitalis	F(AB) fragments
Ethylene glycol/methanol	Ethanol
Iron	Deferoxamine
Lead	Calcium ethylenediaminetetraacetate, British anti-lewisite, dimercaptosuccinic acid
Mecury/arsenic	BAL, D-penicillamine
Methemoglobinemia	Methylene blue
Opiates	Naloxone
Organophosphates	Atropine, 2-pralidoxime
Tricyclic antidepressants	Sodium bicarbonate

If a child presents with a severe overdose that may require dialysis, early consultation with a nephrologist is critical.

Disposition

Disposition of the poisoned pediatric patient depends on the clinical condition of the child, the potential toxicity of the agent, and the reliability of follow-up. Clearly, all children demonstrating clinical instability are best monitored in an intensive care setting. Emergency department observation for 6 to 8 h is adequate if the patient demonstrates no overt signs of toxicity. If the child has ingested a potentially dangerous dose of a toxin, is manifesting mild to moderate toxicity, requires antidotal therapy, or comes from a home environment that is not considered safe, admission is indicated. In the setting of any accidental overdose, the parents are counseled and educated regarding proper poison prevention in the home. If the patient is suicidal, psychiatric consultation is obtained.

For a more detailed discussion, see Erickson T: General principles of poisoning: Diagnosis and management, chap. 78, p. 487, in *Pediatric Emergency Medicine: A Comprehensive Study Guide.*

---

79 Acetaminophen Toxicity

Leon Gussow

Acetaminophen is a common cause of toxic ingestion, though it rarely results in death. Young children are relatively resistant to the hepatotoxic consequences of acetaminophen ingestion. Although *N*-acetylcysteine (NAC) is an effective antidote if given early, initial signs and symptoms of acetaminophen overdose are usually nonspecific, and the therapeutic window within which treatment is effective may be missed unless acetaminophen levels are routinely obtained when any drug ingestion is suspected.

PHARMACOLOGY/PATHOPHYSIOLOGY

Acetaminophen (also called APAP or paracetamol) is a synthetic analgesic and antipyretic that lacks the anti-inflammatory effects found in salicylates and the nonsteroidal agents. Clinical effects are most likely mediated by inhibition of prostaglandin synthesis.

The therapeutic dose of APAP in children is 15 mg/kg every 4 to 6 h, with a maximum recommended daily dose of 80 mg/kg. Therapeutic serum levels are 5 to 20 μg/mL. Following gastrointestinal absorption, APAP is taken up by the liver. Serum half-life is 1 to 3 h after a therapeutic dose but may be prolonged in a hepatotoxic ingestion.

Acetaminophen is eliminated primarily by hepatic pathways. After a therapeutic dose, 90 percent of the drug is metabolized to inactive sulfate and glucuronide conjugates. In young children, unlike adults and adolescents, the sulfate conjugate predominates. Less than 5 percent is excreted unchanged in the urine. A small amount (2 to 4 percent) is metabolized by the cytochrome P_{450} mixed-function oxidase (MFO) system to the toxic intermediate *N*-acetyl-*p*-benzoquinoneimine (NAPQI). In the presence of adequate hepatic stores of glutathione, NAPQI is rapidly converted to nontoxic mercapturic acid and cysteine conjugates. In the overdose setting, the sulfate and glucuronide pathways become saturated, and increased amounts of acetaminophen are shunted through the P_{450}-MFO system. Glutathione becomes depleted, and free NAPQI forms covalent bonds with structures on the hepatocytes, causing hepatic necrosis. Acetaminophen can directly produce toxicity to the kidneys and pancreas; however, this virtually never occurs in children.

The toxic dose of acetaminophen is generally considered to be 140 mg/kg, but susceptibility to hepatotoxicity after acetaminophen overdose varies significantly. Children are more resistant than adults. Certain drugs predispose to toxicity even at therapeutic levels; these include phenobarbital, phenytoin, carbamazepine, rifampicin, and isoniazid. Malnutrition may also predispose to more severe acetaminophen toxicity.

CLINICAL PRESENTATION: THE FOUR STAGES OF ACETAMINOPHEN TOXICITY

Stage 1 (0 to 24h)—Gastrointestinal Irritation

Patients may be asymptomatic, but young children frequently vomit after acetaminophen overdose. In massive overdose or in children on chronic therapy with enzyme-inducing medication, an anion-gap metabolic acidose may rarely occur within hours of ingestion.

Stage 2 (24 to 48 h)—Latent Period

As nausea and vomiting resolve, the patient appears to improve, but rising transaminase levels may reveal evidence of hepatic necrosis. On physical examination, hepatic tenderness and enlargement may be apparent. The incidence of hepatotoxicity is significantly lower in children than in adults with similar acetaminophen levels.

Stage 3 (72 to 96 h)—Hepatic Failure

Severe hepatotoxicity presents with jaundice, hypoglycemia, renewed nausea and vomiting, right upper quadrant pain, coagulopathy, lethargy, coma, hyperbilirubinemia, and markedly elevated transaminases. Renal failure may occur.

Stage 4 (4 to 14 days)—Recovery of Death

Patients who ultimately recover show improvement in laboratory parameters of hepatic function starting at about day 5; they then recover completely. Other patients show progressive encephalopathy, renal failure, bleeding diatheses, and hyperammonemia; they will die unless a liver transplant is performed.

LABORATORY

An acetaminophen level is drawn 4 after an acute ingestion, or immediately if more than 4 h have elapsed since the ingestion. Levels drawn earlier than 4 h may be misleadingly low. In addition to the acetaminophen level, laboratory tests that influence management or indicate prognosis include liver enzymes, amylase, bilirubin, electrolytes, creatinine, and prothrombin time.

MANAGEMENT

Gastric Decontamination

Induction of emesis with syrup of ipecac is contraindicated in known or suspected acetaminophen ingestion, since it is only minimally effective and will delay administration of NAC. Standard doses of activated charcoal can be given if the patient presents within 2 h of ingestion of acetaminophen alone or if other toxic substances may also be involved.

Antidote

N-Acetylcysteine is a glutathione precursor that restores the liver's ability to detoxify NABQI and prevents hepatonecrosis. It is most effective if started within 10 h of ingestion and seems to have decreased efficacy if treatment is delayed beyond that time. However, there is now good evidence that NAC has some benefit even if started very late, possibly up to days after ingestion, when hepatic failure has already ensued. It should not be witheld on the basis of an arbitrary time limit.

The Rumack-Mathew nomogram indicates which patients will require treatment with NAC. Any patient with a level that falls in the range of possible or probable hepatotoxicity is treated with a full course of NAC. If the time of ingestion is unknown or if ingestion of significant amounts of acetaminophen occurred over a prolonged period of time, treatment is started and a repeat level is drawn 4 h after the first. Elevated liver enzymes, elevated prothrombin time, or a serum half-life of acetaminophen greater than 24 h are indications to complete treatment with NAC. If there is any doubt, it is best to administer the full course of therapy.

If the patient is chronically on medication that induces the P_{450} system, the threshold for treatment indicated on the Rumack-Mathew nomogram is reduced. Some advocate treating if the acetaminophen level is more than half that on the algorithm that indicates possible or probable toxicity.

The oral protocol approved by the U.S. Food and Drug Administration requires a loading dose of 140 mg/kg and then 17 additional doses of 70 mg/kg. The commercial 20% solution (Mucomyst, Mead Johnson & Company) is unpalatable and is diluted with three parts fruit juice or soda pop. If vomiting occurs within 1 h of treatment, the dose is repeated. Persistent vomiting that interferes with therapy can be suppressed with metoclopramide or ondansetron. If necessary, NAC can be infused slowly through a nasogastric tube. If activated charcoal has been administered, the usual dose of NAC does not need to be increased, but it should be given at least 30 to 60 min after the charcoal.

Intravenous NAC is commonly used in Europe but has not yet been approved by the U.S. Federal Drug Administration. In cases of significant overdose where oral NAC is either contraindicated or not tolerated, the same NAC preparation used for oral dosing can be given intravenously. In such cases, a poison control center should be consulted.

CHRONIC ACETAMINOPHEN POISONING

The Rumack-Mathew nomogram applies specifically to a single acute overdose taken at a known moment in time. It is now clear that children can develop hepatotoxicity after even moderately supratherapeutic doses of acetaminophen administered over several days. Doses greater than 150 mg/kg/day can cause toxicity. These children often present with lethargy and a history of fever. Liver enzymes are elevated. Renal failure and pancytopenia may also be seen. The differential diagnosis includes Reye's syndrome and hepatitis. These children should be treated with a full course of NAC.

For a more detailed discussion, see Gussow L: Acetaminophen toxicity, chap. 79, p. 493, in *Pediatric Emergency Medicine: A Comprehensive Study Guide.*

80 Toxic Alcohols

Timothy Erickson

ETHANOL

Ethanol is a common toxic ingestion in children. In addition to alcohol-containing beverages such as beer, wine, and hard liquors, children have access to mouthwashes (containing up to 75% ethanol), colognes and perfumes (40 to 60% ethanol), and over 700 medicinal preparations containing ethanol.

The alcohol dehydrogenase pathway is the major metabolic pathway of ethanol. In children under 5 years of age, the ability to metabolize ethanol is diminished.

Ethanol is a selective central nervous system (CNS) depressant at low concentrations and a generalized depressant at high concentrations. It initially produces exhilaration and loss of inhibition, which progress to lack of coordination, ataxia, slurred speech, gait disturbances, drowsiness, and ultimately stupor and coma. The intoxicated child may demonstrate a flushed face, dilated pupils, excessive sweating, gastrointestinal distress, hypoventilation, hypothermia, and hypotension. Severe hypoglycemia due to inhibition of hepatic gluconeogenesis can occur and is most common in children under 5 years of age.

Laboratory

In a symptomatic pediatric patient, the most critical laboratory tests are the serum ethanol and glucose levels. Although blood ethanol levels roughly correlate with clinical signs, treatment is based on symptomatology. If the ethanol level does not correlate with the clinical picture, other ingestions must be considered.

Management

The majority of children with acute ingestions of ethanol respond to supportive care. Attention is directed toward management of the child's airway, circulation, and glucose status. All obtunded patients receive 2 to 4 mL/kg of $D_{25}W$ (one ampole of $D_{50}W$ in older children and adolescents) after a blood glucose level is drawn. If no response is elicited, naloxone 2 mg IV push is indicated to rule out opiate toxicity. Serial glucose levels are followed to avoid hypoglycemia. Unless coingestion of another drug is suspected, gastric decontamination is usually unnecessary unless performed within 1 h of ingestion. Activated charcoal and cathartics are probably not efficacious. Hemodialysis increases ethanol clearance by three to four times and may be indicated with ethanol levels over 500 mg/dL or with evidence of deteriorating vital signs or hepatic function.

Disposition

Any young pediatric patient with significant altered mental status following an acute ethanol ingestion is admitted for observation. Asymptomatic patients may be discharged home.

METHANOL

Methanol is an uncommon but potentially fatal ingestion. It is contained in antifreeze, paint solvents, gasohol, gasoline additives, canned heat products, windshield washer fluid, and duplicating chemicals.

Pharmacokinetics/Pathophysiology

Methanol is rapidly absorbed following ingestion and is primarily metabolized by hepatic alcohol dehydrogenase to the extremely toxic metabolites formaldehyde and formic acid. Ingestion of only 10 mL can lead to blindness.

Clinical Presentation

The onset of symptoms following ingestion varies from 1 to 72 h. The patient commonly presents with visual complaints, abdominal pain, and metabolic acidosis. Eye symptoms include blurring of vision, photophobia, constricted visual fields, snow-field vision, "spots before the eyes," and total blindness. The ophthalmologic examination may reveal dilated pupils with hyperemia of the optic disk, but it can be normal early in the clinical course. Blindness is usually permanent. The patient also typically complains of epigastric pain, nausea, and vomiting and can experience gastrointestinal bleeding and acute pancreatitis. Unlike patients who have ingested the other alcohols, these patients often lack the odor of ethanol on their breath and can have a clear sensorium.

Laboratory

Baseline laboratory data include complete blood count, electrolytes, blood urea nitrogen/creatinine, glucose, amylase, urinanalysis, and arterial blood gas. Classically, the methanol-intoxicated patient presents with an elevated anion gap metabolic acidosis.

The anion gap is calculated using the following equation:

$$\text{Anion gap} = (\text{Na}) - (\text{Cl} + \text{HCO}_3) \qquad (\text{normal } 8\text{–}12)$$

Another valuable clue in establishing the diagnosis is the presence of an elevated osmolal gap. The osmolal gap is the difference between the measured osmolarity and calculated osmolarity and reflects the fact that methanol, a highly osmotic compound not normally found in the serum, is present in a significant quantity. The normal difference is less than 10. The most accurate determination of the measured serum osmolality is made using a freezing point depression method.

Generally, methanol levels below 20 mg/dL result in minimal to no symptoms. Central nervous system symptoms appear with levels over 20 mg/dL, and peak levels over 50 mg/dL indicate serious toxicity. Ocular symptoms occur at levels over 100 mg/dL, and fatalities have been reported in untreated victims with levels over 150 mg/dL.

Management

Gastrointestinal decontamination may be efficacious for patients presenting within 1 h of ingestion. While activated charcoal is of uncertain benefit, 1 g/kg can be administered.

Ethanol competitively binds hepatic alcohol dehydrogenase and delays the formation of formaldehyde and formic acid. If a significant ingestion of methanol is likely, empiric treatment with intravenous ethanol is indicated. Other indications for ethanol therapy include serum methanol levels greater than 20 mg/dL or acidemia (pH <17.20). Ethanol levels are maintained between 100 and 150 mg/dL. An intravenous solution of 10% ethanol in D_5W is optimal, with a loading dose of 0.6 g/kg. A simplified approximation of the loading dose is 1 mL/kg of 10% diluted absolute ethanol. Close monitoring of the ethanol levels every 1 to 2 h is necessary. If intravenous ethanol preparations are unavailable, oral ethanol therapy can be instituted. Continued therapy is recommended until methanol levels fall below 10 mg/dL. Since hypoglycemia is a complication of toxic ethanol levels in young children, serum glucose levels are monitored.

An investigational drug, 4-methyl pyrazole (4-MP), is a direct inibitor of alcohol dehydrogenase and may prove useful. Folate, the active form of folic acid, is a coenzyme indicated in the methanol-intoxicated patient. Up to 50 mg of folate can be given every 4 h intravenously until the acidosis is corrected and methanol levels fall below 20 mg/dL.

Hemodialysis is effective in severe cases. Indications include any visual impairment, severe metabolic acidosis not corrected with bicarbonate administration, renal failure, or methanol levels greater than 50 mg/dL, with or without symptoms. Ethanol is readily dialyzed, so the rate of administration may have to be increased during dialysis.

ETHYLENE GLYCOL

An overdose of ethylene glycol is uncommon but serious. Ethylene glycol is a colorless, odorless, sweet-tasting compound that is found in antifreeze products, coolants, preservatives, and glycerine substitutes.

Pathophysiology/Pharmacokinetics

Ethylene glycol is rapidly absorbed and undergoes hepatic metabolism via alcohol dehydrogenase to form various toxic metabolites, including glycolaldehyde, glycolic acid, and oxalate, which are ultimately excreted through the kidney. The hallmark of ethylene glycol toxicity is a severe anion gap metabolic acidosis due to accumulation of glycolic acid and lactate. Hypocalcemia results from the precipitation of calcium oxalate crystals in the kidney.

Clinical Presentation

The clinical effects of ethylene glycol toxicity can be divided into three distinct stages. Stage 1 occurs within the first 12 h of the ingestion, with CNS symptoms similar to those experienced with ethanol, including slurred speech, nystagmus, ataxia, vomiting, lethargy, and coma. The patient may suffer convulsions, myoclonic jerks, and tetanic contractions due to hypocalcemia. As with methanol toxicity, the patient can demonstrate an anion gap acidosis with an elevated osmolal gap. In approximately one-third of the cases, calcium oxalate crystals will be discovered in the urine, a finding considered pathognomonic for ethylene glycol poisoning. Stage 2 occurs within 12 to 36 h after ingestion and is characterized by rapidly progressive tachypnea, cyanosis, pulmonary edema, adult respiratory distress syndrome (ARDS), and cardiomegaly. Death is most common during this stage. Stage 3 occurs 2 to 3 days postingestion; it is heralded by flank pain, oliguria, proteinuria, anuria, and renal failure. Ethylene glycol poisoning is possible in any inebriated patient lacking an odor of ethanol who has severe acidosis or calcium crystalluria.

Laboratory

Laboratory studies include a complete blood count, electrolytes, glucose, calcium, blood urea nitrogen/creatinine, creatine kinase, serum ethanol and ethylene glycol levels, arterial blood gas, serum osmolarity, and urinanalysis for crystals, protein, and blood. Both anion and osmolal gaps are calculated. Because of the potential for severe cardiopulmonary effects in stage 2, a chest radiograph and electrocardiogram are recommended. Since fluorescein is present in many antifreeze products, fluorescence of the patient's urine under a Wood's lamp may be a valuable diagnostic clue.

Management

Gastric lavage may be useful in a patient presenting within 1 h of ingestion. Syrup of ipecac is contraindicated due to potential CNS depression. Activated charcoal may be effective, but this has not been well studied. Seizures are treated with diazepam, phenobarbital, or phenytoin.

If a strong suspicion of ethylene glycol ingestion exists, the patient is acidotic (pH <17.20), or if the ethylene glycol level is over 20 mg/dL, intravenous ethanol therapy is instituted. Ethanol competes with ethylene glycol for alcohol dehydrogenase and slows the accumulation of toxic metabolites. If an intravenous preparation of ethanol is unavailable, the patient can be loaded orally to achieve an ethanol level of 100 to 150 mg/dL. Since toxic ethanol levels result in profound hypoglycemia in smaller children, serial glucose measurements are monitored.

The alcohol dehydrogenase inhibitor 4-MP has been investigated as a possible antidote for ethylene glycol toxicity. Bicarbonate administration is recommended in patients with pH's under 7.20 to correct the acidosis. Serum calcium levels are monitored, and hypocalcemia is treated with 10% calcium gluconate. Additionally, thiamine and pyridoxine (vitamin B_6) are recommended in ethylene glycol poisonings to shunt or reroute the metabolism of ethylene glycol toward less toxic metabolites (Table 80-1).

Hemodialysis is indicated in the setting of metabolic acidosis not responsive to bicarbonate administration, pulmonary edema, renal failure, and serum ethylene glycol levels over 50 mg/dL.

TABLE 80-1 Toxic Alcohol Antidotes

Methanol	Ethylene Glycol
Ethanol drip	Ethanol drip
Folate	Thiamine, pyridoxine
4-methylpyrazole	4-methylpyrazole

ISOPROPANOL

Exposure to isopropyl alcohol occurs more frequently than ethanol ingestions in children below 6 years of age. Toxicity can result from oral ingestion and from as inhalation and dermal exposures.

Pathophysiology/Pharmacokinetics

Isopropanol is rapidly absorbed from the gastric mucosa. It is metabolized to the CNS depressant acetone. Respiratory elimination of the acetone causes a fruity-acetone odor to the patient's breath similar to that in diabetic ketoacidosis (DKA). A level of 50 mg/dL is comparable to an ethanol level of 100 mg/dL.

Clinical Presentation

Isopropanol-intoxicated patients are classically lethargic or comatose, hypotensive, and tachycardic, with the characteristic breath odor of rubbing alcohol or acetone. Coma develops at levels over 100 mg/dL. Hypotension results from peripheral vasodilation and cardiac depression. Gastrointestinal irritation with acute abdominal pain and hematemesis can also ensue. Severe metabolic acidosis is uncommon, but isopropanol can produce a significant osmolal gap (Table 80-2).

Laboratory

The patient is tested for the presence of acetonemia and acetonuria. Unlike with DKA, the acetone levels are typically found in the absence of glucosuria, hyperglycemia, or acidemia. Laboratory studies include a complete blood count, electrolytes, arterial blood gas, serum osmolarity, glucose, blood urea nitrogen/creatinine,

TABLE 80-2 Comparison of Toxic Alcohols

	Methanol	Ethylene Glycol	Isopropanol
Anion gap acidosis	+	+	−
Osmolal gap	+	+	+
CNS depression	+	+	+
Eye findings	+	−	−
Renal failure	+/−	+	−
Ketones	−	−	+
Oxylate crystals	−	+	−

and serum ethanol and isopropanol levels. Isopropanol levels over 400 mg/dL correspond to severe toxicity.

Management

Initial management addresses the patient's airway. Hypotension is treated with the administration of crystalloid. Gastric decontamination is indicated only if performed within 1 h of ingestion. Induction of emesis is avoided due to the potential for rapid development of altered mental status. Activated charcoal may be administered, although its efficacy in the setting of isopropanol alone is questionable. Hematemesis is managed with gastric lavage.

Hemodialysis is indicated for prolonged coma, refractory hypotension, and isopropanol levels above 400 to 500 mg/dL. Typically, the patient progresses well with supportive care. Ingestion of more than three swallows (15 mL) of 70% isopropyl by a 10-kg child (1.5 mL/kg) is an indication for several hours of observation.

For a more detailed discussion, see Erickson T: Toxic alcohols, chap. 80, p. 498, in *Pediatric Emergency Medicine: A Comprehensive Study Guide.*

---

81 Anticholinergic Poisoning

Steven E. Aks

Anticholinergic poisoning results from both pharmaceutical agents and natural toxins. Common pharmaceuticals include antihistamines and decongestants, while natural toxins include plants and mushrooms. Many of these products are widely available in over-the-counter preparations (Table 81-1).

PHARMACOLOGY AND PATHOPHYSIOLOGY

Anticholinergics inhibit the action of the neurotransmitter acetylcholine, which is found at the sympathetic and parasympathetic ganglia, at parasympathetic nerve endings, at neuromuscular junctions, and in the central nervous system (CNS).

TABLE 81-1 Common Examples of Anticholinergics

Pharmaceuticals	Natural products
Atropine	Jimsonweed
Cyprohepatidine	Deadly nightshade (belladonna)
Diphenhydramine	Mushrooms (*Amanita muscaria*)
Dimenhydrinate	
Astemizole	
Pyrilines	
Other drug categories with anticholinergic properties	
Antipsychotics	
Antispasmotics	
Antiparkinsonian agents	
Cyclic antidepressants	
Phenothiazines	

CLINICAL PRESENTATION

Anticholinergic toxicity is typified by the toxidrome "Hot as a hare, blind as a bat, dry as a bone, red as a beet, and mad as a hatter."

The major CNS manifestations of anticholinergic toxicity range from overstimulation, agitation, delirium, and seizures to depression, lethargy, drowsiness, and coma. Cardiovascular effects include tachycardia and dysrhythmias. Syncope can occur, and either hypotension or hypertension may be present. Electrocardiographic (ECG) changes secondary to anticholinergic poisoning include prolonged QT interval, QRS widening, ventricular dysrhythmias, and heart block. Torsade de pointes has been described after antihistamine (Astemizole) overdose. Mucous membranes are dry, and the skin is flushed. Urinary retention is common, and gastrointestinal mobility may be impaired. Hyperthermia may be severe.

DIAGNOSIS

The diagnosis is generally made by observing the constellation of signs and symptoms of the anticholinergic toxidrome. Occasionally, unusual physical findings give clues to the diagnosis of anticholinergic poisoning. Routine laboratory studies include a complete blood count, electrolytes, blood urea nitrogen/creatinine, and glucose. Creatine phosphokinase is useful to rule out rhabdomyolysis, which may result from seizures or hyperthermia. Twelve-lead ECG is indicated. Routine urine toxicology screens may not include common antihistamines.

MANAGEMENT

As with any toxin that can induce seizures or cause coma, strict attention must be paid to the maintenance of the airway, breathing, and circulation. Continuous cardiac monitoring is essential. Decontamination by lavage is preferred, followed by the administration of activated charcoal. Lavage can be of value several hours after ingestion because of the decreased gut motility seen with anticholinergic poisoning. Ipecac is contraindicated because of the potential for altered mental status and seizures. Multiple dosing of activated charcoal is controversial because of the likelihood of toxin-induced gastric atony.

Supportive care is generally sufficient to treat anticholinergic poisoning. For agitation and seizures, benzodiazepines are useful. Hyperthermia is treated aggressively with cooling measures. Urinary retention is managed symptomatically.

Cardiac dysrhythmias are treated by standard measures. However, wide-complex tachycardia after diphenhydramine has been treated successfully with sodium bicarbonate. Magnesium has been used successfully to treat torsade de pointes after Astemizole overdose.

Physostigmine is an anticholinesterase agent that counteracts the effects of anticholinergic drugs. It is a tertiary amine that crosses the blood-brain barrier and reverses both the central and peripheral effects of the anticholinergic poisoning. It should be used only in cases of pure, severe anticholinergic toxicity that do not respond to supportive care. The dose of physostigmine is 2 mg by slow IV push in adults. In children, it is 0.02 mg/kg (not to exceed 0.5 mg) by slow IV push over 2 min. The dose can be repeated after 20 min if no effect is noted. Complications of physostigmine include nausea, vomiting, seizures, and worsening dysrhythmias. It has been reported to cause cardiac standstill in the setting of atrioventricular block with cyclic antidepressant overdose. Cardiac monitoring is essential during its administration.

A child or toddler with an accidental ingestion exhibiting only minor or no symptoms can be observed in the emergency department for at least 6 h after decontamination and administration of activated charcoal and then be discharged to reliable caretakers.

For a more detailed discussion, see Aks SE: Anticholinergic poisoning, chap. 81, p. 501, in *Pediatric Emergency Medicine: A Comprehensive Study Guide.*

82 Oral Anticoagulants

Jerrold Leikin

Anticoagulants are available in the form of prescription medications such as warfarin (Coumadin) and are the predominant agent in many rodenticides, some of which contain extremely potent and long-acting superwarfarin anticoagulants (Table 82-1). A vast majority of anticoagulant poisonings involve small children ingesting rodenticides.

PATHOPHYSIOLOGY

It is the vitamin K antagonists that cause most of the problems in the pediatric age group. They can be categorized as either hydroxycoumarins, which include warfarin, and indandiones, which include pindone. The hydroxycoumarin group also includes the "superwarfarin" agents, whose toxicity can last for weeks. Each category of anticoagulant inhibits the formation of vitamin K–dependent clotting factors II, VII, IX, and X by inhibiting the action of K_1 reductase and depleting active vitamin K_1.

Acute exposure to more than 0.5 mg/kg of warfarin or about 0.05 mg/kg of the superwarfarins usually requires intervention. Patients who have chronic ingestions may require prolonged observation.

DIAGNOSIS

The clinical toxicity of anticoagulants is almost entirely restricted to bleeding diathesis. Spontaneous emesis, epistaxis, ecchymosis, soft tissue hematomas, gastrointestinal bleeding, hematuria, and hemoptysis can occur. Intracranial hemorrhage is a devastating complication and is possible in any patient with a history of anticoagulant exposure and headache or who develops mental status changes.

In patients who ingest a rodenticide, it is essential to determine whether the compound contained a "normal" anticoagulant or one of the superwarfarins. Ingestion of the lower-toxicity agents usually does not require aggressive intervention, while ingestion of the superwarfarin compounds is cause for concern.

LABORATORY STUDIES

In the acute ingestion, all laboratory studies are likely to be normal. In chronic exposures or in cases where a toxic dose has been

TABLE 82-1 Vitamin K–Antagonist Agents

Coumarin derivatives	
Difenacoum (Ratak)	Phenprocoumon
Bromadiolone (Bromone)	Acenocoumarin
Brodifacoum (Talan)	Sodium Warfarin
Coumatetralyl (Endox)	Prolin (Eraze)
Discoumacetate	Coumafene
Zoocoumarin (Rodex)	Fumarin
Valone (PMP Tracking Powder)	Coumapuryl
Bishydroxy-Coumarin	Tomarin
Indandione derivatives	
Diphacione (Dipazin)	Diphenadione
Pindone (Pival)	Diphacin (Kill-ko Rat Killer)
Chlorphacione (Caid, Drat)	Pival
Valone	Piraldione (Tri-ban)
Anisindione	Radione
Phenindione	

ingested significantly prior to arrival to the emergency department, measurement of the prothrombin time (PT) correlates with the depression of the vitamin K–dependent clotting factors. In cases where the PT is prolonged, a baseline hemoglobin is necessary, as is a platelet count.

MANAGEMENT

Gastric Decontamination

Gut decontamination after ingestion of anticoagulants is controversial. In a patient presenting within 1 h of ingestion, ipecac-induced emesis or, preferably, gastric lavage is indicated, especially when more than 0.05 mg/kg of a superwarfarin has been ingested.

In chronic cases or in situations where arrival to the emergency department has been delayed, emesis or lavage is contraindicated because of the possibility of a coagulopathy and iatrogenically induced gastric hemorrhage. Activated charcoal is indicated in acute ingestions.

Vitamin K_1 is the specific antidote for anticoagulant toxicity and is indicated in the presence of a prolonged PT or in patients who present with bleeding. Vitamins K_3 and K_4 are not useful antidotes. Vitamin K_1 can be administered subcutaneously, intramuscularly, and intravenously. In patients with severe toxicity, the intravenous route is preferred. The major adverse reaction to intravenous administration is anaphylaxis. The intramuscular route is not rec-

TABLE 82-2 Doses of Vitamin K_1

Oral dose	Adult: 15–25 mg
Larger daily amounts for superwarfarin poisoning	
For small ingestion	Child: 5–10 mg
Intravenous dose	Adult: about 10 mg
For rapid correction only; diluted in a saline or glucose at a rate not to exceed 5 percent of total dose per minute	Child: 1–5 mg
Intramuscular dose	Adult: 5–10 mg
Mild ingestions—where risk of hematoma is low	Child: 1–5 mg
Subcutaneous injection	Adult: 5–10 mg Child: 1–5 mg

ommended in patients with severe toxicity because of the risk of hematoma formation (Table 82-2).

Patients with severe bleeding or with evidence of intracranial hemorrhage require rapid reversal of the coagulopathy and are treated with fresh frozen plasma or pooled clotting factors.

Patients ingesting superwarfarin agents have been treated with phenobarbital, which potentially increases the hepatic synthesis of vitamin K–dependent clotting factors. The efficacy of this is unknown. Likewise, cholestyramine has been utilized to increase clearance of warfarin, but this remains experimental.

DISPOSITION

Hospitalization is usually not necessary for children who ingest Coumadin tablets or rodenticides that do not contain superwarfarin compounds. However, they require close outpatient follow-up, with observation for gastrointestinal bleeding and prolongation of PT for up to 5 days after the ingestion. After ingestions of over 0.5 mg/kg of warfarin or 0.05 mg/kg of a superwarfarin compound and in patients with prolonged PT or active bleeding, hospitalization is indicated until the coagulation profile normalizes. In patients who ingest superwarfarin compounds, observation and monitoring of PT continues for several weeks.

For a more detailed discussion, see Leikin J: Oral anticoagulants, chap. 82, p. 503, in *Pediatric Emergency Medicine: A Comprehensive Study Guide.*

83 Antihypertensives, Beta Blockers, and Calcium Antagonists

Ken Bizovi / Timothy Erickson / William Ahrens

BETA BLOCKERS

Beta blockers are used in the treatment of hypertension, thyrotoxicosis, dysrhythmias, angina, migraine headaches, withdrawal states, and glaucoma. The overall mortality of beta-blocker overdose is much lower than that of overdose from calcium channel blockers or digoxin.

Pharmacology

Beta-blocker properties include $beta_1$ antagonist activity, $beta_2$ antagonist activity, intrinsic sympathomimetic activity, and membrane-stabilizing activity. The absorption, distribution, and elimination of beta blockers varies with the various drug preparations. Some beta blockers are available in extended-release preparations.

Because of the rapid absorption of many beta blockers, the onset of symptoms may be as rapid as 30 min after ingestion, but it most commonly occurs within 1 to 2 h. The cardiovascular manifestations include hypotension, bradycardia, heart block, and congestive heart failure. Aside from atrioventricular (AV) block, electrocardiographic manifestations of toxicity include prolongation of the PR and QT intervals, widened QRS complex, and bundle branch block. Respiratory toxicity includes adult respiratory distress syndrome (ARDS), pulmonary edema, exacerbation of asthma, and decreased respiratory drive. Patients may also present with central nervous system (CNS) depression or seizures.

Laboratory Evaluation

All patients with a history of beta-blocker ingestion are placed on a cardiac monitor and receive an electrocardiogram (ECG). Laboratory tests for blood levels are helpful only in confirming exposure. Serum electrolytes and glucose are evaluated. Arterial blood gas may be useful in the patient with respiratory signs or symptoms.

Management

The patient with a history of beta-blocker ingestion is placed on a cardiac monitor, and intravenous access is established.

Absorption can be decreased by gastric emptying and administration of activated charcoal. If the ingestion occurred less than 4 h prior to presentation, gastric emptying is indicated. Ipecac is relatively contraindicated because rapid CNS depression may occur. The airway is protected with endotracheal intubation in patients with altered mental status.

The patient with respiratory compromise is evaluated for the presence of pulmonary edema or bronchospasm. Bronchospasm is treated with oxygen and beta agonists. Aminophylline may be useful. Patients with pulmonary edema are supported with oxygen and, if necessary, intubation.

In patients with symptomatic bradycardia and hypotension, glucagon has been shown to reverse the toxic effects of beta blockers. In adults, an initial bolus of glucagon is administered at a dose of 50 to 150 μg/kg, administered intravenously over 1 min. If symptoms recur, a repeat bolus is given. If symptoms persist, an infusion may be started at 1 to 5 mg/h. Pediatric dosing has not been established. If glucagon is administered multiple times or as an infusion, it is mixed in normal saline or D_5W, since the package diluent contains phenol.

Patients who do not respond to glucagon are treated with aggressive fluid resuscitation and sympathomimetics. Dopamine or dobutamine may be helpful. Isoproterenol, a pure beta agonist, has at least theoretical use, but can cause hypotension and has been associated with myocardial ischemia when used in the treatment of asthma. It is reasonable to try atropine in patients with bradycardia.

In patients with bradycardia and hypotension refractory to pharmacologic intervention, temporary pacing is an option, but it may not reverse the cardiac depression of severe beta-blocker overdose. Interventions such as extracorporeal membrane oxygenation (ECMO) or cardiac bypass are considerations in patients with toxicity refractory to all other therapy.

Hemodialysis and Hemoperfusion

Hemodialysis and hemoperfusion are of limited use, and information is largely limited to case reports. The main indications for hemodialysis are renal failure and hemodynamic instability.

Disposition

A patient with a history of non-sustained-release beta-blocker ingestion is observed on a cardiac monitor for 6 h after ingestion.

Patients who have signs of cardiovascular, respiratory, or CNS toxicity are admitted to a monitored bed. Patients who have a history of ingestion of extended-release preparations are admitted and monitored for 24 h. A patient who has ingested a beta blocker that is not a sustained-release product can be discharged home after the observation period if there are no signs of toxicity.

CALCIUM CHANNEL BLOCKERS

Calcium channel blockers decrease contraction of vascular muscle and myocardium by inhibiting the influx of calcium into the cell. Each drug affects a different subset of calcium channels, leading to a unique set of physiologic effects. In overdose, any of these drugs can cause peripheral vasodilatation, decreased AV conduction, and decreased myocardial contractility. It is extremely important to be aware that sustained-release preparations can have life-threatening sequelae 24 h after ingestion due to their prolonged absorption time.

Clinical Effects

The different pharmacological profile of calcium channel blockers will cause various presentations, but in all cases the cardiovascular effects predominate. Verapamil and diltiazem typically cause bradycardia and hypotension. Hypotension may be due to sinoatrial node depression, atrioventricular node depression leading to AV blocks, or decreased peripheral vascular resistance. Nifedipine primarily affects the arterioles, causing decreased peripheral vascular resistance, which leads to hypotension and reflex tachycardia.

Neurologic and respiratory findings are usually secondary to cardiovascular toxicity and shock. Respiratory effects include decreased respiratory drive, pulmonary edema, and ARDS. Neurologic sequelae include depressed sensorium, cerebral infarction, and seizures. Nausea, vomiting, and constipation can occur.

The most important gastrointestinal consequence to recognize is obstruction due to a concretion of sustained-release capsules. In addition to causing a bowel obstruction, the concretion can be a source of continued toxicity. Early recognition of sustained-release capsules in the gastrointestinal tract and their evacuation can decrease morbidity and mortality. Decreased insulin release can lead to hyperglycemia. Hypoperfusion may lead to profound lactic acidosis. Hypocalcemia is the most frequent electrolyte abnormality. Hypokalemia and hyperkalemia have also been reported.

Drug levels for calcium channel blockers are helpful only in confirming the presence of the agent. An ECG is obtained in any patient with a history of calcium channel blocker overdose and is assessed for blocks, bradycardia, and ischemic changes. When possible, the ECG is compared to previous ECGs. Electrolytes are evaluated, specifically Na^+, Ca^{2+}, Mg^{2+}, and K^+. Sustained-release tablets may be radiopaque. An abdominal radiograph may be useful in patients with signs of obstruction or history of ingesting sustained-release tablets.

Management

In the unstable patient, supportive care and antidotal therapy are instituted immediately. The patient is placed on a cardiac monitor, intravenous access is established, and fluid resuscitation with crystalloid is initiated in hypotensive patients. Intubation may be necessary for airway protection or in patients with respiratory failure secondary to pulmonary edema. Absorption can be decreased by gastric emptying and administration of activated charcoal. If the ingestion occurred less than 4 h prior to presentation, gastric emptying may be helpful. Ipecac is relatively contraindicated because rapid CNS depression can occur. In cases that present early, lavage is indicated.

In patients who have ingested sustained-release preparations, whole bowel irrigation is a consideration. A dose of charcoal is administered prior to initiating whole bowel irrigation, as it can absorb drug that is released while the pills remain in the gastrointestinal (GI) tract.

The primary antidote for an overdose of a calcium channel blocker is calcium. Calcium is indicated in patients with hypotension, bradycardia, or heart blocks.

Two calcium salts are available: calcium gluconate and calcium chloride. The recommended pediatric doses are calcium chloride 10% solution 10 to 20 mg/kg/dose or calcium gluconate 10% solution 0.2 to 0.5 mL/kg/dose by slow IV push. The dose is repeated in 10 to 15 min for persistent hypotension or bradycardia. Calcium gluconate is preferred in patients with acidosis.

The calcium salts primarily reverse hypotension due to vasodilation and may have little or no effect on heart rate or conduction. Bradycardia may respond to atropine. When hypotension persists despite the administration of fluids and calcium salts, therapy with vasopressors is indicated to restore perfusion. Dopamine is a reasonable first-line option. If it is ineffective, therapy with norepinephrine or dobutamine may be helpful. Amrinone, a phosphodiesterase inhibitor, has been reported to be effective in reversing hypotension secondary to calcium channel blocker overdose. In adults, amrinone can be given as an initial bolus of 0.75 mg/kg over 2 to 3 min, followed by an infusion of 5 to 10 μ/kg/min. Pediatric dosing has not been established. Currently, clinical experience with amrinone is limited.

Glucagon is another proposed antidote for calcium channel blocker toxicity. Currently glucagon should be reserved for toxicity refractory to other measures. The adult dose is 150 μ/kg given by slow IV push over 1 min. It can be infused at a rate of 1 to 5 mg/h. Pediatric dosing has not been established. If glucagon is administered multiple times or as an infusion, the package diluent should not be used, since it contains phenol. It can be mixed in normal saline or D_5W.

Hemodialysis and Hemoperfusion

Hemodialysis and hemoperfusion are of limited usefulness in the setting of calcium channel blocker overdose. Dialysis could be considered in a patient who has renal failure. There has been one case of clinical improvement after hemoperfusion in a patient with combined diltiazem and metoprolol ingestion.

Disposition

Children who have signs of cardiovascular, respiratory, or CNS compromise are admitted to an intensive care unit. Children with a history of sustained-release ingestion are observed with cardiac monitoring for at least 24 h. Those patients with no signs of toxicity, no history of sustained-release ingestion, and no ECG abnormalities can be observed for 8 h after the time of ingestion.

CLONIDINE

Clonidine is widely used as an antihypertensive agent and often to treat opiate withdrawal. It is available in tablets and in sustained-release patches, both of which can be ingested by children. Especially in young children, even small doses of clonidine can cause serious toxicity.

Clonidine decreases heart rate, cardiac output, and peripheral vascular resistance. At high doses, it can cause hypertension, although this effect is transitory and is usually followed by hypotension. Clonidine also functions as a CNS depressant. Hypotensive effects can last up to 24 h. Severe toxicity has been reported after an ingestion of as little as 0.1 mg by a child. Clinical manifestations include altered mental status, somnolence, respiratory depression, and, especially in children, recurrent apnea. Central nervous system depression can last for 24 h. Miosis can occur, which, in combination with altered mental status and depressed respiratory drive, can appear exactly like opiate toxicity. In addition to miosis, the neurological examination may reveal hypotonia and decreased reflexes. Seizures are rare. Some patients may develop hypothermia.

Bradycardia and hypotension are the predominant cardiovascular manifestations, though patients can initially be hypertensive. Cardiac arrhythmias can occur. The cardiovascular effects can develop hours after the onset of mental status changes.

Management

The initial management of clonidine overdose focuses on stabilizing the airway and breathing. Respiratory depression may require ventilatory support. Prior to intubation, all patients receive naloxone. This is especially important given the difficulty in distinguishing clonidine ingestion from an opiate overdose. In addition, naloxone may actually be useful in reversing the effects of a clonidine overdose.

After ventilation is stabilized, gastric decontamination is indicated. Lavage is the preferred method, given clonidine's tendency to cause CNS depression and seizures. Ipecac-induced emesis can potentially result in aspiration. Following lavage, activated charcoal is administered.

Clonidine-induced bradycardia is treated with atropine if it is associated with hypotension. Hypotension itself is treated with aggressive fluid resuscitation. For hypotension that does not respond to fluids, moderate-dose dopamine may be useful. Dopamine may also ameliorate bradycardia. In patients with hypertension, it is important to realize that this side effect is transient and should be treated only if there is evidence of end-organ compromise. A short-acting agent such as nitroprusside is used to avoid precipitating profound hypotension, which can occur if a longer-acting agent such as nifedipine is administered.

Naloxone may reverse the opiatelike side effects of clonidine on mental status and respiratory depression, and there is some indication that it can reverse clonidine-mediated hypotension. However, at this point data on this subject are conflicting, and naloxone cannot be considered a specific antidote for clonidine overdose. While there are no contraindications to its use, the administration of naloxone in the setting of clonidine overdose has been associated with hypertension, and blood pressure monitoring is necessary during its administration.

Tolazoline is an alpha-antagonist agent that has been reported to reverse clonidine-mediated hypotension. However, it is not the specific antidote for clonidine. Data on its use are conflicting. It can cause profound hypotension, and its use should be restricted to the most refractory cases.

For a more detailed discussion, see Bizovi K: Antihypertensives, beta blockers, and calcium antagonists, chap. 83, p. 506, in *Pediatric Emergency Medicine: A Comprehensive Study Guide.*

84 Arsenic

Jerrold Leikin

Arsenical pesticide exposures most often occur in small children. Other sources of arsenic include flypapers (Orpiment), Fowler's solution (Liquor Arsenicalis), soil, well water, herbal preparations, and shellfish (usually organic arsenic).

PATHOPHYSIOLOGY

Arsenic combines reversibly with sulfhydryl groups of several enzymes of the Krebs cycle and can disrupt oxidative phosphorylation. A potentially lethal dose of arsenic is 1 to 4 mg/kg. Inorganic compounds are more toxic than organic arsenic (Table 84-1).

CLINICAL MANIFESTATIONS

The initial manifestations of arsenic poisoning include nausea, abdominal pain, vomiting, and diarrhea that is characterized as "rice water." Hypotension can occur. The patient may have a characteristic garlic odor.

Other systemic manifestations are diaphoresis, renal failure, hepatic dysfunction, and cardiac rhythm disturbances, including torsades de pointes. In severe intoxication, seizures and coma can occur. A peripheral neuropathy can develop 10 days to 3 weeks after ingestion; it is characterized by paresthesias of the extremities followed by motor disability. Because of the neuropathy, arsenic toxicity can be confused with Guillain-Barré syndrome.

Chronic arsenic toxicity can have a similar though less fulminant course and is characterized by dermatologic manifestations. Hyperpigmentation in a "raindrops" configuration can occur on the eyelids, on the temples, and in the neck region. Skin desquamation

TABLE 84-1 Arsenical Pesticides

Compound	Preparations
Inorganic	
Trivalent	
Arsenic trioxide	Grant's Ant Control Ant Stakes
Sodium arsenite	Weed control (aqueous solution)
Calcium arsenite	Used on fruit (powder)
Copper arsenite	Wood preservative (powder)
Copper acetoarsenite	Insecticide outside the United States
Pentavalent	Defoliant/herbicide (aqueous)
Arsenic acid	Ant insecticide
Sodium arsenate	Herbicide (powder)
Calcium arsenate	Insecticide (powder)
Lead arsenate	Used on potatoes/tomatoes (powder)
Zinc arsenate	
Organic (pentavalent)	
Cacodylic acid	
Methane arsenic acid	
Monosodium methane arsenate	Herbicide/defoliant
Disodium methane arsenate	Herbicide
Monoammonium methane arsenate	Herbicide/defoliant
	Herbicide/silvicide
Calcium acid methane arsenate	Postemergence herbicide
	Postemergence herbicide

and brittle nails with transverse white striae (Aldrich-Mees lines) can develop after 4 to 5 weeks of exposure. Patchy and diffuse alopecia can develop. Mucosal involvement is generally spared.

DIAGNOSIS

Pancytopenia, elevated liver function tests, and elevated creatinine all may occur from arsenic poisoning.

Urinary arsenic levels above 100 μg/24 h are consistent with poisoning. Arsenic exposure can also be diagnosed by tissue testing of pubic hair or fingernails. Arsenic is radiopaque and in acute ingestions may be visible on plain radiographs.

MANAGEMENT

Gastric decontamination is performed by gastric lavage or, if abdominal radiographs are positive, whole bowel irrigation. Activated charcoal does not adsorb arsenic.

TABLE 84-2 Chelators of Arsenic

	Route	Dose, mg/kg	Dosing interval
Dimercaprol	IM	3–5	4–12 h
D-Penicillamine	PO	25	4 times daily
2,3 Dimercaptosuccinic acid (DMSA or succimer) (Not FDA-approved at the present time)	PO	10	Every 8 h

Chelation is indicated when the 24-h urinary arsenic concentration exceeds 200 μg/L (Table 84-2). Chelation probably must be performed during the first 24 h after exposure to avoid the delayed neuropathy associated with arsenic toxicity.

The management of exposure to arsine gas, which like arsenic has a characteristic garlic odor, is radically different from that of arsenic ingestion. Toxicity from arsine gas results in hemolysis, abdominal pain, jaundice, and hematuria. Chelation is not effective, and the treatment consists of dialysis or exchange transfusion.

For a more detailed discussion, see Leikin J: Arsenic, chap. 84, p. 512, in *Pediatric Emergency Medicine: A Comprehensive Study Guide.*

85 Aspirin

Michele Zell-Kanter

Acetylsalicylic acid continues to be a common cause of toxicity. As an accidental ingestant, it is especially common in children below 5 years of age.

PHARMACOKINETICS

At normal doses, aspirin is rapidly absorbed from the small intestine. If aspirin is taken in large amounts, absorption can be delayed by the formation of concretions. In therapeutic doses, metabolism is first-order; but in the overdose setting, pharmacokinetics change to zero-order. Ingestions of less than 150 mg/kg are generally nontoxic. With ingestions of 150 to 300 mg/kg, mild to moderate toxicity occurs, and overdoses of more than 300 mg/kg can be lethal. Infant aspirin bottles are limited to 36 tablets of 81 mg each. Oil of wintergreen, on the other hand, contains 100% methyl-salicylate and can be lethal in extremely small amounts.

PATHOPHYSIOLOGY AND CLINICAL PRESENTATION

After an ingestion, children have a quicker onset and exhibit more severe signs of toxicity than do adults. Patients may complain of tinnitus and decreased hearing. Direct stimulation of respiratory centers causes tachypnea and early respiratory alkalosis. Uncoupling of the Krebs cycle results in anaerobic metabolism and ketonemia, which causes an anion gap metabolic acidosis. Hypovolemia results from vomiting, increased insensible losses from tachypnea and perspiration, and an osmotic diuresis. Fluid losses are especially severe in young children. In pediatric patients, the onset of metabolic acidosis tends to occur more rapidly than in adults and is often not preceded by a respiratory alkalosis.

Central nervous system toxicity can cause agitation, delirium, seizures, and coma. Rhabdomyolysis can occur and can cause acute renal failure. Patients can develop noncardiogenic pulmonary edema. Risk factors for this include central nervous system toxicity, metabolic acidosis, and chronic ingestion. Hyperthermia indicates significant toxicity.

Commonly observed electrolyte abnormalities include hypo- and hypernatremia, hypokalemia, and hypocalcemia. In children, hypoglycemia is more common than hyperglycemia.

LABORATORY STUDIES

Initial laboratory studies include a complete blood count, electrolytes, and an arterial blood gas. Serum salicylate levels are best drawn 6 h postingestion, when they reflect peak concentration. The Done nomogram is useful in acute, isolated ingestions of an immediate-release preparation. It must always be correlated with the patient's condition. In patients with chronic ingestions, clinical findings are more predictive of toxicity than the nomogram.

Some simple bedside tests can confirm the presence of salicylate. Thirty minutes after ingestion, 2 to 3 drops of ferric chloride added to 1 mL of the patient's urine will turn purple in the presence of salicylate. In the presence of salicylate at serum concentrations as low as 20 mg/dL, Phenistix will turn a brownish purple.

MANAGEMENT

Goals in the management of the salicylate-intoxicated patient are the correction of dehydration and metabolic disturbances, the prevention of further absorption of the toxin, and the enhancement of its elimation.

Intravascular volume is restored by boluses of crystalloid. After urine output is established, potassium is added to the intravenous fluid in patients who are hypokalemic.

In patients who present within 1 h of ingestion, syrup of ipecac may be useful. Patients with altered mental status are best managed by gastric lavage. Large amounts of aspirin have a tendency to form concretions in the stomach; thus patients with significant ingestions may benefit from gastric evacuation for several hours after ingestion. Whole bowel irrigation is indicated in patients in whom a concretion is observed on radiograph and in those who have ingested sustained-release preparations.

Activated charcoal is effective in adsorbing aspirin and is administered as soon as gastric evacuation is accomplished. While studies evaluating multiple doses of charcoal are at this point inconclusive, multiple doses are indicated in significant ingestions. The efficacy of whole bowel irrigation with activated charcoal is unknown.

Elimination of salicylate is enhanced by systemic alkalinization. As the urine becomes alkaline, an increased fraction of salicylate in the tubular fluid becomes ionized and unreabsorbable and is excreted. As urine pH increases from 5 to 8, renal clearance of salicylate increases by a factor of 10 to 20.

The goal of alkalinization is to increase the urine pH to 7.5 to 8. This is accomplished by administering sodium bicarbonate in an initial bolus of 1 to 2 meg/kg, followed by a bicarbonate drip titrated to the urine pH. Serial arterial blood gases are obtained to assure that the patient is not overalkalinized.

Hypokalemia is common in salicylism and can impair attempts to alkalinize the urine, since potassium is exchanged for hydrogen in the tubular fluid when serum potassium is low.

Complications of alkalinization include congestive heart failure secondary to volume load, excessive alkalemia, and hypernatremia.

Hemodialysis removes salicylates three to five times faster than systemic alkalinization. Indications for its use include congestive heart failure, noncardiogenic pulmonary edema, central nervous system depression, seizures, metabolic acidosis refractory to alkalinization, hepatic failure, and coagulopathy. The salicylate level is not useful as a sole criterion for dialysis unless it exceeds 80 mg/dL in an acute ingestion. The threshold for dialysis is lower in a chronic ingestion than in acute overdose, since toxicity is more severe.

An investigational modality in salicylate poisoning involves the use of glycine, which may act as a substrate in enhancing the excretion of salicylate.

For a more detailed discussion, see Zell-Kanter M: Aspirin, chap. 85, p. 514, in *Pediatric Emergency Medicine: A Comprehensive Study Guide.*

86 Carbon Monoxide

Timothy Turnbull

Carbon monoxide (CO) is the most common cause of death due to poisoning. It is a colorless, odorless gas formed as a by-product of incomplete combustion in fossil fuels. Carbon monoxide poisoning is most commonly due to smoke inhalation.

Carbon monoxide binds to hemoglobin with 250 times the affinity of oxygen. It also alters the hemoglobin molecule so that the remaining oxygen is bound with greater affinity. The result is a reduction in the oxygen-carrying capacity of the hemoglobin molecule and impairment of its ability to provide oxygen to the tissues. Carbon monoxide also binds to cytochrome enzymes and to myoglobin, and inhibits cellular respiration.

The central nervous system and heart are most susceptible to the effects of CO poisoning. Children are presumed to be more vulnerable to central nervous system damage at lower levels of CO than are adults. The developing fetus appears to be particularly vulnerable to CO toxicity. Carboxyhemoglobin (COHb) levels attained in the fetus are routinely 10 to 15 percent higher than those in the maternal circulation, and the elimination phase of CO in the fetus is markedly prolonged compared to that of the mother.

CLINICAL PRESENTATION

Clinical signs and symptoms of CO poisoning are notoriously nonspecific and correlate only roughly with the carboxyhemoglobin

TABLE 86-1 Relationships of COHgB Level and Clinical Manifestations of Carbon Monoxide Toxicity

Carboxyhemoglobin level, %	Signs and symptoms
0–10	None
10–20	Mild headache, dyspnea on exertion
20–30	More severe headache, dyspnea
30–40	Severe headache, dizziness, nausea, vomiting, fatigue, poor judgment, dim vision
40–50	Confusion, tachypnea, tachycardia
50–60	Syncope, seizures, coma
60–70	Coma, hypotension, respiratory failure, death
>70	Rapidly fatal

level at the scene (Table 86-1). The longer the interval between exposure and evaluation, the more likely it is that the symptoms and level will be discordant. A careful history and high index of suspician are keys to the diagnosis.

Many patients with "occult" CO intoxication complain of flulike symptoms, with headache, nausea, and fatigue. In more severe cases, there may be a history of syncope, or the victim's recollection of events may differ from that of the person who has brought the patient to the hospital. Infants may be irritable or have difficulty feeding.

It is axiomatic that any illness affecting more than one victim of a family or group from a common environment requires that CO poisoning be ruled out.

The physical examination is usually normal. Vital sign abnormalities are nonspecific. The "cherry red" skin commonly associated with CO poisoning is usually a postmortem finding. Retinal hemorrhages suggest CO poisoning but are infrequent. Cardiac toxicity most commonly manifests as arrhythmias, but in older patients it can precipitate angina or an acute myocardial infarction. Neurologic abnormalities vary widely, from a normal examination to fulminant coma. Pulmonary edema, rhabdomyolysis, and renal failure occur rarely.

LABORATORY STUDIES

The diagnosis of CO poisoning is confirmed by measurement of the carboxyhemoglobin level. Normal carboxyhemoglobin is less than 1 percent. Levels are as high as 5 percent in nonsmoking urban residents, and heavy smokers can have levels between 5 and 15%.

The carboxyhemoglobin level and the severity of toxicity correlate poorly. The degree of toxicity depends on duration of exposure, concentration of CO, and the activity level of the victim. Since CO does not affect the P_{O_2}, it will be normal, but measured oxygen saturation will be decreased.

An electrocardiogram is recommended to detect ischemic changes in adults, but its value in children is unknown. Urine myoglobin is indicated in patients with prolonged unconsciousness or who are otherwise at risk for rhabdomyolysis.

Computed tomography and magnetic resonance imaging may reveal characteristic changes in the globus pallidis and white matter in cases of CO poisoning. The utility of these tests in the acute phase of intoxication is unknown.

TREATMENT

The cornerstone of treatment is supplemental oxygen. While the half-time of carboxyhemoglobin is about 5½ h in room air, it is decreased to 40 to 90 min at an F_{IO_2} of 100 percent. An F_{IO_2} of 100 percent can be approached with a tight-fitting nonrebreathing mask with a reservoir. Obtunded patients may require intubation.

In cases of mild to moderate intoxication, treatment with supplemental oxygen at atmospheric pressure is sufficient. It can be terminated when the carboxyhemoglobin level falls below 5 percent. Pregnant women must be treated five times longer than usual because of the more avid binding and prolonged elimination of CO by fetal hemoglobin.

In more severely intoxicated patients or those at high risk for central nervous system toxicity, hyperbaric oxygen (HBO) therapy is indicated. Hyperbaric oxygen can reduce the half-time of carboxyhemoglobin to 20 min while increasing the amount of dissolved oxygen in the plasma by 2 vol percent for every atmosphere. In patients with cerebral edema, HBO seems to lower intracranial pressure. Aggressive use of HBO in the treatment of CO poisoning may reduce early morbidity and mortality and the incidence of delayed neuropsychiatric complications.

Indications for HBO vary among centers with hyperbaric chambers. Generally accepted clinical indications include coma or other signs of neurologic impairment, any period of unconsciousness including syncope, and evidence of myocardial ischemia. Also included is any pregnant patient with a carboxyhemoglobin greater than 20 percent or with evidence of fetal distress. Aggressive use of HBO should also be considered in neonates and infants.

The use of the carboxyhemoglobin level as an indication for HBO in nonpregnant patients or those with mild to moderate symptoms is controversial. Some centers use a level of 40 percent or more. Those with levels below 40 percent and minimal symptoms undergo acute psychometric testing and are treated with HBO or atmospheric oxygen according to the results. Other centers simply treat every patient with a carboxyhemoglobin level above 20 or 25 percent with HBO. The nearest HBO facility can be located by contacting Divers Alert Network at Duke University in North Carolina (telephone number 1-919-684-8111).

DISPOSITION

Children with mild poisoning, whose carboxyhemoglobin level falls below 5 percent and who are no longer symptomatic can be discharged. Parents and caretakers are advised of the potential for delayed neuropsychiatric sequelae, including persistent headaches, memory lapses, irritability, and personality changes. It may be useful to recommend psychometric testing 3 to 4 weeks after exposure for any patient with a history of significant toxicity. Although most delayed sequelae will resolve, the course may take years.

For a more detailed discussion, see Turnbull T: Carbon monoxide, chap. 86, p. 516, in *Pediatric Emergency Medicine: A Comprehensive Study Guide.*

87 Caustics

Bonnie McManus

Caustics are chemicals that cause injury on contact. They account for approximately 5 percent of all accidental toxic exposures, with small children being the most frequently affected. Lye is the most frequent reported exposure. Acids are also frequently ingested, but the severe pain caused on initial contact usually limits accidental ingestion in small children.

PATHOPHYSIOLOGY

Regardless of whether the caustic is an acid or alkali, the severity of injury depends on the following factors: (1) the nature, volume, and concentration of the agent, (2) contact time, (3) presence or absence of stomach contents, (4) tonicity of the pyloric sphincter, and (5) esophageal reflux after the ingestion. Solid products tend to produce intense localized upper esophogael injury, while liquids, especially strong bases, tend to produce circumferential lesions in the distal esophagus. Areas of anatomic narrowing, such as at the cricopharyngeus or the carina, are associated with more severe injury. Theoretically, the presence of stomach contents will decrease tissue injury by exerting a buffering effect. Pylorospasm can increase contact time of the corrosive with the stomach and result in more severe gastric injury. Reflux of ingested material back into the esophagus can exacerbate tissue injury.

ALKALI BURNS

Alkali burns cause liquefaction necrosis, a deep-penetration injury associated with a pronounced exothermic reaction. Tissue destruction continues until the compound is significantly neutralized by tissue or the concentration is greatly decreased. Chemicals with a pH greater than 12.5 usually cause severe injury and frequently lead to esophageal stricturing, whereas those with a pH less than 11.4 rarely cause more than superficial mucosal burns. Most household bleaches have a pH of 11 to 12 and cause superficial burns.

Solid alkalais tend to cause perioral, oropharyngeal, and upper esophageal injury. The injury may be severe, with deep, irregular linear burns. Of special concern are Clinitest tablets, which may cause minimal symptoms but, when lodged in the esophagus, can cause catastrophic complications. Penetration into the aorta has been reported.

Liquid lye can cause severe esophageal injury with minimal oropharyngeal findings. The complications following liquid lye ingestion tend to be more severe than those following solid ingestions because the injury is circumferential and leads to stricturing. The stomach is involved about 20 percent of the time that there is esophageal injury. The relatively low incidence of stomach injury occurs because most of the lye is neutralized in the esophagus. Small quantities of ingested base can cause severe esophageal damage and never reach the stomach. The total amount of gastric acid in the stomach is insignificant in neutralizing a strong base.

There are three major phases of caustic esophageal injury. Phase 1 is an acute inflammatory stage in which vascular thrombosis and cellular necrosis peak at 1 to 2 days, followed by sloughing of the necrotic tissue at approximately 3 to 4 days, resulting in an area of ulceration. Phase 2 is the latent granulation phase, in which fibroplasia begins to fill in the ulcer with granulation tissue in the middle of the first week. By the end of the first week, collagen starts to replace the granulation tissue. Perforation is most likely during the second week, when the esophageal wall is the weakest. The third phase is the chronic cicatrization phase. It begins during weeks 2 to 4, producing variable degrees of scar formation and contractures.

ACID BURNS

Acid burns cause coagulation necrosis, with severe injury to superficial tissues, but penetration is avoided by the formation of an eschar that limits damage to deeper tissues. Unlike liquid alkali, which tends to produce injury very rapidly, acid injury may continue to evolve for up to 90 min after the ingestion. The nature of the injury is such that acid tends to reach the stomach without being buffered in the esophagus and can cause severe gastric injury, including perforation. Thus, esophageal injury associated with severe gastric injury is rare, and esophageal perforation has not been reported. If the pyloric sphincter is relaxed at the time of ingestion, injury to the small bowel can occur.

PRESENTATION AND STABILIZATION

The presentation of a child with a caustic ingestion varies from completely asymptomatic to fulminant respiratory distress or shock. Many caustics, including highly alkaline laundry detergents, can cause life-threatening airway edema, which must be urgently addressed. Stridor, dyspnea, and dysphonia all indicate upper airway compromise that requires intervention. Patients with upper airway obstruction are intubated under direct visualization or may need a surgical airway. Blind nasotracheal intubation is contraindicated.

Patients with a history of caustic ingestion but without signs of airway compromise are observed for excessive crying, drooling, or refusal to eat or drink, all of which indicate a significant injury. The mouth is examined for signs of intraoral burns and the chest for retractions, wheezes, or rhonchi, which indicate potential aspiration. The abdomen is examined for tenderness, which in cases of acid ingestion suggests the possibility of gastric perforation. In cases of suspected perforation, the patient is monitored carefully for the presence of intraabdominal hemorrhage and hypovolemic shock.

In patients with signs of respiratory distress, oxygen saturation or arterial blood gases are critical in assessing lung function. Many caustics are powerful emetics and, if aspirated, can cause severe pneumonitis or noncardiogenic pulmonary edema. Household bleach, when combined with acid or ammonia, produces chlorine or chloramine gas, respectively. Exposure to either in a closed area can result in severe respiratory compromise.

Laboratory studies include a complete blood count, serum electrolytes, blood urea nitrogen, creatinine, and glucose. A chest radiograph is indicated in patients with signs of a significant ingestion or respiratory distress. Patients with abdominal pain or tenderness require an abdominal radiograph to exclude the presence of free air, which indicates a perforation.

MANAGEMENT

Symptomatic patients require special attention to the airway. After it is stabilized, an intravenous catheter is indicated in the event that volume resuscitation is required. In the event of a large acid ingestion, a nasogastric tube is placed in an attempt to remove pooled acid and reduce injury.

DILUENTS/BUFFERS

Currently, attempting to buffer a strong acid is not recommended because an extraordinary exothermic reaction can occur that can increase tissue destruction. Diluents may have a role in weak acid ingestion because injury is purely caustic and does not have the risk of thermal injury. There are, however, no controlled studies to support this. Milk or water may be indicated in the ingestion of solid alkali in an attempt to move particulate material out of the oropharynx and esophagus. The amount given should be easily tolerated by the child without inducing emesis. There is no value in administering diluents in the case of liquid lye ingestion because the injury is complete in a very short time and the risk of inducing emesis is great.

EMESIS

Induction of emesis in caustic ingestions is contraindicated. Increased tissue damage occurs as the esophagus is reexposed to the offending agent. With violent emesis, there is an increased risk of perforation as well as an increased risk of aspiration. In acid ingestion, emesis worsens the overall contact time and increases injury; in alkali ingestions, the injury is usually complete prior to arrival at the emergency department.

GASTRIC ASPIRATION AND LAVAGE

In general, gastric aspiration and lavage are not indicated in alkali injury because of the rapidity of the injury. Although there are no studies showing an advantage or disadvantage of gastric aspiration in strong acid ingestion, it is recommended that gastric contents be removed through a soft catheter if the patient is seen within 90 min of ingestion. While concern exists regarding the possibility of inducing a gastric perforation by placing a catheter, this is not supported by studies.

CHARCOAL AND CATHARTICS

The administration of charcoal and cathartics is contraindicated because caustics are poorly adsorbed by charcoal, the injury tends to occur prior to arrival to the emergency department, and charcoal creates a problem with visualization for the endoscopist.

ENDOSCOPY

The challenge in managing the child with a caustic ingestion is in identifying the patient who is at risk for a serious injury, since many patients have minimal clinical findings. While there may be a greater risk of a higher-grade lesion if there are significant injuries to the oral mucosa, clinical criteria are not reliable in identifying the presence or severity of burns. If two of the three symptoms of vomiting, drooling, and stridor are present, the likelihood of gastrointestinal burns is high. Of the three, vomiting is the most powerful predictor of severe esophageal injury.

Endoscopy helps to define the extent of the injury and to develop a prognosis. Because of the unreliability of clinical findings in predicting significant esophageal injury, the threshold for endoscopy is low. Any child with a history of significant ingestion, with oral lesions, or who is otherwise symptomatic deserves endoscopy. The optimal time frame for the procedure is 12 to 24 h after the injury. If done too early, endoscopy can underestimate the extent of the injury. Endoscopy is not indicated for asymptomatic ingestion of household bleach, ammonia, and nonphosphate detergents. Evidence of perforation and shock is a contraindication to endoscopy.

Glucocorticoids are controversial in caustic ingestions. They may decrease the incidence of esophageal strictures in patients with severe burns. Risks of glucocorticoids include suppurative complications and an increased possibility of perforation.

SPECIAL CONCERNS

Caustic Eye Injuries

Caustic eye injury can have devastating consequences, with blindness frequently resulting from extensive exposure. Excessive tearing, refusal to open the eye, or holding the eye closed indicate ocular involvement that requires immediate attention. The eyes are irrigated with several liters of normal saline or another balanced salt solution. Both upper and lower cul-de-sacs are flushed copiously by retracting the eyelids, with lid retractors if necessary. At least 30 min of irrigation is recommended, after which the pH of the cul-de-sacs is checked. Irrigation may need to continue for up to 90 min. A complete eye examination is then performed, including visual acuity and slit-lamp examination. If perforation is possible, the eye is covered with a rigid shield. The full extent of ocular damage may not be evident for 48 to 72 h.

Button Batteries

Button batteries contain various combinations of zinc, cadmium, mercury, silver, nickel, or lithium in a concentrated alkaline medium, usually sodium or potassium hydroxide. Although the vast majority of patients do well, this ingestion poses a unique risk of caustic injury, and deaths have occurred. If the battery breaks open, the caustic contents may cause local injury and perforation. A battery lodged in the esophagus requires urgent removal. Burns have been reported as early as 4 h after ingestion, and perforation as early as 6 h. The preferred method of extraction is endoscopy. Emetics are usually unsuccessful in expelling a battery, and the use of a Foley catheter poses the risk of aspiration and does not allow for direct visualization of any injury.

If the battery is intact and has passed through the esophagus, it does not need to be retrieved unless there are indications of intraabdominal injury. A large battery ingested by a small child may also require removal. If a battery larger than 15 mm ingested by a child below 6 years of age has not passed the pylorus within 48 h it is unlikely to do so. Stool discoloration without signs of gastrointestinal injury is not an indication for battery removal.

An asymptomatic patient with a gastrointestinal battery not lodged in the esophagus can be discharged and followed as an outpatient. Whole bowel irrigation is an alternative easily performed in the emergency department; it will promote passage of the battery in 4 to 8 h.

Hydrofluoric acid

Hydrofluoric acid is an extremely powerful substance that can have grave consequences despite minimal exposure. External contact can result in severe dermal or ocular injury. Death has been reported with exposures affecting as little as 2.5 percent of the body surface area. Severe pain and deep penetration despite minimal skin findings are the hallmark of a hydrofluoric acid burn. The mechanism of injury involves liquefaction necrosis and the formation of insoluble calcium and magnesium salts. Oral ingestions are frequently fatal.

In cases of significant burns, systemic acidosis, hypocalcemia, hypomagnesemia, and hyperkalemia are common. Renal failure and hemolysis have been reported to occur.

En route to the emergency department, copious irrigation is indicated. A gel of 3.5 g of calcium gluconate and 5 oz of water-soluble jelly or 25% magnesium sulfate soak (Epsom salts) will provide pain relief. Pain can also be alleviated by intradermal injection of calcium gluconate. In cases of oral ingestion, calcium and magnesium are given on a milliequivalent-per-milliequivalent basis via nasogastric tube.

For a more detailed discussion, see McManus B: Caustics, chap. 87, p. 519, in *Pediatric Emergency Medicine: A Comprehensive Study Guide.*

---

88 Cocaine Toxicity

Steven E. Aks

Cocaine abuse and toxicity continue to be pervasive problems. Children usually suffer toxicity when exposed to cocaine being used by others. Seizures have been reported in children who accidentally ingest cocaine, and toxicity has occured in toddlers who inhale freebase cocaine being smoked in close proximity by adults.

PHARMACOLOGY AND PATHOPHYSIOLOGY

Chemically, cocaine is derived from the plant *Erythroxylum coca.* It is rapidly absorbed from mucous membranes, lung tissue, and the gastrointestinal tract.

Pharmacologically, cocaine is a sympathomimetic whose primary target organs are the central nervous system (CNS), cardiovascular system, lungs, gastrointestinal tract, skin, and thermoregulatory center.

Clinically, cocaine causes CNS stimulation that can result in agitation, hallucinations, abnormal movements, and convulsions. Paradoxically, children may present with lethargy.

Cardiovascular manifestations of cocaine toxicity include sinus tachycardia and both supraventricular and ventricular dysrhythmias. Elevations in blood pressure can range from mild to fulminant hypertension associated with strokes. Myocardial ischemia, including myocardial infarction, has occurred in individuals as young as 17 years of age.

Multiple pulmonary effects from inhalation of cocaine include exacerbation of asthma, pulmonary infarction, pneumomediastinum, pneumothorax, and respiratory failure.

Orally ingested cocaine can cause ischemic complications in the gastrointestinal tract that include acute abdominal pain, hemorrhagic diarrhea, and shock.

In association with agitation and hypertension, cocaine-induced hyperthermia can occur. A potential complication of hyperthermia is acute rhabdomyolysis. Cocaine-induced rhabdomyolysis can also occur in the absence of hyperthermia.

DIAGNOSIS

Cocaine toxicity is likely in a patient who exhibits signs and symptoms of sympathomimetic stimulation. Occasionally the sympathomimetic toxidrome is difficult to distinguish from that caused by anticholinergic toxicity. Unlike sympathomimetic toxicity, however, anticholinergics will cause urinary retention and decreased bowel sounds. Also, sympathomimetic toxicity is often associated with diaphoresis, whereas anticholinergic overdose is associated with dry skin.

LABORATORY STUDIES

A toxicology screen can confirm cocaine ingestion. Electrocardiographic monitoring is essential to evaluate the patient for dysrhythmias. Patients who complain of chest pain require a 12-lead electrocardiogram. In these patients, a radiograph is useful in order to exclude a pneumothorax, pneumomediastinum, or infiltrate.

Laboratory studies help to establish a baseline and are useful in patients with significant toxicity. They include a complete blood count, serum electrolytes, glucose, and blood urea nitrogen, and creatinine. If a urine dipstick is positive for blood but microscopy is negative for red blood cells, the patient is evaluated for rhabdomyolysis with a serum creatine kinase and urine myoglobin.

Computed tomography (CT) of the brain is indicated in patients with a severe headache or neurological deficit to rule out the possibility of a cocaine-induced cerebrovascular accident.

MANAGEMENT

Mildly toxic patients generally require no specific therapy. Moderate to severe agitation responds to benzodiazepines, which are also the drug of choice for seizures. Persistent seizure activity may require treatment with dilantin or phenobarbital. Rarely, status epilepticus requires paralysis. Patients with persistent seizures may suffer from a structural CNS lesion or toxicity from a coingestant.

Benzodiazepines are also effective treatment for most patients with mild to moderate hypertension. In more severe cases, labetalol, which has both alpha- and beta-blocking characteristics, has been effective, as has sodium nitroprusside. Beta blockers are contraindicated, since unopposed alpha stimulation can exacerbate hypertension.

Patients with severe hyperthermia are treated with aggressive cooling, and the urine is alkalinized in patients with rhabdomyolysis. Activated charcoal absorbs unpackaged orally ingested cocaine and is useful for gastric contamination.

BODY STUFFERS

Body stuffers may swallow cocaine in an attempt to illegally transport the drug. Even carefully packaged packets can rupture, with fatal results. Types of packages that are likely to rupture are those made of paper and poorly secured plastic bags. The physician may be able to gather enough information regarding the amount of cocaine ingested and the type of packaging used to assess the potential for toxicity.

Abdominal radiographs may be useful if the ingested packets are radiopaque. A Gastrografin swallow or CT of the abdomen may reveal ingested packets in cases where plain radiographs are negative but the suspicion for an ingestion is high.

In body stuffers, gastric decontamination with syrup of ipecac or gastic lavage is contraindicated, since both may cause rupture of the packets. Whole bowel irrigation with polyethylene glycol electrolyte lavage solution can be used to enhance transit through the gastrointestinal tract. It is important to be sure that all ingested packets pass before the patient is discharged. To do so may require a Gastrografin swallow or abdominal CT. In symptomatic body stuffers, a surgical consultation is indicated, since laparotomy may be necessary.

In asymptomatic or mild cases of cocaine toxicity, 4 to 6 h of observation in the emergency department is adequate. Patients with moderate to severe symptoms are admitted to a monitored bed. Body stuffers are observed in a monitored setting until all packets have passed.

For a more detailed discussion, see Aks SE: Cocaine toxicity, chap. 88, p. 523, in *Pediatric Emergency Medicine: A Comprehensive Study Guide.*

89 Cyanide Poisoning

Anne Krantz

Cyanide poisoning is unusual in the United States and very rare among children, although its contribution to toxicity and death may be underestimated in victims of smoke inhalation. There are a variety of sources of cyanide exposure in the pediatric population. These are summarized in Table 89-1.

PATHOPHYSIOLOGY

The primary mechanism of toxicity in cyanide poisoning is cellular hypoxia caused by the inhibition of mitochondrial cytochrome oxidase. There is a shift to anaerobic metabolism, resulting in a severe lactic acidosis. Cyanide also shifts the oxyhemoglobin dissociation curve to the left, further impairing oxygen delivery to the tissues. The critical targets of cyanide are the brain and heart. Initial symptoms of toxicity include nausea, vomiting, headache, giddiness, anxiety, and confusion. With progression of toxicity, patients may experience a feeling of neck constriction, suffocation, and unsteadiness. Alternatively, victims of cyanide poisoning may be overcome quickly and present with coma, seizures, and cardiovascular collapse.

Initial physical signs include bradycardia, tachypnea, mild hypertension, and anxiety. Later, hypotension, tachycardia, bradypnea, dysrhythmias, seizures, and coma occur. Pupils may be dilated. Retinal veins may appear as red as arteries due to the lack of tissue abstraction of oxygen. There may be a musty odor, similar to that of the bitter almond plant, to the breath, although the ability to detect this is a genetically determined trait. Pulmonary edema may occur. The absence of cyanosis in a patient otherwise

TABLE 89-1 Sources of Cyanide Exposure

Cyanogenic plants
Prunus species (leaves, stem, bark, seed pits)
American plum, wild plum
Apricot
Cherry laurel, Carolina cherry laurel
Cultivated cherry
Peach
Wild black cherry
Chokecherry
Bitter almond
Other
Apple (seeds)
Pear (seeds)
Crabapple (seed)
Elderberry (leaves and shoots)
Hydrangea (leaves and buds)
Cassava (beans and roots)
Household agents
HCN-containing fumigants
Rodenticides
Insecticides (aliphatic thiocyanates: Lethane 60, Lethane 302, Thanite)
Sculpted nail removers containing acetonitrile (e.g., Nailene Glue Remover)
Silver and metal polish
Combustion products
Silk, wool
Polyurethane
Polyacrylonitrile
Other
Nitroprusside

showing clinical evidence of severe hypoxia suggests the diagnosis of cyanide poisoning.

LABORATORY EVALUATION

Arterial blood gases will typically show a metabolic acidosis. An elevated anion gap will be evident on electrolyte determination, due to the presence of a lactic acidosis. There may be a diminished arterial venous O_2 difference ($a_{O_2} - v_{O_2}$ approaching zero) due to the inability of tissues to utilize oxygen. When the arterial oxygenation is normal, a comparison of the calculated $\%O_2$ saturation and the measured $\%O_2$ saturation obtained from cooximetry may reveal an "O_2 saturation gap" greater than or equal to 5 percentage points. This occurs because some cyanide combines with hemoglobin, forming cyanhemoglobin, which cannot carry oxygen. The calculated O_2 saturation will be falsely elevated, whereas the more accurate measured value will be lower. Numerous electrocardiographic changes may occur in cyanide toxicity.

TREATMENT

Initial supportive care includes 100% oxygen, maintenance of pulse and blood pressure, and assisted ventilation if necessary. Severe acidosis may be partially corrected with sodium bicarbonate. Mouth-to-mouth resuscitation is avoided because of the risk of secondary cyanide exposure to rescue personnel. Gastric and skin decontamination are performed when indicated, although antidotal therapy takes precedence.

Cyanide Antidotes

Antidotal therapy clearly improves survival and shortens the recovery period. The only antidote currently approved for use in the United States is the Lilly Cyanide Antidote Kit, which contains amyl nitrite perles, sodium nitrite solution, and sodium thiosulfate.

The recommended regimen and pediatric doses for the Lilly Kit components are summarized in Table 89-2. Amyl nitrite perles are administered first, prior to the insertion of an intravenous line or while the sodium nitrite solution is being prepared. Amyl nitrite administration will produce a methemoglobin level of 3 to 7 percent. Once an intravenous line is established and the sodium nitrite solution prepared, amyl nitrite administration may be stopped.

Sodium nitrite (9 mg/kg or 0.3 mL/kg of a 3% solution, not to exceed 10 mL) is administered at a rate of 2.5 mL/min. In an unstable or hypotensive patient or when there is concomitant carbon monoxide poisoning, the dose may be given more slowly, over 30 min. The methemoglobin level peaks about 35 to 70 min following the dose at the slower rate and rises to roughly 10 to 15 percent. This level is lower than the 25 percent recommended in earlier literature as a goal of therapy. However, the lower level is therapeutic and avoids further impairment of tissue oxygen delivery due to a high methemoglobin level. Methemoglobin levels are monitored periodically following the end of the infusion.

Side effects of nitrite administration include headache, blurred vision, nausea, vomiting, and hypotension.

Following the nitrite administration, sodium thiosulfate is given to enhance clearance of cyanide as thiocyanate. Alternatively, the thiosulfate may be administered concurrently with the sodium

TABLE 89-2 Recommended Usage of Lilly Cyanide Antidote Kit

Antidote	Quantity/form	Pediatric dose
Amyl nitrite	12 perles (0.3 mL/perle)	Crush 1 to 2 perles in gauze and hold under patient's nose or over ET tube for 15 s/min[a]
Sodium nitrite	2 ampules of 3% solution (300 mg/10 mL)	0.3 mL/kg (9 mg/kg), not to exceed 10 mL (300 mg), IV at 2.5 mL/min, or over 30 min in fire victims with CO poisoning[b]
Sodium thiosulfate	2 ampules of 25% solution (12.5 g/50 mL)	1.6 mL/kg (400 mg/kg) up to 50 mL (12.5 g) at rate of 3–5 mL/min

[a] Check expiration date of all components. Shelf life for amyl nitrite is 1 year.

[b] Infuse more slowly when hypotension occurs. Monitor for blood pressure and be prepared to treat severe hypotension with fluids and vasopressors as needed. Monitor methemoglobin levels.

nitrite, at a separate intravenous site, when the latter is being given at the slower rate. The pediatric dose is 1.65 mL/kg of a 25% solution, up to 50 mL (12.5 g). Thiosulfate appears to have few if any side effects. Thiocyanate levels above 10 mg/dL may be associated with nausea, vomiting, arthralgias, and psychosis and may occur in the setting of renal failure resulting in impaired thiocyanate excretion.

Typically, symptoms and signs of cyanide poisoning begin to respond within minutes of the administration of nitrites. When symptoms recur following antidote administration, both the sodium nitrite and sodium thiosulfate may be given again at half their original doses.

Because there is no diagnostic test for cyanide poisoning that can be obtained in a timely manner, the diagnosis in the acute setting is made clinically. When the likelihood of cyanide poisoning is uncertain, the clinician may be reluctant to use nitrites. In this situation, the use of sodium thiosulfate alone may be considered. However, there are few published data on the efficacy of this approach. When a patient is treated with nitrites but shows no clinical response, the diagnosis of acute cyanide toxicity should be reconsidered.

In fire victims who require intubation or who have a persistent metabolic acidosis, abnormal mental status, or cardiovascular instability not resolving with therapy for carbon monoxide poisoning, treatment for cyanide poisoning should be strongly considered.

DISPOSITION

Patients who are asymptomatic and whose exposure has apparently been minimal are observed for 4 to 6 h. Those who have ingested cyanogenic glycosides are observed for at least 6 h for evidence of the onset of toxicity. Those ingesting acetonitrile-containing compounds are observed for 12 to 24 h. Patients requiring antidotal treatment are cared for in an intensive care unit. Following recovery, patients are observed for 24 to 48 h. Rarely, late neurologic syndromes have been reported following cyanide toxicity, and periodic outpatient follow-up is advised.

For a more detailed discussion, see Krantz A: Cyanide poisoning, chap. 89, p. 525, in *Pediatric Emergency Medicine: A Comprehensive Study Guide.*

---

90 Cyclic Antidepressant Overdose

Steven E. Aks

Cyclic antidepressants are a relatively common cause of accidental poisoning in children and occasionally result in fatalities. The greatest number of major effects was with amitriptyline, followed by imipramine and desipramine.

PHARMACOLOGY

Amitriptyline and imipramine are prototypical tricyclic antidepressants. The effect of each cyclic antidepressant depends on its specific pharmacologic site of action. The major toxicities involve the cardiovascular and central nervous systems. Toxic effects can be grouped as follows:

1. *Anticholinergic side effects* cause tachycardia and the anticholinergic overdose syndrome of mydriasis, dry mucous membranes,

hyperthermia, decreased gastrointestinal motility, and urinary retention. Mental status changes range from agitation to stupor and coma.

2. *Blockade of norepinephrine reuptake* augments tachycardia and can cause hypertension. Upon depletion of norepinephrine stores, hypotension can occur.
3. *A "quinidinelike effect"* accounts for cardiac dysrhythmias by inducing conduction blocks that manifest clinically with a widened QRS complex and QT abnormalities.
4. *Alpha blockade* causes hypotension by decreasing peripheral vasomotor tone.

In therapeutic doses, cyclic antidepressants are rapidly and almost completely absorbed. In toxic doses, absorption can be delayed because anticholinergic effects delay gastrointestinal motility.

CLINICAL PRESENTATION

The clinical presentation of cyclic antidepressant overdose is related primarily to the effects on the central nervous and cardiovascular systems.

Patients can present to the emergency department with mental status changes that range from anxiety and agitation to confusion, delirium, and coma. Seizures can occur and are of ominous clinical significance.

Tachycardia is the most common cardiovascular manifestation of cyclic antidepressant toxicity. Other abnormal rhythms include ventricular dysrhythmias, bradydysrhythmias, and cardiac arrest. The patient's blood pressure can be high or low.

Other possible manifestations of toxicity are hyperthermia, rhabdomyolysis, renal failure, pancreatitis, and hepatitis.

A hallmark of cyclic antidepressant overdose is the proclivity of the patient to arrive at the emergency department appearing clinically stable, then suddenly deteriorate. Most patients who develop life-threatening problems do so within 2 h of arrival in the emergency department.

DIAGNOSIS

When the diagnosis of cyclic antidepressant overdose is entertained, cardiac monitoring is essential. Persistent tachycardia is consistent with an overdose and raises the suspicion that toxicity will progress. The QRS duration has received a great deal of attention as a marker for overdose. In adults, a QRS duration less than 100 ms is correlated with a low risk of developing toxicity, while a QRS interval between 100 and 160 ms is at times associated with seizures and dysrhythmias. A QRS interval greater than 160 ms is associated with a high risk of seizures and dysrhythmias. In children, however, the QRS duration has not been well studied. Likewise, in adults, a frontal plane terminal 40-ms QRS that has a rightward deviation is correlated with toxicity, but the significance of this parameter in children is unknown.

Because of the large volume of distribution of cyclic antidepressants, the serum level does not accurately reflect clinical toxicity. Only when very high levels are present (>1000 ng/mL) do they correlate with life-threatening toxicity.

In children, arterial blood gas monitoring is critical to the treatment of cyclic antidepressant overdose. Acidemia may increase the proportion of drug released from binding sites and contributes significantly to the propensity toward dysrhythmias.

MANAGEMENT

Stabilization

Intubation is necessary in patients with depressed mental status. It is also justified in patients who appear to be deteriorating clinically and in patients with altered mental status in whom gastric lavage is necessary.

In intubated patients, hyperventilation is indicated, since alkalemia can potentially reverse the cardiac toxicity of cyclic antidepressant overdose. In all patients, hypoxia is avoided, since it can worsen metabolic acidosis.

Hypotension is treated initially with boluses of crystalloid. If fluid resuscitation does not stabilize the blood pressure, pharmacologic support is indicated. Norepinephrine has theoretical advantages over dopamine because of its potential to directly reverse the alpha blockade caused by cyclic antidepressants, but dopamine has been shown to be similarly effective.

Gastric Decontamination

In all patients with suspected cyclic antidepressant overdose, the induction of emesis with ipecac is contraindicated because of the potential for sudden deterioration, which can lead to airway compromise if the patient vomits while unconscious.

Activated charcoal is administered, along with a single dose of sorbitol. Multiple doses are probably useful because charcoal binds to the drug still present in the gut and inhibits absorption. The contribution of multiple doses of activated charcoal to interrupting enterohepatic circulation is probably negligible.

Treatment of Severe Toxicity

If the QRS interval is greater than 100 ms, most authors agree that alkalinization is indicated. This is accomplished by administering sodium bicarbonate as a 1- to 2-meq/kg bolus, followed by an infusion in which sodium bicarbonate is added to D_5W. If the child is intubated, alkalinization can be obtained by a combination of bicarbonate administration and hyperventilation.

Alkalinization is believed to work by reversing the "quinidinelike" effects of cyclic antidepressants. The administration of sodium bicarbonate also has an effect on reversing sodium channel blockade. Alkalinization may increase the percentage of the drug that is protein-bound and therefore may protect from toxicity.

Supraventricular dysrhythmias usually do not require intervention. Ventricular dysrhythmias unresponsive to boluses of bicarbonate are treated with lidocaine. Because of the quinidinelike effect of the cyclic antidepressants, other type Ia antidysrhythmics are contraindicated. Phenytoin (Dilantin), a type Ib antidysrhythmic, may be of value but has not been shown to be uniformly effective. If the patient is hypotensive with a tachydysrhythmia, cardioversion is appropriate. Bradydysrhythmias may respond to overdrive pacing.

Seizures are an ominous sign in the setting of a cyclic antidepressant overdose. While generally short, seizures have been associated with incipient cardiac dysrhythmias. Seizures usually require no treatment, but benzodiazepines are effective. Phenytoin is useful in prolonged seizures but is not useful prophylactically.

Physostigmine has been suggested as an antidote for anticholinergic toxicity. However, its use in association with atrioventricular blocks, QRS widening, and bradycardia has resulted in asystole and death. Physostigmine should be viewed as a last line of therapy in cases of uncontrolled seizures, supraventricular dysrhythmia, and severe hypotension.

DISPOSITION

Patients with signs and symptoms of overdose are treated aggressively. Patients who are symptomatic or who appear to be progressing are admitted to an intensive care unit. Patients who do not develop tachycardia, QRS widening, anticholinergic symptoms, or drowsiness can be discharged after 6 h of monitoring in the emergency department.

For a more detailed discussion, see Aks SE: Cyclic antidepressant overdose, chap. 90, p. 529, in *Pediatric Emergency Medicine: A Comprehensive Study Guide.*

91 Digoxin Toxicity

Steven E. Aks / Jerrold Leikin

Digoxin is in use today for the treatment of congestive heart failure and supraventricular dysrhythmias. In addition, there are several plants that contain cardiac glycosides, including foxglove, oleander, lily of the valley, and red squill. Prior to the development of antibody therapy, deaths from digoxin toxicity were not rare.

PHARMACOLOGY/PATHOPHYSIOLOGY

Digoxin is a positive inotrope that increases the force and velocity of myocardial contractions. On the cellular level, digoxin presumably functions by binding to and inactivating the Na^{+*}, K^+-ATPase in the heart. This results in increased intracellular sodium concentration. In addition, enhanced contractility depends on intracellular ionized calcium concentrations during systole. At toxic concentrations, it is felt that intracellular calcium concentrations are markedly increased and that the membrane potential is unstable, which leads to dysrhythmias.

There are numerous factors that predispose the patient to digoxin toxicity. Hyperkalemia, in particular, can result in significant conduction delays. Hypokalemia is common in patients on diuretic therapy and can predispose them to the effects of chronic digoxin toxicity. Hypomagnesemia, hypercalcemia, renal insufficiency, and underlying heart disease all predispose to digoxin toxicity.

CLINICAL PRESENTATION

The presentation of digoxin toxicity is highly varied and depends largely on whether it results from an acute overdose or is a manifestation of chronic toxicity.

In the acute setting, patients tend to have more dramatic clinical and laboratory parameters than in chronic toxicity. Symptoms can be abrupt, with severe nausea, vomiting, and diarrhea. Other complaints include weakness, headache, paresthesias, and altered color perception. Cardiovascular symptoms include palpitations and dizziness secondary to hypotension.

Patients with chronic toxicity tend to have more vague complaints, though many of the symptoms of acute overdose also occur. Malaise, anorexia, and low-grade nausea and vomiting are common. Patients with chronic toxicity tend to be more symptomatic at lower levels than patients with acute overdose.

Cardiovascular toxicity is the most important factor in determining morbidity and mortality. A myriad of abnormal rhythms are associated with digoxin toxicity, the most common being frequent ventricular premature beats. Other dysrhythmias can be supraventricular, nodal, or ventricular. Common disturbances are junctional escape beats and accelerated junctional rhythm, paroxysmal atrial tachycardia with atrioventricular (AV) block, and AV block of varying degrees. There is no single pathognomonic rhythm.

DIAGNOSIS

A history of the exact amount of digoxin ingested is extremely helpful. A dose greater than 0.1 mg/kg has been suggested as an indication for the use of digoxin-specific Fab fragments.

A digoxin level is indicated whenever there is clinical suspicion of toxicity. A level is best obtained 6 h after ingestion. Therapeutic digoxin levels are usually considered to be between 0.8 and 1.8 ng/mL. Toxicity can occur at levels greater than 2 ng/mL in the chronic setting. In the acute setting, for children, a level of 2.6 ng/mL does not correlate well with toxicity. One author has recently suggested a cutoff level of 5 ng/mL alone as an indication for Fab therapy. However, drug levels may not correlate with toxicity, and the treatment is guided by the clinical picture.

Other necessary laboratory studies include a complete blood count, serum electrolytes, calcium, magnesium, and blood urea nitrogen and creatinine. Cardiac monitoring is essential, as is a 12-lead electrocardiogram.

MANAGEMENT

Digoxin-intoxicated patients can be highly unstable. All patients require a secure airway, intravenous access, and cardiac monitoring.

Gastric Decontamination

Syrup of ipecac is relatively contraindicated in the asymptomatic child because of the potential for sudden hemodynamic instability and deterioration of consciousness, which can lead to vomiting and aspiration. It is absolutely contraindicated in any patient who presents with abnormal vital signs or altered mental status. Gastric lavage is indicated after an adequate airway is assured; this may require intubation. A single dose of activated charcoal along with a cathartic is indicated. Multiple doses of charcoal have been reported to be of value for digitoxin preparations where there is avid enterohepatic circulation, but they are probably of little value for digoxin.

Antidotal Therapy

Digoxin immune Fab fragments are specific antidigoxin antibodies raised in sheep. Only the Fab fragment is used in order to decrease the risk of immunogenicity. Use of the Fab fragments is indicated in cases of severe digitalis intoxication manifested by a significant history, a high level, or signs and symptoms of toxicity. Specific indications include an ingestion of greater than 0.1 mg/kg, a digoxin level of greater than 5.0 ng/mL, or the presence of a life-threatening dysrhythmia or conduction delay. The antidote is also given in any patient whose condition appears to be deteriorating. In the case of chronic toxicity, this can occur at relatively low levels. Hyperkalemia greater than 5.0 meq/L is another indication to consider the use of Fab fragments. Standard modalities to treat hyperkalemia may also be used, with the exception of calcium salts. In the face of digoxin toxicity, the administration of calcium may exacerbate the development of dysrhythmias.

The dose of Fab fragments is based on either the amount ingested or the serum level. Guidelines are available in the package insert. Each vial of Fab fragments contains 40 mg of drug, which will bind approximately 0.6 mg of digoxin (see Table 91-1).

Allergic reactions to Fab fragments are rare. Skin testing is usually not necessary. In cases where Fab fragments have been effective, results have been achieved 30 min to 4 h after administration.

After administration of Fab fragments, subsequent digoxin levels will be falsely elevated for several days because the bound digoxin is measured along with the free drug.

In addition to the administration of Fab fragments, standard treatment of dysrhythmias or AV blocks is indicated. Atropine or temporary pacing may be necessary as a temporizing measure while Fab fragments are taking effect. Cardioversion and lidocaine

TABLE 91-1 Dose Estimates of Digibind

$$\text{Dose (number of vials)} = \frac{\text{total digitalis body load (mg)}}{\text{0.6 mg of digitalis bound/vial}}$$

If the digoxin serum level is available, the following formula can be used to *estimate* the dose in adults:

$$\text{Dose (number of vials)} = \frac{\text{serum digoxin concentration (ng/mL)} \times \text{weight (kg)}}{100}$$

	Serum digoxin concentration, ng/mL						
Weight, kg	1	2	4	8	12	16	20
1	0.4 mg	1.0 mg	1.5 mg	3.0 mg	5.0 mg	7.0 mg	8.0 mg
3	1.0 mg	3.0 mg	5.0 mg	10 mg	15 mg	19 mg	24 mg
5	2.0 mg	4.0 mg	8.0 mg	16 mg	24 mg	32 mg	40 mg
10	4.0 mg	8.0 mg	16 mg	32 mg	48 mg	64 mg	80 mg
20	8.0 mg	16 mg	32 mg	64 mg	96 mg	128 mg	160 mg

For very small doses, the drug should be diluted. A reconstituted vial containing 40 mg can be diluted with 36 mL of sterile isotonic saline to achieve a concentration of 1 mg/mL. The required dose can be administered with a tuberculin syringe.

Source: Reproduced from Burroughs Wellcome: *Dosing for Infant and Small Children Dose Estimates of Digibind (in mg) from Steady-State Serum Digoxin Concentration.*

are appropriate in the event of ventricular tachycardia or fibrillation.

Hemodialysis and hemoperfusion do not aid in the removal of digoxin or digitoxin.

DISPOSITION

Children with trivial ingestions who are asymptomatic and have no detectable levels of digoxin 4 h after the ingestion can be discharged from the emergency department after 6 h of observation.

Any child with signs or symptoms of toxicity is admitted to a monitored bed, preferably in a pediatric intensive care unit.

For a more detailed discussion, see Aks SE, Leikin J: Digoxin toxicity, chap. 91, p. 532, in *Pediatric Emergency Medicine: A Comprehensive Study Guide.*

---

92 Fish Poisoning

Timothy Erickson

Marine food-borne poisonings are divided into those induced by fish harboring ciguatoxin, scombrotoxin, paralytic shellfish saxitoxin, or tetrodotoxin. As a result of the wide availability of fresh and frozen fish, there is an increasing frequency of toxic ingestions in North America.

CIGUATERA

Pathophysiology

Ciguatera fish poisoning is a serious public health problem in the Caribbean and Indo-Pacific regions. Ciguatoxin is produced by the dinoflagellate *Gambierdiscus toxicus* and concentrated in the food chain of predator reef fish such as barracuda, grouper, red snapper, parrotfish, jacks, and moray eels. When contaminated fish are ingested by humans, poisoning can cause distinct neurologic and gastrointestinal symptomatology due to the toxin's anticholinesterase activity.

Clinical Presentation

In nonepidemic areas, the diagnosis of cigutera poisoning is made only by a high index of suspicion combined with a recent ingestion history of a specific fish. Within hours of ingestion, the patient may complain of neurologic symptoms such as circumoral tingling, headache, tremor, diffuse paresthesias, and, classically, reversal of hot and cold sensation. Younger children may present with only discomfort and irritability. Other signs such as miosis, ptosis, and muscular spasm are more objective but occur much less frequently. The patient also commonly suffers watery diarrhea, vomiting, and abdominal cramping. Because of their smaller size, children are potentially at a higher risk for greater concentration of the toxin. Potentially fatal cardiovascular manifestations such as severe bradycardia, hypotension, and respiratory depression are possible but uncommon. Mortality from poisoning is 0.1 percent. The neurologic symptoms can become chronic and may persist for several weeks to months.

Management

Treatment of ciguatera poisoning is primarily supportive care. If the child presents within 2 h of ingestion of the suspected fish and has not already vomited, gastric decontamination with either ipecac or gastric lavage followed by activated charcoal is indicated. If the patient is already experiencing watery diarrhea, cathartics are not recommended, as they only exacerbate fluid losses and electrolyte disturbances. To date, specific treatment of ciguatera has been limited. Several agents such as amitriptyline and nifedipine have been advocated but are of unproven efficacy. Recently, there has been some success with mannitol administration.

Disposition

If the child is experiencing significant fluid losses, electrolyte imbalance, or neurologic manifestations, admission for observation and fluid resuscitation is recommended.

SCOMBROTOXIN

Pathophysiology

Scombroid poisoning is a food-borne illness associated with the consumption of improperly handled dark-meated fish such as tuna, bonito, skipjack, mackerel, and mahi-mahi (dolphin fish). Scombrotoxin is contracted from the flesh of fish that has undergone bacterial decomposition. The symptoms of scombroid poisoning are a toxic response to exogenous histamine.

Clinical Presentation

Within minutes to hours following ingestion of a fish containing scombrotoxin, the patient experiences a histaminelike syndrome, with diffuse erythema, pruritus, urticaria, dysphagia, and headache. Palpitations and dysrhythmias have been reported but are rare. The symptoms usually last about 4 h, and occasionally may persist for 1 or 2 days.

Management

Supportive measures and fluid resuscitation are indicated, as is gastric decontamination if the ingestion was recent. Diphenhydramine has been reported to shorten the duration of symptoms, but the benefit is inconsistent. Intravenous infusion of a histamine H_2-receptor antagonist such as cimetidine has proven effective in patients with inadequate responses to diphenhydramine.

Disposition

If the vital signs are stable and there is a good response to antihistamine agents, patients can be safely discharged home on diphenhydramine and oral cimetidine for 2 to 3 days. If there is an immediate threat of anaphylaxis or angioneurotic edema, aggressive therapy, including proper airway management and admission, is recommended.

PARALYTIC SHELLFISH POISONING

Pathophysiology

Specific neurotoxic species of the dinoflagellate *Gonyaulax* form red tides and concentrate the toxin saxitoxin in bivalve shellfish such as mussels, clams, and scallops. Humans who consume contaminated shellfish can develop profound muscle weakness via a curarelike effect.

Clinical Presentation

Gastrointestinal symptoms may develop minutes to hours after ingestion, with vomiting, diarrhea, and abdominal cramping. Additionally, the patient may experience headache, ataxia, facial paresthesias, and, on rare occasions, muscle paralysis resulting in respiratory paralysis up to 12 h after ingestion.

Management

Supportive care includes fluid resuscitation and, in recent ingestions, gastric decontamination. If paralytic shellfish poisoning is suspected, the patient is admitted for a 24-h period to observe for respiratory depression.

TETRODOTOXIN

Pathophysiology

Tetrodotoxin results from the ingestion of the puffer fish, California newt, Eastern salamander, or blue-ringed octopus. Intoxication produces profound neurologic symptoms and muscle weakness due to blockade of neuromuscular transmission. Mortality may approach 60 percent.

Clinical Presentation

Symptoms following ingestion of tetrodotoxin begin within 30 min and include circumoral and throat paresthesias. These findings are followed by vomiting and abdominal cramping. If a large amount has been ingested, patients may experience a "feeling of doom" heralded by ascending paralysis, respiratory depression, dilated pupils, hypotension, bradycardia, and a classic "locked-in" or "zombieism" syndrome. Death results from respiratory paralysis or cardiovascular collapse. If the patient survives beyond 24 h, recovery typically occurs.

Management

Treatment includes rapid stabilization and gastric decontamination with gastric lavage. Syrup of ipecac is contraindicated due to potentially rapid central nervous system depression. Atropine has been recommended for bradycardia and hypotension. Edrophonium and neostigmine may be beneficial in restoring motor strength. Most importantly, the patient's airway and respiratory status must be supported aggressively.

Disposition

Any patient with suspected poisoning from tetrodotoxin should be admitted to the intensive care unit for a minimum observation period of 24 h.

For a more detailed discussion, see Erickson T: Fish poisoning, chap. 92, p. 535, in *Pediatric Emergency Medicine: A Comprehensive Study Guide.*

93 Hydrocarbons

Bonnie McManus

Of all accidental childhood poisonings, 5 percent are from hydrocarbons, with gasoline, kerosene, lighter fluid, mineral seal oil, and turpentine being the most frequently ingested compounds. Young children most frequently ingest hydrocarbons accidentally, while adolescents typically abuse volatile substances or deliberately ingest hydrocarbons in suicidal gestures or attempts.

CLASSIFICATION AND PROPERTIES

There are three major classes of hydrocarbons. The straight-chain, or aliphatic, hydrocarbons include kerosene, mineral seal oil, gasoline, solvents, and paint thinners. Aliphatic compounds include halogenated hydrocarbons such as carbon tetrachloride and trichloroethane, which are typically found in industrial settings as solvents. The cyclics, or aromatic compounds, contain a benzene ring and are widely used as industrial solvents. The terpene compounds consist mainly of cyclic terpene rings and include compounds such as turpentine and pine oil.

Viscosity, volatility, and surface tension are the physical properties that determine the type and extent of toxicity. Viscosity is the resistance to flow and is the most important property in determining the risk of aspiration. Volatility is the ability of the substance to vaporize. Highly volatile substances include the aromatic hydrocarbons, which are capable of giving off gas and replacing alveolar air, causing hypoxia. Surface tension is the compound's ability to adhere to itself at the liquid's surface. Low surface tension allows easy spread over a wide surface area. A substance with low surface tension may easily spread from the oropharynx to the trachea, promoting aspiration. Compounds that have low viscosity and low surface tension carry the highest risk of aspiration.

Hydrocarbons that exist as gases, such as methane and butane, can act as asphyxiants by displacing air in the lung and causing hypoxia. They are also capable of crossing the capillary membrane and directly causing central nervous system (CNS) depression. Gasoline and naphtha have relatively high volatilities and can cause primary CNS depression after inhalation of fumes, with minimal pulmonary damage.

Of the aromatics, benzene is the most toxic, with death reported after an oral ingestion of as little as 15 mL. The aromatics are highly volatile, and, unlike the straight-chain hydrocarbons, benzene and its major derivatives toluene and xylene are well absorbed from the gastrointestinal (GI) tract.

The halogenated hydrocarbons are well absorbed by the lungs and gut, making them particularly dangerous. Centrilobular hepatic necrosis and renal failure are associated with the ingestion of halogenated hydrocarbons such as carbon tetrachloride.

PATHOPHYSIOLOGY

The principal concern after most hydrocarbon ingestions is pulmonary toxicity. The lungs are spared unless there is direct contact with the hydrocarbon via aspiration. Gastrointestinal absorption by itself does not result in pulmonary toxicity. Chemical pneumonitis may be due to direct destruction of lung tissue itself, depending on the type of hydrocarbon, or to an aggressive inflammatory reaction. Later findings may be due to the destruction of surfactant, which results in decreased lung compliance and can cause significant atelectasis. Adult respiratory distress syndrome (ARDS) and bacterial superinfection can occur. Hemorrhagic pulmonary edema and respiratory arrest can occur within 24 h. Following resolution of the acute insult, pulmonary dysfunction can persist for years. At the time of ingestion, there may be only minimal coughing or choking.

A lipoid pneumonia is seen frequently with high-viscosity hydrocarbons such as mineral oil and liquid paraffin. This lesion is more localized and less inflammatory than the reaction produced by low-viscosity petroleum distillates like kerosene. A hemorrhagic pneumonitis does not occur. Despite the less aggressive inflammatory response, lipoid pneumonitis can take several weeks to resolve.

Central nervous system compromise is frequently seen, but the factors responsible for this are controversial. Neurologic injury may be due to the chemical properties of an orally absorbed hydrocarbon and a direct effect on the CNS, but most authorities agree that asphyxiation and hypoxia are major contributors to CNS lesions. The aromatic hydrocarbons have a high potential for causing major CNS depression. The terpenes are more easily absorbed than petroleum distillates and typically cause mild CNS depression. The halogenated and volatile hydrocarbons may produce a euphoric state similar to that of alcohol intoxication. These products rapidly attain high concentrations in the CNS and can suppress ventilatory drive. This is most commonly seen in the adolescent glue sniffer who appears intoxicated. In situations of chronic exposure or abuse, neurologic lesions may be severe and irreversible.

Gastrointestinal symptoms include nausea, vomiting, abdominal pain, and diarrhea. These symptoms are frequent but are usually mild. Vomiting increases the risk of aspiration pneumonitis; therefore, it is important to attempt to limit emesis. Ingestion or chronic inhalation abuse can cause hematemesis. Absorption of aliphatic hydrocarbons from the GI tract is limited, but aromatic or halogenated hydrocarbons may be readily absorbed. In general, ingestion of most petroleum distillates in a volume less than 1 to 2 mL/kg does not cause systemic toxicity.

When skin is exposed to hydrocarbons for an extended time, an eczematoid dermatitis develops due to the drying and defatting action of these compounds. This is typically seen in adolescents abusing volatile substances, and is known as the "glue-sniffer's rash." It is predominantly located in the perioral area or midface. There may be significant skin erythema, inflammation, and pruritis. Gasoline and other hydrocarbons can cause full-thickness burns.

Fever is seen on presentation in 30 percent of the cases. It does not correlate with clinical symptoms and is possibly of central origin. Three-fourths of patients defervesce within 24 h. If fever persists for more than 48 to 72 h, bacterial superinfection is possible.

Many anticholinesterase pesticides are combined with kerosene vehicles. A cholinergic crisis is likely in patients, with excessive bronchorrhea, salivation, lacrimation, or urinary incontinence. The classic bradycardia and miosis may be obscured by the tachycardia and mydriasis from hydrocarbon-induced hypoxia.

CLINICAL PRESENTATION

On presentation to the emergency department, patients may be completely asymptomatic or may suffer severe respiratory distress and CNS depression. A history of coughing or gagging is consistent with aspiration. In addition to cough, early signs of pulmonary toxicity include gasping, choking, tachypnea, and wheezing. Bronchospasm may contribute to ventilation-perfusion mismatch and exacerbate hypoxia. Cyanosis may be present. In the early stages, cyanosis is usually due to replacement of alveolar air by volatilized hydrocarbon, but in the later stages, it is due to direct pulmonary toxicity. Central nervous system symptoms range from irritability, which can be a sign of hypoxia, to lethargy and coma. After a significant oral ingestion, gastrointestinal disturbance is common.

In any patient with a history of hydrocarbon ingestion, it is essential to try to identify the compound, since this information can have profound implications for management and prognosis.

MANAGEMENT

The mainstay of treatment for hydrocarbon exposure is supportive care. It essential to realize that patients with respiratory compromise on presentation to the emergency department can suffer rapid deterioration.

Airway patency is evaluated and established. Any patient with respiratory symptoms, including grunting, tachypnea, or cyanosis, is treated with humidified oxygen and requires an arterial blood gas. An alveolar-arterial gradient is frequently present in serious exposures. Nebulized $beta_2$ agonists are the drugs of choice in patients with bronchospasm. Patients with respiratory failure require artificial ventilation. Because hydrocarbons solubilize surfactant, continuous positive airway pressure (CPAP) or positive end expiratory pressure (PEEP) may be needed as a ventilatory adjunct in patients with significant respiratory distress. Extracorporeal membrane oxygenation has been reported to be successful in pediatric patients suffering hydrocarbon-induced pneumonitis who fail to respond to conventional ventilatory support.

Cyanosis is usually due to hypoxia but may occur secondary to methemoglobinemia in cases where aniline or nitrobenzene has been ingested. Exposure to methylene chloride, which is frequently found in paint strippers and is metabolized to carbon monoxide, must be considered in patients with persistent symptoms of hypoxia. Treatment consists of 100% oxygen and, depending on the degree of toxicity and the carboxyhemoglobin level, hyperbaric oxygen (see Chap. 86).

In the event of a cutaneous exposure, all contaminated clothing is removed and the skin is irrigated and washed twice with soap and water. Appropriate precaution is taken by the staff to avoid being contaminated.

Fluid administration is restricted to maintenance requirements to minimize the risk of pulmonary edema.

Gastric Evacuation

Most authors discourage the use of gastric decontamination procedures in the case of accidental ingestions. Usually the risk of aspiration is higher than the risk of systemic absorption in the accidental ingestion. It is recommended that in accidental ingestions of a pure petroleum distillate or turpentine in patients with minimal or no symptoms, removal not be attempted. Gastric evacuation is reserved for massive ingestions, which usually occur in the adult population after suicide attempts. While this is still controversial, ingestions of greater than 4 to 5 mL/kg of naphtha, gasoline, kerosene, or turpentine should probably be removed. Other ingestions in which gastric evacuation is indicated are those that contain dangerous additives such as benzene, toluene, halogenated hydrocarbons, heavy metals, camphor, pesticides, aniline, or other toxic compounds.

Currently there is no overwhelming support for either emesis with ipecac or gastric lavage as a superior mode of gastric evacuation. In the awake, alert patient with an intact gag reflex, ipecac is appropriate. Emesis is contraindicated if there is previous unprovoked emesis or there is any degree of neurologic, respiratory, or cardiac compromise. In these cases, gastric lavage is indicated after endotracheal intubation. A cuffed tube is used. If the child is under 8 years old, the cuff is inflated only during lavage. A nasogastric tube may be adequate to remove liquid ingestants, but if there is a concomitant solid ingestant, this would be insufficient. Orogastric tubes without the added protection of the airway by an endotracheal tube are extremely controversial because they usually induce gagging and vomiting, which promote aspiration.

Activated charcoal is not indicated in the vast majority of hydrocarbon ingestions unless there is known to be an adsorbable coingestant.

Ancillary Therapy

Glucocorticoids do not affect outcome, and their use is not indicated. Antibiotics are reserved for patients with definite evidence of infection.

LABORATORY STUDIES

A chest radiograph is indicated in all patients with a history of hydrocarbon ingestion. In about 90 percent of patients with respiratory symptoms on presentation, the initial chest radiograph will be abnormal. Radiographic abnormalities can occur as early as 20 min or as late as 24 h after ingestion. Typical findings include increased bronchovascular markings and bibasilar and perihilar infiltrates. Lobar consolidation is uncommon. Pneumothorax, pneumediastinum, and pleural effusion are rare. Pneumatoceles can occur and resolve over weeks.

Depending on the severity of the ingestion, the patient's acid-base status, electrolyte balance, complete blood count, and hepatic profile are followed.

DISPOSITION

A patient who accidentaly ingests a hydrocarbon and presents to the emergency department without symptoms is observed for 6 h. If the patient remains asymptomatic during that time and oxygen saturation is normal, discharge is appropriate. If symptoms develop during the 6-h period of observation, hospital admission is indicated.

All patients who are symptomatic on presentation are admitted to the hospital. If respiratory compromise or hypoxia is present, admission to a pediatric intensive care unit is advised. Hospital admission is also indicated when there is a risk for significant delayed organ toxicity, as in the case of ingestion of carbon tetrachloride or other toxic additives.

VOLATILE SUBSTANCE ABUSE

Among adolescents, inhalation abuse of volatile hydrocarbons is a significant health hazard. Typically, solvent-containing fluids such as typewriter correction fluid (trichloroethane/trichloroethylene), adhesives (toluene), and other halogenated hydrocarbons, such as those found in gasoline and cigarette-lighter fluid (butane), are abused. These substances are inexpensive and easily obtained. Typically, deep inhalations are taken after the substance is poured into a plastic bag (known as *bagging*) or a cloth is saturated and held to the face (known as *huffing*).

The acute risk of inhalation abuse has commonly been referred to as "sudden sniffing death." It is believed that the myocardium is hypersensitized and a sudden outpouring of sympathetic stimulation leads to fatal cardiac dysrhythmias. There have been numerous case reports of patients abusing solvents and then collapsing shortly after beginning marked physical exertion or being startled.

Indirect effects of volatile substance abuse include trauma due to impaired judgment, aspiration of vomit, or asphyxia associated with plastic bags.

Acute poisoning with volatile substances involves an initial period of euphoria and disinhibition, with further intoxication leading to dysphoria, ataxia, confusion, and hallucinations. There is rapid onset and recovery, but repeated inhalations can prolong the altered state. Because of the short half-life, patients rarely present acutely intoxicated. Treatment of the intoxicated patient consists of supportive measures. If resuscitation is necessary, standard advanced cardiac life support measures are indicated.

For a more detailed discussion, see McManus B: Hydrocarbons, chap. 93, p. 538, in *Pediatric Emergency Medicine: A Comprehensive Study Guide.*

94 Iron Poisoning

Steven E. Aks

Iron is an extremely common cause of poisoning and has a high potential for morbidity and mortality. From 1983 to 1990, iron was the most common cause of pediatric unintentional ingestion death, accounting for 30.2 percent of reported cases.

PATHOPHYSIOLOGY

Iron is absorbed through the gastrointestinal mucosa in the ferrous (Fe^{2+}) state. It is oxidized to the ferric (Fe^{3+}) state and attaches to ferritin. Toxicity occurs when ferritin and transferrin are saturated and serum iron exceeds the total iron binding capacity (TIBC). Circulating free iron can damage blood vessels and can cause transudation of fluids from the intravascular space, resulting in hypotension. Other target organs include the gastrointestinal tract, heart, and lungs.

CLINICAL PRESENTATION

Patients commonly present to the emergency department with a history of having ingested iron tablets or vitamins containing iron. It is useful to attempt to identify the exact preparation, since the content of elemental iron, which is the toxic ingredient, varies. If the preparation is identified, the number of pills ingested is important information, since the ratio of elemental iron ingested to the weight of the patient is critical in estimating the potential for toxicity (see Table 94-1). If the amount of elemental iron ingested cannot be closely approximated, a worst-case scenario is assumed.

It is useful to describe iron overdose in terms of the known stages of toxicity. The stages are generally sequential, although there can be overlap.

Stage 1

This stage begins at the time of ingestion and lasts for about 6 h. In mild cases there is nausea and vomiting. In more severe ingestions, there is vomiting, diarrhea, hematemesis, altered mental status, and possibly hypotension.

Stage 2

Stage 2 lasts from about 6 to 12 h postingestion and is referred to as the quiescent or "danger" phase. A meticulous history is

TABLE 94-1 Iron Preparations

Iron preparation	Percent elemental iron
Ferrous sulfate	20
Ferrous fumarate	33
Ferrous gluconate	12
Ingested dose, mg/kg	**Treatment recommendation**
<20	Dilute and observe
20–40	Ipecac at home and observe
>40	Refer to health care facility

vital to diagnosing a patient in this stage, with emphasis on stage 1 symptoms, especially vomiting and diarrhea.

Stage 3

The period from 12 to 24 h postingestion marks stage 3, in which the patient can exhibit major signs of toxicity. Gastrointestinal hemorrhage and cardiovascular collapse can occur. Patients may develop altered mental status ranging from lethargy to coma. Both renal and hepatic failure can occur, and patients can develop a severe metabolic acidosis.

Stage 4

This is a latent phase in which the patient has recovered from the acute insult. It occurs 4 to 6 weeks after the ingestion when the patient develops symptoms from strictures that develop in the gastrointestinal tract as a result of scar formation.

DIAGNOSIS

The easiest way to assess the potential of an iron ingestion to result in toxicity is to quantitate the amount ingested (see Table 94-1).

Certain laboratory tests support the diagnosis of iron toxicity. A white blood cell count (WBC) greater than 15,000/mm^3 and a serum glucose greater than 150 mg/dL have been correlated with serum iron levels greater than 300 μg/dL. While more recent studies have cast doubt on the predictive value of these markers, they are considered suggestive of a toxic ingestion. Normal WBC and serum glucose do not rule out iron toxicity.

Iron level is optimally drawn at 4 h postingestion. A level greater than 300 to 350 μg/dL is considered toxic. Levels greater than 500 μg/dL suggest potentially life-threatening toxicity.

Measurement of the TIBC has been used to determine the presence of a toxic ingestion, based on the assumption that toxicity occurs when serum iron exceeds the TIBC. A recent study has indicated that this is not a reliable indicator, since ingesting iron will raise the measured TIBC level when the measurement is done by standard colorimetric methods.

Deferoxamine is a compound that chelates free iron. The "deferoxamine challenge test" can be administered to patients who have ingested an unknown or borderline quantity of iron. The challenge is conducted by administering 40 to 90 mg/kg of deferoxamine intramuscularly, up to a maximum of 1 g in children and 2 g in adults. A positive test is indicated by the patient's urine developing a "*vin rosé*" color 4 to 6 h after receiving deferoxamine. However, this classic appearance is seen in a minority of patients. A subtle change in the color of the urine may be more easily detected by obtaining a baseline urine specimin prior to administering the challenge. Even a slight change in color to an orange or red indicates a positive test. The test must be correlated with the history and physical.

TREATMENT

Gastric Emptying

Since neither activated charcoal nor any other substance is capable of absorbing iron in the gastrointestinal tract, gastric emptying is the sole method of gut decontamination. There is a trend toward gastric lavage in patients in whom it is technically feasible. Lavage is performed with saline. Previous recommendations included adding bicarbonate to the lavage solution, since it was felt that it would bind iron and make it insoluble and easier to remove. This has not been shown to be effective in the clinical setting. In addition, both deferoxamine and phosphate have been suggested as additives to the lavage solution. Neither is currently recommended. Deferoxamine may actually enhance the absorption of iron, and phosphate may worsen the clinical course by causing significant hyperphosphatemia and hypocalcemia.

It is currently recommended that whole bowel irrigation with polyethylene glycol electrolyte lavage solution be initiated if pills are noted on abdominal radiographs after gastric lavage. The end point of therapy is the disappearance of pills seen on radiograph. Active gastrointestinal bleeding, ileus, or bowel obstruction are contraindications to whole bowel irrigation. In the absence of pill fragments seen on radiograph, whole bowel irrigation is probably not helpful.

Chelation

Chelation with deferoxamine is used for significant iron ingestions. Standard indications for therapy include a peak iron level of 300 to 350 μg/dL or a patient who exhibits signs of toxicity in the absence of an available iron level.

Deferoxamine can be administered intramuxcularly or intravenously. Intramuscular administration is appropriate for a deferoxamine challenge test or in patients who exhibit mild toxicity. Deferoxamine is administered at 6-h intervals. The intramuscular dose is 90 mg/kg/dose, with a maximum single dose in children not to exceed 1 g.

Intravenous administration is indicated in patients with moderate to severe toxicity. Hypotension is the most common side effect of intravenous therapy and can usually be treated by slowing down the drip or making the solution more dilute. Allergic reactions are rare. The dose of intravenous deferoxamine is 10 to 15 mg/kg/h.

The end point of chelation is reached when the color of the patient's urine returns to normal. Significant cases can require chelation for 12 to 16 h or longer. Chelation should not exceed 24 h, and, in general, the total dose of deferoxamine should not exceed 6 to 8 g. Delayed pulmonary toxicity with symptoms resembling those of acute respiratory distress syndrome has been reported in patients who received prolonged chelation.

A proposed end point of chelation therapy that is not yet clinically available is the measurement of the ratio of urinary iron to creatinine. This could be a more reliable end point than the change in urine color.

DISPOSITION

Children with peak serum iron levels below 300 μg/kg approximately 4 h postingestion and without symptoms of toxicity may be discharged to reliable caretakers. Children with symptoms of toxicity, iron levels greater than 350 μg/kg, or positive deferoxamine challenge tests require hospital admission. Mild overdoses can be managed on the floor. Any child who requires intravenous chelation is admitted to an intensive care unit.

For a more detailed discussion, see Aks SE: Iron poisoning, chap. 94, p. 542, in *Pediatric Emergency Medicine: A Comprehensive Study Guide.*

95 Isoniazid Toxicity

T. J. Rittenberry / Michael Green

Isoniazid (INH) is a fundamental treatment for tuberculosis, a growing public health problem in the United States. Its structure is similar to the metabolic cofactors nicotinic acid, nicotinamide adenine dinucleotide (NAD), and pyridoxine. The metabolic degradation of INH is complex and occurs primarily via hepatic acetylation. The ability to inactivate INH via acetylation is genetically determined, resulting in two groups of patients, fast acetylators and slow acetylators. Slow acetylators are more prone to develop toxicity.

PATHOPHYSIOLOGY

Isoniazid impairs conversion of pyridoxine to pyridoxal phosphate, a necessary cofactor in the formation of the inhibitory brain peptide gamma aminobutyric acid (GABA). Pyridoxine depletion and reduced GABA levels in the brain lead to the lower seizure threshold seen in acute INH toxicity.

The toxic dose of INH is highly variable. Patients with an underlying seizure disorder may suffer toxicity at doses as low as 10 mg/kg. Otherwise healthy patients may develop seizures at doses above 30 mg/kg. High mortality is associated with doses of 80 to 150 mg/kg.

Symptoms can occur within 30 min of INH ingestion. Nausea, vomiting, dizziness, and slurred speech may be quickly followed by metabolic acidosis, generalized seizures, and coma. Suspicion of toxic INH ingestion in the pediatric patient is typically delayed until overt signs are apparent. The triad of seizures, coma, and acidosis should alert the emergency physician to the possibility of INH ingestion.

In the acute ingestion, quantitative INH levels are typically unavailable. The laboratory workup must encompass any cause of coma, seizures, and anion gap acidosis of unknown etiology.

TREATMENT

In the patient presenting with protracted seizures or coma, endotracheal intubation is indicated. Seizures are controlled with standard anticonvulsants. Even in asymptomatic patients, the induction of emesis is not recommended, since seizures may occur without warning. Gastric lavage is performed to achieve gut decontamination. Activated charcoal and a cathartic such as sorbitol are administered.

Antidotal Therapy

The mainstay of treatment in INH toxicity is pyridoxine. Commercially available in 1 g/10 mL vials, it is mixed in a 5% or 10% solution with D_5W. If the INH dose is known, an equal dose of pyridoxine on a gram-per-gram basis is administered over 15 min. If the dose of INH is unknown, pyridoxine is given initially at 70 mg/kg and repeated in 15 min for the persistently comatose or convulsing patient. The therapeutic window for pyridoxine is large, and the cumulative dose is arbitrarily limited at 40 g in the adolescent and 20 g in the child. The severe acidosis seen in INH overdose may require sodium bicarbonate administration, but, in most cases, control of seizures with anticonvulsants and pyridoxine and adequate fluid resuscitation will reverse acidemia. Bicarbonate therapy is reserved for severe, persistent acidosis.

If seizures continue despite appropriate use of pyridoxine and diazepam, short-acting barbiturates or inhaled anesthetics may be considered.

Hemodialysis, hemoperfusion, and exchange transfusion have all been described as useful but are reserved for only the most severe, refractory cases or for patients with renal failure.

DISPOSITION

Patients with suspected INH poisoning who remain asymptomatic beyond 6 h following ingestion and patients without a seizure disorder who have ingested less than 20 mg/kg may be discharged from the emergency department. Symptomatic patients require hospital admission to a monitored bed.

CHRONIC TOXICITY

Chronic INH toxicity is extremely rare in the normal pediatric population and is usually restricted to children receiving active or prophylactic treatment. The appearance of nausea and vomiting may herald hepatic insult, which, if not treated, can progress to fulminant hepatitis.

For a more detailed discussion, see Rittenberry TJ, Green M: Isoniazid toxicity, chap. 95, p. 545, in *Pediatric Emergency Medicine: A Comprehensive Study Guide.*

96 Lead Poisoning

Yona Amitai / Daniel Hryhorczuk

While the prevalence of lead poisoning is highest in inner-city populations, the toxin affects millions of American children. In 1991, the Centers for Disease Control revised the 1985 blood lead intervention level of 25 μg/dL downward to 10 μg/dL. Interventions for individual children begin at blood lead levels of 15 μg/dL.

SOURCES

Ingestion of leaded paint is associated with the most clinically severe lead poisoning. A small paint chip containing 50% lead can produce acute lead poisoning in a toddler. Renovation of old buildings and poorly controlled lead abatement pose a risk for lead poisoning through inhalation and ingestion of contaminated dust and soil. Lead exposure can occur through ingestion of drinking water contaminated by lead in plumbing. Children living in close proximity to stationary air pollution sources such as lead smelters are at risk of lead poisoning. Other potential sources of exposure include secondary exposure to lead brought home from workplaces, drinking from improperly fired lead-glazed pottery, some folk remedies, bullets lodged in joint spaces, and other unusual sources. The phaseout of leaded gasoline has had a major impact in reducing exposure to lead.

PHARMACOKINETICS/PATHOPHYSIOLOGY

The absorption rate of lead through the gastrointestinal tract in infants and children is about 50%. Iron deficiency and dietary calcium deficiency increase the absorption of lead in the gut. Lead dust and fumes can also be absorbed through the respiratory tract. Percutaneous absorption of lead is less than 0.1% of the applied quantity. Lead readily crosses the placental barrier, and fetal exposure is cumulative until birth. The distribution of absorbed lead in the body can be modeled using three compartments: blood, soft tissue, and bone. Under steady-state conditions, 99% of the lead in blood is attached to red blood cells. Under chronic exposure conditions, bone serves as a storage organ and can release lead back into the blood and soft tissues.

The major target organs of lead are the bone marrow, central nervous system, peripheral nervous system, and kidney. Lead inhibits heme synthesis through inhibition of ALA-dehydratase, coproporphyrin utilization, and ferrochelatase, resulting in the buildup of aminolevulonic acid, coproporphyrins, and free erythrocyte protoporphyrin. Clinically, inhibition of heme synthesis is manifested as microcytic anemia. The pathophysiology of lead encephalopathy is demyelinization and precipitation of ribonucleoprotein, with resulting cell death, tissue necrosis, vascular damage, and cerebral edema. There is an increase in cerebrospinal fluid protein and pressure. The central nervous system is the primary target organ in the fetus.

CLINICAL MANIFESTATIONS

Symptoms and signs of lead toxicity may be subtle and nonspecific. In the United States, the most likely cause for referral to the emergency department (ED) in such children is a high blood lead level (BLL) found during a screening program. Symptomatic lead poisoning is characterized by decrease in play activity, irritability, drowsiness, anorexia, sporadic vomiting, intermittent abdominal pain, constipation, regression in newly acquired skills (particularly speech), sensorineural hearing loss, clumsiness, and slight attenuation of growth. Lead toxicity is grossly correlated with BLL (Table 96-1) but is more pronounced in young children and in those with a prolonged exposure to lead.

Overt lead encephalopathy may ensue after days or weeks of symptoms and present with ataxia, forceful vomiting, lethargy, or stupor; it can progress to coma and seizures. It may occur with BLL > 70 μg/dL but is generally associated with BLL in excess of 100 μg/dL. Permanent brain damage may result in 70 to 80 percent of children with lead encephalopathy. Peripheral neuropathy is rare under the age of 5.

Lead nephropathy can result in Fanconi syndrome and acute tubular necrosis but is rare in children. Mild elevation in liver transaminases may occur. Microcytic anemia frequently coexists with lead poisoning.

The differential diagnosis of lead poisoning includes iron deficiency, behavioral and emotional disorders, abdominal colic and constipation, mental retardation, afebrile seizures, subdural hematoma, central nervous system neoplasms, sickle cell anemia, and Fanconi syndrome. The definitive diagnosis of lead poisoning and assessment of its severity and chronicity depend on laboratory tests. The most important test is a venous BLL (see Table 96-1). Since 99 percent of the lead in blood is in the red cells, lead assay is done in whole blood collected in tubes with heparin or ethylenediaminetetraacetic acid (EDTA). Definitions of lead poisoning class, the toxic effects of lead at various levels, and the

TABLE 96-1 Class of Child, Toxic Effect, and Recommended Action According to Blood Lead Measurement

Class	Blood lead, μg/dL[a]	Toxicity: lowest observed effect level	Recommended action
I	0–5	No noticeable effect	
	5–9	Inhibition of ALAD[b]	
IIA	10–14		Rescreen every 3–4 months
IIB	15–19	Inhibition of ferrochelatase	Retest in 3–4 months, nutritional and educational intervention, environmental investigation
III	20–24	↓ Growth, ↓ hearing, ↓ nerve conduction	All of the above plus pharmacological treatment (optional)
	25–44	Neuropsychological deficits, ↓ heme synthetase, ↑ EP,[c] ↑ urine d-ALA[d]	Treatment with penicillamine or DMSA or $CaNa_2$-EDTA (following a positive lead mobilization test)
IV	45–69	Anemia, abdominal colic, ↓ IQ "lead lines" in x-ray	Immediate chelation: $CaNa_2$-EDTA or DMSA
V	>70	Encephalopathy risk, nephropathy (>100 μg/dL)	Medical emergency chelate: BAL + EDTA, ↑ ICP precaution

[a] Conversion factor 1.0 μg/dL = 0.04826 mmol/L.
[b] ALAD = aminolevulonic acid dehydratase.
[c] EP = erythrocyte protoporphyrin.
[d] ALA = aminolevulinic acid.
Source: Centers for Disease Control, Bethesda, MD, 1991.

recommended action are outlined in Table 96-1. Elevation in BLL is followed by a rise in the free erythrocyte protoporphyrin (EP), whose conversion to heme by heme synthetase is inhibited by lead. This effect occurs at BLL >25 μg/dL and lags 2 to 3 weeks after the initial rise in BLL, because it affects only the newly formed red blood cells (RBC) and reflects exposure to lead over the preceding 120 days of the RBC life cycle.

Radiographic evidence of lead poisoning consists of bands of increased density at the metaphyses of long bones; these are best seen in radiographs of the distal femur and proximal tibia and fibula. The increased radiopacity is caused by abnormal calcification from the disrupted metabolism of bone matrix. The formation of lead lines requires a few months of elevated BLL (greater than 45 μg/dL). Radiopaque foreign material seen in the intestine by a flat abdominal film suggests a recent (<148 h) ingestion of lead-containing paint chips.

Other essential tests are measurement of hemoglobin and hematocrit, evaluation of the patient's iron status, examination of the blood smear for basophilic stippling of the erythrocytes, and a urinalysis to exclude glycosuria or proteinuria. A spinal tap is avoided in children with lead encephalopathy due to the concern of herniation.

A new method for evaluating the total body lead burden by x-ray fluorometry (XRF) of bone lead has been introduced in adults and is being studied in children. With further reduction in radiation, this technique may eventually supersede blood lead screening in populations with low blood levels.

MANAGEMENT

The principles of individual case management in lead poisoning include identification and removal of the lead source, correction of dietary deficiencies that enhance lead absorption, chelation and supportive therapy, and long-term follow-up.

For patients with lead levels below 20 μg/dL, treatment consists of environmental management and repeated screening. In many cases, this involves removing the child from the home until the source of lead exposure is identified and removed.

The removal of lead-based paint from the home is done by professional deleaders. Nutritional intervention consists of a review of the child's diet and correction of deficiencies of iron, calcium, and zinc. If there is evidence of recent ingestion of lead paint on an abdominal film, cathartics are given for several days.

For patients with a BLL between 20 and 25 μg/dL, pharmacologic intervention is optional. Asymptomatic patients with a BLL between 25 and 44 μg/dL can usually be treated with chelation therapy on an ambulatory basis, along with environmental management. The decision to treat may be aided by a $CaNa_2$-EDTA immobilization test. This drug is administered in a dose of 500 mg/m^2 in 5% dextrose infused IV over 1 h, or the same dose may be given intramuscularly. The amount of lead is measured in urine collected over the next 8 h. A ratio of lead excreted (in micrograms) to the $CaNa_2$-EDTA dose (in milligrams) greater than 0.6 is considered positive.

Outpatient treatment is possible with oral D-penicillamine (Cuprimine), which must be given for weeks to months. Currently penicillamine is not approved by the FDA for the treatment of lead poisoning, but it is approved for other uses. Side effects include leukopenia, thrombocytopenia, transient elevation of liver enzymes, vomiting, and, rarely, nephrotoxicity. It must not be given to patients allergic to penicillin. Iron supplements are avoided in patients treated with D-penicillamine, since they can block its absorption.

Another option is outpatient chelation with $CaNa_2$-EDTA, administered intramuscularly over 3 to 5 days.

Multicenter trials are currently investigating the effectiveness of oral dimercapto-succinic acid (DMSA) in children with a BLL between 25 and 45 μg/dL. Chemically similar to dimercaprol British antilewisite (BAL) DMSA produces a lead diuresis comparable to that produced by $CaNa_2$-EDTA without depletion of other metals. It has a bad odor and may cause nausea and vomiting, rashes (4 percent), and transient elevation of liver enzymes. It is currently approved for patients with a BLL $>$ 45 μg/dL.

Children with asymptomatic lead poisoning and a BLL of 45 to 69 μg/dL are admitted to the hospital for chelation therapy with either $CaNa_2$-EDTA or DMSA. Children with *symptomatic* lead poisoning with or without encephalopathy who have a BLL $>$ 45 μg/dL and all patients with a BLL $>$ 70 μg/dL are treated with BAL at a dose of 450 mg/m^2/day in divided doses every 4 h, given by deep intramuscular injection. Once the first dose is given and adequate urine flow is established, $CaNa_2$-EDTA is added as a continuous intravenous infusion in dextrose or saline. In treating a child with encephalopathy, the intramuscular route for $CaNa_2$-EDTA with procaine 0.5% is preferred to reduce the amount of fluid administrated. This combined treatment is given for 5 days, with daily monitoring of blood urea nitrogen (BUN), creatinine, liver enzymes, and electrolytes. In the event of rebound of BLL after chelation, a second course of $CaNa_2$-EDTA alone (at a BLL of 45 to 70 μg/dL) or combined with BAL (at a BLL $>$ 70 μg/dL) may be required after a 2-day interval from the end of the first course. Side effects of $CaNa_2$-EDTA include fever and transient renal dysfunction, resulting in a rise in BUN, proteinuria, and hematuria. Also, BAL may cause nausea and vomiting, transient hypertension, fever, transient elevation in liver enzymes, and hemolysis in glucose-6-phosphate dehydrogenase (G6PD)-deficient patients. Iron can form a toxic complex with BAL and is not administered simultaneously.

Lead encephalopathy is treated with fluid restriction, mechanical hyperventilation, and furosemide. Mannitol is avoided because it may leak from the compromised vessels into the cerebellar interstitial spaces and cause a rebound intracranial pressure. Dexamethasome may have a salutary effect in improving the vascular integrity. Seizures are controlled with diazepam. When treating encephalopathy, $CaNa_2$-EDTA is administered intramuscularly to reduce the amount of fluid administered. Patients with lead encephalopathy are best managed in an intensive care unit.

Due to the chronic nature of lead poisoning, the rebound elevation of BLL after each course of chelation therapy, and the problem of environmental control, children with lead poisoning should be followed for prolonged periods by clinicians who are familiar with the multiple aspects of this disease and can provide a multidisciplinary team approach. The importance of removing the child from the source of lead exposure cannot be overemphasized.

For a more detailed discussion, see Amitai Y, Hryhorczuk D: Lead poisoning, chap. 96, p. 548, in *Pediatric Emergency Medicine: A Comprehensive Study Guide.*

---

97 Methemoglobinemia

Timothy Erickson / Michele Zell-Kanter

Methemoglobin is formed when iron in hemoglobin is oxidized from the ferrous (Fe^{2+}) state to the ferric (Fe^{3+}) state. Under normal physiologic conditions, methemoglobin is present in red blood cells at concentrations of 1 to 2 percent. Because the oxygen in methemoglobin is so tightly bound, it is not available for tissue use; thus methemoglobin is not an oxygen-transporting pigment. The oxygen-hemoglobin dissociation curve is also shifted to the left, causing an increase in hemoglobin's affinity for oxygen.

TABLE 97-1 Causes of Acquired Methemoglobinemia

Acetanilid	Lidocaine	Phenacetin
Aminophenols	Menthol	Phenols
Aniline compounds	Nitrates	Phenylazopyridine
Antimalarials	Nitrites	Phenylhydroxyamine
Benzocaine	Nitrofurans	Prilocaine
Bismuth subnitrite	Nitroglycerin	Pyridine
Chlorates	Nitrous oxide (contaminated)	Quinones
Cobalt preparations		Resorcinol
Copper sulfate	Para-aminosalicylic acid	Shoe polish
Dapsone	Paratoluidine	Sulfonamides
Dinitrobenzene	Pesticides (propham, fenuron)	Sulfones
Fuel additives		Trinitroluene

Two conditions of hereditary methemoglobinemia are (1) a deficiency in NADH-dependent methemoglobin reductase and (2) hemoglobin M, which is a structural abnormality in hemoglobin. Acquired methemoglobinemia results from exposure to drugs or chemicals that accelerate the oxidation of hemoglobin beyond the cell's capacity to reduce it (Table 97-1).

Infants are more sensitive than adults to methemoglobin-producing agents such as nitrites, nitrates, or contaminated foods. Other populations with increased risk of developing methemoglobinemia include individuals with NADH-dependent methemoglobin reductase, uremic patients, and patients with underlying hypoxic states from disorders.

CLINICAL PRESENTATION

The clinical symptoms induced by methemoglobinemia are dependent on the amount of hemoglobin oxidized into methemoglobin. Concentrations ranging from 30% to 40% may produce generalized symptoms such as poor feeding, lethargy, and irritability. The older child may complain of fatigue, dizziness, headaches, and weakness. At levels above 55%, patients may experience respiratory depression, cardiac arrhythmias, seizures, and coma. Concentrations over 70% are potentially lethal.

The diagnosis of methemoglobinemia is possible in any child presenting with a history of exposure to any of the agents listed in Table 97-1 and in patients with central cyanosis that is unresponsive to oxygen therapy. A rapid bedside test that may help to confirm a clinical suspicion of methemoglobinemia consists of placing a drop of the patient's blood on a filter paper alongside a normal control sample. If the concentration of methemoglobin exceeds 15%, the patient's blood will appear chocolate brown in color. Another screening test involves bubbling 100% oxygen through a sample of the patient's venous blood. Normal hemoglobin should turn bright red, while methemoglobin will be unaltered. In addition, an arterial blood gas may provide a diagnostic clue if a normal P_{O_2} is noted in the presence of decreased measured oxygen saturation. Finally, methemoglobin concentrations can be directly measured using a spectrophotometric method available to most hospital laboratories.

MANAGEMENT

Initial treatment of any drug or chemically induced methemoglobinemia involves supportive care consisting of airway control, supplemental oxygen, and removal of the patient from the source of exposure. Children with altered mental status, dyspnea, cyanosis, or unstable vital signs require immediate intervention. Oral exposure is managed with gastric emptying and charcoal administration. The skin is decontaminated if dermal absorption is suspected. If methemoglobin levels exceed 30% or the patient exhibits clinical signs of hypoxia, administration of methylene blue is recommended. The initial dose is 1 to 2 mg/kg of a 1% solution given intravenously over 5 min. If clinical signs persist, the dose is repeated in 1 h and every 4 h thereafter to a maximum dose of 7 mg/kg. Above this dose, methylene blue can induce hemolysis and act as an oxidizing agent, thereby exacerbating the underlying methemoglobinemic state. During administration of methylene blue, the child's response is monitored by following the oxygen saturation. Patients with methemoglobin levels above 70% who are unresponsive to methylene blue are candidates for exchange transfusions or hyperbaric oxygenation.

DISPOSITION

Patients who have methemoglobin concentrations below 20% and are asymptomatic require only admission and close observation. Any symptomatic pediatric patients with levels over 20% or those requiring methylene blue administration should be monitored in an intensive care setting.

For a more detailed discussion, see Erickson T, Zell-Kanter M: Methemoglobinemia, chap. 97, p. 552, in *Pediatric Emergency Medicine: A Comprehensive Study Guide.*

---

98 Mushroom Poisoning

T. J. Rittenberry / Jaime Rivas

Mushrooms are responsible for approximately 2 percent of all poisonings. Of these, 70 percent involve children. In approximately 96 percent of reported cases, the actual identity of the mushroom involved was not determined.

IDENTIFICATION

Exact mushroom identification is difficult or unlikely in most cases and is not critical to initiating emergency care. The key to success is the participation of the local poison control center and an experienced mycologist. Even when identification is accomplished, toxin concentrations can be highly variable depending on species, season, locale, and the specific part of the mushroom ingested. Few actual antidotes exist. The prognosis is also dependent on age, with infants and small children most likely to suffer morbidity or mortality, time from ingestion to appearance of symptoms, and rapidity with which aggressive treatment is instituted.

CLASSIFICATION

Categorization based on the predominant toxin conveniently classifies North American mushrooms into seven groups: the gastroenteric irritants, the cyclopeptides, the gyromitrin group, the muscarine group, the coprine-containing group, those containing ibotenic acid and muscimol, and the hallucinogenic indole containing mushrooms.

GASTROENTERIC IRRITANTS

The gastroenteric irritants represent the most commonly encountered pediatric mushroom ingestion. These include the "little brown mushrooms'' found commonly in yards and *Chlorophyllium molybdides,* probably the most frequently reported toxic mushroom exposure in North America. Onset of symptoms for the gastroenteric irritants is rapid and provides a key characteristic to diagnosis. Symptoms begin in 30 min to 2 h, with a duration of 3 to 6 h, and include nausea, vomiting, abdominal pains, and diarrhea that can be bloody and can contain fecal leukocytes. One should ensure gut decontamination with gastric lavage and administer activated charcoal early. Further treatment consists of support of fluid and electrolytes. Symptomatic patients are hospitalized for observation and possibly serial charcoal administrations until symptomatology and laboratory data can rule out a potentially lethal ingestion.

CYCLOPEPTIDES

The cyclopeptide group of mushrooms is responsible for most North American deaths. It includes the *Amanita* species and related groups containing amatoxins, which cause severe hepatorenal dysfunction and gastritis. *Amanita phalloides,* known as ''the death cap,'' is responsible for more than 50 percent of all serious mushroom poisonings, with several other *Amanita* such as *virosa* (''destroying angel'') also involved. These mushrooms share in common the production of large amounts of cyclopeptide amatoxins, the most toxic of which is alpha-amanitin, capable of causing death in doses of 0.1 mg/kg. Probably due to the enterohepatic circulation of amatoxins, the liver is typically profoundly affected.

The clinical presentation of the ingestion of the cyclopeptide group of mushrooms occurs in four stages. The initial latent phase is characterized by a 6- to 12-h asymptomatic period, during which time protein synthesis is being disrupted. A gastroenteritislike phase follows, at which time phalloidin-induced gastrointestinal disturbances such as nausea, vomiting, bloody diarrhea, and abdominal pain predominate; this may last up to 24 hours. The following latent phase is marked by an apparent remission of 6 to 24 h, as overt symptomatology is absent but hepatocellular damage continues. The final hepatorenal phase follows within 36 to 72 h of ingestion, during which jaundice, hypoglycemia, confusion, coagulopathy, and hepatorenal failure develop.

The diagnosis of *Amanita* ingestion relies on a high level of suspicion supported by the characteristic symptom profile. A delay in the development of gastrointestinal symptoms after ingestion is an ominous finding. Radioimmune assay and thin-layer chromatography can identify amatoxin but are typically unavailable. Very early on, laboratory studies are normal. A rising serum ammonia level and deteriorating coagulation profile are harbingers of fulminant hepatic failure.

The keystone to treatment is early gut decontamination. The immediate home use of ipecac in the pediatric patient is important in all suspected mushroom ingestions. Gastric lavage is employed, with the aspirate saved for possible use in identification. Activated charcoal is administered, with or without a cathartic. Repeated doses of activated charcoal and duodenal drainage may be useful during the first 24 to 72 h to enhance elimination and interrupt enterohepatic circulation. Hemoperfusion has anecdotally been reported useful when initiated in the first 24 h. Although several antidotes have been proposed for poisoning with the cyclopeptide group of mushrooms, no agent is recognized as clearly efficacious. Severe ingestion may require liver transplantation. The fatality rate in one case series was almost 50 percent for children less than 10 years of age.

INDOLE-CONTAINING MUSHROOMS

These psilocybin-psilocin–containing mushrooms are sought out for recreational use. When they are ingested by children, severe symptoms may result. Laboratory findings are not useful in identification of an indole-containing hallucinogenic mushroom ingestion.

Treatment consists of gut decontamination and supportive care. Hospitalization for observation in a low-stimulus environment, with repeated doses of activated charcoal, is appropriate. The severe complications of hyperpyrexia, seizures, and coma are treated with cooling, anticonvulsants, and supportive care.

MONOMETHYLHYDRAZINE GROUP

Gyromitrin is a toxic hydrazone that is a hemolysin, neurotoxin, and hepatotoxin that inhibits reactions requiring pyridoxal phosphate in a manner similar to isoniazid. The mechanisms resulting in its renal and hepatic effects are unclear. In severe cases, methemoglobinemia, hemolysis with hemoglobinuria, confusion, lethargy, seizures, acidosis, and hypoglycemia may develop. Laboratory findings are nonspecific, as in most ingestions of the monomethylhydrazine group of mushrooms. Baseline laboratory studies, including complete blood count, electrolytes, blood urea nitrogen creatinine, glucose, liver function tests, urinalysis, and methemoglobin are useful.

Treatment is elimination and supportive care. Gastric lavage may be useful with an early presentation. Ipecac-induced emesis is potentially dangerous in light of an increased likelihood of seizures.

Activated charcoal is indicated. Seizures are treated with pyridoxine in a manner similar to isoniazid toxicity. Pyridoxine is administered parenterally at an initial dose of 25 mg/kg and increased to a maximum dose of 300 mg/kg or until seizures resolve. Anticonvulsants are indicated if seizure activity continues. Severe hypoglycemia, fluid loss, and electrolyte imbalance are the most likely causes of morbidity. Mortality approaches 10 percent in those patients who develop symptoms.

MUSCARINE

Muscarine is found in the *Clitocybe, Inocybe,* and *Amanita* genera. Although *A. muscaria* has trace amounts of muscarine present, its toxicity is *not* due to this agent. Ingestion results in a muscarine-induced cholingeric crisis.

Symptoms occur rapidly, usually within 15 to 60 min, and are those expected of cholinergic stimulation. Salivation, lacrimation, urinary frequency, increased gastroenteric motility, diarrhea, diaphoresis, miosis, blurred vision, bronchospasm, bronchorrhea, bradycardia, and even hypotension may occur. Symptoms are typically mild and short-lived, lasting up to 6 h.

Treatment consists of gut decontamination using gastric lavage, followed by activated charcoal. Cardiac monitoring is necessary because of the potential for bradyarrhythmias. The use of atropine in the face of severe cholinergic crisis is indicated, with an initial dose of 0.01 mg/kg IV. The total dose is titrated based on the drying of secretions, rather than on pupillary dilation.

COPRINE GROUP

The common "alcohol inky" (*Coprinus atramentarius*) is an edible mushroom without toxic effects when eaten in the absence of ethanol. However, when ethanol is coingested, a disulfiramlike reaction may occur. The prolonged effects of coprine may hinder any connection being made between mushroom ingestion and that of ethanol.

Patients presenting acutely after coprine exposure and ethanol use exhibit facial flushing, paresthesias, diaphoresis, headache, nausea, and vomiting. Severe reactions may result in hypotension or acidosis. Arrhythmias have been reported in adults. Gastric lavage may be useful in the event that mushroom ingestion was recent or that ethanol ingestion was recent and excessive. Activated charcoal is indicated only if toxicity from other mushrooms is entertained, since this disulfiramlike reaction will resolve spontaneously in a few hours as serum alcohol levels decrease. Severe reactions may require aggressive fluid resuscitation.

IBOTENIC ACID AND MUSCIMOL

Amanita muscaria and *A. pantherina* contain the psychoactive isoxazoles, which are responsible for the toxicologic profile of this ingestant. In spite of its name, *A. muscaria* carries insignificant amounts of muscarine and does not result in a syndrome of cholinergic excess.

Within 30 min to 2 h of ingestion of mushrooms of this group, symptoms resembling ethanol intoxication occur, with ataxia, confusion, irritability, bizarre behavior, euphoria, hyperkinetic activity, and the sparing of speech and articulation. More severe ingestion may progress to varying degrees of obtundation, hallucinosis, myoclonic jerking, or seizures. Vomiting is rare.

Supportive care is the mainstay of treatment. Gastric lavage followed by activated charcoal is followed by observation. The use of atropine is not indicated. Seizure activity is treated with anticonvulsants as necessary. Symptoms typically resolve in 4 to 6 h.

For a more detailed discussion, see Rittenberry TJ, Rivas J: Mushroom poisoning, chap. 98, p. 554, in *Pediatric Emergency Medicine: A Comprehensive Study Guide.*

---

99 Neuroleptics

Timothy Erickson

Neuroleptics, or phenothiazines, are a group of major tranquilizers or antipsychotic drugs that are therapeutically designed to treat schizophrenia and other psychiatric disorders.

PHARMACOLOGY

Five classes of neuroleptics exist, all of which have the same basic three-ringed structure. Although all classes exhibit similar therapeutic and adverse effects, modification of the basic structure results in variable degrees of toxicity.

PATHOPHYSIOLOGY

Neuroleptics act by blocking dopaminergic, alpha-adrenergic, muscarinic, histaminic, and serotoninergic neuroreceptors. Blockade of the dopamine receptors results in the desired behavior modification but also produces extrapyramidal side effects, such as dystonic reactions. Alpha-adrenergic blockade produces peripheral vasodilation and orthostatic hypotension. Muscarinic blockade results in anticholinergic properties such as sedation, tachycardia, flushed or dry skin, urinary retention, and delayed gastrointestinal (GI) motility. Neuroleptics also cause a membrane depressant action or quinidinelike effect that alters myocardial contractility and can result in conduction defects. Although the mechanism of toxicity in neuroleptics resembles that of tricyclic antidepressants, serious cardiac dysrhythmias, refractory hypotension, respiratory depression, and seizures are uncommon.

DYSTONIC REACTIONS

Clinical Presentation

Acute dystonia is an unpredictable side effect of neuroleptics and is present in approximately 10 percent of overdoses. It can also occur as an idiosyncratic reaction following a single therapeutic dose of a neuroleptic. Dystonic reactions are characterized by slurred speech, dysarthria, confusion, difficulty swallowing, hypertonicity, tremors, and muscle restlessness. Other reactions or dyskinesias include oculogyric crisis (upward gaze), torticollis (neck twisting), facial grimacing, opisthotonos (scoliosis), and tortipelvic gait disturbances. Symptoms usually begin within the first 5 to 30 h after ingestion. Dystonic reactions are relatively common in infants and adolescents. Of the neuroleptics, prochlorperazine most often causes acute dystonia, limiting its use as an antiemetic agent in children.

Management

If a child exhibits signs of acute muscular dystonia, intravenous diphenhydramine (2 mg/kg up to 50 mg over several minutes) is rapidly administered. Alternatively, the patient can be given benztropine intramuscularly in a dose of 0.05 to 0.1 mg/kg (up to 2 mg). Improvement usually occurs within 15 min. Doses exceeding 8 mg over a 24-h period can result in severe anticholinergic symptoms.

ACUTE OVERDOSE

Clinical Presentation

Following an acute overdose of neuroleptics, mild central nervous system (CNS) depression is common, usually occurring within

1 to 2 h of the ingestion. Children are more susceptible to these sedative effects than adults. In the overdose setting, respiratory depression can occur but rarely requires aggressive airway management. Neuroleptics tend to lower a patient's seizure threshold, though the actual incidence of seizures in acute overdose is low.

Like poisoning from the tricyclic antidepressants, poisoning from neuroleptics can result in orthostatic hypotension and cardiac dysrhythmias, particularly with the piperidine and aliphatic phenothiazines. Sinus tachycardia is the most common dysrhythmia, but prolongation of the QT interval as well as QRS widening can be noted on electrocardiography. Other clinical effects in the acute overdose setting include pupillary miosis, which in one study was observed in 72 percent of children with high-grade coma following ingestion of a phenothiazine. Due to the anticholinergic properties of the neuroleptics, the patient may also exhibit decreased GI motility, urinary retention, hyperthermia, and dry, flushed skin. Hypothermia can be noted but is rarely clinically significant.

Laboratory

Although serum phenothiazine levels can be obtained to confirm an ingestion, they correlate poorly with clinical effects. Baseline laboratory tests include a complete blood count, electrolytes, blood urea nitrogen/creatinine, and glucose. Urine should be collected for myoglobin, particularly if the patient is hyperthermic. The urine can be tested qualitatively with a 10% ferric chloride solution. Some 10 to 15 drops of ferric chloride will change the color of the urine to a deep burgundy if phenothiazines are present. Due to potential neuroleptic-induced cardiotoxicity, an electrocardiogram is indicated. Since phenothiazines tend to delay GI motility and can be radiopaque, a flat plate of the abdomen may confirm the ingestion.

Management

Initial management of an acute neuroleptic overdose includes stabilizing the airway and circulation. If the patient remains hypotensive despite adequate amounts of intravenous fluid, an alpha-adrenergic agonist like norepinephrine should be considered. Vasopressors with both alpha- and beta-agonist activity, such as dopamine, may actually exacerbate hypotension because of unopposed beta-adrenergic stimulation, during which alpha receptors are being blocked by the neuroleptic. Because of the potential cardiotoxicity of phenothiazines, patients require close cardiac monitoring. Since phenothiazine toxicity classically demonstrates central nervous system depression and pupillary miosis, adequate doses of naloxone should be given to treat potential concomitant opioid toxicity. Since the anticholinergic properties of neuroleptics tend to slow GI motility, gastric lavage is recommended up to 6 h postingestion. Activated charcoal is administered following lavage in a multiple-dose regimen. Syrup of ipecac is relatively contraindicated in the setting of phenothiazine overdose because the patient has potential for CNS and respiratory depression. No specific antidote exists for acute neuroleptic poisoning, and hemodialysis is not efficacious. Most children presenting after acute neuroleptic toxicity do well with supportive care alone.

NEUROLEPTIC MALIGNANT SYNDROME

Clinical Presentation

Less than 1 percent of the patients exhibit life-threatening extrapyramidal dysfunction known as the *neuroleptic malignant syndrome,* characterized by skeletal muscle rigidity, coma, and severe hyperthermia following the use of phenothiazines or haloperidol. This syndrome can occur following acute overdose, chronic therapy, or idiosyncratically following a single dose of a neuroleptic.

Management

The neuroleptic malignant syndrome results in a high mortality rate and is treated aggressively, with rapid cooling and administration of dantrolene at 0.8 to 3.0 mg/kg intravenously every 6 h, up to 10 mg/kg/day. Dantrolene acts peripherally by treating skeletal muscle rigidity. Bromocriptine, a direct dopamine agonist, has been used successfully alone and in conjunction with dantrolene to treat adult patients with neuroleptic malignant syndrome.

Disposition

Any symptomatic child presenting with acute neuroleptic poisoning should be admitted and observed for CNS and respiratory depression as well as for cardiotoxicity or thermoregulatory problems. Patients with minor, asymptomatic ingestions can be observed for up to 6 h. If the patient is discharged, parents should be advised to watch for signs of delayed dystonic reactions. If the child has been treated successfully for acute dystonia with either diphenhydramine or benztropine, a 2- to 3-day course of oral diphenhydramine is indicated, since many of the neuroleptics have a long duration of action.

For a more detailed discussion, see Erickson T: Neuroleptics, chap. 99, p. 558, in *Pediatric Emergency Medicine: A Comprehensive Study Guide.*

---

100 Nonsteroidal Anti-Inflammatory Drugs

Michele Zell-Kanter

There are many drugs in use today that are categorized as nonsteroidal anti-inflammatory agents (NSAIDs). In the overdose setting, NSAIDs are relatively devoid of toxicity.

CLINICAL PRESENTATION

The typical ingestion of an NSAID results in only central nervous system (CNS) or gastrointestinal (GI) toxicity. Common symptoms of CNS toxicity can include drowsiness, dizziness, and lethargy. Ponstel has a propensity to cause seizures, as do piroxicam, naproxen, and ketoprofen. Headache is more likely to occur after ingestion of indomethacin than after ingestion of other NSAIDs.

Symptoms of gastrointestinal toxicity include nausea, vomiting, and epigastric pain, all of which can occur at therapeutic doses. The gastritis associated with NSAIDs probably occurs secondary to inhibition of prostaglandin synthesis.

Cardiovascular complications of NSAID overdose are generally limited to tachycardia and hypotension secondary to volume depletion. Rare respiratory complications are hyperventilation and apnea.

Long-term use of NSAIDs is associated with nephrotoxicity, including acute tubular necrosis, acute interstitial nephritis, and acute renal failure. Renal papillary necrosis has been reported in children being treated with NSAIDs for juvenile rheumatoid arthritis. Renal toxicity is not associated with acute overdose.

Other long-term complications of NSAID use include hepatocellular injury and cholestatic jaundice.

LABORATORY STUDIES

In symptomatic patients, indicated laboratory tests include a complete blood count, electrolytes, glucose, creatinine, and coagulation profile. Drug levels correlate poorly with toxicity.

Infrequently, overdose of NSAIDs has been associated with an anion-gap acidosis. In patients with severe clinical symptoms, an arterial blood gas is indicated.

MANAGEMENT

After the patient is stabilized, gastric decontamination procedures are indicated. In a patient who presents within 1 h of ingestion, syrup of ipecac can be used. It is relatively contraindicated in ingestions of NSAIDs known to cause seizures. Gastric lavage is the preferred method of elimination in patients who arrive at the emergency department more than 1 h after ingestion.

Activated charcoal is administered after ipecac-induced emesis ceases or lavage is terminated. Multiple-dose charcoal should be considered in any serious overdose in which charcoal is indicated.

The high protein binding of NSAIDs renders extracorporeal methods of elimination ineffective. Likewise, forced diuresis is of no value.

For a more detailed discussion, see Zell-Kanter M: Nonsteroidal anti-inflammatory drugs, chap. 100, p. 561, in *Pediatric Emergency Medicine: A Comprehensive Study Guide.*

---

101 Opioids

Timothy Erickson

Opioids are naturally occurring or synthetic drugs that have opium- or morphinelike activity. Although most opioids have an onset of action within 1 h, many of the oral agents, such as methadone, codeine, and diphenoxylate-atropine (Lomotil), demonstrate a delayed effect of up to 4 to 12 h and a half-life as long as 24 h. The toxic effects are mediated through the mu and kappa opioid receptors located in the central and peripheral nervous systems.

CLINICAL PRESENTATION

The classic triad of acute toxicity consists of central nervous system (CNS) depression, respiratory depression, and pupillary constriction (miosis). Central nervous system depression ranges from mild sedation to stupor and coma. In massive overdoses, the respiratory toxicity can also manifest as noncardiogenic pulmonary edema. Patients are typically hypotensive, hypothermic, bradycardic, and hyporeflexic, with diminished bowel sounds. Less common effects of opioid toxicity include generalized seizure activity following overdose of propoxyphene, meperidine, or pentazocine. Propoxyhene can cause cardiotoxicity via conduction dysfunction.

MANAGEMENT

The management of opioid poisoning includes maintaining the airway and administration of the pure opioid antagonist naloxone. The onset of action for naloxone is usually within 1 min after administration. In addition to intravenous administration, naloxone can be given via the endotracheal tube or intralingually with a comparably rapid onset of action. In the overdose setting, the dose of naloxone is 0.1 mg/kg from birth until age 5 years or 20 kg of weight, at which time a dose of at least 2 mg is given. If there is no response, repeat doses of 2 mg are given to older children and adolescents, up to a maximum of 10 mg. Even with large doses of naloxone, minimal to no adverse side effects have been noted. An exception to this rule is the opioid-dependent patient, in whom a withdrawal syndrome can be precipitated. Because of the short half-life of naloxone (20 to 30 min), repeated doses may be indicated in the overdose setting, particularly in the case of those opioids with longer durations of action, such as codeine, methadone, and Lomotil. If repeat doses of naloxone are required, a continuous intravenous infusion of naloxone is instituted.

Since opioids tend to slow gastrointestinal motility, gastric decontamination several hours following oral ingestions may still prove efficacious. This is particularly true of Lomotil, which contains atropine. Gastric lavage is preferred over ipecac, since the patient has the potential for CNS and respiratory depression. A dose of activated charcoal with cathartic is advised following an oral ingestion.

DISPOSITION

Any pediatric patient presenting with CNS and respiratory depression from opioid poisoning responsive to naloxone is admitted, since most of the opioids demonstrate longer durations of action than naloxone and require repetitive administration or continuous naloxone infusion.

For a more detailed discussion, see Erickson T: Opioids, chap. 101, p. 563, in *Pediatric Emergency Medicine: A Comprehensive Study Guide.*

---

102 Organophosphates and Carbamates

Jerrold Leikin

The organophosphates, and to a lesser extent the carbamate compounds, are widely distributed throughout industry, agriculture, and the home, where they are used predominantly as pesticides. Organophosphates are usually found in No-Pest Strips (Vapona) and roach killers.

ORGANOPHOSPHATES

Pathophysiology

Organophosphates exert their toxicity by inactivating acetylcholinesterase. In the case of organophosphates, the inactivation is essentially permanent. The inactivation of acetylcholinesterase leads to the accumulation of acetylcholine at cholinergic receptor sites. Excess acetylcholine initially stimulates and then paralyzes cholinergic transmission at parasympathetic nerve endings, certain sympathetic nerve endings, and the neuromuscular junction. Organophosphates penetrate the central nervous system (CNS), where they paralyze cholinergic transmission.

Clinical Presentation

The initial signs and symptoms of cholinergic excess are usually muscarinic in nature (Table 102-1). Gastrointestinal symptoms include abdominal cramps, vomiting, and diarrhea. Pulmonary findings include increased bronchial secretions, bronchoconstriction, dyspnea, and in some cases pulmonary edema. Lacrimation

TABLE 102-1 Clinical Effects of Organophosphate/Carbamate Intoxication

Muscarinic effects (organophosphate/carbamate)	
Salivation	Bradycardia
Diaphoresis	Miosis (late finding)
Lacrimation	Bronchorrhea
Defecation	Bronchospasm
Abdominal cramps	
Rhinorrhea	
Nicotinic effects (organophosphate only)	
Fasciculations/twitching	Tachycardia
Weakness	Hypertension
Tremors	Pallor
Areflexia	Cramps
Central nervous system effects (carbamates rarely, organophosphate predominantly)	
Headache	Seizures
Restlessness	Coma
Confusion	Respiratory depression
Bizarre behavior	Ataxia
Intermediate syndrome (organophosphate only)	
Paralysis of head, neck, and extremity muscles 3½ to 7 days after resolution of cholinergic synchrony.	

and salivation are increased. Miosis occurs, occasionally preceded by mydriasis. Bradycardia can occur, as can urinary incontinence. This constellation of findings is characterized by the mnemonic SLUDGE, which stands for salivation, lacrimation, urination, defecation, gastrointestinal cramps, and emesis. The mnemonic does not include the pulmonary findings, which can cause life-threatening hypoxia and require urgent intervention.

Nicotinic manifestations noted include hypertension, pallor, and tachycardia. Striated muscle can be severely affected. Initially cholinergic excess stimulates fasciculations, which are followed by weakness; this can range from very mild to full paralysis. The combination of increased airway secretions and weakness of the respiratory musculature can rapidly produce respiratory failure and often necessitates urgent intubation.

Central nervous system toxicity ranges from agitation to full delirium and coma. Seizures can also occur.

An intermediate syndrome has been described that is manifested by neck and extremity paralysis at an interval of 12 h to 7 days after exposure to some organophosphate agents. This syndrome may occur due to lack of administration of an oxime during treatment.

Diagnosis

Exposure to an organophosphate is in the differential diagnosis for any patient presenting with the characteristic SLUDGE symptom complex. Muscle fasciculations with or without CNS abnormalities make an organophosphate exposure highly likely. Patients exposed to agricultural or other occupational pesticides are at particularly high risk.

Laboratory Studies

In the acute phase, there is no test that can identify organophosphate toxicity, and the initial management of the patient is based on clinical findings.

Organophosphates cause depression of red blood cell cholinesterase and plasma pseudocholinesterase. Red blood cell cholinesterase represents cholinesterase found in nerve tissue, brain, and erythrocytes. It is a better indicator of toxicity than plasma pseudocholinesterase, which is a liver protein. Measured depressions of 50 percent or more of red blood cell cholinesterase correlate with mild toxicity, while a 90 percent depression indicates severe poisoning. In untreated organophosphate poisoning, regeneration of the enzyme takes 1 to 3 months.

Laboratory studies useful in the acutely ill patient include electrolytes in patients with vomiting and diarrhea and, in those with pulmonary symptoms, an arterial blood gas or percutaneous oxygen saturation. A chest radiograph is indicated in patients with evidence of pulmonary involvement.

Treatment

Stabilization

The most important aspect of stabilization is to assure adequate oxygenation and ventilation. In cases where there is severe bronchospasm, copious secretions, or marked weakness of respiratory muscles, urgent intubation and ventilation is indicated until antidotal therapy takes effect. Patients with marked CNS involvement may also require intubation to assure protection of the airway.

Fluid resuscitation may be required in patients who have suffered significant volume loss from the gastrointestinal tract.

Decontamination

The patient is completely undressed, including any jewelry, and the skin cleansed with soap and water. Contaminated clothing is discarded. The hospital staff must take care that they are not contaminated by contact with patients with dermal exposure.

Since emesis and diarrhea are common in organophosphate and carbamate intoxication, ipecac or lavage is rarely useful. Activated charcoal is indicated to adsorb toxin remaining in the gastrointestinal tract.

Antidotal Therapy

Atropine is the antidote for the muscarinic effects of organophosphate toxicity. It also relieves the CNS manifestations. An initial dose of 0.05 mg/kg is indicated; this may be doubled every 5 to 10 min until symptoms are relieved. The goal of therapy is the drying of airway secretions, so that oxygenation and ventilation are maintained. Pupillary dilation can occur before secretions are alleviated and is not an indication of adequate atropinization. In some cases, massive doses of atropine are required. Tachycardia is not a contraindication to its use. Treatment with atropine must usually continue for at least 24 h. Endotracheal or nebulized administration of ipratropium bromide (0.5 mg every 6 h) may also assist in drying secretions.

The specific antidote for the nicotinic manifestations of organophosphate toxicity is pralidoxime (2-PAM or Protopam). It also relieves the CNS effects. Pralidoxime works by restoring the activity of acetylcholinesterase. It is most effective when administered early, but should be used at any point at which organophosphate poisoning with nicotinic or CNS manifestations is considered. Pregnancy is not a contraindication to its use.

Pralidoxime is administered at a dose of 25 to 50 mg/kg diluted to a 5% concentration in normal saline and infused over a 5- to 30-min period. It is repeated at 6- to 12-h intervals until there is relief of muscle weakness. Continuous infusion of 9 to 19 mg/kg/h following the loading dose of 25 to 50 mg/kg is indicated if breakthrough nicotinic symptoms occur or if there is continued absorption of poison. Treatment is generally necessary for at least 48 h. Side effects of pralidoxime include nausea, tachycardia, lethargy, and diplopia. There may be mild elevation of liver enzymes.

Charcoal hemoperfusion is effective in removing parathion, demeton-S-methyl sulfoxide, dimethioate, and malathion. Exchange transfusion also has been utilized in parathion toxicity. Newer modalities, such as the use of exogenous plasma cholinesterase to act as a scavenger agent in organophosphate toxicity, or dextetimide or scopolamine as anticholinergic agents, are investigational.

CARBAMATES

Carbamates are commonly found in flea and tick powders and in ant killers. Like organophosphates, carbamates inactivate acetylcholinesterase. Unlike that caused by organophosphates, however, inactivation is not permanent, and functional activity of the enzyme is often largely restored within 8 h. Red blood cell cholinesterase usually is completely restored within 48 h.

Toxicity with carbamates is mainly restricted to muscarinic effects, which are often the only manifestations of poisoning (Table 102-1). Carbamates are much less likely than organophosphates to cause CNS effects, since they do not penetrate the blood-brain barrier well. However, children with severe carbamate poisoning can develop CNS depression and, on occasion, seizures. Nicotinic manifestations are also uncommon.

The initial management of the muscarinic effects of carbamate toxicity is the same as for organophosphates, with stabilization of the airway and breathing and complete decontamination of the patient. The skin is washed, although dermal exposure is less likely with carbamates than with organophosphates. Atropine is administered as antidotal therapy. Because the inactivation of acetylcholinesterase by carbamates is relatively short, pralidoxime is unlikely to be of benefit.

For a more detailed discussion, see Leikin J: Organophosphates and carbamates, chap. 102, p. 565, in *Pediatric Emergency Medicine: A Comprehensive Study Guide.*

---

103 Phencyclidine Toxicity

Steven E. Aks

INTRODUCTION/EPIDEMIOLOGY

Phencyclidine (PCP) is a common drug that is used for recreational purposes by adolescents and adults. Toddlers and infants have been exposed via passive inhalation, which has resulted in significant clinical toxicity. Phencyclidine should be included on every clinician's list of drugs that can cause altered mental status in children of all ages.

Phencyclidine is a cyclohexylamine that is structurally related to ketamine. The mechanism of action of PCP is severalfold. It is felt to inhibit the uptake of dopamine and norepinephrine; in addition, it has some anticholinergic and alpha-adrenergic properties. Angel dust, peace pill, wickey weed, wacky weed, Sherman, monkey tranquilizer, embalming fluid, Cadillac, and rocket fuel are all terms that characterize this drug.

The neurologic effects of PCP overdose include excitation, hyperreflexia, blank stares, nystagmus, hallucinations, seizures, and psychosis. Phencyclidine can cause acute behavioral toxicity. A hallmark is its ability to cause a fluctuating level of consciousness, characterized by periods of lethargy and coma alternating with aggressive or assaultive activity. The combination of psychotic and aggressive behavior places the PCP user at great risk for traumatic injury. As with opioid toxicity, the pupils are often pinpoint, although mydriasis may be seen.

Young children exposed to PCP can present with the rapid onset of lethargy, coma, staring spells, ataxia, opisthotonos, and nystagmus. Side effects have been described in patients as young as 2 months of age.

Cardiovascular side effects include hypertension, which may be severe enough to create a hypertensive crisis, tachycardia, and dysrhythmias.

In PCP overdose, the skin can be flushed and diaphoretic. Hyperthermia and muscle hyperactivity can occur, as can rhabdomyolysis and renal failure.

LABORATORY

Useful laboratory studies include a complete blood count, electrolytes, and renal function tests. A blood glucose is indicated to rule out hypoglycemia. A urinalysis is obtained to screen for rhabdomyolysis. Measurement of serum creatine kinase and sequential monitoring of renal function are indicated. Electrocardiographic monitoring is important. Phencyclidine is included in standard toxicology screens.

MANAGEMENT

The mainstay of management of the patient with PCP intoxication is supportive care. The patient is placed in a dark, quiet room. Attempts to "talk the patient down" are generally ineffective. Physical and appropriate chemical restraints are used as necessary.

If multiple drugs are ingested, lavage with subsequent administration of activated charcoal is appropriate. However, in some cases this may agitate the patient and increase the risk of self-injury or injury to the staff. Nasogastric aspiration of gastric fluid has been suggested as a means of removing PCP that is ionized in the stomach, but this is generally not realistic in the agitated patient.

Pharmacologic agents such as benzodiazepines and haldol have been used successfully in cases of PCP intoxication. Phenothiazines are contraindicated in the setting of PCP intoxication because of their potential to lower the seizure threshold and cause hypotension. Antihypertensives are generally not required in PCP overdose, but if they are necessary, a short-acting agent such as nitroprusside is useful.

Although acidification of the urine has been reported to enhance elimination of PCP, it is contraindicated because of the potential for rhabdomyolysis.

DISPOSITION

Patients with prolonged coma, seizures, hyperthermia, rhabdomyolysis, or unstable vital signs are admitted to an intensive care unit for monitoring and supportive care. Patients with minor manifestations of toxicity can be observed in the emergency department for 6 to 8 h and discharged in the care of responsible family members when their mental status returns to baseline.

For a more detailed discussion, see Aks SE: Phencyclidine toxicity, chap. 103, p. 568, in *Pediatric Emergency Medicine: A Comprehensive Study Guide.*

104 Poisonous Plants

Kimberly Sing

Plants are commonly ingested by children. Although the vast majority of plants are nontoxic, a small number are mildly toxic and a few are harmful or fatal with even a small exposure. It is useful to classify plants according to the most serious manifestations of toxicity.

GASTROINTESTINAL IRRITANTS

A majority of plants cause primarily nausea, vomiting, and diarrhea. The *Solanum* spp. cause gastrointestinal symptoms and an anticholinergic syndrome. Children usually eat the brightly colored berries, with two to three berries causing significant symptoms in adults. The phytolaccine alkaloid found in the pokeweed affects cells with the most rapid growth, especially those in the gastrointestinal tract. The green berries contain more toxin than the purple berries. The toxalbumins of the rosary pea and the castor bean are the most toxic substances known. Decontamination should be attempted even 4 h after ingestion.

During the Christmas holidays, children are often exposed to mistletoe and holly. The leaves are more toxic than the berries and cause mainly gastroenteritis, although symptoms are usually not severe. The European variety, also found in Sonoma County, California, contains a toxin that is similar to cobra venom and is reported to cause cardiotoxicity in animal studies.

The *Arum* species Dieffenbachia and Philodendron are houseplants and are the most common cause of symptomatic plant ingestions. They can cause severe oral and pharyngeal burns secondary to insoluble calcium oxylate crystals. Usually the upper airway is most affected. When there is severe exposure, the patient may need to be intubated to protect the airway. These plants do not cause gastroenteritis. Children who are not in extremis should be encouraged to drink milk or water. At home, application of oral numbing gels may be helpful. Respiratory obstruction usually progresses within the first 6 h after exposure.

CARDIOVASCULAR TOXINS

Historically, plants that contain cardiac glycosides have been used for various cardiac ailments. Each of the following plants contain glycosides in increasing potency: lily of the valley, foxglove, oleander, and yellow oleander.

Toxicity can consist predominantly of gastrointestinal symptoms, with vomiting and diarrhea. Some patients may complain of seeing yellow halos around lights. In severe cases, cardiac toxicity results, mainly in the form of arrythmias that include first-, second-, and third-degree heart block.

In patients who have not vomited, gastric decontamination is indicated. In patients with bradydysrhythmias, atropine and cardiac pacing are indicated. If cardiac instability is noted, a trial of Digibind is given. Although it has proven useful in dog studies, there is only one reported human case of Digibind being used in oleander toxicity.

Digoxin levels are not a reliable predictor of cardiac toxicity, and symptomatic patients are treated regardless of laboratory results.

NEUROLOGIC TOXINS

Water hemlock is easily confused with the wild carrot or Jerusalem artichoke. Patients may progress to status epilepticus, respiratory distress, and death. Rhabdomyolysis may develop. Treatment is primarily supportive. There is controversy over whether patients benefit from barbiturates. Patients who exhibit any central nervous system (CNS) symptoms or cardiac instability require hospital admission. Patients who are asymptomatic are observed for 4 to 6 h before discharge. Other plants thought to cause seizures are podophyllum resin, trematol, pennyroyal oil, margosa oil, and eucalyptus oil. Occasionally, *Aconitum* (monkshood), *Taxus* spp., and *Veratrum* spp. cause convulsions.

NICOTINELIKE TOXINS

Plants that contain nicotinelike toxins cause a toxidrome consisting of nausea, vomiting, salivation, abdominal cramps, confusion, tachycardia, mydriasis, and fever. Seizures may occur in this initial stimulatory stage. This progresses to CNS depression and may result in respiratory failure.

Poison hemlock contains coniine, which causes a curarelike paralysis at the neuromuscular junction and a strychninelike convulsant activity. Death occurs from respiratory paralysis. Whole bowel irrigation may prove helpful if large amounts have been ingested. The *Nicotinia* and *Lobelia* species contain nicotine or nicotiniclike alkaloids. Mild intoxication may resolve in a few hours, with severe poisonings requiring 24 h to resolve. Treatment of cigarette ingestion in children is controversial. Ingestion of one-half to one cigarette may cause symptoms, and two cigarettes will cause serious symptoms. Gastric decontamination is indicated in these children. Atropine may improve the bradycardia and hypotension but does not alter the neuromuscular weakness.

ANTICHOLINGERGIC TOXINS

Jimsonweed, black henbane, and mandrake all contain varying amounts of both hyoscyamine and scopolamine. Decontamination is attempted even 12 to 24 h after ingestion because there is delayed gastric emptying. Physostigmine is reserved for patients with seizures, severe hallucinations, hypertension, or arrhythmias. Physostigmine can be given at 0.02 mg/kg up to 0.5 mg over several minutes. If there is no improvement, readministration after 5 min may be attempted, not to exceed 2 mg. Because of the short half-life, it may need to be readministered after 30 to 40 min. The *lowest* effective dose is utilized. This antidote cannot be given as an infusion. Symptoms usually resolve after 24 to 48 h.

RENAL TOXINS

The stalk of the rhubarb is edible, but the leaves are toxic because of the high content of soluble calcium oxalate, which can cause renal failure. Symptoms usually begin 6 to 12 h after ingestion but may be delayed 24 h. Because of the precipitation of calcium, patients may develop hypocalcemia, resulting in electrocardiographic changes, paresthesias, tetany, hyperreflexia, muscle twitches, muscle cramps, and seizures. Calcium gluconate may be required to reverse the hypocalcemia. Poison hemlock has also been reported to cause renal failure, probably through the development of rhabdomyolysis.

For a more detailed discussion, see Sing K: Poisonous plants, chap. 104, p. 570, in *Pediatric Emergency Medicine: A Comprehensive Study Guide.*

---

105 Sedative Hypnotics

Timothy Erickson / Will Ignatoff

There are several agents that are classified as sedative hypnotic drugs. Agents commonly encountered in the pediatric include barbiturates, benzodiazepines, and chloral hydrate.

BARBITURATES

Pharmacology/Pathophysiology

The barbiturates are classified as either ultrashort-acting (thiopental), short-acting (pentobarbital), or long-acting (phenobarbital). These agents are primary used as anticonvulsants and for induction of anesthesia. Barbiturates are primarily central nervous system (CNS) depressants. Toxicity can result in suppression of skeletal, smooth, and cardiac muscle, leading to depressed myocardial contractility, bradycardia, vasodilation, and hypotension.

Clinical Presentation

In the overdose setting, the pediatric patient will present with sedation and coma, often accompanied by respiratory depression. Vital signs may reveal hypotension, bradycardia, and hypothermia. Pupils are constricted early in the clinical course but can be dilated in later stages of coma. Noncardiogenic pulmonary edema has been described in severely toxic patients. Phenobarbital-induced hepatotoxicity has also been described in children.

Laboratory

Aside from routine baseline laboratory studies, a quantitative serum phenobarbital level is obtained. Patients with levels above 50 μg/mL will exhibit mild toxicity, while those with levels over 100 μg/mL are typically unresponsive to pain and suffer from respiratory and cardiac depression.

Treatment

The primary management in barbiturate toxicity is support and stabilization of the airway and circulation. Hypotensive patients are managed with fluid resuscitation and, if necessary, pressors. As a result of the delayed gut motility, gastric lavage may be useful up to 6 h postingestion. Since most barbiturate ingestions cause CNS depression, syrup of ipecac is contraindicated. Several investigations have demonstrated the efficacy of multidose activated charcoal in children.

Urinary alkalinization with sodium bicarbonate to a pH of 7.5 to 8.0 can hasten the renal excretion of phenobarbital and is recommended in severe toxicity. Alkalinization is not effective in treating toxicity from shorter-acting agents. Fluid overload is avoided because of the potential for pulmonary and cerebral edema. In unstable patients or in those with renal failure, hemodialysis is indicated for long-acting barbiturates. Charcoal hemoperfusion seems more efficacious for shorter-acting agents.

BENZODIAZEPINES

Benzodiazepines cause the majority of sedative hypnotic overdoses. They are used for their anxiolytic, muscle relaxant, and anticonvulsant properties. The benzodiazepines act by facilitating the neurotransmission in gamma-aminobutyric acid (GABA). Overdoses result in a mild to moderate CNS depression. Deep coma requiring assisted ventilation is uncommon. In severe overdoses, benzodiazepines can induce cardiovascular and pulmonary toxicity. Fatalities from benzodiazepine overdoses are rare.

Clinical Presentation

Following an acute overdose, the patient presents with sedation, somnolence, ataxia, and slurred speech. Coma is rare. Very young children are more susceptible to CNS depression. Benzodiazepines can also induce paradoxical reactions such as anxiety, delirium, combativeness, and hallucinations, particularly in children. Pupils are typically dilated, and the patient may be hypothermic. Benzodiazepines rarely cause significant cardiovascular changes. Quantitative benzodiazepine concentrations in the blood correlate poorly with toxicity.

Treatment

The most critical management intervention is stabilization of the child's respiratory status. Ipecac is contraindicated due to the CNS effects of these agents. Gastric lavage is indicated in patients presenting within 1 h of ingestion, and activated charcoal is recommended in all significant overdoses. Forced diuresis is not efficacious. Because benzodiazepines are highly bound to plasma proteins, hemodialysis and hemoperfusion are ineffective.

Flumazenil is an antidotal agent that competes with benzodiazepines at CNS GABA sites. In children, an initial dose of 0.01 mg/kg intravenously is recommended. If no response is elicited, this dose can be repeated. In neonates, the intravenous loading dose is 0.02 mg/kg. The duration of flumazenil is less than 1 h, often necessitating subsequent doses or an infusion. Contraindications to flumazenil include seizure disorders, chronical use of benzodiazepines, and coingestion with agents like tricyclic antidepressants or isoniazid. It is not prudent to administer flumazenil in coma of unknown cause.

CHLORAL HYDRATE

Although an uncommon cause of overdose, chloral hydrate is frequently used in the pediatric population for sedation prior to procedures or radiologic testing. Chloral hydrate is a sedative hypnotic that produces minimal respiratory depression when given in therapeutic doses. Doses up to 80 to 100 mg/kg have been reported as safe for pediatric sedation.

Clinical Presentation

Signs and symptoms of chloral hydrate toxicity include respiratory, CNS, and cardiovascular manifestations. Pupils are typically miotic early in the clinical course but dilate in later stages of coma. The child may have a classic "pearlike" odor to the breath. Gastrointestinal upset with vomiting and abdominal pain is common. Cardiac dysrhythmias include atrial fibrillation, multifocal premature ventricular contractions, and ventricular tachycardia and fibrillation progressing to torsade de pointes. In severe overdose, the pediatric patient can exhibit hypothermia, hypotension, and noncardiogenic pulmonary edema. Choral hydrate levels correlate poorly with toxicity. If the ingestion is recent, an abdominal radiograph may confirm the diagnosis, since chloral hydrate is radiopaque.

Treatment

The airway is stabilized. Attention is directed to the cardiovascular status because of chloral hydrate's potential cardiotoxicity. Gastric decontamination considerations are similar to those for the other sedative hypnotic agents. Ventricular dysrhythmias have responded to lidocaine, beta-blocker, and magnesium administration; however, cases have been anecdotal. If the patient is unstable, hemodialysis is effective.

DISPOSITION

Any pediatric patient who is symptomatic following any sedative hypnotic overdose should be admitted and monitored for both respiratory and cardiovascular stability.

For a more detailed discussion, see Erickson T, Ignatoff W: Sedative hypnotics, chap. 105, p. 577, in *Pediatric Emergency Medicine: A Comprehensive Study Guide.*

---

106 Theophylline

Frank P. Paloucek

Theophylline toxicity is one of the ten most frequent causes of reported fatalities for all age groups. Important factors contributing to the toxicity of theophylline are its widespread use, narrow therapeutic index, proliferation of dosage forms, availability as a nonprescription product, and multiple drug-drug, drug-disease, and drug-food interactions.

It is useful to classify theophylline toxicity as either acute, acute on chronic, or chronic. For this discussion, *acute* toxicity refers to ingestion of one or more excessive doses within an 8-h interval, *acute on chronic* refers to a single acute exposure in a patient ingesting theophylline for >24 h, and *chronic* toxicity is that occurring in the presence of maintenance drug therapy for at least 24 h.

PHARMACOLOGY/PHARMACOKINETICS

The exact mechanism of action of theophylline is unknown. It is known to stimulate the central nervous system and medullary vomiting center, have positive inotropic and chronotropic effects, reduce peripheral arteriolar resistance, increase renal blood flow and glomerular filtration rate, and stimulate secretion of gastric acid and pepsin. Many of these effects are mediated via stimulation of the beta$_2$-adrenergic receptors, which are also responsible for theophylline-induced cellular shifts in electrolytes.

Theophylline is readily absorbed (80 to 100 percent). It is predominantly marketed and used in sustained-release dosage forms. For most ingestions of the parenteral and immediate-release dosage forms of theophylline, the worst-case scenario estimates peak serum concentration following an overdose at twice the mg/kg exposure dose. Although the sustained-release products rarely act like the immediate-release forms, a more accurate estimation of the peak concentration following an overdose is equal to the mg/kg ingested dose. Multiple factors such as diseases, drugs, age, sex, and diet can either enhance or impair theophylline metabolism. Common factors contributing to chronic toxicity include age <2 or >60 years, symptomatic congestive heart failure, hepatic disease, acute viral infections, and concomitant treatment with erythromycins, H_2 histamine antagonists, fluoroquinolones, and allopurinol.

ACUTE THEOPHYLLINE TOXICITY

The clinical manifestations of acute theophylline toxicity are primarily gastrointestinal, cardiovascular, and neurologic. Disturbances in serum electrolytes also occur.

Gastrointestinal manifestations include nausea, vomiting, and gastrointestinal bleeding. Nausea and vomiting are nonspecific and can occur at therapeutic levels. Vomiting can be severe and limits the use of activated charcoal. Gastrointestinal bleeding has been reported in acute pediatric overdoses but is not clinically significant. Concretions or bezoars should be suspected with markedly prolonged increases or unchanged serum concentrations (>24 h).

Cardiovascular manifestations include sinus and supraventricular tachycardias. These are not life-threatening in the absence of other underlying cardiac disease. Specific to acute or acute-on-chronic toxicity are multifocal atrial tachycardias. Ventricular ectopy is reasonably common, but significant ventricular arrhythmias are very rare. Hypotension secondary to theophylline toxicity is unique to acute overdoses and is associated with serum concentrations >100 mg/L. It is due to peripheral $beta_2$-receptor-mediated vasodilatation. Cardiac arrests are exceedingly rare.

Neurologic manifestations include mental status changes, tremor, seizures, and coma. Acute toxicity generally presents with one to three generalized tonic-clonic seizures. Status epilepticus can occur and is associated with more significant morbidity and mortality than status epilepticus from other causes in children. Seizures are associated with serum theophylline concentration >100 mg/L. Up to 20 percent of patients with theophylline-induced seizures die. Death may be a direct consequence of seizures, but more commonly secondary complications result in fatality. Coma has been reported in theophylline toxicity. This has always occurred postictally and is probably not a direct consequence of theophylline toxicity.

Electrolyte disturbances include hypokalemia, hypophosphatemia, and hypercalcemia. When due to theophylline effects alone, they are not associated with any significant pathology. All forms of acid:base disorders have been reported for theophylline, consistent with underlying diseases and concomitant ingestant. Theophylline-induced lactic acidosis has rarely occurred in severe acute toxicity.

Miscellaneous manifestations of theophylline toxicity include diuresis secondary to transient increase in renal blood flow in the acute pediatric exposure, rhabdomyolysis, and tachypnea. Hyperglycemia can also occur.

Increased mortality is associated with age <2 or serum theophylline concentrations >100 mg/L in acute pediatric overdoses.

The single most important laboratory evaluation for a suspected theophylline toxicity is a serum theophylline concentration. The "normal" range is 10 to 20 mg/L, and the "toxic" range is >20 mg/L, although toxic symptoms can occur at concentrations of 10 to 20 mg/L. Significant toxicity is likely with concentrations >100 mg/L for acute overdoses. Theophylline concentrations of 100 mg/L can be expected to occur with ingestion of 50 mg/kg of immediate-release tablets or 100 mg/kg of sustained-release tablets. It is critical, especially in known sustained-release overdoses, that serial concentrations be measured every 2 h until two consecutive decreasing theophylline concentrations are obtained. This allows for appropriate monitoring of the absorption phase of these products as well as potential concretion formation and identification.

Additional laboratory testing includes finger-stick glucose, serum electrolytes, arterial blood gas, and 12-lead electrocardiogram. Both ultrasound and KUB (kidney, ureter, bladder) x-ray can identify intact sustained-release dosage forms or concretions in the gastrointestinal tract.

MANAGEMENT

Gastric decontamination is indicated in the acute presentation. Ipecac is generally not indicated due to the emetogenic nature of theophylline and the need to administer activated charcoal. Its use is limited to the prehospital setting. Gastric lavage is indicated within 1 h of large ingestions (>50 mg/kg). The use of the largest-bore tube available is critical, given the size of most sustained-release theophylline products. Activated charcoal is the gastric decontamination treatment of choice. The initial dose is calculated to deliver 10 g of charcoal for every 1 g of ingested theophylline, up to a maximum of 100 g of charcoal. This may require multiple doses. This initial therapy is separate from subsequent elimination enhancement achieved by gastrointestinal dialysis with multiple-dose activated charcoal. The initial dose is administered with sorbitol in a 1.5 g/kg dose for children and alert adults and 3 g/kg for the obtunded adult. Charcoal can reduce apparent theophylline half-life to 2 h even in the absorption phase.

An alternative to gastric decontamination with charcoal is whole bowel irrigation with high-molecular-weight polyethylene glycol (such as Golytely) dosed at 15 to 40 mL/kg/h in children and 1 to 2 L/h in adults. This is not effective in late presentations of acute ingestions, in which charcoal is the treatment of choice. To date, there is no evidence of benefit from combining these two therapies.

Elimination enhancement is an important consideration for theophylline toxicity. Effective modalities include multiple-dose oral activated charcoal, hemodialysis, charcoal hemoperfusion, exchange transfusions, and plasmapheresis. For any significant ingestion (theophylline concentrations >30 mg/L), oral activated charcoal at 25 g every 2 h is initiated and continued until concentrations are <120 mg/L or gastrointestinal complications occur. This can be administered as boluses or as a continuous nasogastric infusion. In this setting it is critical to monitor concomitant sorbitol administration, since this can lead to severe diarrhea, dehydration, and electrolyte imbalance. Also, several of the initial doses of multidose regimens may in fact be adsorbing theophylline from tablets still in the gastrointestinal tract if the initial dose failed to achieve the preferred 10:1 dosing ratio.

Hemodialysis and charcoal hemoperfusion are indicated prophylactically in patients with theophylline concentrations >100 mg/L in an overdose. Hemoperfusion is preferred to hemodialysis, as it achieves higher clearance rates. Both hemodialysis and charcoal hemoperfusion have been used simultaneously, although there are no comparative clinical data suggesting a benefit to this procedure.

There has been limited experience with exchange transfusion or plasmapheresis in neonatal and infant intoxications where dialysis or hemoperfusion was not feasible.

The treatment of choice for seizures is a benzodiazepine. Barbiturates are second-line therapy. Phenytoin is absolutely contraindicated, as it lowers the seizure threshold in vitro and has not been effective clinically. The development of repetitive seizures or status epilepticus is an indication for barbiturate coma with or without paralysis. Single isolated seizure activity does not require long-term maintenance anticonvulsant therapy.

Arrhythmias are treated with beta blockade or calcium channel blockade. Verapamil is avoided, as it can inhibit theophylline metabolism. Short-acting agents such as esmolol are preferred. Ventricular arrhythmias and cardiac arrests are managed conventionally. Hypotension is initially managed by conventional supportive therapy. If the patient fails to respond, a trial with beta blockade to reverse the probable $beta_2$-mediated hypotension is considered. Again, the shortest-acting agent available is chosen.

Persistent vomiting may be treated with metoclopramide, which is effective in approximately 50 percent of cases.

Electrolyte disturbances in acute overdoses without other potential causes for the imbalance are managed expectantly. The cellular shifts of electrolyte are transient, and serial monitoring is essential.

ACUTE-ON-CHRONIC THEOPHYLLINE TOXICITY

Patients with acute-on-chronic theophylline toxicity present with the same clinical manifestations as those with acute toxicity, but toxicity develops at lower levels. Acute-on-chronic toxicity is likely in patients taking theophylline who develop multifocal atrial tachycardias, hypotension, or hypokalemia. Seizures occur with the same frequency as in acute presentations but can occur at concentrations >30 mg/L. Significant toxicity is likely with concentrations >60 mg/L in acute-on-chronic and chronic patients, as opposed to >100 mg/L for acute overdoses. Worst-case estimates can be calculated as for acute toxicity, with the addition of 20 mg/L to represent the chronic maintenance level.

Management is similar to that for the acute toxic overdose.

The only variation occurs with the use of elimination-enhancing treatment. The end point of multiple-dose activated charcoal is 30 mg/L, not 20 mg/L. Hemodialysis and charcoal hemoperfusion are indicated prophylactically in patients with theophylline concentrations >100 mg/L in an acute or acute-on-chronic overdose.

CHRONIC THEOPHYLLINE TOXICITY

Chronically theophylline-toxic patients do not present with gastrointestinal bleeding, multifocal atrial tachycardias, hypotension, or hypokalemia. All remaining toxic manifestations of theophylline occur in chronic patients at much lower serum levels.

Seizures in chronic patients present as either one to three partial complex seizures or as generalized tonic-clonic seizures. Status epilepticus is associated with more significant morbidity and mortality. Seizures have been reported in chronic patients with theophylline concentrations >20 mg/L, and the incidence increases significantly with serum concentrations >60 mg/L. Age above 60 years is the sole prognostic factor for chronic toxicities. Serum theophylline concentrations >60 mg/L in chronic overdose may be associated with an increase in morbidity or mortality.

Gastric decontamination is not indicated for the chronic patient. For theophylline concentrations >30 mg/L, oral activated charcoal at 25 g every 2 h is initiated and continued until concentrations are <30 mg/L. Either hemodialysis or charcoal hemoperfusion is indicated in the chronic patient whose serum theophylline concentration is greater than 60 mg/L, especially if the patient is over 60 years of age.

Electrolyte disturbances are treated conventionally in the chronic overdose patient.

For a more detailed discussion, see Paloucek FP: Theophylline, chap. 106, p. 580, in *Pediatric Emergency Medicine: A Comprehensive Study Guide.*

107 Lethal Toxins in Small Doses

Leon Gussow

There are a number of prescription and over-the-counter preparations that are extremely toxic in small amounts. Familiarity with these is essential for the emergency physician.

CAMPHOR

Camphor is present in many over-the-counter linements and cold preparations. Campho-Phenique is 10.80% camphor, Ben-Gay Children's Rub is 5%, and Vicks Vaporub is 4.18%. Camphor has a strong odor and a pungent taste that some children find attractive. It is a rapidly acting neurotoxin that produces both excitation and depression of the central nervous system (CNS). Major toxicity has not been reported for ingestions of less than 30 mg/kg and is rare in ingestions of less than 50 mg/kg. Ingestions of less than 1 tsp of topical liniments or cold preparations should not cause toxicity.

Clinical symptoms begin rapidly. A feeling of generalized warmth progresses to pharyngeal and epigastric burning. Mental status changes can follow, with confusion, restlessness, delirium, and hallucinations. Muscle twitching and fasciculations may herald the onset of seizures, which have also been reported to occur suddenly, without preceding symptoms.

Management of an ingestion of camphor consists of supportive care and gastric decontamination. Gastric lavage is the preferred method. The use of ipecac is discouraged because of the potential for seizures. Lavage is followed by the administration of activated charcoal. Seizures are managed with benzodiazepines. The drug of choice for status epilepticus is phenobarbital.

BENZOCAINE

Benzocaine is present in many local anesthetics, including first-aid ointments and infant teething formulas. Baby Orajel contains 7.5% benzocaine, Baby Orajel Nighttime Formula 10%, and Americaine Topical Anesthetic First Aid Ointment 20%. Exposure can be from oral ingestion or dermal absorption. Benzocaine is metabolized to aniline and nitrosobenzene, both of which can cause methemoglobinemia, especially in infants less than 4 months of age. Methemoglobinemia has occurred in an infant after an ingestion of 100 mg of benzocaine, the amount in 1/4 tsp of Baby Orajel.

Clinical signs and symptoms begin 30 min to 6 h after ingestion, with tachycardia, tachypnea, and cyanosis that does not respond to oxygen. In more severe exposures, agitation, hypoxia, metabolic acidosis, lethargy, stupor, and coma may supervene. Seizures can occur.

Treatment of toxicity consists of gastric emptying, general support, and, in selected cases, the administration of antidote. Gastric emptying is indicated in patients presenting within approximately 30 min of ingestion who have ingested more than 1/4 tsp of a benzocaine-containing substance. Gastric lavage is the preferred method. Ipecac-induced emesis is used with caution due to the risk of seizures. Activated charcoal is administered, along with a cathartic.

The antidote for patients with methemoglobinemia is methylene blue. Indications for its use include methemoglobin levels over 30%, respiratory distress, or altered mental status. The dose is repeated in 1 to 2 h if symptoms persist. Isolated cyanosis is not an indication for methylene blue, since it occurs at low methemoglobin levels, is often well tolerated, and resolves spontaneously. There is a further discussion of the use of methylene blue in Chap. 97.

LOMOTIL

Lomotil is an antidiarrheal preparation that combines an opiate (diphenoxylate) with an anticholinergic (atropine). Several unique properties make Lomotil poisoning extremely dangerous in the pediatric population.

Each tablet or 5 mL of liquid Lomotil contains 2.5 mg diphenoxylate hydrochloride and 0.025 mg atropine sulfate. Ingestions of ½ tablet to 2 tablets have been reported to cause toxic signs and symptoms. Both atropine and diphenoxylate are rapidly absorbed from the gastrointestinal tract, but since the anticholinergic effect from atropine can delay gastric emptying, intact tablets have been recovered on lavage as long as 27 h after ingestion.

Although patients often present with a confusing mixture of opioid and anticholinergic signs and symptoms, opioid effects are always seen in overdose and often predominate. Anticholinergic symptoms can occur before, during, or after opioid manifestations, or they may not occur at all. Initial manifestations of Lomotil overdose in children include drowsiness, lethargy or excitement, dyspnea, irritability, miosis, hypotonia or rigidity, and urinary retention. In severe cases, the patient may present with coma, respiratory depression, hypoxia, and seizures. Symptoms may not be dose-related and can recur as late as 24 h after ingestion. Death is often accompanied by cerebral edema.

Treatment of Lomotil poisoning includes admission of all patients and close monitoring for a minimum of 24 h. Syrup of ipecac is contraindicated. In any patient with CNS or respiratory depression, gastric lavage is indicated even if many hours have passed since ingestion. Multiple-dose activated charcoal (1 g/kg every 4 h) is recommended. A cathartic can be given with the first dose of charcoal. Excessive hydration is avoided to minimize the risk of cerebral edema. Respiratory depression or coma is treated with intravenous naloxone (0.1 mg/kg). When naloxone is given, anticholinergic symptoms may emerge.

CHLOROQUINE

Chloroquine is a powerful, rapidly acting cardiotoxin capable of causing sudden cardiorespiratory collapse. The interval between ingestion and cardiac arrest is often less than 2 h. Chloroquine is used for the treatment and prophylaxis of malaria and also to treat certain connective tissue diseases. Even only a slightly supratherapeutic dose can be toxic in a child; deaths have been associated with ingestions of 0.75 to 1 g.

Chloroquine causes myocardial depression and vasodilatation, producing sudden profound hypotension. The automaticity and conductivity of heart muscle are also decreased, resulting in bradycardia and ventricular escape rhythms. The electrocardiogram can show sinus bradycardia, widened QRS, prolonged intraventricular conduction time, T-wave changes, ST depression, prolonged QT, complete heart block, ventricular tachycardia, or ventricular fibrillation. Neurotoxicity secondary to chloroquine often presents as drowsiness and lethargy, followed by excitability. Dysphagia, facial paresthesia, tremor, slurred speech, hyporeflexia, seizures, and coma can occur.

Treatment is supportive. Intubation, ventilation, defibrillation, and cardiac pacing may be required. Blood pressure is maintained with intravenous fluids and pressors. Class IA antiarrhythmics (quinidine, procainamide, disopyramide) are contraindicated. Gastric lavage is the preferred method of gastric emptying. Activated charcoal (1 g/kg) and a cathartic are given by mouth or via orogastric tube. Recent evidence suggests that early mechanical ventilation with high-dose diazepam and epinephrine may be lifesaving in severe cases. A poison control center should be consulted on any case of significant chloroquine ingestion.

METHYL SALICYLATE

Methyl salicylate is a concentrated liquid that can produce severe salicylate toxicity. It is found in many topical liniments (Ben Gay,

Icy Hot Balm) and in oil of wintergreen food flavoring. One teaspoon of oil of wintergreen contains 7 g of salicylate (equivalent to 21 aspirin tablets). Ingestion of less than a teaspoon has killed a child. Therefore, any ingestion of these preparations is potentially serious. Clinical presentation and treatment of this overdose are similar to those for other salicylate poisoning.

For a more detailed discussion, see Gussow L: Lethal toxins in small doses, chap. 107, p. 584, in *Pediatric Emergency Medicine: A Comprehensive Study Guide.*

SECTION XVIII
ENVIRONMENTAL EMERGENCIES

108 Human and Animal Bites

David A. Townes / Gary R. Strange

In evaluating a bite wound, it is important to determine what type of animal caused the wound and how old the wound is. One must also elicit host factors that may affect wound healing, such as diabetes, peripheral vascular disease, glucocorticoid use, or other immunocompromised states.

The physical examination should include a full exploration of the wound. The type of wound (laceration, crush, or puncture) and the extent of involvement of deep structures must be determined. One should keep in mind that the canine jaw may generate forces up to 450 psi, a force that is sufficient to penetrate the cranium of a child. If the wound occurs over a joint, the joint should be examined through the full range of motion. When appropriate, radiographs should be obtained to look for fractures, foreign bodies, and air in the joint or soft tissues. For bite wounds to the scalp, computed tomography of the head should be considered.

During the physical examination, careful attention should be paid to signs of infection, such as erythema, swelling, discharge, lymphadenopathy, or pain on passive range of motion.

WOUND CARE

The most common complication associated with bite wounds is wound infection. Infection rates run as high as 30 percent for dog bites, 50 percent for cat bites, and 60 percent for human bites.

One of the best ways to reduce the risk of infection is to adequately irrigate the wound. An acceptable method is to irrigate the wound with 1 to 2 L of normal saline through a 19- or 20-gauge vascular catheter. The wound should be debrided as needed. Some authorities recommend extending puncture wounds to allow better irrigation.

The decision on whether to close the wound depends on the type, age, and location of the wound. Under no circumstances should a wound that appears infected be closed. Dog bites may be safely closed if they are not more than 8 to 12 h old and are not located on the hand. In general, cat bites, which are usually puncture wounds, should not be closed. Human bites may be closed if they can be adequately cleaned and are not located on the hand. In most cases, bite wounds on the hand should be left open. Wounds that are more than 8 to 12 h old should also be left open. The exception to this rule is a potentially disfiguring wound on the face, which may be closed even when more than 12 h old. These patients must be followed very carefully for evidence of infection. Surgical consultation should be obtained if there are questions concerning the management of these wounds.

The decision to close any bite wound primarily must come after adequate cleaning of the wound. All bite wounds treated on an outpatient basis should be reevaluated in 48 h.

ANTIBIOTICS

Wounds that have evidence of infection should be treated with antibiotics. The use of antibiotics in prophylaxis remains controversial. The type of animal, location of the wound, and host factors must be considered. Bite wounds caused by cats and humans should be treated prophylactically, while those caused by dogs and rodents may not require treatment with antibiotics. Wounds on the hands and feet should receive antibiotics, while those of the face and scalp are less likely to become infected and do not usually require antibiotics. If the decision to treat with prophylactic antibiotics is made, the initial treatment should be for 3 days. If, at the end of this time, there is no evidence of infection, the wound is very unlikely to become infected.

In general, the organisms responsible for bite wound infections are from the animal's oral flora rather than from the host's skin flora. About one-third of wound infections demonstrate multiple organisms. Dog bites tend to become infected with *Staphylococcus aureus, Streptococcus* sp., and *Pasteurella multocida,* but *Psuedomonas* sp., *Enterobacter cloacae,* and many others have been identified. Cat bites are more likely to become infected with *P. multocida.* This is a rapidly developing infection, with signs and symptoms apparent in less than 24 h. Delay in these findings for more than 24 h should lead the physician to consider other etiologic agents. Human saliva contains 10^8 bacterial per milliliter, with over forty species represented. Human bite wounds tend to become infected with *S. aureus, Streptococcus* sp., and *Eikenella corrodens. Pasteurella multocida* is an unlikely infectious agent in human bite wounds.

Antibiotic choice should be aimed at the most likely infective organisms. *Staphylococcus* and *Streptococcus* spp. may be covered with dicloxacillin or a first-generation cephalosporin. *Pasteurella* coverage is obtained with penicillin, amoxicillin, amoxicillin/clavulanic acid, first-generation cephalosporins, or erythromycin in the penicillin-allergic patient. For human bite wounds, *E. corrodens* may be covered with penicillin or amoxicillin/clavulanic acid, and dicloxacillin can be used to cover *Staphylococcus* and *Streptococcus*. It may be necessary to use a two-antibiotic regimen for human bite wounds.

RABIES PROPHYLAXIS

A special consideration in animal bite wounds is rabies infection. Rabies is caused by the rhabdovirus group and may lead to an atypical encephalomyelitis. The disease is almost universally fatal but, fortunately, rare.

In considering rabies prophylaxis, the physician must consider the type of animal and the prevalence of rabies in the region. If rabies is not suspected, no treatment is necessary. If rabies is suspected, the animal should be captured and quarantined for 10 days. If the animal remains healthy, no treatment is necessary. If the animal becomes ill or if the suspicion of rabies is high, the animal should be sacrificed and the brain examined for evidence of rabies. If the animal proves to be infected, the child should be treated. If the animal cannot be located, decisions regarding prophylaxis must be based solely on the prevalence of rabies in the area and the species of the biting animal. Local animal-control authorities may be helpful in obtaining this information.

The treatment includes human diploid cell vaccine (HDCV), which is given in five 1-mL IM (deltoid or anterolateral thigh) injections on days 1, 3, 7, and 14. The patient should also receive human rabies immune globulin (HRIG). This is dosed at 20 IU/kg, with half being administered IM and the other half infiltrated around the wound.

TETANUS PROPHYLAXIS

Tetanus immunoprophylaxis should also be considered (see Chap. 21).

For a more detailed discussion, see Townes DA, Strange GR: Human and animal bites, chap. 108, p. 587, in *Pediatric Emergency Medicine: A Comprehensive Study Guide.*

109 Snake Envenomations

Timothy Erickson / Bruce E. Herman / Mary Jo A. Bowman

Families of venomous snakes indigenous to the United States include the Crotalidae (pit vipers) and Elapidae (coral snakes). The pit vipers account for over 95 percent of all envenomations and are divided into the genuses *Crotalus* (rattlesnakes), *Agkistrodon* (cottonmouths, copperheads), and *Sistrusus* (pigmy rattlesnakes, massasaugas). Snake envenomation rarely results in death.

PIT VIPERS

Anatomy

Pit vipers classically possess a triangular or arrow-shaped head, whereas nonpoisonous snakes have a smooth, tapered body and narrow head. Crotalids have facial pits between the nostril and eye that serve as heat and vibration sensors, enabling the snake to locate prey. While nonpoisonous snakes typically possess round pupils, pit vipers have vertical or elliptical pupils. The genus *Crotalus* is further characterized by tail rattles.

Pathophysiology

Because of their small body weight, infants and young children are vulnerable to severe envenomation. The severity of envenomation also depends on the location of the bite. Bites on the head or trunk are two to three times more severe than those on the extremities. Bites on the upper extremities are most common and are more dangerous than those on the lower extremities.

The venom itself is a complex mixture of enzymes that primarily function to immobilize, digest, and kill the snake's prey. The major toxic effects occur within the surrounding tissue, blood vessels, and blood components.

Clinical Presentation

Local cutaneous changes classically include one or two puncture marks with pain and swelling at the site, while nonvenomous snakes usually leave a horseshoe-shaped row of multiple teeth marks. If the envenomation is severe, swelling and edema may involve the entire extremity within an hour. Ecchymosis, hemorrhagic vesicles, and petechiae may appear within several hours. Systemic signs and symptoms include parethesias of the scalp, periorbital fasciculations, weakness, diaphoresis, nausea, dizziness, and a minty or metallic taste in the mouth. Severe bites can result in coagulopathies and disseminated intravascular coagulation (DIC). Rapid hypotension and shock, with pulmonary edema and renal and cardiac dysfunction, can also result, particularly if the victim suffers a direct intravenous envenomation.

Management

The bitten extremity is immobilized and physical activity minimized. To maintain renal flow and intravascular volume, oral fluids are vigorously administered. Anecdotal first aid measures can actually be dangerous. Incision and suction of the bite wound with the human mouth may result in tissue damage or infection. Mechanical suction devices exist; however, no human clinical trials support their use. Cryotherapy can lead to further wound necrosis and is not currently recommended. Recently, electric shock therapy was highly publicized as a first aid treatment of snake bites. Case reports and animal studies have not documented any improvement with this technique. Wounds are graded as minimal, with local cutaneous swelling and tenderness at the bite site; moderate, with significant extremity swelling and evidence of systemic toxicity; and severe, with obvious systemic findings, unstable vital signs, and laboratory evidence of coagulopathy.

Laboratory tests include a complete blood count, platelet count, prothrombin time/partial thromboplastin time, fibrin split products, electrolytes, blood urea nitrogen/creatinine, creatine phosphokinase, blood type, and cross-matched blood products. The patient's tetanus prophylaxis is updated, and broad-spectrum antibiotics are administered in moderate or severe envenomations. The progression of the edema and swelling is carefully monitored. If evidence of compartment syndrome in the involved extremity exists, orthopedic consultation is obtained.

Aside from supportive care, Crotalidae antivenin is the fundamental treatment of pit viper envenomation. The antivenin is a high-affinity antibody that binds to the venom proteins and enhances elimination. It is effective against envenomations from rattlesnakes, cottonmouths, copperheads, fer-de-lance, cantiles, and South American bushmasters. The amount of antivenin administered depends on the severity of the envenomation. Antivenin is packaged in vials of 10 mL each. In general, if the envenomation is rated as minimal, 5 vials are administered; in moderate cases, 10 vials; and in severe cases, 15 vials. Compared with adults, pediatric patients are given proportionately more antivenin, since children receive a greater amount of venom per kilogram of body weight. Antivenin is most efficacious if given within 4 to 6 h of the bite. It is of less value if delayed for 8 h and is of questionable value after 24 h. Prior to any antivenin administration, skin testing is done with dilute horse serum given subcutaneously (usually available in the antivenin kit). In the setting of a severe envenomation, patients with positive skin reactions can still receive the antivenin, although only with close monitoring for anaphylaxis and pretreatment with diphenhydramine and glucocorticoids.

Complications of the antivenin therapy include anaphylaxis and serum sickness. Serum sickness usually develops 1 to 20 days after antivenin administration and correlates with the number of vials given. It is generally self-limited and effectively treated with antihistamines and a short course of glucocorticoids.

Disposition

The prognosis following pit viper envenomation is generally good, with an overall mortality rate of less than 1 percent if the antivenin is given in adequate amounts without delay. Even when the antivenin is withheld due to severe allergic reactions, the morbidity and mortality are low. If a pediatric patient only has a suspected bite, develops no signs or symptoms of envenomation during 6 h of observation, and has normal laboratory studies, the child can be discharged. Exceptions to the rule are bites from the Mojave rattlesnake, which can cause delayed neurologic and respiratory depression several hours after envenomation. If the child exhibits moderate to severe envenomation, has evidence of coagulopathy, or requires antivenin administration, admission is indicated.

CORAL SNAKES

Micrurus euryxanthus (western coral snake) is located in Arizona and New Mexico, and *Micrurus fulvius* (eastern coral snake) is found in the Carolinas and the Gulf states. An informative quote that differentiates the coral snakes from other nonpoisonous snakes is "red on yellow, kill a fellow; red on black, venom lack," which refers to the colored bands that run vertically down the body of the coral snake. Coral snakes account for only 1 to 2 percent of annual snake bites in the United States.

Clinical Presentation

The venom of the coral snake is primarily neurotoxic. The bite site will initially exhibit local cutaneous edema, swelling, and tenderness. However, there have been reports of envenomation without evidence of actual teeth marks. Within several hours, the patient may experience parethesias, vomiting, weakness, diplopia, fasciculations, confusion, and occasionally respiratory depression. Convulsions have been observed in smaller children. The fatality rate from eastern coral snake bites is as high as 10 percent.

Management

Coral snake bites are treated aggressively, since a significant bite can lead to neurologic and respiratory depression within the first 24 h. The antivenin is administered early in the treatment course. The coral snake antivenin is effective against bites of the eastern coral snake. It is not efficacious against western coral snake envenomations. Three to five vials of the antivenin are generally recommended following skin testing. As with the *Crotalid* antivenin, adverse side effects include anaphylaxis and serum sickness.

Disposition

Any child who has sustained a documented bite from a coral snake is admitted to the intensive care unit for airway management and appropriate antivenin administration for a 24- to 48-h period.

EXOTIC SNAKES

Several bites occur each year from nonindigenous snakes. Physicians encountering victims of exotic snake envenomation may receive assistance in treatment by calling the Antivenom Index at 602-626-6016 in Tucson, Arizona. The general approach is local wound care and supportive treatment.

For a more detailed discussion, see Erickson T, Herman BE, Bowman MJA: Snake envenomations, chap. 109, p. 590, in *Pediatric Emergency Medicine: A Comprehensive Study Guide.*

---

110 Spider Bites

Bruce E. Herman / Timothy Erickson / Mary Jo A. Bowman

At least 50 to 60 species of spiders in the United States are known to bite humans, although in most cases the diagnosis is not suspected and no treatment is necessary. Only the black widow and brown recluse spiders are known to cause significant wounds and, rarely, death.

BLACK WIDOW SPIDERS

Anatomy

Widow spiders, or the genus *Latrodectus,* are found throughout the temperate and tropical zones of the earth. *Latrodectus mactans,* the black widow spider of North America, is a shiny black spider with eight eyes, eight legs, fangs, and poison glands, with a recognizable red hourglass configuration on the ventral surface of its abdomen.

Black widow spiders normally bite only as a feeding or defense mechanism. Only the female is toxic. The most common envenomation site is the hand.

Latrodectus venom is a potent toxin. Physiologically, the venom of the black widow facilitates exocytosis of synaptic vesicles and the release of the neurotransmitters norepinephrine, gamma-aminobutyric acid, and acetylcholine. The toxin also causes degeneration of motor endplates, resulting in denervation. The venom destablilizes nerve cell membranes by opening ionic channels, causing a massive influx of calcium into the cell, which results in hypocalcemia.

Clinical Presentation

Latrodectus bites produce a characteristic syndrome. The bite typically produces a pinprick or a burning sensation and frequently goes unnoticed. Within the first few hours, the bite site may develop redness, cyanosis, urticaria, or a characteristic halo-target lesion. This is followed by more generalized symptoms consisting of pain in the regional lymph nodes, chest, abdomen, and lower back. The pain classically descends down the lower extremities, with burning of the soles of the feet. Abdominal rigidity, along with vomiting, is often severe enough to be mistaken for a surgical emergency. Flexor spasm of the limbs will cause the patient to assume a fetal position while writhing in pain. Patients may also demonstrate hypertension, sweating, salivation, dyspnea with increased bronchosecretions, and convulsions. If untreated, symptoms may last for up to 7 days, with persistent muscle weakness and pain for several weeks. Although uncommon, death can result from respiratory or cardiac failure, with overall mortality rates of 4 to 5 percent.

Management

For local pain relief, early application of ice to the bitten area may be effective. Tetanus prophylaxis should be updated, but antibiotics are not routinely indicated unless there is evidence of wound infection. For pain control, opiates are useful but are often suboptimal, particularly if administered orally. A parenteral opiate such as morphine is recommended. Muscle relaxants such as diazepam have been commonly administered; these provide some, but limited pain relief. Because of the relative hypocalcemia induced by black widow spider bites, many recommend 10% calcium gluconate at 1 to 2 mL/kg up to 10 mL/dose given slowly with careful cardiac monitoring as the first-line treatment in symptomatic patients. However, many of the reports regarding the use of calcium have been anecdotal, and more recent studies refute its effectiveness; these studies strongly recommend administration of *Latrodectus*-specific antivenin with severe envenomations. The antivenin is available in Australia and Arizona, where these envenomations most commonly occur. Since the antivenin is derived from horse serum, the patient should be skin tested by injecting a 1 : 10 dilution subcutaneously prior to full administration of the antivenin to avoid anaphylactic reactions. The use of *Latrodectus*-specific antivenin is restricted to patients with severe envenomation and no allergic contraindications in whom opioids and benzodiazepines are ineffective. Patients who should receive the antivenin early include the very young and the elderly as well as those with hypertensive and cardiac disease. The antivenin provides relief within 1 to 2 h, and readministration is rarely indicated. Patients receiving the antivenin may experience flulike symptoms or serum sickness 1 to 3 weeks following treatment. This entity is generally self-limited and responsive to antihistamines and steroids.

Disposition

Any symptomatic pediatric patient who has suffered a bite from a black widow spider is admitted for observation and pain control. If there is cardiopulmonary compromise or convulsions, the child is admitted to the intensive care unit for stabilization and antivenin administration.

The venom acts directly on the cell wall, causing immediate injury and death. Following cell wall damage, an intravascular coagulation process causes a cascade of clotting abnormalities and local polymorphonuclear leukocyte infiltration, culminating in a necrotic ulcer.

BROWN RECLUSE SPIDERS

Anatomy

The brown recluse spider, or *Loxosceles reclusa,* is a brown- to fawn-colored spider 1 to 5 cm in length with a characteristic violin or fiddle-shaped area on the dorsal cephalothorax (also nicknamed "fiddleback spider"). They have long, slender legs, and have six eyes instead of the eight typical of most spiders.

Clinical Presentation

The clinical response of loxoscelism ranges from a cutaneous irritation (necrotic arachnidism) to a life-threatening systemic reaction, although there have been no proven fatalities in North America. Signs and symptoms of envenomation are most often localized to the bite area. Normally, there is little pain at the time of the bite. Within a few hours, the patient will experience itching, swelling, erythema, and tenderness over the bite. Classically, erythema surrounds a dull blue-grey macule circumscribed by a ring or halo of pallor. This color difference is important in identifying necrotic arachnidism. Gradually, within 3 to 4 days, the wound forms a necrotic base with a central black eschar. Within 7 to 14 days, the wound develops a full necrotic ulceration.

The systemic reaction, which is much less common than the cutaneous reaction, is associated with a higher morbidity. The reaction rarely correlates with the severity of the cutaneous lesion. Within 24 to 72 h following the envenomation, the patient experiences fever, chills, myalgias, and arthralgias. If the systemic reaction is severe, the patient may suffer coagulopathies, disseminated intravascular coagulation (DIC), convulsions, renal failure, and hemolytic anemia, heralded by the passage of dark urine.

Management

The proper management of envenomation by the brown recluse spider depends on whether the reaction is local or systemic. Since it is difficult to predict which types of wound will eventually progress to a disfiguring necrotic ulcer, the wound should be cleaned, tetanus immunization updated, and the involved extremity immobilized to reduce pain and swelling. Early application of ice to the bite area lessens the local wound reaction, whereas heat will exacerbate the symptoms. Antibiotic treatment is indicated only in secondary wound infections. Antihistamines may prove beneficial, particularly in children. Many experts advocate the use of a polymorphonuclear leukocyte inhibitor such as dapsone to diminish the amount of scarring and subsequent surgical complications. However, because of limited human studies and the potential for dapsone to induce methemoglobinemia, cautious administration is recommended in the pediatric population. Although supported in the early literature, early excisional treatment can cause complications such as recurrent wound breakdown and hand dysfunction.

A better approach is to wait until the necrotic process has subsided (usually within several weeks) and perform secondary closure with skin grafting as indicated. The systemic effects of brown recluse spider envenomation can be life-threatening and should be treated aggressively. Although not proven in clinical trials, glucocorticoids may provide a protective effect on the red blood cell (RBC) membrane, thus slowing the hemolysis. The patient must be monitored closely for the development of DIC. Transfusion of RBCs and platelets may be necessary. Urine alkalinization with bicarbonate may lessen renal damage if the patient is experiencing acute hemolysis. Although it is not commercially available in the United States, there is ongoing research with a brown recluse antivenin.

Disposition

Patients with a rapidly expanding lesion or necrotic area with evidence of hemolysis are hospitalized. Patients who are asymptomatic following a period of observation in the emergency department and have normal baseline laboratory data may be discharged home with close outpatient follow-up and wound care within 24 to 48 h.

TARANTULAS

Tarantulas are widely feared because they are the largest of all spiders. Found in the deserts of the western United States, these large, hairy spiders are relatively harmless. They are extremely shy and bite only when vigorously provoked or roughly handled. Their bite produces only local pain and edema. Treatment consists of local wound care and tetanus prophylaxis. Of more concern are hairs on their abdomen, which, when flicked off in defense, are capable of producing urticaria and pruritis that may persist for several weeks. Treatment includes antihistamines and topical glucocorticoids.

SCORPIONS

Worldwide, scorpions are responsible for thousands of deaths annually. In the United States, there have been no reported deaths from scorpion stings in more than 25 years. Nevertheless, they remain a public health concern throughout the South and Southwest. Only the southwestern desert scorpion, *Centruroides exilicauda* (formerly *C. sculpturatus*), poses a serious health concern in the United States. *Centruroides* venoms cause spontaneous depolarization of nerves of both the sympathetic and parasympathetic nervous systems.

Most victims will have only local pain, tenderness, and tingling; however, younger children and those who suffer more serious envenomations may manifest the venom effects as overstimulation of the sympathetic, parasympathetic, and central nervous systems. Elevation of all the vital signs usually occurs within an hour of envenomation, and tachydysrhythmias may develop during this time. Dysconjugate, roving eye movements are very common in children, along with other neurologic findings that include muscle fasciculations, weakness, agitation, and opisthotonos. Less common findings are ataxia, respiratory distress, and seizures.

The treatment of *Centruroides* envenomations is supportive. Cool compresses and analgesics are used for the local symptoms and pain. Wound care and tetanus prophylaxis are indicated. Tachydysrhythmias and hypertension may be treated with intravenous beta blockers; esmolol or labetolol is preferable to propranolol. Benzodiazepines may be helpful for agitation and muscle spasms. Advanced life support and airway control are essential for more severe envenomations. A hyperimmune goat serum antivenin has been used with success for more severe envenomations with potentially life-threatening symptoms; however, it is available only in Arizona. Consultation for treatment is available through the Arizona Poison Control System at 602-626-6016.

HYMENOPTERA

The order Hymenoptera includes bees, vespids (hornets and wasps), and fire ants. While Hymenoptera venoms possess intrinsic toxicity, it is their ability to sensitize the victim and cause subsequent anaphylactic reactions that makes them so lethal.

Bees and Vespids

Honey bees (*Apis mellifera*) are fuzzy insects with alternating black and tan body stripes. Not intrinsically aggressive, they usually sting defensively when stepped on. The stinger can be removed manually but should be scraped off with lateral pressure rather than grasped to avoid injecting more venom.

African "killer" bees (*Apis mellifera scutellata*) are present in the United States in areas where winter temperatures average more than 60°F. They attack in swarms, and death has occurred as a result of the large amount of venom injected.

The most common hornets in the United States are the yellow jackets (*Vespa pennsylvanica*). They are extremely aggressive and sting with little provocation.

Wasps (*Polistes annularis,* the paper wasp) have thin, smooth bodies and a formidable sting. The vespids are "carnivorous," able to use their smooth stingers multiple times to kill smaller insects and worms.

Although their enzymes are similar, there is little immunologic cross-reactivity between bee and vespid venoms. While a bee sting may not sensitize a person to yellow jackets, a yellow jacket sting would more likely sensitize one to wasps.

Sting reactions are usually classified as local, toxic, or systemic. Local reactions are generally mild. There is variable edema and erythema associated with pain at the sting site. Treatment is symptomatic, with ice or cold compresses and an antihistamine. In more severe local reactions, there is a more sustained inflammatory response; the swelling may spread to the entire extremity and persist for several days. A short course of prednisone (1 mg/kg/day for 5 days) may decrease the duration of symptoms. Toxic reactions reflect the effects of multiple stings. Gastrointestinal symptoms are the principal features; urticaria and bronchospasm are not usually present. Treatment is supportive.

Systemic reactions occur in approximately 1 percent of Hymenoptera stings. They range from mild, non-life-threatening cutaneous reactions to classic anaphylactic shock. These reactions are generally IgE-mediated and reflect previous sensitization. However, 50 to 80 percent of patients who die from insect stings have no prior history of hypersensitivity. Sensitivity causes degranulation and the release of mediators of anaphylaxis. The majority (70 percent) of systemic reactions in children consist of generalized urticaria, pruritus, or angioedema. More severe reactions are manifested as bronchospasm, laryngeal edema, and hypotensive shock secondary to massive vasodilation.

In all but the mildest of systemic reactions, the mainstay of treatment is epinephrine. Epinephrine counteracts the bronchospastic and vasodilatory effects of histamine. Epinephrine can be given as a subcutaneous injection (0.01 mL/kg of 1:1000 solution). In more severe reactions, the intravenous or endotracheal route is preferred (0.1 mL/kg of 1:10,000 solution). The dose may be repeated at 15-min intervals as needed. Early intubation is indicated for evidence of severe laryngeal edema or stridor, as airway obstruction is the leading cause of death in anaphylaxis. Antihistamines should be given early, but not as a substitute for epinephrine. An H_2-receptor blocker (e.g., cimetidine or ranitidine), in addition to an H_1-receptor blocker (diphenhydramine), may aid in inhibiting the vasodilatory effects of histamine. Adjunctive therapy for bronchospasm might include inhaled $beta_2$ agonists (e.g., albuterol) and intravenous aminophylline. When hypotension is present, vigorous isotonic fluid resuscitation should be instituted. The use of MAST (military anti-shock trousers) may be helpful while

TABLE 110-1 Epinephrine Injection Kits for Emergency Self-Treatment of Systemic Reactions to Insect Stings

Injection kit	Dose delivered
Epi Pen Auto-Injector[a] (0.3 mg)	0.3 mL of 1 : 1000 epinephrine
Epi Pen Jr. Auto-Injector[a] (0.5 mg)	0.3 mL of 1 : 2000 epinephrine
Ana-Kit[b]	Up to 0.6 mL of 1 : 1000 epinephrine (0.3 mL at one time, total of 0.6 mg)

[a] Epi Pen and Epi Pen Jr. are spring-loaded automatic injectors distributed by Center Laboratories, 35 Channel Drive, Port Washington, NY 11050.

[b] Ana-Kit can deliver fractional doses; it is distributed by Hollister-Stein Pharmaceutical Division, Spokane, WA 99207. The kit also contains four chewable antihistamine tablets.

Source: Adapted from Graft DF: Stinging insect allergy: How management has changed. *Postgrad Med* 85:175, 1987.

fluid repletion is underway. Glucocorticoids should be given for their anti-inflammatory effects as well as their effect on preventing the late-phase response. An effort should be made to look for the presence of any stingers still in the skin and to remove them by scraping. A delayed serum sickness–like reaction may appear 10 to 14 days following the initial sting. This immune complex disorder may be treated with a short course of prednisone.

Patients who have had a systemic reaction should be instructed to avoid Hymenoptera habitats. Portable epinephrine kits are available (see Table 110-1). They should be prescribed prior to the patient's leaving the emergency department. The patient should be urged to carry the kit at all times and to use epinephrine with any systemic symptoms. Even if symptoms are mild, the patient should still seek emergency care. The patient should also be instructed to wear a medical alert tag.

Venom immunotherapy desensitization is very effective in preventing further systemic reactions, with 95 to 100 percent protection after 3 months of treatment. Referral to an allergist is indicated for any child who has life-threatening respiratory symptoms (e.g., stridor or wheezing) or hypotension. Children less than 16 years old who have only urticaria and/or angioedema do not require venom immunotherapy. Only 10 percent of these children will have systemic reactions with subsequent stings.

Imported Fire Ants

Two species of fire ants have been imported into the United States: the red fire ant (*Solenopsis invicta*) and the black fire ant (*Sole-*

nopsis richteri), of which *S. invicta* is the predominant species. They are presently found in 13 southern states, from Florida to Texas, their geographic range apparently limited by soil, temperature, and moisture.

Fire ants tend to attack in swarms, with multiple stings the norm. Stings are more common among children and occur most frequently on their ankles and feet during the summer months.

Fire ants first bite the victim with powerful mandibles, then, if undisturbed, will arch the body and swivel around the attached mandibles to sting the victim repeatedly with the stinger. This produces a characteristic circular pattern of papules/stings around two central punctures.

Fire ant venoms produce a sharp, burning sensation, hence the name "fire" ant. The venoms have cytotoxic, bactericidal, insecticidal, and hemolytic properties. They also activate the complement pathway and promote histamine release. Fire ant venoms are immunogenic and result in sensitization of the sting victim and the risk of future anaphylaxis.

The initial bites and stings cause burning pain associated with circular wheals or papules around the central hemorrhagic punctures. The wheal-and-flare reactions resolve within 1 h but then develop into sterile pustules within 24 h. The pustules slough off over 48 to 72 h, leaving shallow ulcerated lesions. The pustules are intensely pruritic and often become contaminated after the victim scratches the lesions. These secondary infections are usually minor but may cause considerable morbidity. No intervention has been shown to prevent or resolve the pustules, and treatment consists of local conservative measures: application of ice or cool compresses for symptomatic relief and gentle, frequent cleansing of the affected areas to prevent secondary infections. An oral antihistamine may be helpful for the pruritus.

Between 15 and 50 percent of victims develop more severe local reactions, characterized by an exaggerated wheal-and-flare response followed by the development of erythema, edema, and induration greater than 5 cm in diameter. These lesions are intensely pruritic, may resemble cellulitis, and persist for 24 to 72 h before subsiding. Topical glucocorticoid ointments, local anesthetic creams, and oral antihistamines may be useful for the itching associated with these reactions.

Anaphylactic reactions have been estimated to occur after as many as 1 percent of fire ant stings. Anaphylaxis may occur several hours after a sting, and is known to occur more frequently in children than in adults.

Immunotherapy may be appropriate for persons with severe hypersensitivity to fire ant venom, or who have had a previous anaphylactic reaction to a fire ant sting. The efficacy of immunotherapy has been variable, but it has been reported to provide as high as 98 percent protection.

For a more detailed discussion, see Herman BE, Erickson T, Bowman MJA: Spider bites, chap. 110, p. 593, in *Pediatric Emergency Medicine: A Comprehensive Study Guide.*

111 Marine Envenomations

Bruce E. Herman / Mary Jo A. Bowman

COELENTERATES

Coelenterates include jellyfish, sea anemones, and corals. They envenomate through venom-coated threads that are found in specialized epithelial cells that cover the tentacles. Upon contact or when encountering a change in osmolality, these threads are injected through the epidermis to the nerve- and vascular-rich dermis. Both living and dead coelenterates can envenomate.

Jellyfish envenomations are the most common marine envenomations. The most feared jellyfish is the Portuguese man-of-war (*Physalia physalis*). This jellyfish is most commonly found in the Gulf of Mexico and off the Florida coasts. Envenomation causes characteristic linear, spiral, painful urticarial lesions. The pain occurs almost instantly, peaks within a few hours, and persists for many more. Systemic symptoms may include nausea, vomiting, muscle cramps, diaphoresis, weakness, hemolysis, and, rarely, vascular collapse and death.

The most commonly encountered jellyfish is the sea nettle (*Chrysacra quinquecirrha*), which is widely distributed in temperate and tropical waters. Sea nettles cause predominantly local effects consisting of painful urticarial lesions. Treatment includes reassurance of the patient and immobilization of the injured part. Ice may provide some analgesia. The area is rinsed with sterile saline or seawater to maintain isosmolar conditions and wash off unfired nematocysts. Fresh water is not used because it is hyposmolar and will activate unfired nematocysts. To inactivate nematocysts remaining on the skin, various remedies such as vinegar (5% acetic acid solution), baking soda pastes, shaving cream, or Adolph's

Meat Tenderizer (papain) are useful. The inactivated nematocysts are then removed by gentle scraping or shaving. Analgesics and antihistamines are helpful. Tetanus immunization is indicated, but prophylactic antibiotics are not.

Sea anemones and corals are sessile creatures that cause local urticarial reactions upon contact. Contact with hard corals may cause lacerations that are treated with vigorous local wound care, tetanus prophylaxis, and a broad-spectrum antibiotic.

VENOMOUS FISH

Stingrays are the most commonly encountered venomous fish, with over 2000 stings reported annually. When startled or stepped on, the stingray drives its venom-laden sting into the victim. Parts of the sheath may be torn away and remain in the wound. The venom is short-acting, is heat-labile, and causes varying degrees of neurologic and cardiovascular disturbance. Intense pain out of proportion to the injury is the initial finding, peaking within 1 h but lasting up to 48 h. Signs and symptoms are usually limited to the injured area, but weakness, nausea, anxiety, and syncope in response to the severe pain have been reported. Treatment of the wound includes irrigation with sterile saline or seawater to dilute the venom and remove sheath fragments. The injured part is immersed in hot water at no more than 113°F for 30 to 90 min to inactivate the heat-labile venom. Analgesics are usually required. Because of the penetrating nature of the envenomation, wounds are debrided and left open. Tetanus immunization is updated, and broad-spectrum prophylactic antibiotics—trimethoprim/sulfamethoxazole (TMP/SMX) or a third-generation cephalosporin—administered.

Scorpion fish include scorpion fish (*Scorpaena*), zebrafish (*Pterois*), lionfish, and stonefish (*Synanceja*), in increasing order of venom toxicity. The venoms are heat-labile and cause immediate intense pain that peaks within 60 to 90 min and persists for up to 12 h. Local erythema or blanching, edema, and paresthesias may persist for weeks. Systemic findings include nausea and vomiting, weakness, dizziness, and respiratory distress. Treatment is immersion of the affected limb in hot water (113°F) for 30 to 90 min, or until pain is relieved. Wounds are irrigated with sterile saline, explored, and cleaned of debris. The wound is left open and treated with prophylactic antibiotics (TMP/SMX or a third-generation cephalosporin) in addition to tetanus prophylaxis.

Stonefish envenomations can cause dyspnea, hypotension, and cardiovascular collapse within 1 h and death within 6 h. They can also cause local necrosis and severe pain that may persist for days.

Treatment of stonefish envenomations is the same as that for envenomations of other scorpion fish, with special attention given to maintaining cardiovascular support.

Catfish

More than 1000 species of *catfish* are found in both fresh and salt water. Stings occur from spines contained within an integumentary sheath on their dorsal or pectoral fins. The heat-labile venoms contain dermatonecrotic, vasoconstrictive, and other bioactive agents and produce symptoms similar to those of mild stingray envenomations. A stinging, burning, throbbing sensation occurs immediately and usually resolves within 60 to 90 min, but will occasionally last up to 48 h. Treatment is immediate immersion in hot water (no more than 113°F) for pain relief. Catfish spines may penetrate the skin and break off. The spines can be seen on radiographs. The wound should be explored and debrided, and any retained catfish spines should be removed. The puncture wound should be left open and treated with prophylactic broad-spectrum antibiotics, in addition to tetanus prophylaxis.

ECHINODERMS

Echinoderms are spiny invertebrates that include sea urchins, starfish, sand dollars, and sea cucumbers. Of these, sea urchins are the only ones that regularly cause medically significant envenomations. Their venom can cause local pain that may persist for days. Treatment is immediate immersion in hot water (no more than 113°F), careful removal of pedicellariae and radiopaque spines, and vigorous local wound care. Tetanus immunization and broad-spectrum antibiotic prophylaxis are indicated.

For a more detailed discussion, see Herman BE, Bowman MJA: Marine envenomations, chap. 111, p. 599, in *Pediatric Emergency Medicine: A Comprehensive Study Guide.*

112 Near Drowning

Simon Ros

Drowning is to die from suffocation in water, and near drowning is to survive, at least temporarily, after suffocation by submersion in water. *Secondary drowning* refers to delayed death (>24 h after submersion) due to rapid deterioration of respiratory status. *Immersion syndrome* refers to sudden death following contact with icy-cold water.

The primary injury following submersion occurs in the lung. Hypoxemia, the result of the pulmonary dysfunction, is the cause of the secondary injuries to the brain and heart. Fluid aspiration occurs in 90 percent of drowning victims, but it is unusual for large quantities of water to be aspirated during drowning. Laryngospasm prevents aspiration in 10 percent of the cases and results in a "dry" drowning.

The pathophysiology of lung injury following drowning is dependent on the characteristics of the aspirated fluid. Aspiration of fresh water inactivates surfactant and damages the alveolar basement membrane. The loss of surfactant's surface tension activity results in alveolar collapse and a ventilation-perfusion mismatch. The hypotonic water is rapidly absorbed into the pulmonary circulation. Aspiration of hypertonic seawater results in the movement of intravascular fluid into the alveoli, with subsequent edema and shunting.

Hypothermia appears to exert a protective effect on drowning victims. Low body temperature decreases oxygen requirements, thus enabling organs to survive without oxygen for prolonged periods of time. The diving reflex, which results in preferential shunting of blood to the brain and the heart, has been suggested as an additional contributing factor to intact survival following extended submersion in very cold (≤40°F) water (see Chap. 116).

MANAGEMENT

Prehospital Care

Early initiation of cardiopulmonary resuscitation in a submersion victim is of paramount importance. As cardiopulmonary resuscitation in the water is not effective, the patient must be extricated as soon as possible. In view of the possibility of neck injury, cervical spine precautions are maintained throughout the patient's management.

Once the patient is on firm land, the ABCs (airway, breathing, and circulation) are attended to. Oxygen is administered to all patients. Airway maintenance and copious secretions are among the indications for endotracheal intubation. Postural drainage maneuvers are not recommended and may delay cardiopulmonary resuscitation. Cardiac monitoring is begun as soon as possible. Wet clothing is removed to minimize heat loss. Prolonged delay in transport in order to obtain IV access must be avoided. All submersion victims are taken to a hospital for evaluation regardless of their clinical condition following initial stabilization.

Hospital Management

Reevaluation of the ABCs is in the initial hospital management of a submersion victim. All patients are placed on a cardiopulmonary monitor and pulse oximeter, and 100% oxygen is administered by mask or endotracheal tube. Persistent hypoxemia suggests the need for continuous positive airway pressure (CPAP) or positive end-expiratory pressure (PEEP). Patients who have an arterial $P_{O_2} < 50$ mmHg or $P_{CO_2} > 50$ mmHg while on 100% oxygen are intubated. Apnea, unstable airway, and prevention of aspiration represent some of the other indications for intubation. A chest radiograph and an arterial blood gas are obtained as soon as possible.

Bronchospasm in submersion victims is treated with selective beta agonists, such as albuterol. Glucocorticoids and prophylactic antibiotics have not been proven to be of benefit.

A nasogastric tube is inserted in all submersion victims in order to prevent gastric dilatation. Intravenous access must be established promptly and poor perfusion treated with intravenous fluids. Repeated boluses of normal saline or Ringer's lactate (20 mL/kg) are administered until the patient's circulation is stable. Pressor agents, such as dopamine or dobutamine, are used if fluid volume management is ineffective. A Foley catheter is inserted in order to monitor urine output.

Hypothermia is managed by preventing additional heat loss (heat lamps and the removal of wet clothes) and by core rewarming. Hypothermia merits lengthier resuscitative efforts in view of the reports of survivors following prolonged submersion in icy water.

The management of patients with suspected hypoxic cerebral injury includes hyperventilation, head elevation (in the absence of cervical spine injury), furosemide, and muscle relaxants. The use of intracranial pressure (ICP) monitoring, dexamethasone, mannitol, and high-dose barbiturates is no longer recommended.

Hypoxic seizures are controlled with intravenous diazepam (0.3 mg/kg) and phenytoin (20 mg/kg). Emergent computed tomography of the head is indicated in all patients with suspected intracranial injury.

Toxicologic studies should be considered in all victims of submersion.

DISPOSITION

Asymptomatic patients with normal arterial blood gases and chest radiography may be discharged after a 6-h period of observation. All other patients are admitted to the hospital. Near-drowning victims must not be discharged from the emergency department without observation because of the possibility of delayed pulmonary complications.

For a more detailed discussion, see Ros S: Near drowning, chap. 112, p. 601, in *Pediatric Emergency Medicine: A Comprehensive Study Guide.*

---

113 Burns

Donald Scott Hill / Gary R. Strange

Burns are described in terms of location, depth, and body surface area involved. *Location* is an important determinant of disposition. Burns of the hands, feet, and perineum should always be considered serious, and all significant burns in these locations should initially be managed in the hospital, preferably in a burn center. *Depth* of the burn is estimated by clinical criteria, which are used to classify the burn by degrees.

1. *First-degree burns* involve only the epidermis. The skin is erythematous, but there are no blisters. Sensation is preserved. A common example is sunburn. First-degree burns heal within 1 week and require only symptomatic treatment.
2. *Second-degree burns* are partial-thickness burns that involve the dermis to a variable degree. The dermal appendages are always preserved and provide a source for regeneration. Second-degree burns are characterized by the presence of marked

edema, erythema, blistering, and weeping from the wound. There is usually marked tenderness to palpation. Deep partial-thickness burns may be difficult to distinguish from full-thickness burns. The most common causes of second-degree burns are exposure to hot liquids and flames. Healing requires 2 to 3 weeks.

3. *Third-degree burns* are full-thickness injuries. The dermis and dermal appendages are destroyed. The skin appears whitish or leathery. The surface is dry and nontender to palpation. Third-degree burns result when there is prolonged exposure to fire or hot liquids.

The *body surface area* (BSA) involved is also important in determining treatment and disposition. The percentage surface area involved in the burn is estimated by the "rule of nines" in adults, but in children the proportion of body surface area made up by anatomic parts, especially the head, varies considerably with age (Fig. 113-1).

DIAGNOSTIC EVALUATION

History and Physical Examination

The history of the events leading to the burn may be helpful in assessing the degree of injury and the likelihood of other injuries, such as smoke inhalation and blunt trauma. Concomitant medical problems, medications, allergies, and tetanus immunization status should be ascertained.

Primary Survey

The airway is assessed immediately on presentation. The most common cause of death during the first hour after a burn injury is respiratory impairment. Inhalation injury produces upper airway edema, which can proceed with alarming speed to complete airway obstruction. As edema develops, successful intubation becomes increasingly difficult. Therefore, intubation is indicated early in the emergency department course of patients who have signs of upper airway involvement (Table 113-1).

Humidified oxygen is used to maintain oxygenation. Positive end-expiratory pressure (PEEP) or continuous positive airway pressure (CPAP) may be useful to improve oxygenation when there is pulmonary involvement. Bronchospasm is treated with beta-adrenergic agonists. Close monitoring of oxygen saturation by pulse oximetry, supplemented by arterial blood gases, is indicated.

Patients with greater than 15 percent BSA burns require a large-bore intravenous line for isotonic fluid administration. A second

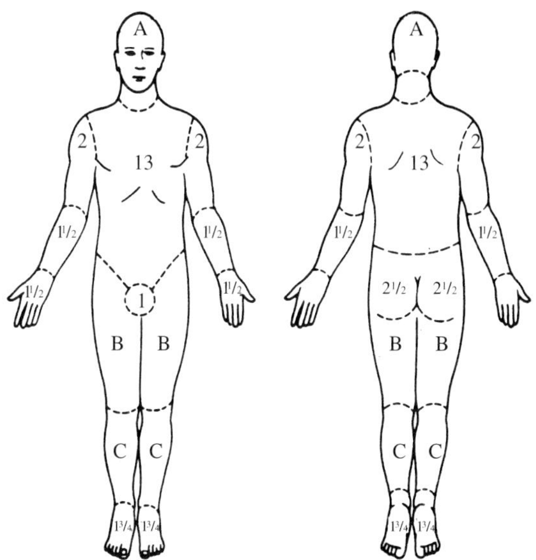

Relative Percentages of Areas Affected by Growth (Age in Years)

	0	1	5	10	15	Adult
A: half of head	$9\frac{1}{2}$	$8\frac{1}{2}$	$6\frac{1}{2}$	$5\frac{1}{2}$	$4\frac{1}{2}$	$3\frac{1}{2}$
B: half of thigh	$2\frac{3}{4}$	$3\frac{1}{4}$	4	$4\frac{1}{4}$	$4\frac{1}{2}$	$4\frac{3}{4}$
C: half of leg	$2\frac{1}{2}$	$2\frac{1}{2}$	$2\frac{3}{4}$	3	$3\frac{1}{4}$	$3\frac{1}{2}$

Second degree ________ and
Third degree __________ =
Total percent burned ___

FIG. 113-1 Classic Lund and Browder chart. Reproduced with permission from Dimick AR: Burns, in Tintinalli JE, Krome RL, Ruiz E: *Emergency Medicine: A Comprehensive Study Guide*. New York: McGraw-Hill, 1992, p 692.

TABLE 113-1 Indications for Early Intubation in Burn Patients

Stridor
Hoarseness
Rales
Wheezing
Singed nasal hairs
Carbonized sputum
Cyanosis
Altered mental status

line is advisable for extensive burns and is essential if there are signs of cardiovascular instability.

Secondary Survey

After stabilization, a thorough physical examination is needed to assess the burn injury completely and to evaluate for concomitant injury. Particular attention to the vascular status of extremities is imperative. Circumferential burns may result in vascular compromise and require escharotomy to prevent limb loss.

Laboratory Evaluation

A *complete blood count* is indicated to establish baseline characteristics. The hematocrit will often be elevated secondary to fluid loss, and the white blood cell count is often elevated as a result of an acute-phase reaction. Later in the course, elevation of the white blood cell count is an indicator of infection, which must be diagnosed early and treated aggressively. *Serum electrolytes* will often reveal an elevated potassium level, due to the breakdown of cells, and depressed bicarbonate level, due to metabolic acidosis resulting from fluid loss and hypovolemic shock. *Renal function tests* (blood urea nitrogen and creatinine) are used to assess renal and overall tissue perfusion. On *urinalysis,* the urine specific gravity is helpful in assessing the hydration status. The presence of myoglobin is important to detect. Myoglobin is indicated by a positive dip test for blood in the absence of red blood cells on the microscopic examination. When myoglobinuria is suspected, aggressive hydration is initiated and potent diuretics, such as furosemide and mannitol, are considered in efforts to maintain high urine flow and prevent tubular necrosis. Baseline *clotting studies* are indicated. *Typing and crossmatching for blood* is indicated if there is associated trauma or if surgical intervention, such as grafting, is considered. *Pulse oximetry, arterial blood gases,* and *chest radiography* are indicated in the management of the patient with airway involvement or with vascular instability. *Carboxyhemoglobin level* is indicated in all burns that occur in a closed space (see Chap. 86).

MANAGEMENT

After assurance of airway integrity, the primary guiding principle in burn management is the restoration or maintenance of tissue perfusion. Fluid resuscitation in burns is most often guided by the Parkland formula: Isotonic crystalloid is administered to a total amount of 4 mL/kg/%BSA over the first 24 h. Half of this amount is administered over the first 8 h and the remainder over 16 h. Maintenance fluid requirements must be added to the fluid amounts calculated by the Parkland formula (see Chap. 49).

It must be remembered that burn fluid calculations provide only an estimation of fluid requirements. Sufficient fluid should be administered to maintain a urine flow of 1 mL/kg/h. Patients in shock require aggressive fluid resuscitation and may require hemodynamic monitoring as a guide (see Chap. 3).

Initial wound care consists of sterile saline–soaked dressings. Room-temperature solutions are sufficient; the application of ice or cold solutions is contraindicated due to the possibility of developing hypothermia in extensively burned patients and of the addition of cold injury to the burned surface. The burned surface can be cleaned with povidone-iodine solution and debris and devitalized tissue removed. If the patient is to be transferred to a burn unit, care should be taken to be in compliance with the burn unit protocol. Often this will include simply covering the burn wound surface with dry sterile sheets after initial cleaning. Most burn units will not want the surface covered with any kind of ointment or cream, since this will impair their assessment of the patient.

It must also be remembered that burns are often extremely painful. Once the patient is hemodynamically stabilized, consideration for analgesia with a potent narcotic analgesic, such as morphine, is indicated.

Tetanus prophylaxis should be considered for all burns. Guidelines are given in Chap. 21.

Minor burns can be soaked in sterile saline, cleaned gently with povidone-iodine solution, and dressed with a topical antibiotic preparation. Silver sulfadiazine is commonly used. Management on an outpatient basis should include periodic reevaluation until healing is clearly under way without evidence of infection. In outpatient management, it is reasonable to leave stable blisters

TABLE 113-2 Guidelines for Burn Triage and Disposition

Outpatient Management
Partial-thickness burn—less than 10% body surface
Full-thickness burn—less than 2% body surface
Inpatient Management
Hospital (other than burn center)
Partial-thickness burn—less than 25% body surface
Full-thickness burn—less than 15% body surface
Partial-thickness burn—face, hands, feet, perineum
Questionable burn wound depth or extent
Chemical burn, minor
Significant coexisting illness or trauma
Inadequate family support
Suspected abuse
Fire in an enclosed space
Burn center
Partial-thickness burn—more than 25% body surface
Full-thickness burn—more than 15% body surface
Full-thickness burn—face, hands, feet, perineum
Respiratory tract injury
Associated major trauma
Major chemical and electrical burns

Reproduced with permission from Burns: Thermal and electrical trauma, in Silverman BK (ed): *APLS: The Pediatric Emergency Medicine Course.* American Academy of Pediatrics, Elk Grove Village, IL/American College of Emergency Physicians, Dallas, 1993, p 122.

intact. Flaccid blisters and those already broken should be debrided carefully and the surface covered with antibiotic cream and a sterile dressing.

DISPOSITION

Criteria for outpatient management, admission, and transfer to a burn center are outlined in Table 113-2.

For a more detailed discussion, see Hill DS, Strange GR: Burns, chap. 113, p. 603, in *Pediatric Emergency Medicine: A Comprehensive Study Guide.*

114 Electrical and Lightning Injuries

Barbara Pawel

Electrophysiology

The factors that determine the extent of electrical injuries are voltage, current (amperage), resistance, current type, duration, and pathway.

1. *Voltage.* Voltage is a measurement of the electrical "pressure" in a system. Injuries are divided into low (less than 1000 V) and high (greater than 1000 V) voltage. The latter usually produces greater tissue destruction.
2. *Current (Amperage).* Amperage is a measure of the rate of flow of electrons. There is a direct relationship between current and damage. The margin between the household amperage (0.001 to 0.01 A) and that capable of causing respiratory arrest (0.02 to 0.05 A) and ventricular fibrillation (0.05 to 0.10 A) is narrow.
3. *Resistance.* Resistance is a measure of the difficulty of electron flow. Specific tissues have defined resistances. Resistance increases in the following order: nerve, blood, muscle, skin, tendon, fat, and bone. The skin is the primary resistor to electric current. Its resistance is affected by thickness, age, moisture, and cleanliness. This explains more serious injuries in bathtub accidents or when a person is sweating. In general, skin with high resistance will sustain greater thermal damage at the site of contact but impede the intensity of current. Skin with lower resistance will have less local thermal damage and greater internal damage.
4. *Current Type.* Alternating current is much more dangerous than direct current at the same voltage. Household circuits (110/220 V) operate at 60 cycles per second (cps), a frequency at which neuromuscular function remains refractory indefinitely, leading to tetany. These tetanic muscle contractions "freeze" the victim to the current course, increasing the duration of contact and the amount of tissue destruction. In addition, alternating current is often associated with local diaphoresis, which further reduces skin resistance.
5. *Current Duration.* Increased duration results in increased damage.
6. *Current Pathway.* The current pathway will determine the nature of injuries and complications. Once surface resistance is overcome, low-voltage current follows the path of least resis-

tance. High-voltage current follows a direct course to ground regardless of tissue type and resistance.

Types of Injuries

Electrical injuries are often classified under burns but are more closely related to crush injuries. Victims of electrical injury may have very little external damage while sustaining serious underlying tissue damage.

Skin and Underlying Tissues

Entry and exit burns are found commonly in all non-water-related electrical injuries. The most common entry points are the hands and skull. The most common exit points are the heels. The different types of burns are as follows:

1. *Contact Burns.* These result from direct contact with an electrical source.
2. *Localized Arc Burns.* The victim becomes part of a circuit as the current arcs to him or her from a high-voltage line. These often generate temperatures up to 2500°C and are accompanied by extensive deep tissue damage.
3. *Flash Burns.* A current courses outside of the body from a contact point to the ground. An example is lightning injury.
4. *Flame-Type Burns.* These are secondary to ignition of clothes or flammable chemicals in the environment and are often extensive.

Very young children often bite on electrical cords, sustaining severe orofacial injuries. Burns are often full-thickness, involving the lips and oral commissure. These burns are initially bloodless and painless. As the eschar separates in 2 to 3 weeks, severe bleeding can occur from damage to the labial, facial, or even carotid arteries. There can be mandibular damage, devitalization of teeth, and microstomia from extensive scarring.

Cardiovascular System

Current passing directly through the heart can induce ventricular fibrillation. Lightning injury will frequently induce asystole. A wide variety of arrythmias can occur, including supraventricular tachycardia, extrasystoles, right bundle branch block, and complete heart block. The most common electrocardiographic (ECG) abnormalities are sinus tachycardia and nonspecific ST-T changes. Most rhythm disturbances are temporary and rhythms return to normal. Myocardial infarction and ventricular perforation have been reported.

Vascular injuries include thrombosis, vasculitis with necrosis of large vessels, vasospasm, and late aneurysm formation. Maximal decrease in blood flow will occur in the first 36 h. Strong peripheral pulses do not guarantee vascular integrity.

Kidney

Acute renal failure may occur from rhabdomyolysis. Kidney damage may also occur from blunt trauma, hypoxic ischemic injury, cardiac arrest, and hypovolemia. Oliguria, albuminuria, hemoglobinuria, and renal casts may be seen transiently.

Neurologic Effects

Immediate CNS effects include loss of consciousness, agitation, amnesia, deafness, seizures, visual disturbance, and sensory complaints. Vascular damage may result in epidural, subdural, or intraventricular hemorrhage. Peripheral nerve injury from vascular damage, thermal effect, or direct action of current may occur and be progressive. A variety of autonomic disturbances also occur.

Eyes

Cataracts can be seen in any electrical injury involving the head or neck.

Gastrointestinal Tract

Passage of current through the abdominal wall can cause Curling's ulcers in the stomach or duodenum. Other injuries described include evisceration, stomach and intestinal perforation, esophageal stricture, and electrocoagulation of the liver and pancreas.

Skeletal System

Blunt trauma or tetanic muscle contractions can cause fractures or dislocations. Amputation of an extremity is necessary in 35 to 60 percent of survivors due to extensive underlying injuries.

Psychological Sequelae

Victims often display depression, flashbacks, and general psychosocial dysfunction.

Management

Prehospital Care

Extrication is extremely dangerous until the power source is disconnected. Victims should be treated as multiple blunt trauma patients with special attention given to spinal immobilization. Attention is first paid to the ABCs (airway, breathing, circulation), with standard protocols for arrest victims followed. Aggressive fluid therapy is essential to sustain circulation and begin diluting myoglobin. Transport to a health care facility should not be delayed.

Emergency Department Care

Any victim of electrical injury should be approached in the same way as a victim of blunt trauma with a crush injury. The greatest threats to life include cardiac arrythmias, renal failure, and hyperkalemia. A thorough search for entry and exit wounds and hidden skeletal injuries is necessary. Laboratory tests should include arterial blood gases, blood count, serum electrolytes, blood urea nitrogen, glucose, creatinine, creatine kinase (CK), blood type and crossmatch, and urinalysis for myoglobin. Radiographs of the cervical spine, chest, and pelvis may be done in addition to areas dictated by physical exam. Baseline electrocardiography (ECG) is indicated. Although CK-MB (muscle brain) isoenzyme elevations can be seen, they may be from damaged skeletal muscle. If the ECG is consistent with cardiac injury, further evaluation with echocardiography or nuclear scanning may be necessary.

The usual fluid replacement formulas utilized in burn patients underestimate fluid requirements in electrical burn patients. Fluids should maintain a urine output of 1 to 2 mL/kg/h. Accurate measurement requires Foley catheter placement. Alkalinization of the urine with bicarbonate and administration of mannitol or furosemide may be needed to treat myoglobinuria. Overzealous use of bicarbonate can result in metabolic alkalosis or hypernatremia. Any unexplained coma, lateralizing signs, or change in mental status necessitates cranial computed tomography (CT).

Extensive muscle damage frequently requires fasciotomy. Debridement is best left to a burn surgeon. Tetanus prophylaxis should be evaluated and given as needed in the emergency department.

Nasogastric intubation may be required and antacids and cimetidine should be administered.

Consultations may be required, depending on the severity and type of injury. All children with oral injuries require plastic surgical or dental consults. Neurosurgical, ophthalmological, and ear-nose-throat consults may also be necessary. Transfer to a burn center may be indicated.

Infection remains the most common cause of death after electrical injury. Despite aggressive debridement and decompression, digit or limb loss may be unavoidable.

Recommendations for admission are varied. It is generally agreed that admission is not required for nontransthoracic low-voltage injuries in the asymptomatic child without ECG abnormalities. All other patients require admission and close observation. A multidisciplinary approach—including medical, psychiatric, and social services—is required.

LIGHTNING INJURIES

Mechanism of Injury

There are several mechanisms by which lightning can cause injury.

1. *Direct Strike.* This is the most serious form of lightning injury. The likelihood of direct strike is increased when one is carrying or wearing metal objects such as golf clubs, umbrellas, or hairpins.
2. *Side Flash, or "Splash."* In this form of lightning injury, the victim is near an object that is struck, with object resistance greater than air resistance between the object and the person.
3. *Ground Current.* In ground-current injury, lightning strikes the ground close to a victim, with the result that the ground current passes through the victim. When the victim stands with feet apart, a potential difference between the feet allows current to flow through the body to the ground (stride potential or step current).
4. *Thermal Flash.* Temperatures between 8000 and 30,000°C of short duration (0.001 to 0.010 s) can cause burns. These are generally not as severe as household or industrial electrical burns.
5. *Blunt Injury.* The cylindrical shock wave emanating from the axis of the lightning channel can cause perforation of the tympanic membrane or damage to internal organs. This shock wave can also throw a victim, causing secondary blunt injury.

Substantial differences in lightning-strike properties account for variability in the type and severity of injury. Lightning acts as a direct-current countershock, with higher voltage and amperage than seen in high-voltage electrical accidents. The extremely short duration of lightning shock accounts for the small amount of skin damage usually seen. Most of the lightning energy flows around the outside of the body, with less energy actually flowing through the victim.

Types of Injuries

Skin

Skin damage is decreased by the short duration of contact and by lower skin resistance from rain or sweat. Entry wounds, exit wounds, and deep muscle damage are rare. Major types of burns include the following:

1. *Feathering burns.* These are arborescent, spidery, erythematous streaks which are pathognomonic of lightning injury. They appear up to several hours after injury and disappear within 24 h.
2. *Linear Burns.* Linear burns are partial-thickness burns in areas of high sweat concentration.
3. *Punctate Burns.* These are multiple, discrete, circular burns in groups. They can be full or partial thickness.
4. *Thermal Burns.* Heating of metal objects or ignition of clothing can cause secondary thermal burns.

Over 60 percent of patients have multiple burns, while approximately 10 percent are not burned at all.

Cardiopulmonary Effects

Asystole can result from the massive direct-current countershock produced by a lightning strike. Respiratory arrest may occur from effects on the medullary respiratory center. Although the heart usually resumes an organized rhythm spontaneously, prolonged respiratory arrest leads to hypoxia and ventricular fibrillation. Myocardial infarction occurs secondary to hypoxia or direct cardiac damage and has been reported as late as 30 days after injury in adults. Congestive heart failure, cardiac contusions, and rupture have also been reported.

Electrocardiographic changes include nonspecific ST-T changes, T-wave changes, axis shift, QT prolongation, and ST-segment elevation. These often resolve gradually. Lung injuries reported include pulmonary contusion, hemorrhage, pneumothorax, pulmonary edema, and aspiration secondary to altered mental status.

Vascular Effects

Arterial spasm and vasomotor instability result in cool, mottled, pulseless extremities. This usually resolves in several hours.

Neurologic Effects

Transient loss of consciousness, retrograde amnesia, transient paralysis, and paresthesias are common. Keraunoparalysis (from the Greek *Keraunos,* meaning lightning) is a flaccid paralysis accompanied by vasomotor changes, which may last up to 24 h. Other possible neurologic findings include seizures, skull fractures, intracerebral hemorrhages and hematomas, elevated intracranial pressure, cerebellar ataxia, Horner's syndrome, SIADH, and peripheral nerve damage. Cerebral edema may occur late. Direct or blunt injury to the spinal cord should always be ruled out, especially if symptoms do not resolve.

Kidneys

Myoglobinuria is rare; however, hypovolemia and prolonged cardiac arrest can lead to acute tubular necrosis. The kidneys may also be damaged by direct blunt trauma from a shock wave or other object.

Eyes

Cataracts are the most common injury and may develop immediately or over a prolonged period. Some resolve spontaneously. Fixed and dilated pupils are often seen after lightning strike and are not a prognostic factor. Other eye injuries reported include uveitis, hyphema, vitreous hemorrhage, retinal detachment, and optic atrophy.

Ears

Tympanic membrane rupture is common. Other complications include hearing loss, tinnitus, vertigo, and nystagmus.

Gastrointestinal Tract

Gastric dilatation is common. Hematoma or perforations can occur secondary to blunt trauma.

Psychological Sequelae

Anxiety, sleep disturbances, nocturnal enuresis, depression, and hysteria-related phenomena have all been reported.

Management

Prehospital Care

Lightning injury victims should be approached as blunt multiple trauma patients with attention to advanced life-support protocols and cervical spine protection. Due to the unusual findings of transient fixed and dilated pupils from autonomic abnormalities and transient asystole with prolonged apnea, standard triage procedures should be ignored. Victims who appear to be dead should be treated aggressively. If the history of lightning strike is unclear, protocols for altered mental status should be followed (i.e., glucose, naloxone). Bystanders may be helpful in providing history.

It should be noted that, contrary to popular belief, lightning can strike twice in the same area. Emergency personnel should exhibit caution if the threat of lightning strike still exists at the time of their arrival.

Emergency Department Care

Treatment follows the same guidelines as for all severely injured patients. Amnesia suffered by the victim and lack of available bystanders may limit history taking. Clues that may lead to the diagnosis of lightning strike include recent thunderstorm, outdoor occurrence, clothing disintegration, typical arborescent burn pattern, tympanic membrane injury, and magnetization of metallic objects on the victim's body. A complete physical exam with priority to ABCs and cervical spine control is indicated. A thorough search for blunt trauma injuries is necessary, as are baseline ECG and continued cardiac monitoring. Any arrythmia should be treated by standard protocols. Routine lab tests include complete blood count, creatine phosphokinase with isoenzymes, renal function tests, and urinanalysis for myoglobin. The patient's status may necessitate arterial blood gas, serum chemistries, and blood type and crossmatch. Urine and blood should be sent for toxicology. Radiographs are done as indicated but include cranial CT in all unconscious patients.

Fluid resuscitation must be approached cautiously; central monitoring lines may be helpful.

Burns should be treated by protocol. Fasciotomy is rarely indicated, as the mottled, pulseless extremity associated with lightning injury often improves over several hours. Eye and ear exams should not be overlooked. Careful attention to tetanus prophylaxis is necessary.

Disposition

Some authorities suggest admission for all victims of lightning injuries. Others suggest admission for all except those children with a completely normal exam, normal lab tests and ECG, plus adequate home supervision and close follow-up care. Appropriate consultation and documentation is necessary.

Sequelae

Long-term sequelae may include paralysis, dysesthesia, and disturbances in mood, affect, and memory. Supportive psychotherapy may be necessary.

For a more detailed discussion, see Pawel B: Electrical and lightning injuries, chap. 114, p. 607, in *Pediatric Emergency Medicine: A Comprehensive Study Guide.*

115 Heat Illness

Gary R. Strange

The spectrum of heat illness varies from mild, self-limited problems, such as heat cramps, to major, life-threatening problems, such as heat stroke. Infants are predisposed to the development of heat illness due to their poorly developed thermoregulatory systems. Older children and adolescents are susceptible to heat illness when they exercise vigorously under hot, humid conditions. Adolescent zeal for competitive athletics, coupled with an often held belief among the young in their invulnerability, can lead to serious heat illness.

Heat illness is the second leading cause of death in athletes, after head and spinal injuries. Drug-related heat illness (see Table 78-1) is also seen with increasing incidence in the adolescent population. Other factors associated with the development of heat illness in pediatric patients are obesity, dehydration, excessive clothing/bundling, and infections. An especially tragic situation, which is entirely preventable through parental education, is the development of heat illness in small children left in closed cars on hot days. Children with cystic fibrosis (see Chap. 28) are prone to develop a form of heat illness characterized by excessive electrolyte loss with sweating. Any patient who has had a previous episode of heat stroke is markedly predisposed to recurrence.

Acclimatization to a hot, humid environment allows the individual to perform harder and longer without developing heat illness. Full acclimatization takes 3 to 4 weeks, during which the individual must limit exertion. Children take longer to acclimatize than adults.

TYPES OF HEAT ILLNESS

Heat Cramps

With heavy exertion, the muscles that are working hardest may begin to go into spasm. The cause is dilutional hyponatremia, which usually occurs in conditioned athletes who replace fluid losses with water. The body temperature remains normal, and there is associated sweating. There are no central nervous system signs.

Heat Exhaustion

Heat exhaustion is a syndrome of dizziness, nausea, vomiting, weakness, and, occasionally, syncope, which may be associated with normal temperature or moderate temperature elevation (39 to 41.1°C). There is no sustained change in mentation. The skin is usually wet from profuse sweating. The associated morbidity is low.

The cause of heat exhaustion may be either salt or water depletion. Salt depletion and hyponatremia occur when fluid losses are replaced by water or other hypotonic solutions. Water depletion occurs when victims are unable to replace fluid losses, resulting in hypernatremic dehydration. This can occur in infants or mentally retarded children, who cannot communicate their thirst.

Heat Stroke

Heat stroke is the most severe form of heat illness, with reported mortality between 17 and 80 percent. Patients with heat stroke present with disorientation, seizures, or coma. In classic heat stroke, which is typically seen in the elderly, the skin is usually hot and dry. With exertional heat stroke, which is much more likely in the pediatric population, the skin may be dry or sweating may continue. The temperature ranges from 41.1 to 42.2°C.

Complications are common, leading to the high mortality rate. Rhabdomyolysis and renal failure may occur in up to 25 percent of patients with exertional heat stroke. Hypotension, hepatic failure, and disseminated intravascular coagulation are other relatively common complications.

MANAGEMENT

Heat cramps are treated by removing the patient to a cool environment and providing rest and oral electrolyte solutions. Salt tablets may cause gastrointestinal cramping and are not recommended. A solution of 1 tsp of table salt in 500 mL of water can be used if no prepared solutions are available.

Heat exhaustion is also treated by removal to a cool environment and providing rest. Intravenous rehydration is recommended, starting with 20 mL/kg of normal saline over 30 min and continuing rehydration as outlined in Chap. 49. If hypernatremic dehydration is suspected on clinical or laboratory grounds, slower replacement is indicated.

Victims of heat exhaustion may require observation in the hospital. However, if all symptoms have resolved during emergency department treatment and observation, the patient may be released to continue rest and rehydration in a cool environment.

Heat stroke is an immediately life-threatening entity and must be treated vigorously. After assessment and stabilization of the airway, breathing, and circulation, cooling should be immediately instituted. Spraying the skin with room-temperature water and directing an electric fan onto the patient's skin will usually result in rapid reduction of the core temperature. Ice packs may be used in the groin and axilla, but ice water applied widely to the skin may cause vasoconstriction and impair the dissipation of heat. Submersion in cold water is very effective in lowering the temperature but makes other resuscitative efforts practically impossible. Invasive lavage to lower the body temperature has not been adequately studied and is not currently recommended. Antipyretics are also ineffective. Core temperature should be monitored continuously during treatment, and active cooling should continue until the core temperature falls to 39°C.

Diazepam, 0.2 to 0.3 mg/kg/dose IV, may be required to prevent shivering.

Intravenous fluids are required and should initially be given as isotonic crystalloid at a rate of 20 mL/kg over the first hour. Central venous or pulmonary artery catheters are frequently needed for adequate monitoring of the fluid resuscitation.

Since the effects of heat stroke are widespread throughout essentially every system of the body and the differential diagnosis is broad (Table 115-1), extensive diagnostic evaluation is indicated. *Arterial blood gases* are helpful in evaluating oxygenation, ventilation, and acid-base status. Changes in body temperature alter blood gas values, but whether corrections in the values are helpful before making treatment decisions is controversial. The *complete blood count* will usually show an elevated white blood cell count. Counts >20,000/mm^3 and elevated band counts are more consistent with an underlying infection and should prompt a complete septic workup. Hemoglobin/hematocrit values are usually elevated due to dehydration. *Electrolyte studies* may reveal abnormal sodium levels. Elevated potassium levels may indicate the development of rhabdomyolysis. *Renal function tests* may initially be elevated due to dehydration but may rise later as renal failure develops. *Urinalysis* will often show a high specific gravity as a reflection of the hydration status. If the urine is positive for hemoglobin in the absence of red blood cells on the microscopic evaluation, rhabdomyolysis should be suspected. *Liver enzymes* may be elevated, since the liver is very sensitive to heat stress. Transminase levels peak in 24 to 48 h and correlate well with the severity of injury. Very high levels (aspartate transaminase >1000 IU) are predictive of severe illness and complications. *Serum glucose levels* are variable but should be monitored to assess need for replacement or control. *Coagulation studies* are needed to detect the development of disseminated intravascular coagulation. Cultures

TABLE 115-1 Differential Diagnosis of Heat Stroke—Symptom Complex: Altered Mental Status, Hyperthermia

Potential diagnosis	Pertinent history	Pertinent findings on physical examination	Pertinent laboratory data
Encephalitis/meningitis	Fever, prodromal illness, severe headache, chills	Temperature, neck stiffness (Kernig and Brudzinski signs)	Lumbar puncture: elevated WBCs, positive Gram's stain, cultures
Malaria	Exposure, travel history, previous history	Fever pattern, confusion	Peripheral blood smear
Typhoid fever, typhus	Exposure, travel history	Fever pattern	Titers: Weil-Felix reaction, complement fixation
Sepsis	Fever, age extreme, immunocompromised	Fever, confusion, coma, focal infection	Chest x-ray WBC: elevated; cultures: blood, urine, spinal fluid
Hypothalamic hemorrhage	Hypertension, anticoagulant therapy	Coma and fever, focal neurologic findings	Brain CT: hemorrhage

Thyroid storm	Preexisting hyperthyroidism (e.g., Graves' disease); risk factors include stress or surgery, trauma, infection, failure to take antithyroid medication	Goiter, tachycardia, seizures, hypotension	Thyroid function studies: T_3 and T_4
Malignant hyperthermia	Inhalation anesthetic, succinylcholine	Muscle fasciculations	Arterial blood gases: acidosis Electrolytes: hyperkalemia, hypermagnesemia
Heat stroke	Risk factors, exposure to heat load, exercise	Hot, flushed skin, confusion, agitation, seizures, tachycardia, hypotension, vomiting, diarrhea, muscle tenderness	AST: elevated WBC: elevated Electrolytes: hyper- or hypokalemia, hyponatremia, hypocalcemia, hypophosphatemia Arterial blood gases: metabolic acidosis Urine: myoglobin; clotting factors: decreased; blood glucose: variable

Reproduced with permission from Barreca RS: Heat illness, in Hamilton GC, Sanders AB, Strange GR, Trott AT: *Emergency Medicine: An Approach to Clinical Problem-Solving*. Philadelphia, Saunders, 1991, p 402.

are an integral part of the sepsis workup, which is essential to rule out an infectious etiology.

Radiologic studies will usually include a chest radiograph as part of the sepsis workup. Computed tomographic scanning of the brain is indicated to rule out intracranial pathology, especially if the mental status does not promptly improve with lowering of the temperature.

An *electrocardiogram* is indicated to evaluate for myocardial ischemia, which can result from severe cardiovascular stress.

After evaluation and stabilization, patients with heat stroke are admitted to an intensive care setting for continued monitoring and aggressive treatment.

For a more detailed discussion, see Strange GR: Heat illness, chap. 115, p. 613, in *Pediatric Emergency Medicine: A Comprehensive Study Guide.*

---

116 Cold Illness

Gary R. Strange / Mary Ann Cooper

Hypothermia is defined as a core temperature of less than 35°C. A low body temperature may develop as a result of exposure to low ambient temperature or may be secondary to a disease process (Table 116-1).

Age is an important factor in determining the susceptibility to hypothermia and the morbidity and mortality associated with it. Neonates are at high risk for developing hypothermia due to their large surface area compared to body mass and the relative paucity of subcutaneous tissue. They have also been postulated to have poorly developed thermoregulatory systems. The evaporation of warm amniotic fluid from the skin of the newborn is a major source of heat loss that must be guarded against in all cases. Throughout infancy and young childhood, children remain susceptible to hypothermia with exposure to cold, although less so with advancing age. Most cases of accidental hypothermia in older children and adolescents are associated with near drowning in cold water. However, in recent years there has been an increase in exposure-related hypothermia in older children and adolescents that is believed

TABLE 116-1 Causes of Hypothermia in Infants and Children

Environmental factors
Exposure
Near drowning
Infections
Meningitis
Encephalitis
Sepsis
Pneumonia
Metabolic/endocrine factors
Hypoglycemia
Diabetic ketoacidosis
Hypopituitarism
Myxedema
Addison's disease
Uremia
Malnutrition
Toxicologic factors
Alcohol
Anesthetic agents
Barbiturates
Carbon monoxide
Cyclic antidepressants
Narcotics
Phenothiazines
CNS disorders
Degenerative diseases
Head trauma
Spinal cord trauma
Subarachnoid hemorrhage
Cerebrovascular accidents
Intracranial neoplasm
Vascular factors
Shock
Pulmonary embolism
Gastrointestinal hemorrhage
Dermatologic factors
Burns
Erythrodermas
Iatrogenic factors
Cold fluid infusion
Exposure during treatment or postdelivery
Prolonged extrications

to be associated with the increased popularity of winter sports. Inexperience and lack of caution, which are common characteristics of adolescents, increase the likelihood of becoming a victim of hypothermia.

DIAGNOSIS

The diagnosis of hypothermia may be obvious when a history of exposure is known. However, hypothermia may develop insidiously due to causes other than exposure or due to exposure in relatively warm environments.

The hypothermic patient is often not able to give an adequate history, and other sources of information should be sought. Family, friends, police, and paramedics are all valuable sources of information.

Once hypothermia is known or suspected, a history of exposure is sought, including the circumstances, location, ambient temperature, length of exposure, and presence or absence of submersion or wet skin/clothing.

If significant exposure is unlikely, an extensive history is required to search for clues to other causes of hypothermia (Table 116-1).

The key physical findings in patients with hypothermia and the temperature level at which they occur are depicted in Table 116-2. The core temperature defines the presence and severity of hypothermia. Most thermometers for routine clinical use will record a temperature only down to 34.4°C. Special glass or electronic thermometers are required for accurate measurement of temperature in hypothermic patients. Continuous monitoring of rectal, esophageal, or tympanic temperature is very useful during treatment.

Shivering will often be present in the older child or adolescent but ceases by the time the temperature reaches 31°C. The skin is typically cold, firm, pale, or mottled. Localized damage due to frostbite may be present.

Early neurologic signs of hypothermia include confusion, apathy, poor judgment, slurred speech, and ataxia. Coma usually supervenes by the time the temperature reaches 27°C. Focal neurologic defects may be present. The Glasgow Coma Scale can serve as a useful quantitative means of following the patient's response to treatment, but it is not as useful with the nonverbal infant.

Since hypothermia affects multiple systems, other pathology can be masked. Signs of trauma, toxic ingestion, and endocrine disturbance should be sought, and the complete physical examination must be repeated at intervals during treatment in order to discover clues to problems that were initially masked by the hypothermia.

TABLE 116-2 Pathophysiologic Changes during Hypothermia

Centigrade	Fahrenheit	Findings
37.6	99.6	Normal rectal temperature
37	98.6	Normal oral temperature
35	95.0	Maximal shivering; increased metabolic rate
33	91.4	Apathy, ataxia, amnesia, dysarthria
31	87.8	Progressive decrease in level of consciousness, pulse, blood pressure, respiratory rate. Shivering stops
29	85.2	Dysrhythmias may occur, insulin not effective, pupils dilated; poikilothermia
27	80.6	Reflexes absent, no response to pain, comatose
25	77	Cerebral blood flow one-third normal, cardiac output one-half normal, significant hypotension
23	73.4	No corneal reflex, ventricular fibrillation risk is maximal
19	66.2	Asystole, flat electroencephalogram
16	60.8	Lowest temperature survived from accidental hypothermia
9	48.2	Lowest temperature survived from therapeutic hypothermia

Reproduced with permission from Cooper MA, Danzl DF: Hypothermia, in Hamilton GC, Sanders AB, Strange GR, Trott AT: *Emergency Medicine: An Approach to Clinical Problem-Solving*. Philadelphia, Saunders, 1991, p 415.

In patients with hypothermia not related to exposure and in those exposure-related cases who present with temperatures below 32°C, extensive diagnostic testing is indicated.

Arterial blood gases These are useful for evaluation of oxygenation, ventilation, and acid-base status. In hypothermia, there is decreased tissue perfusion, and the oxyhemoglobin dissociation curve is shifted to the left. While some authorities have recommended correcting blood gas results for body temperature, correction can lead to false elevation of P_{O_2} and subsequent undertreatment. Metabolic acidosis is usually present, and the buffering capacity of the blood is markedly reduced.

Complete blood count Hematocrit increases 2 percent for each 1°C drop in temperature. Hemoglobin may be decreased due to blood loss or chronic illness. The white blood count is reduced by sequestration and bone marrow depression. Even in the presence of severe infection, leukocytosis may not be seen.

Serum electrolytes These should be monitored during the rewarming process to assess the need for intervention. There are no consistent effects of hypothermia on electrolyte concentrations, but hypokalemia is the most common finding.

Renal function tests These tests are useful for establishing baseline renal function but are poor indicators of fluid status in hypothermia. Acute tubular necrosis may develop after rewarming.

Serum glucose concentration This value may be elevated due to catecholamine effect and insulin inactivity below 30°C. Persistently elevated levels suggest pancreatitis or diabetic ketoacidosis. Hypoglycemia may develop due to inadequate glycogen stores in neonates and malnourished children.

Hemostatic studies Studies of prothrombin time, partial thromboplastin time, platelet count, and fibrinogen are indicated in cases of moderate to severe hypothermia. Cold induces thrombocytopenia and prolongs clotting times. Persistent changes after rewarming suggest the development of disseminated intravascular coagulation.

Pancreatic enzymes Amylase and lipase may be elevated and, due to the unreliability of the abdominal examination, may be the only indicators of the development of pancreatitis. Pancreatitis in hypothermia is associated with poor outcome.

Toxicologic studies These are frequently indicated to detect causative or predisposing agents.

Urinalysis This will demonstrate a low specific gravity due to cold diuresis. There are no other consistent findings.

Cultures of urine, sputum, and blood These cultures are indicated in all cases of moderate to severe hypothermia. Cultures from other body sites may also be indicated, based on the history and physical findings. Sepsis is a common cause of hypothermia in the infant and may also develop as a complication of hypothermia due to other causes.

Radiologic imaging These studies will include a chest radiograph in all cases of significant hypothermia. Pulmonary edema may develop during rewarming, and aspiration is relatively common.

Cervical spine films may be indicated if there is suspicion of trauma. Cranial computed tomographic scanning may be indicated in the setting of trauma or to search for other etiologic factors, especially when mental status does not clear along with rewarming.

Electrocardiography This procedure is indicated for all patients with core temperature below 32°C to detect dysrhythmias or evidence of myocardial ischemia. The J wave (Fig. 116-1) is usually seen when the temperature falls below 32°C.

PREHOSPITAL CARE

Great caution is needed to prevent hypothermia or to initiate its early treatment in neonates. The neonate should immediately be dried and wrapped in warm blankets. Alternatively, the neonate can be placed against the body of the mother and then covered.

For other potentially hypothermic patients, wet clothing should be removed and dry blankets applied. When prolonged extrications are required, hypothermia is particularly likely to develop. Protection should be provided whenever possible. Likewise, resuscitation fluids should be warmed whenever possible.

Ventilation should be supported as indicated and oxygenation maintained. Cardiac monitoring is indicated to detect dysrhythmias. Since "pulselessness" may be due to marked vasoconstriction and bradycardia, cardiopulmonary resuscitation (CPR) is initiated only when there is cardiac monitor evidence of asystole or ventricular fibrillation.

EMERGENCY DEPARTMENT MANAGEMENT

The initial approach to the patient with hypothermia is the same as that for any seriously ill patient, with evaluation and stabilization of the airway, breathing, and circulation before moving to other aspects of treatment. Obtunded patients without protective airway reflexes require endotracheal intubation after preoxygenation. Intravenous lines are started, and fluid resuscitation is guided by vital signs, urinary output, and pulmonary status. Cardiac monitoring is initiated. In addition, continuous monitoring of rectal, esophageal, or tympanic temperature is very helpful during treatment. A urinary catheter and nasogastric tube are inserted. A bedside glucose determination is done to assess the need for glucose supplementation. If narcotic intoxication is a possibility, naloxone, 2 mg IV, is administered.

Cardiopulmonary resuscitation is begun when asystole or ventricular fibrillation is diagnosed by cardiac monitor. The cold myo-

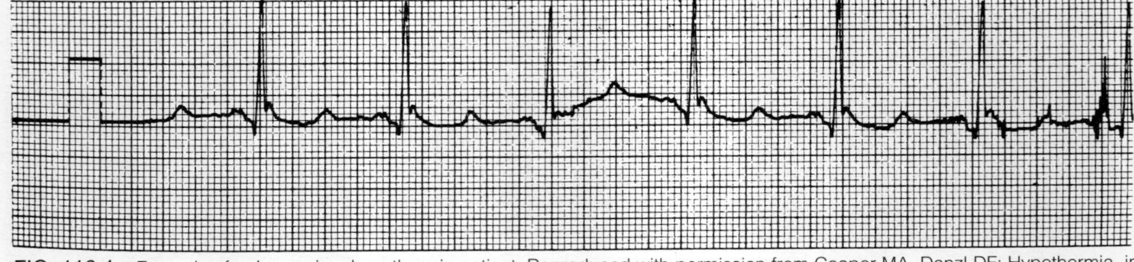

FIG. 116-1 Example of a J wave in a hypothermic patient. Reproduced with permission from Cooper MA, Danzl DF: Hypothermia, in Hamilton GC, Sanders AB, Strange GR, Trott AT: *Emergency Medicine: An Approach to Clinical Problem-Solving*. Philadelphia, Saunders, 1991, p 411.

cardium is resistant to defibrillation and to pharmacologic agents. If initial defibrillation fails to establish a rhythm, CPR is resumed and the patient is rewarmed to 30°C before defibrillation is repeated. Many patients spontaneously convert to an organized rhythm at a core temperature of 32 to 35°C. During hypothermia, protein binding of drugs is increased, and most drugs will be ineffective in normal doses. Pharmacologic attempts to alter the pulse or blood pressure are to be avoided. Lidocaine and procainamide are largely ineffective at cold temperatures, but bretylium may be effective for ventricular fibrillation even at low temperatures. It is important to remember that infants and children who have sustained prolonged hypothermic cardiac arrest have recovered with little or no neurologic impairment. In general, resuscitative efforts should continue until the hypothermic child is warmed to at least 30°C.

In moderate to severe cases of hypothermia, active rewarming is started as soon as possible (Fig. 116-2). Heated, humidified oxygen and intravenous fluids heated to 40°C are used from the beginning. For neonates and infants, radiant warmers are used to prevent further heat loss. The older child and adolescent should be covered with dry blankets. Active external rewarming, as with hot packs and electric blankets, can be dangerous. The rewarming of cold extremities can result in the mobilization of cold peripheral blood to the central circulation, resulting in core-temperature afterdrop. Immersion in warm water has been used, but this makes monitoring and resuscitation difficult. Cold, vasoconstricted skin is also very susceptible to thermal injury. Because of these concerns, active core rewarming is used in most cases of moderate to severe hypothemia.

In addition to heated humidified oxygen and heated intravenous fluids, active core rewarming may be accomplished by irrigation of the stomach, bladder, and colon. Heat transfer by these techniques is somewhat limited. Peritoneal lavage with heated fluid (40 to 45°C) is probably the preferred method of active core rewarming. Extracorporeal rewarming is the most rapid method of rewarming and is indicated in hypothermic cardiac arrest and with patients who present with completely frozen extremities.

Previously healthy patients who are only mildly hypothermic (35 to 33°C) will usually reheat themselves safely if they are placed in a warm environment and given dry insulating coverings (passive external rewarming).

Beyond the neonatal period, sepsis is the most common cause of hypothermia in infants. All hypothermic patients should have a thorough evaluation to search for a source of infection and should have broad-spectrum antibiotics initiated early. An amino-

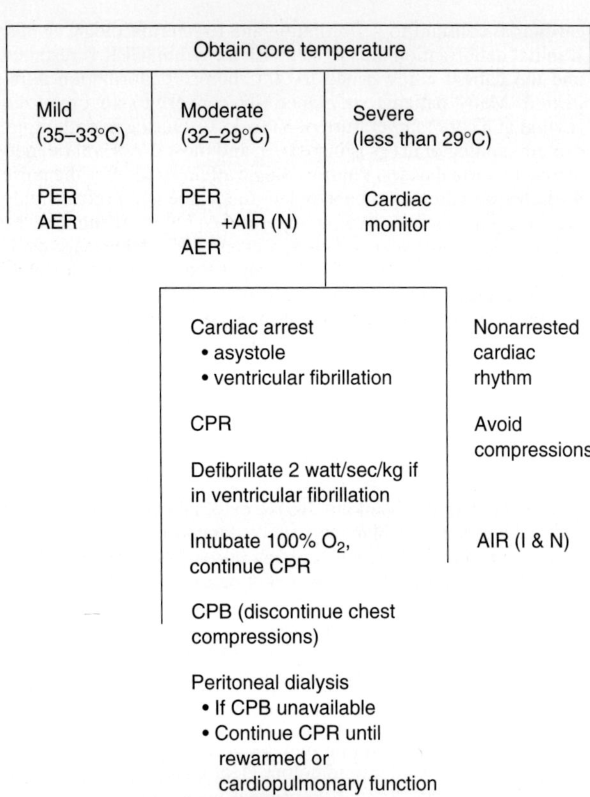

FIG. 116-2 Management of hypothermia. *Abbreviations:* PER = passive external rewarming; AER = active external rewarming (incubators, radiant warmers—to be used with infants only); AIR = Active internal rewarming; N = Noninvasive (warm humidified oxygen/warmed IV fluids); I = Invasive (peritoneal lavage/pleural lavage/cardiopulmonary bypass); CPR = cardiopulmonary resuscitation; CPB = cardiopulmonary bypass. Reproduced with permission from Jackson SC: Pediatric hypothermia, in Surpure JS (ed): *Synopsis of Pediatric Emergency Care.* Boston, Andover Medical Publishers, 1993, p 408.

glycoside combined with ampicillin or a third-generation cephalosporin is generally recommended.

A special consideration in pediatric hypothermia is near drowning in cold water. This entity is discussed in Chap. 112.

Another special consideration is frostbite, which may occur in conjunction with hypothermia or as an isolated localized injury. Localized hypothermia is described in terms similar to those used for burns. First-degree frostbite is limited to the superficial epidermis. Erythema and edema occur and resolve without sequelae. Second-degree frostbite results in deeper epidermal involvement and presents with large, clear bullae. Third-degree injury consists of full-thickness skin injury.

The treatment of frostbite is rapid rewarming. The preferred technique is immersion of the affected part in circulating warm water (40 to 42°C). Narcotic analgesics are often required to control pain during rewarming. It is very difficult to determine tissue viability after significant hypothermic injury. Debridement of nonviable tissue is best delayed for several days to weeks in order to preserve as much tissue as possible. Topical aloe vera cream and ibuprofen may be used for outpatient treatment after rewarming. More extensively injured patients will require continued inpatient treatment and pain control.

Rewarmed body parts are highly susceptible to refreezing, leading to even greater tissue loss. If reexposure is anticipated, it is better not to rewarm the tissue.

DISPOSITION

Most patients with hypothermia will require hospitalization for further treatment and evaluation. Those patients with a core temperature of less than 32°C will require cardiac monitoring. Profoundly hypothermic patients with cardiac arrest and those with completely frozen extremities are candidates for extracorporeal rewarming and may require transfer to a tertiary care facility with this capability.

Patients with mild accidental hypothermia (35 to 32°C) may be rewarmed and discharged to a safe environment if there is no evidence of underlying disease.

For a more detailed discussion, see Strange GR, Cooper MA: Cold illness, chap. 116, p. 616, in *Pediatric Emergency Medicine: A Comprehensive Study Guide*.

117 High-Altitude Illness and Dysbaric Injuries

Ira J. Blumen / Jeffrey J. Leinen

HIGH-ALTITUDE ILLNESS

High-altitude illness most often affects young and otherwise healthy individuals. There is a broad spectrum of disease. It progresses from the mildest form of acute mountain sickness (AMS) into the potentially life-threatening forms as high-altitude pulmonary edema (HAPE) and high-altitude cerebral edema (HACE). Symptoms of high-altitude illness may develop within hours or days of ascent. In contrast, hypoxemia occurs within minutes to hours and results in the initiation of the cascade of physiologic events that lead to AMS, HAPE, and HACE.

Three major factors influence the incidence, onset, and severity of high-altitude illness: rate of ascent, altitude achieved, and length of stay. High-altitude illness of varying severity will occur when any of these factors, or a combination of them, exceeds the individual's ability to adapt to the new environment. Children, because of their physiologic differences, are at greater risk for developing both AMS and HAPE. The highest incidence of AMS occurs betrween the ages of 1 and 20 years. The severity of symptoms decreases with increasing age.

High altitude is generally considered to be 8000 ft (2439 m) or more. At this altitude, arterial oxygen saturation falls below 90% (Pa_{O_2} 60%). Acclimatization is necessary to prevent illness. While severe altitude illness is uncommon below 8000 ft, medically compromised individuals may become symptomatic at *moderate* altitude (5000 to 8000 ft). At *extreme* altitude, which is generally greater than 18,000 ft (approximately 5500 m), acclimatization is not possible and altitude illness is inevitable.

Acute Mountain Sickness

Acute mountain sickness (AMS) is the most common and mildest form of high-altitude illness. Up to 25 percent of individuals traveling to 8000 ft will become symptomatic, while nearly everyone who rapidly ascends to 11,000 ft will develop AMS.

The onset of AMS may be exacerbated by a decreased vital capacity, increased cerebrospinal fluid (CSF) pressure, proteinuria, fluid retention, recent weight gain, or relative hypoventilation. It is postulated that children are more susceptible to AMS, as they are more sensitive to cerebral hypoxemia. Physical fitness does not affect susceptibility to AMS.

Clinical Presentation

The onset of AMS symptoms is usually within 4 to 8 h of a rapid ascent, but it can be delayed up to four days. Symptoms develop following strenuous activity or sleeping at high altitude. In most cases, symptoms peak in 24 to 48 h and resolve by the third or fourth day. If the individual proceeds to a higher altitude after the onset of AMS, symptoms may last considerably longer.

The signs and symptoms of AMS, in order of prevalence, include headache, sleep disturbance, fatigue, shortness of breath, dizziness, anorexia, nausea, and vomiting. Acute mountain sickness should be considered the etiology in any individual at altitude who develops the onset of at least three of these symptoms. Headache occurs in approximately two-thirds of individuals with AMS. It is throbbing in nature and worse after exercise, at night, or on awakening. Nausea and vomiting are common in children. Other symptoms associated with AMS include oliguria, mild peripheral edema, weakness, lassitude, malaise, irritability, decreased concentration, poor judgment, palpitations, deep inner chill, and a dull pain in the posterolateral chest wall.

The differential diagnosis of these symptoms includes an alcohol hangover, exhaustion, dehydration, and viral syndrome. In addition, respiratory and central nervous system (CNS) infections, exhaustion, hypothermia, gastritis, and carbon monoxide poisoning should be considered. However, if the symptoms occur shortly after arrival at high altitude, they must be considered AMS until proven otherwise.

Treatment

Treatment is initially directed toward prevention. Symptoms of AMS are most often mild and self-limiting, lasting only a few days. Once symptoms do occur, activity should be minimized, and ascent should be halted until signs and symptoms have resolved. Proceeding to a lower altitude is indicated for any individual who shows no signs of improvement within 1 to 2 days or who worsens. Immediate descent is indicated if ataxia, decreased level of consciousness, confusion, dyspnea at rest, rales, or cyanosis are present. A descent of 1000 to 3000 ft is recommended. In some situation, a descent of as little as 500 ft may result in improvement.

If descent is not an option, the use of supplementary oxygen will relieve most of the signs and symptoms of AMS. During sleep, 1 to 2 L/min can be of significant benefit.

A Gamow bag is a portable fabric hyperbaric bag that has been shown to relieve the central effects of acute mountain sickness. Using a foot pump, it can be pressurized in excess of 100 torr for the physiologic equivalent of a 4000- to 5000-ft descent.

Symptomatic treatment for the headache is with acetaminophen, which will have no impact on the hypoxic ventilatory response. Victims of AMS are to refrain from using narcotics, which depress this response. Prochlorperazine, given for nausea and vomiting, is also effective in *increasing* the respiratory drive. The dosage of prochlorperazine for children over 10 kg in weight or over 2 years old is 0.1 to 0.15 mg/kg/dose IM, PO, or PR.

The carbonic anhydrase inhibitor acetazolamide may be used in the treatment or prophylaxis of AMS. It decreases the reabsorption of bicarbonate, forcing a renal bicarbonate diuresis that results in a mild metabolic acidosis. This increases the ventilation rate and arterial P_{O_2}. Low-dose acetazolamide is a particularly effective respiratory stimulant in the treatment of sleep apnea. The pediatric dosage for acetazolamide is 5 to 10 mg/kg/day given every 12 h. Side effects include peripheral paresthesias, nausea, vomiting, polyuria, an unpleasant taste in carbonated beverages, drowsiness, and confusion. Acetazolamide is contraindicated for those with sulfur sensitivities. When acetazolamide is used for prophylaxis, it should be started 24 h before ascent and continued for 2 to 3 days after arriving at the planned altitude.

Dexamethasone is also used to treat AMS, although its mechanism of action is unknown. Dexamethasone minimizes the symptoms of AMS but does not affect acclimatization. Its use is reserved for those with sulfur allergies or intolerance to acetazolamide. A dose of 4 mg orally taken four times daily can be started 48 h prior to ascent and continued for 2 days while at high altitude. Care must be taken to avoid a rebound effect when the drug is discontinued.

High-Altitude Cerebral Edema

High-altitude cerebral edema (HACE) is the most severe, life-threatening form of high-altitude illness. It is uncommon, affecting less than 1 to 2 percent of individuals who ascend without acclimatization. It is rare below altitudes of 12,000 ft but has resulted in death at elevations as low as 8200 ft. A common problem is the difficulty of differentiating between AMS and early HACE.

Clinical Presentation

High-altitude cerebral edema commonly begins with the symptoms of AMS and progresses to diffuse neurologic dysfunction. Onset of severe symptoms occurs 1 to 3 days after ascent to altitude, but early signs of AMS may rapidly deteriorate to severe HACE in as few as 12 h. Evidence of high-altitude pulmonary edema (HAPE) may also be present.

Severe headaches, nausea, vomiting, and altered mental status are common symptoms associated with HACE. Truncal ataxia is the cardinal sign of HACE. This alone warrants immediate descent. If not recognized, HACE will proceed to include confusion, slurred speech, diplopia, hallucinations, seizures, impaired judgment, cranial nerve palsies (third and sixth), abnormal reflexes, paresthesias, decreased level of consciousness, coma, and finally death. A 60 percent mortality is associated with HACE once coma is present.

Treatment

Definitive treatment of HACE is descent. This must be done as quickly as possible. High-flow oxygen is indicated as soon as symptoms are recognized. Dexamethasone can produce dramatic improvement. An initial dose of 4 to 8 mg IV (or PO in mild cases) is followed by 4 mg IV every 6 h. Acetazolamide has not been shown to be effective in the treatment of HACE. Hyperbaric therapy with the Gamow bag has been reported to be useful in mild HACE and may be lifesaving if descent is impossible.

For severe cases, intubation and hyperventilation are indicated to decrease intracranial pressure. Furosemide and mannitol are second-line treatments.

Acute episodes of HACE may result in long-term neurologic deficits. Coma may persist for days. Persistent ataxia, impaired judgment, and behavioral changes have been reported to last as long as 1 year. For this reason, it is essential that any evidence of HACE be recognized and treated early and that other etiologies be ruled out if symptoms persist.

High-Altitude Pulmonary Edema

High-altitude pulmonary edema (HAPE) is a life-threatening manifestation of high-altitude illness and represents a unique form of noncardiogenic pulmonary edema. It is estimated that HAPE affects 0.5 to 15 percent of those who ascend rapidly to high altitudes. Other than trauma, it is the most common cause of death at altitude. This condition rarely occurs below 8000 ft and is more commonly associated with altitudes above 14,500 ft. At altitudes between 8000 to 10,000 ft, HAPE may develop after strenuous activity; at higher elevations, it may occur at rest.

High-altitude pulmonary edema is exacerbated by rapid ascent, cold stressors, a past history of HAPE, excessive exertion, and an inability to acclimatize. History of a recent upper respiratory tract infection has also been thought to be contributory.

Children and young adults are more susceptible to HAPE. Individuals under 20 years of age may be 10 to 13 times more prone to develop HAPE. Children are also more susceptible to a special form of this high-altitude illness identified as *reentry HAPE.* This occurs in individuals who are living at higher altitudes and return to this high elevation after spending as little as 24 h at lower altitude.

Clinical Presentation

The onset of HAPE usually occurs within 1 to 4 days after ascent to high altitude, most commonly during the second night. However, initial symptoms may develop within hours following ascent.

Early in the course, the victim will develop a dry cough, fatigue, and dyspnea on exertion. Symptoms of AMS often accompany these initial signs. A few localized rales may be audible in the right middle lobe auscultated over the right axilla. Rales increase with exercise.

As HAPE progresses, the patient will have a productive clear cough, orthopnea, weakness, and altered mental status. This intensifies to severe dyspnea at rest, a cardinal sign of HAPE. The patient may be tachycardic, tachypneic, and febrile to 102°F. Rales become bilateral. Peripheral cyanosis advances to central cyanosis if treatment is not initiated. Dyspnea at rest while at altitude is HAPE until proven otherwise.

A chest radiograph reveals bilateral, fluffy, asymmetric infiltrates and dilated pulmonary arteries. Cardiomegaly, butterfly pattern of infiltrates, and Kerley B lines, commonly seen in cardiogenic pulmonary edema, are not seen in HAPE. An electrocardiogram (ECG) may show sinus tachycardia, right ventricular strain, right axis deviation, P-wave abnormalities, prominent R waves in the right chest leads, and S waves in the left chest leads.

Without treatment, florid pulmonary edema and respiratory failure will develop. Dysfunction of the CNS will ensue, leading to coma and death.

Treatment

As with any form of high-altitude illness, immediate descent may be lifesaving and is not to be delayed. There is a delicate balance, however, between rapid descent and the amount of energy the victim expends to descend quickly. Individuals may deteriorate from overexertion as they proceed to a lower altitude. Therefore, care must be taken to minimize the effort while maximizing the effect. A descent of 1000 to 2000 ft is usually adequate for symptomatic relief.

In addition to rapid descent, bed rest, supplemental oxygen, and prevention of heat loss are necessary. Physical activity and exposure to cold increase catecholamine response, which increases pulmonary pressure. Supplemental oxygen effectively lowers pulmonary arterial pressure, which raises arterial oxygen saturation. As a result, heart rate and respiratory rate will decrease. High-flow oxygen at 6 to 8 L/min by mask is administered to anyone with significant symptoms. It may be possible to reverse symptoms with oxygen alone (without descent) over a period of 2 to 3 days.

An end-positive airway pressure (EPAP) mask that can deliver 5 to 10 cm H_2O of EPAP can be used to improve oxygen delivery. When oxygen is not available and descent is not possible, the portable Gamow bag may be used for hyperbaric treatment and has been shown to be effective in patients with HAPE.

Pharmacologic agents play a limited role in the treatment of HAPE. Acetazolamide may be useful in the prevention of HAPE. While furosemide has been shown to be helpful, caution must be taken due to the prevalence of hypovolemia and dehydration. Nifedipine has been shown to decrease pulmonary arterial pressure. Again, caution must be exercised in its use in a potentially hypovolemic dehydrated patient.

Rapid improvement and resolution of symptoms usually follows descent to a lower altitude. If oxygen saturation is below 90%, hospitalization is indicated. In very severe cases of HAPE, intubation and ventilation with positive end-expiratory pressure (PEEP) may be needed.

The overall mortality of HAPE is 11 percent. Without treatment (descent or supplemental oxygen), the mortality increases to 44 percent.

An episode of HAPE is not a contraindication to further attempts to reach altitude. However, there is a higher incidence for recurrent symptoms with subsequent ascents.

DYSBARIC INJURIES

Dysbaric injuries may be caused by an altitude-related event (e.g., the rapid ascent or descent during airplane transport or sudden cabin decompression at an altitude above 25,000 ft), an underwater diving accident, or a blast injury.

Several terms are often used when discussing this topic. *Dysbarisms* represents the general topic of pressure-related injuries. *Barotrauma* refers to the injuries that are a direct result of the mechanical effects of a pressure differential. The complications related to the partial pressure of gases and dissolved gases are called *decompression sickness.*

Barotrauma: Dysbarisms from Trapped Gases

Barotrauma is the direct result of a pressure difference between the body's air-filled cavities, which are subject to the effects of Boyle's law, and the surrounding environment. During scuba diving, the majority of symptoms will develop during a descent. On descent, a negative pressure develops within these enclosed air spaces relative to the ambient surrounding pressure. If air is unable to enter these structures, equalization does not take place and the air-filled cavities collapse. If the cavity is a rigid structure and unable to collapse, the negative pressure may result in fluid being displaced from the blood vessels of the surrounding mucosa into the intravascular space. The resulting injury pattern can include pain, hemorrhage, edema, vascular engorgement, and tissue damage.

If air is unable to escape on ascent, an expansion of gas within these enclosed air spaces causes a positive pressure. This may result in the rupture of such spaces or the compression of adjacent structures.

Many of the symptoms of barotrauma result in "squeeze" phenomena. These trapped gas disorders are differentiated by the gas-filled part of the body that is affected.

Barotitis

Changes in barometric pressure can result in disturbances of the external, middle, and inner ear. The tympanic membrane (TM) separates the middle ear from the outer ear. The eustachian tube usually functions as a one-way valve that allows gas to escape from but not return to the middle ear.

There are three types of barotitis, with barotitis media the most common.

Barotitis media (middle-ear squeeze) commonly develops on descent between 10 and 20 ft below the surface. The symptoms include a fullness in the ears, severe pain, tinnitus, vertigo, nausea, disorientation, and transient conductive hearing loss. Up to 10 percent of divers may have no pain during descent but will become symptomatic after the dive. If the diver is unable to equalize the pressure and continues to descend, the tympanic membrane may rupture and bleed. With perforation, the caloric stimulation of cold water entering the middle ear will cause vertigo, nausea, and disorientation.

The physical examination may reveal erythema or retraction of the tympanic membrane (TM), blood behind the TM, a ruptured TM, or a bloody nasal discharge.

If pain persists after the dive, decongestants and analgesics may be used. Any patient with barotitis media should be instructed to refrain from diving until all signs and symptoms have resolved. Erythema resolves within 1 to 3 days; however, it will take 2 to 4 weeks when there is blood behind the TM. A perforated tympanic membrane must heal before any further diving is attempted. A 10-day course of antibiotics is indicated if the TM is perforated, but ear drops are to be avoided. Follow-up by an ear, nose, and throat specialist upon discharge from the emergency department is recommended.

Barosinusitis

Normally, air can pass in and out of the sinus cavities without difficulty. However, if a person has a cold or sinus infection, air may become trapped and thus be subject to the barometric pressure changes.

Failure of the air-filled frontal or maxillary sinuses to equilibrate results in pain or pressure above, behind, or below the eyes, which is commonly referred to as *sinus squeeze.* The pain may persist for hours and may be accompanied by a bloody nasal discharge. The ethmoid and sphenoid sinuses rarely contribute to this type of barotrauma.

The treatment of barosinusitis is similar to the treatment of barotitis media. Patients may use a vasoconstrictor nasal spray before initiating a dive or before starting a descent from altitude in an airplane. Antibiotics should be started and continued for 14 to 21 days.

Air Embolism

Air embolism is the most serious dysbaric injury. Due to the buoyancy of air and the fact that scuba divers are usually upright during ascent, the brain is most commonly affected. Symptoms appear immediately on ascent or within 10 to 20 min of surfacing. Neurologic symptoms that develop later than this are more likely due to decompression sickness.

These victims require aggressive care, which includes 100% oxygen, IV fluids, and hyperbaric treatment. They are placed in the Trendelenburg or left lateral decubitus position to minimize the passage of air emboli to the brain.

Pneumothorax and Emphysema

The patient with a pneumothorax, pneumopericardium, pneumomediastinum, or subcutaneous emphysema should not be exposed to any further changes in barometric pressure. This is a significant problem if a pneumothorax develops during a dive. On ascent, a simple pneumothorax may progress to a tension pneumothorax, shock, and loss of consciousness. These complications may also occur during air transport in an unpressurized aircraft. Treatment of a scuba diving pneumothorax is the same as the treatment of other traumatic or nontraumatic pneumothoraxes. Hyperbaric (recompression) treatment is avoided since it can convert a simple pneumothorax into a tension pneumothorax. If hyperbaric treatment will be necessary, chest tubes must be placed before recompression is initiated.

Decompression Sickness: Dysbarisms from Evolved Gases

A diver breathing compressed air is exposed to nitrogen, oxygen, and carbon dioxide. Approximately four-fifths of the air is nitrogen. Under normal circumstances, additional nitrogen gas will not be absorbed by the body during inhalation. However, when a person is exposed to a varying ambient pressure, there is uptake or removal of nitrogen gas from the blood.

As ambient pressure increases, the positive pressure gradient between the alveoli and the blood will result in more nitrogen being dissolved. As a dive progresses, the gas in the blood will quickly equilibrate with the gas in the alveoli. Nitrogen gas, however, is almost five times more soluble in fat. It will take longer to saturate these tissues. Therefore, the body will absorb more nitrogen gas at a rate that is dependent upon the depth and duration of the dive. The longer and deeper the dive, the more nitrogen gas will be accumulated within the body.

Since nitrogen is not metabolized, it remains dissolved until the nitrogen gas pressure in the lungs decreases and the nitrogen can be removed. During a slow ascent, as the surrounding pressure decreases, the nitrogen that is absorbed into the tissues is released into the blood and alveoli. If the ascent is too quick, nitrogen levels do not have the opportunity to equalize between the tissues, blood, and alveoli. The pressure outside the body will drop significantly below the sum of the partial pressures of the gases inside the body. This causes the gas to come out of solution and form gas bubbles. Due to the increased dissolved nitrogen, it has a disproportionately higher partial pressure. Therefore, a significant difference in partial pressure occurs. It is the release of these nitrogen bubbles from solution that results in decompression sickness.

Bends

The term *bends* is often used to identify any form of decompression sickness. When correctly used, however, the term refers to a musculoskeletal syndrome involving the joints, which is a very common dysbarism. The bends occurs in up to 75 percent of all decompression injuries and is caused by the release of nitrogen gas bubbles from the blood into the tissues surrounding the joint.

Symptoms usually develop within 6 to 12 h after the conclusion of a dive. A sharp, throbbing, or dull achy pain is common. There may also be associated numbness or tingling (paresthesias). The joints most often affected are the knees, shoulders, and elbows.

Symptomatic relief may be obtained by splinting the extremity or by applying pressure over the affected joint. Massaging or moving the affected extremity often exacerbates the pain.

The physical examination is usually unremarkable. On occasion, crepitus, edema, or tenderness is noted.

Chokes

The decompression illness that affects the pulmonary system is referred to as the *chokes*. It is caused by arterial or venous nitrogen gas embolization that obstructs the pulmonary vasculature. The symptoms may begin immediately after a dive but often take up to 12 h to develop. They last between 12 and 48 h but can progress to a rapid deterioration.

The classic triad of symptoms includes shortness of breath, cough, and substernal chest pain or tightness. The shortness of breath is described as a feeling of suffocation. The individual becomes tachycardiac and tachypneic. There is a nonproductive, often uncontrollable paroxysmal cough that is exacerbated by deep inspiration. The chest pain is most frequently appreciated with deep inspiration, increased activity, and smoking. There is no radiation of the pain to the neck, arms, or abdomen.

Neurologic Decompression Sickness

Nitrogen gas embolism is the most serious decompression sickness. Venous gas emboli can result in venous obstruction, while arterial gas emboli can cause ischemia as a result of arterial obstruction or induced vasospasm.

As with air embolus, the brain is most commonly affected. The onset of symptoms, however, will usually be delayed and develop within 1 to 6 h after a dive is concluded. These victims require aggressive care, which includes 100% oxygen, intravenous fluids, and hyperbaric treatment. They are placed in the Trendelenburg or left lateral decubitus position to minimize embolization to the brain.

Treatment of Decompression Sickness and Air Embolus

The morbidity and mortality for dysbaric injuries are dependent upon the severity of the injury, rapid identification of the illness, and timely access to appropriate medical care. When the "system" works, the recovery rate is as high as 90 percent.

The treatment of choice for most air emboli and decompression illnesses is hyperbaric (recompression) therapy. This is initiated as soon as possible, ideally within 6 h of the onset of symptoms. In some cases, hyperbaric therapy has been effective in patients who are not treated until 10 to 14 days after the onset of their symptoms.

The goal is to reduce the size of the liberated gas bubbles, facilitate the reabsorption of air bubbles, prevent the formation of new bubbles, and improve oxygenation. Before hyperbaric treatment is initiated, certain procedures should be followed. Endotracheal tube cuffs and Foley catheter balloons should be filled with saline rather than air. It is essential to identify any pneumothorax and insert a chest tube prior to recompression.

In addition to hyperbaric therapy, patients should be dried off immediately and kept warm to prevent hypothermia. The pediatric patient's urine output should be maintained between 1 to 2 mL/kg/h. Intravenous fluids that are packaged in plastic bags, not glass bottles, should be used.

Dysbarisms Caused by Abnormal Gas Concentration

Nitrogen Narcosis

The inhalation of nitrogen gas at elevated partial pressures may cause interference with nerve conduction. As a result, nitrogen narcosis can produce a narcotic or intoxicating effect during a dive. Symptoms can include euphoria, uncontrollable laughter, impaired judgment, memory loss, light-headedness, hallucinations, loss of coordination, and impaired reflexes.

The greatest risk of nitrogen narcosis is drowning. With any evidence or suspicion of confusion, disorientation, or altered mental status, the dive should be terminated. The affected diver should be escorted slowly to the surface by a second diver. No other treatment is required.

For a more detailed discussion, see Blumen IJ, Leinen JJ: High-altitude illness and hyperbaric injuries, chap. 117, p. 623, in *Pediatric Emergency Medicine: A Comprehensive Study Guide.*

118 Radiation Emergencies

Ira J. Blumen / David A. Arai

RADIATION ACCIDENTS

Accidental radiation exposure is a rare occurrence. According to the International Radiation Accident Registry, 331 accidents occurred worldwide between the years 1944 and 1990. These accidents resulted in significant radiation exposure to 3001 individuals and in 103 deaths. A significant percentage of these accidents (63 percent) occurred in the United States, resulting in 31 percent of the deaths (32/103) worldwide.

There are two categories of radiation injuries with which the emergency physician should be familiar. The first type is an *exposure* injury, which generally represents no threat to emergency care providers. *Contamination,* the second type of radiation injury, *may* represent a potential risk to emergency personnel.

Exposure

Exposure radiation injuries may be classified into two categories: a person may be the victim of a *localized radiation injury* or may have suffered a *whole-body exposure.*

Localized Radiation Injuries

A large dose of radiation exposure to a small part of the body will result in a local radiation injury. These injuries often occur over months or even years, but they may occur over a shorter amount of time.

Localized radiation injuries most commonly affect the upper extremities, with the buttocks and thighs representing the next most common sites. Typically these injuries occur in the occupational setting. In addition, adults and children may unknowingly come into direct contact with a radiation source by handling an unknown object or by putting it into their pockets. Localized radiation accidents may also result from an inadvertent exposure to an intense radiation beam.

The dose of radiation that may result in a local radiation injury varies greatly. Larger doses are often better tolerated than if there were a whole-body exposure. Accidental exposure from radioactive sources with a surface dose of nearly 20,000 rad/min have been reported to have caused localized radiation injuries.

The initial clinical picture of a localized radiation injury depicts a thermal injury to the skin. While thermal burns develop soon after an exposure, erythema from a local radiation injury is delayed. Radiation injury should be considered in the differential diagnosis for any patient who presents with a "burn" but who does not remember a thermal or chemical insult.

Prolonged radiation exposure causes blood vessel fibrosis, leading to tissue necrosis. The outcome will be determined by the degree of blood vessel and tissue damage. Classification of these localized injuries can be divided into four types, differentiated by increasing epidermal and dermal injury.

Whole-Body Exposure

Acute Radiation Syndrome may develop following a whole-body exposure of 100 rad or more that occurs over a relatively short period of time. Organ systems with rapidly dividing cells (bone marrow, gastrointestinal tract) are the most vulnerable to radiation injury. With greater doses of radiation, however, all organ systems may become involved, including the central nervous system.

Estimating the exposure (in rads) of a whole-body radiation victim may be difficult when the patient presents to the emergency department. Dosimeters and Geiger counters are not standard equipment in many emergency departments and are often of little help in determining the total radiation dose or duration of exposure. A mechanical dosimetry monitoring device worn by the victim during the time of exposure would be helpful but is rarely available. Instead, the emergency physician's history and physical, along with baseline laboratory values, are essential in estimating the whole-body exposure. This technique is referred to as *biological dosimetry*. For this purpose, the primary indicators include the time of onset of symptoms and depression of absolute lymphocyte count. The earlier signs and symptoms develop, the higher the dose and the worse the prognosis.

A progressive sequence of signs and symptoms following a whole-body exposure can be divided into four stages: the *prodromal stage*, the *latent stage*, the *manifest illness stage*, and the *recovery stage*. An individual's susceptibility, the dose of radiation, dose rate, and dose distribution will dictate the onset, duration, and character of symptoms in a predictable representation. The prodromal stage can begin minutes to hours after exposure and is dose-dependent. The most common symptoms of this stage include nausea, vomiting, and fatigue. Exposure to less than 100 rad rarely causes symptoms, and patients who do not exhibit nausea or vomiting within 6 h of a radiation accident are unlikely to have been subject to a significant whole-body exposure. Prodromal markers beginning within 6 h suggest an exposure in excess of 100 rad. Higher doses will result in a more rapid onset of these initial signs and symptoms, probably due to acute tissue injury and the subsequent release of vasoactive substances, including histamine and bradykinin.

A lower-dose exposure will yield a resolution of the prodromal symptoms over a period of days to weeks, during the latent stage. Progressively higher radiation doses will prolong the prodromal stage while limiting the latent period until a point is reached when it appears that the prodromal stage proceeds directly to the manifest illness stage without any resolution of the prodromal symptoms.

During the manifest illness stage, specific organ symptoms develop and the patient is at the greatest risk for infection and bleeding. Three syndromes may develop during this stage, depending on the total amount of radiation exposure: the hematopoietic syndrome (220 to 600 rad), the gastrointestinal syndrome (600 to 1000 rad), and the neurovascular syndrome (>1000 rad).

Although the effect of radiation on the hematopoietic system is characterized by pancytopenia, the *absolute lymphocyte count* represents the best way to estimate exposure hematologically. Leukocyte counts may be elevated initially due to demargination, but the lymphocyte portion of the differential will quickly start to decrease. A 48-h check will suggest the severity of the exposure. A lymphocyte count greater than 1200/mm^3 indicates a 100- to 200-rad exposure and most often a good prognosis. An absolute lymphocyte count of 300 to 1200/mm^3 suggests a 200- to 400-rad exposure, which promises a fair outcome. Exposure to more than 400 rad is marked by a poor prognosis and is expected with counts below 300/mm^3. Pancytopenia may develop after a latent period lasting a few days to three weeks. The patient will subsequently suffer from dyspnea, malaise, purpura, bleeding and opportunistic infection.

Gastrointestinal illness will be most evident with total-body exposures of 600 to 1000 rad. The prodromal phase is abrupt and is marked by severe vomiting and diarrhea. The latent stage may be quite short and is followed by continued GI symptoms, leading to relentless fluid loss, fever, and prostration. The radiosensitive mucosal cells of the small bowel begin to slough, which—combined with the coexistent hematopoietic abnormalities—produces severe, bloody diarrhea. Even with intense supportive care, the patient rarely survives.

Total-body irradiation with more than 1000 rad results in a neurovascular syndrome. At such high radiation levels, even cells that are relatively resistant to injury are damaged. Ataxia and confusion quickly develop and there is direct vascular damage, with resultant circulatory collapse. The patient usually expires within hours.

Patients with lower levels of exposure or those fortunate enough to respond to aggressive supportive management will enter the recovery stage. Further management is guided by specific organ system insults. For these survivors, the long-term risks of exposure to ionizing radiation include cataracts, leukemia, and development of carcinomas. It should be noted that the median lethal dose of total-body irradiation is estimated at 400 rad.

Contamination

Contamination is the second type of radiation accident. Radioactive particles, solid or liquid, may remain on the surface of the victim, resulting in an external contamination. Internal contamination may be the result of inhaled, ingested, or absorbed radioactive particles. Neutrons, alpha particles, and beta particles are most commonly responsible for contamination. Unlike an exposure victim, the contaminated patient does represent an additional challenge and potential risk to hospital and prehospital personnel.

In most situations, and if the patient's condition permits, decontamination should begin in the prehospital setting. This will reduce the potential spread of radioactive material and will decrease the potential contamination of hospital workers or other rescuers. Fortunately, if appropriate management steps are taken, the radiation-contaminated patient should present little danger to hospital staff, even if decontamination was incomplete prior to arrival at the hospital.

MANAGEMENT

General Concepts

It is important to realize that the general principles of patient care for radiation victims are no different than those for other medical problems. The initial assessment and management is directed toward the routine attention to the ABCs (airway, breathing, circulation). There are no acute, life-threatening complications of a survivable radiation injury that require immediate intervention. Emergency treatment should be supportive and directed toward the prevention of complications.

It will be important to determine, quickly, whether the patients are victims of a radiation exposure or a contamination. Radiation *contamination* requires that decontamination begin promptly after stabilization. The radiation *exposure* patient who is not contaminated represents no danger to the hospital staff or other patients. These victims can be managed in the emergency department and require no immediate intervention related to the radiation exposure.

While both prehospital and hospital workers may be at risk, it is the prehospital personnel and other rescuers, who respond to the site of a radiation accident, who are more often exposed to significant radiation. A threshold of 5000 mrem (5 rem) should be the exposure limit except to save a life. A once-in-a-lifetime exposure to 100,000 mrem (100 rem) to save a life has been established by the National Council on Radiation Protection as acceptable and will not result in any undue morbidity.

Prehospital Management

The history obtained by prehospital personnel is of paramount importance in management decisions regarding radiation victims. When possible, rescuers must gather details regarding the exact type, location, and duration of exposure. For internal exposure, the route of entry, type, and quantity of radioactive material should be determined. If the incident has occurred in an industrial or laboratory setting, initial decontamination procedures may be instituted by on-site personnel according to their established protocol before EMS personnel arrive. A quick response in decontamination will limit the exposure to the victim and decrease the amount of further contamination of both the ambulance and the emergency department. For unstable patients, the minimal action performed prior to rapid transport is the removal of contaminated clothing.

After transport of the patient to the hospital, EMS personnel and their vehicles must be inspected for the presence of radioactive contamination before they leave the facility. This must also be done at the scene for any ambulance and personnel who respond to the accident site and provide field assessment and stabilization without patient transport.

Emergency Department Management

Few hospitals will be called on to treat victims of life-threatening radiation accidents. The exceptions are hospitals in close proximity to nuclear power plants or in the event of a nuclear war. It is more likely, however, that hospitals will be called on to attend victims of a minor industrial accident or an accident involving the transportation of radioactive materials. The end result will be a patient with "routine injuries," whose treatment may be complicated by an inadvertent radiation exposure with or without low-level radioactive contamination.

Radiation Accident Plan

The Joint Commission on Accreditation of Healthcare Organizations (JCAHO) requires each emergency department to have a radiation accident plan. In the event of a medically significant radiation accident, a well-prepared—and practiced—plan will supply emergency care providers with an appropriate knowledge base, management protocols, and additional resources that can be called upon.

A major part of a well-prepared plan facilitates the identification of *significant* versus *perceived* radiation dangers. The incidence of significant radiation accidents may be rare for some hospitals, but the incidence of perceived radiation accidents may be much greater. A vehicular accident involving a truck or train carrying radioactive material near a school may send dozens (or hundreds) of anxious parents and their children to the emergency department. The staff of a well-prepared emergency department can assess the potential risks and, when appropriate, correct any misconceptions and ease the fears the general public may have.

A lack of experience, an incomplete knowledge base, and a significant degree of fear among health care providers often result in the mismanagement of radiation victims. Therefore, it is essential that an emergency department develop protocols for dealing with both the radiation exposure itself and the medical management of these victims.

External Contamination

The process of decontamination, or cleaning the patient of particulate radioactive debris, should be initiated as soon as possible following the event. Rescue personnel must wear protective clothing, including rubber gloves, shoe covers, masks, and film badges. This protective clothing does not reduce the exposure to penetrating radiation. Rather, it serves to prevent any radioactive particles from coming in contact with the personnel or their clothing and to facilitate cleanup and disposal.

Initially any open wounds are covered and the patient's clothing is removed; all articles are placed in clearly labeled plastic bags. Up to 70 to 90 percent of external contamination can be eliminated by this action alone. Any open wound is considered contaminated until proven otherwise, and decontamination should precede the irrigation of intact skin surfaces. The skin is then washed with copious amounts of water and soap, with particular attention to skin folds, ears, and fingernails. The use of damp washcloths rather than rinsing with running water may be more practical for some emergency departments. The disposal of contaminated washcloths in plastic bags may be easier than the collection of contaminated wash water. All waste must be captured in sealed containers labeled "*Radioactive Waste.*"

Shaving of the patient's hair is to be avoided, along with excessive rubbing of the skin. Both of these maneuvers cause an increased risk of transdermal uptake. Open, uncontaminated wounds are covered with sterile dressings, and contaminated wounds are then cleaned aggressively, like other dirty wounds.

Whenever possible, a dosimeter should be used to determine the completeness of the decontamination. The goal is to get the radiation level "as low as reasonably achievable"; this is commonly referred to as the ALARA principle. When dealing with an external contamination, it is important to prevent it from becoming an internal contamination.

Internal Contamination

Radioactive particles that are ingested or inhaled or that contaminate open wounds can cause significant cellular damage. These particles will continue to irradiate tissues until they are eliminated, neutralized, or blocked or until they decay naturally. In general, there is a 1- to 2-h window of time during which absorption of these particles occurs. Therefore it is crucial that any interventions be performed during this period and as soon as possible.

At times it may be difficult to determine the presence of an internal contaminant, especially if an external contaminant still clouds the picture. In addition, special treatment considerations will be determined by the type of radionucleotide involved. Therefore, it is extremely important to identify the offending agent as early as possible, so that the appropriate chelating or blocking agent may be used.

Ideally, chelating agents are administered within 1 h of exposure. Chelating agents provide an ion-exchange matrix that binds metals. This prevents tissue uptake and promotes urinary excretion of a stable complex containing the radioactivity. Diethylenetriamine-pentaacetic acid (DTPA) is an effective chelating agent for many heavy metals. A solution of DTPA is often found in hospital nuclear medicine departments, but this may be too dilute to be used as a chelating agent. Other examples of chelating agents are calcium disodium edetate (EDTA), succimer, and penicillamine. These are recommended when radioactive lead is the cause of an internal contamination.

A blocking agent reduces radioactive uptake by saturating the tissues with a nonradioactive element. Lugol's solution (potassium iodine) is a blocking agent that reduces the uptake of radioactive iodine (^{131}I) by the thyroid gland. An exposure of 10 to 30 rem warrants the initiation of this treatment within a few hours. If the diagnosis has not yet been confirmed, there is little harm in administering a first dose of potassium iodine.

Ingestion

Initial stabilization and decontamination of radiation ingestions are the same as those for "routine" ingestions. The goal is to prevent absorption and enhance elimination. Lavage and activated charcoal are used in the usual manner and cathartics may be used to shorten the GI transit time. All bodily excretions (lavage fluid, emesis, urine, feces) are saved and labeled for radioactive evaluation and proper disposal.

Inhalation

Acute inhalation of radionucleotides is much less common than chronic low-level exposure. An acute inhalation contamination can occur in the event of a radioactive accident in conjunction with a fire or explosion. Radioactive iodine, for example, is highly volatile and likely to be inhaled.

When an inhalation contamination is suspected, a moistened cotton-tipped applicator can be used to swab the nasal passages and check for radioactivity. Bronchopulmonary lavage is performed for removal of particulate matter. Specific blocking and chelating agents may also be given by nebulizer.

Open Wounds

Wounds that undergo successful decontamination may be surgically closed. Wounds that remain contaminated despite aggressive irrigation are left open for 24 h. Debridement of these wounds may become necessary for further decontamination. Contaminated surgical instruments must be replaced to prevent further wound contamination.

Amputation of contaminated extremities is rarely indicated. Two situations may warrant this aggressive management. In the first, the amount of persistent contamination is so high that severe radiation-induced necrosis is anticipated. In the second, the degree of traumatic injury is so severe that functional recovery is doubtful.

Exposure

Despite the significant illness and injury that can result from either a local radiation injury or whole-body exposure, an emergency physician can offer only limited treatment. Fluid resuscitation for severe vomiting and diarrhea, baseline laboratory values, the initiation of antibiotics for infection, and burn management may be all there is to do for the "exposure" patient in the emergency department. The patient will face the greatest risks and management problems several days to several weeks later, at the onset of the manifest illness stage.

In some cases, nothing will alter the patient's outcome. Victims with a whole-body exposure of more than 1000 rad have a mortality rate of 99 to 100 percent. For triage purposes, these patients should be classified as *expectant* or *impending.* Death ensues from the complications affecting the hematopoietic as well as the gastrointestinal and central nervous systems. Emergency department management should consist of appropriate sedation, analgesics, and supportive care.

Based on the presenting symptoms, patients can be classified into three major prognostic classifications: *survivor probable, survivor possible,* and *survivor improbable.*

Survivor Probable

This group includes individuals who are asymptomatic or who have minimal complaints that resolve within hours. Initial and subsequent leukocyte counts are not affected and estimated exposure is less than 200 rad (2 Gy). Following satisfactory decontamination, inpatient care is rarely needed.

Survivor Possible

This group consists of patients with relatively brief gastrointestinal sequelae, usually lasting less than 48 h. After initial presentation and the latent period, patients develop characteristic pancytopenia. Estimated exposure for this group is between 200 and 800 rad (2 to 8 Gy). An exposure of 400 rad represents the median lethal dose.

Survival in this group is influenced by the aggressiveness of supportive therapy, hematologic intervention, antecedent health of the victim, and the response to bone marrow transplantation when indicated.

Survivor Improbable

In these patients the estimated whole-body exposure exceeds 800 rad (8 Gy). The prognosis is dismal despite aggressive supportive therapy and even the implementation of bone marrow transplantation. If severe nausea, vomiting, and diarrhea begin within 1 h of exposure and CNS symptoms appear early, a relatively early death can be expected.

For a more detailed discussion, see Blumen IJ, Arai DA: Radiation emergencies, chap. 118, p. 640, in *Pediatric Emergency Medicine: A Comprehensive Study Guide.*

SECTION XIX
PSYCHOSOCIAL EMERGENCIES

119 Child Maltreatment

Paula Kienberger Jaudes

The spectrum of child maltreatment includes physical abuse, sexual abuse, and emotional abuse. It also encompasses neglect, which can be medical, supervisional, educational, physical, nutritional, or fetal. For some children, recognition of maltreatment can mean the difference between life and death. Approximately one-quarter of substantiated reports of child maltreatment originate from health professionals.

PHYSICAL ABUSE

Physical abuse in a child results when an injury is inflicted by an older caretaker. It commonly results in bruises, burns, fractures, and head or visceral injury. Some cases result from poisoning. In many patients, abuse is recurrent, and a search will reveal multiple old injuries. It is common for physical abuse to be discovered when the child is brought to the emergency department (ED) for treatment of a seemingly innocuous medical condition.

The history is vital in distinguishing abuse from noninflicted injury. The mechanism of injury must adequately explain the lesion and must correlate with normal childhood development. Important clues that can help distinguish noninflicted injury from inflicted injury include a changing or inconsistent history or a different history given by different caretakers. If the child is verbal, he or she should be questioned about the injury. Inappropriate delay in seeking medical treatment is always a cause for grave concern and raises the issue of medical neglect. Another clue to abuse is an inappropriate interaction between child and caretaker. A withdrawn or extremely nonverbal child with an acute injury is cause for concern. Some abused children try to protect the abusing parent. Caretakers who are inappropriately hostile, threatening, or demanding may be trying to deflect questioning away from the nature of the child's injury. In cases where more than one caretaker is with the child, it is important to try to obtain separate histories from each.

The physical examination of the potentially abused child focuses on detecting acute injuries as well as old lesions. The medicolegal ramifications of abuse are such that the examination must be extremely thorough and the documentation meticulous. Describing injuries on predrawn silhouettes may aid in thorough documentation.

The examination of the skin is particularly important, since cutaneous manifestations of physical abuse are usually the most easily recognized signs of maltreatment. It is important to note the location, shape, number, and ages of lesions.

Noninflicted bruises tend to be found on prominent bony areas, such as shins, knees, elbows, and the forehead of a toddler. Inflicted bruises may be found on fleshy areas, such as the face, back, abdomen, thighs, or buttocks, or on relatively protected areas of the neck, chest, or genitalia. Common lesions include a handprint, loop marks from a cordlike object, marks produced by striking with a belt buckle or hanger, circumferential marks caused by restraints, or well-demarcated bruises caused by striking with a blunt instrument. Bruises in various stages of healing are highly suspicious of abuse if there is no underlying bleeding diathesis. In general, bruises 1 to 5 days old are reddish-blue, while those 5 to 7 days old develop a green color. Bruises 7 to 10 days old are yellow, while at 10 to 14 days after the injury, the lesion becomes brown.

Human bites are common abuse-related injuries. In infants they tend to occur around the genitalia or buttocks, while in older children multiple lesions are often found randomly around the body. Human bite marks are oval or elliptical lesions caused by a crushing injury, while animal bites cause punctures and tears of the skin. Human bite marks should be photographed in both color and black-and-white film, with a centimeter ruler placed in the photographed field. The skin should be swabbed for saliva with a cotton swab moistened in saline and then labeled, bottled, and placed in the refrigerator.

Approximately 20 percent of all burns in children are inflicted. Abusive burns are usually contact or immersion in nature. Common objects used to burn children include cigarettes, irons, grids, hot plates, space heaters, and light bulbs. Spills or splash-scald burns are often caused when a child pulls down a container filled with a hot liquid from a countertop or stove. The pattern of these burns is typically arrow shaped, with separate small satellite splash burns. An immersion burn characteristically leaves a stocking or glovelike pattern, usually on the extremities or buttocks.

The vast majority of children who suffer inflicted skeletal trauma are under 2 years of age. In patients with fractures, it is absolutely crucial that the history provide a mechanism of injury that adequately explains the type of fracture. In many cases of abuse, the caretaker blames a fall for the lesion. Skeletal fractures in children who have been maltreated can be divided into those involving the metaphyseal-epiphyseal region and those involving the diaphysis. Bucket-handle fractures, corner fractures, and metaphyseal lucency represent varying appearances of the same injury and are highly suggestive of abuse. They result when twisting forces avulse bone attached to the tightly adherent periostium. Diaphyseal fractures that are spiral or transverse are less specific for abuse but are more commonly found in children who have been abused than are accidental fractures. Fractures of the ribs, sternum, scapula, medial and lateral clavicle, vertebral body, and spinous process should heighten the suspicion of possible abuse. Subperiosteal elevation may indicate an old subperiosteal hematoma caused by trauma. Multiple fractures in different stages of healing are highly indicative of abuse, but underlying conditions that predispose to fractures, such as osteogenesis imperfecta and rickets, must be considered and excluded. The radiographic skeletal survey is the principal imaging study for suspected child maltreatment.

Head injuries are the leading cause of death and morbidity from child maltreatment. The shaken-impact syndrome is especially common in children less than 2 years of age. It results from repetitive, violent shaking of the infant's relatively large head, and in many cases is associated with blunt trauma. Infants with brain injury and increased intracranial pressure may present with vomiting and lethargy, which may be confused with gastroenteritis. The physical examination may reveal bruising around the head, face, ear, scalp, or neck. In infants with increased intracranial pressure, the fontanelle may be full, the cranial sutures widely split, and the head circumference increased. Retinal hemorrhages may be present. Subdural hematomas and subarachnoid hemorrhage are common in the shaken-impact syndrome. Computed tomography (CT) is the best initial study. In most cases, magnetic resonance imaging (MRI) is eventually indicated to differentiate between acute, subacute, and chronic hemorrhages. Children with head injuries often have associated skeletal injuries. Multiple skull fractures are highly correlated with abuse.

Visceral injuries are the second leading cause of death from child abuse. Blunt trauma causes crushing of solid viscera or compression of hollow viscera against the vertebral column, or shearing of the posterior attachments or vascular supply of viscera. Any and all of the thoracic or abdominal viscera have been known to be avulsed, torn, ruptured, or injured due to physical abuse. An especially common lesion is a duodenal hematoma, which can present with bilious vomiting. Lacerations of the liver or spleen can result in hypovolemic shock. Management is predicated on the nature of the injury.

Child abuse can also result from intentional poisoning. Accidental poisonings often occur in children between 1 and 3 years of age. Children 1 to 2 years of age usually ingest household products, while children 2 to 3 years of age swallow drugs. Intentional poisoning should be suspected in cases in which older or very young children ingest a drug. Other clues of intentional poisoning are an unexplained history of ingestion, a previous history of a child or sibling with poisoning, recurrent illnesses unexplained by medical workups, or serious illness or death caused by poisonings. Common agents include ipecac, laxatives, pepper, and drugs such as cocaine and alcohol. Toxicology screens should be performed if poisoning is suspected.

The laboratory evaluation of the potentially abused child varies according to the presentation. However, any patient with significant bruising or hemorrhage is evaluated with a complete blood count, including platelets, and a prothrombin and partial thromboplastin time to exclude a bleeding diathesis. Patients with abdominal complaints should have liver enzymes and amylase evaluated. Plain films or an abdominal CT may be necessary. A skeletal survey of the body is indicated if cutaneous lesions suggest physical abuse or in cases where there is a suspicious fracture or head injury. Patients with multiple fractures should have serum levels of calcium, phosphate, and alkaline phosphatase evaluated to exclude underlying bone disease.

The major decision in the emergency department is whether to admit the child to the hospital for protection or discharge the child to a caretaker. Many hospitals involve an abuse team in this process, which permits a multidisciplinary approach to the family.

SEXUAL ABUSE

It is estimated that between 1 in 5 and 1 in 10 children have been sexually misused. Typically, sexual abuse is repetitive and is performed by a family member. In the vast majority of sexual abuse cases, the perpetrators are known to the child prior to the offense. Approximately 80 percent of the victims are females, but an increasing number of male children are being identified.

The history is the key to establishing the diagnosis of sexual abuse. Sexually abused children can present to the ED with a number of complaints, including an outcry of sexual abuse, abdominal complaints, urogenital symptoms or injuries, altered or sexual behavior that raises concern in an adult, or medical reasons unrelated to abuse. Ideally, the interview in the ED constitutes a screening history that establishes suspicion of sexual abuse but does not provide a detailed account of the process. The screening history should be well documented, using direct quotations from the child whenever possible. Open-ended questions and the child's own words in connection with anatomic body parts should be used. Leading questions are inappropriate. Care is taken to be supportive and empathetic. Expressions of shock are avoided. The family is interviewed separately to ascertain their knowledge of the abuse and to assess whether the child can safely be discharged to the care of the family. A more in-depth forensic interview occurs outside the ED by professionals trained to interview child victims of sexual abuse.

A complete physical examination is performed, leaving the genital and perianal examination for last. External inspection of the vaginal and perianal area is usually sufficient. Magnification with a hand-held magnifying glass or an otoscope aids in the visualization of the genital area. Speculums may be used for the examination of adolescents. The physician examines the genital area of the female child for any abnormalities, including discharge, bruises, and lacerations. The shape, contour, and intact state of the hymen is evaluated, especially in the 3- to 9-o'clock position. The size of the vaginal opening is evaluated, as is the posterior forchette. For the perianal examination, the physician looks for bruising, abrasions, anal fissures, skin tags, or irregular skin folds not in the 6- or 12-o'clock position, and for gaping dilatation of the rectal ampulla without the presence of stool. In the evaluation of the male child, the physician examines for signs of trauma around the penis, the scrotum, and the perianal area. In over half of all sexual abuse cases, the physical examination is normal.

Studies are performed to collect forensic evidence if the sexual assault occurred within 72 h of the child's presentation to the ED. Cultures to be considered include throat, vagina/urethral meatus, and rectal cultures for *Chlamydia trachomatis* and *Neisseria gonorrhoeae.* Enzyme-linked assay tests are not used in the detection of *Chlamydia* because the potential for false-positive results renders them legally useless. Blood is drawn for serologic evaluation of syphilis. Vesicular lesions should be cultured to exclude herpes simplex. In patients with a vaginal discharge, a wet mount is performed to screen for *Trichomonas vaginalis* or bacterial vaginosis. Patients with condylomata may require biopsy for papillomavirus. In selected cases of sexual abuse, serologic screening for human immunodeficiency virus (HIV) should be considered. Documented infection with *N. gonorrhoeae* and syphilis is considered to be unequivocal evidence of abuse, while infection with *Chlamydia,* herpes simplex, and *Trichomonas* is highly suggestive of sexual maltreatment.

In the event that sexual abuse is suspected, the physician is mandated to report the case to the child protection service agency. In cases of sexual abuse, the law enforcement agency is also contacted. The decision on disposition from the ED is usually made with the help of social services. Follow-up referrals for psychological counseling for the child and family are important. In selected cases, prophylactic therapy for sexually transmitted disease is indicated. Young children cannot take doxycycline; the drug of choice for *Chlamydia* is erythromycin. Pregnancy prophylaxis should be considered in cases of rape.

NEGLECT

Neglect is the most common type of maltreatment reported to state agencies, and it causes the greatest morbidity and mortality in children. Child neglect can be categorized as medical, supervisional, physical, abandonment, and failure to thrive.

Medical neglect encompasses a spectrum of behaviors, ranging from the caretaker who refuses or denies treatment for serious acute illnesses to caretakers who do not seek basic medical care. A common result of medical neglect is the exacerbation of a chronic medical problem that the child's caretaker has ignored. The overutilization of the ED to care for children whose chronic diseases could be controlled by compliance with prescribed medical treatment is a cause of great morbidity.

Supervisional neglect is expressed in the morbidity and mortality of potentially avoidable childhood "accidents." The ED is in a position to provide injury prevention counseling and education to many of these caretakers.

Physical neglect is the failure to provide adequate food, clothing, or shelter. Abandonment is the ultimate form of physical neglect, which occurs when a parent cannot or will not care for a child. Typically, the child is left with a relative or baby-sitter.

Failure to thrive is the failure of an infant to grow and develop properly in the absence of organic medical problems. Infants, usually under 2 years of age, often present with acute medical problems such as a rash or an infectious illness. The physical examination reveals little subcutaneous tissue, protruding ribs, and loose folds of skin. Muscle tone may be either hyper- or hypotonic. The children are often passive, irritable, or wary. The patient's height, weight, head circumference, and weight for height should be plotted on standardized growth charts. The weight is disproportionally decreased compared to the height or head circumference. The weight-for-height measurement falls below the fifth percentile.

The ED laboratory evaluation of the child with failure to thrive includes a complete blood count, urinalysis, and serum electrolytes.

These infants usually require admission. Neglect as the etiology of failure to thrive is confirmed when the patient gains weight on an appropriate diet. Hospitalization also allows further evaluation for an organic etiology and permits multidisciplinary involvement in educating and counseling the caretaker.

Management of Neglect

Management of the various causes of neglect is individualized. Occasionally, children need to be admitted for medical reasons and for protection. Emergency departments without specialized abuse services may consider referral to an appropriate pediatric center.

CHILD PROTECTION SERVICES AND THE LEGAL SYSTEMS

In all 50 states, child protection laws require all professionals who interact with children to notify the state child protection services if there is a suspicion of child maltreatment. All health professionals working in the emergency department are mandated reporters.

The physician has an obligation to inform the parents of the mandated requirement to notify the state child protection services. Mandated reporters are protected from legal retribution by alleged abusers. Health professionals in the ED may be subpoenaed to testify in court.

For a more detailed discussion, see Jaudes PK: Child maltreatment, chap. 119, p. 657, in *Pediatric Emergency Medicine: A Comprehensive Study Guide.*

120 Psychiatric Emergencies

Elizabeth Schwarz / Tom Wright

A psychiatric emergency exists when a situation arises in which patients have become dangerous to themselves or others or in which symptoms or problems escalate to the point where either patients or their support systems (i.e., family or school) are overwhelmed and seek additional services. A psychiatric crisis often provides a window of opportunity to reach a patient and/or family system that has been resistant to intervention in the past and to connect them with the appropriate services. The emergency physician can identify a patient's weaknesses and strengths so as to help shape the treatment plan for the current crisis.

GENERAL APPROACH

The assessment of pediatric patients is similar to that of adults (Table 120-1). However, it is necessary to modify the source of

TABLE 120-1 Emergency Assessment and Management

Identifying data Age, sex, race, occupation, referral source
Chief complaint
History of present illness Presenting problem, time course, precipitants, previous episodes, previous and current treatments
Past psychiatric history Psychosis, depression, suicide attempts, aggression, medications, therapy
Past medical history
Medications Neuroleptics, antidepressants, steroids, anticonvulsants, tranquilizers
Developmental history Mental retardation, autism, developmental delays or regression
Social history Family constellation, alcohol and drug use, school, abuse and neglect, social interaction
Family psychiatric history
Mental status exam General appearance and behavior, level of consciousness and orientation, speech, mood, affect, thought process, thought content (suicidal, homicidal, delusions, paranoia, hallucinations), memory, concentration, judgment, insight, impulse control
Diagnostic tests Chemistry, toxicology, CT, EEG, LP, diagnostic rating scales (Beck Depression Inventory, Conners Suicide Intent Rating Scale)
Dispositions Psychiatric hospitalization, medical hospitalization with consultation, partial hospitalization, child welfare agency, outpatient referral (individual, group, family, psychopharmacology, community mental health center, school counselor), return to emergency room, court system

TABLE 120-2 Restraining a Child

A minimum of four people are needed to put a child in restraints (more may be necessary depending on size of child)
Keep hands away from patient's mouth to prevent being bitten
Explain to patient what is going on even if patient does not appear to understand
Monitor patient frequently for comfort and safety
As patient calms down, remove one restraint at a time

information and the style of gathering it. The ability to give a coherent history will depend on the child's attitude toward the interview, mental status, and intellectual and developmental level. Although it is important to obtain as much history as possible from the patient, it is necessary to obtain collateral history from parents, teachers, law officers, or other contacts. Children should be interviewed separately from their parents.

Certain steps are applicable across diagnostic categories in managing out-of-control behavior. The continuum of interventions begins with placing the child in a quiet, private area. Efforts are made to calm the child with supportive, reassuring statements indicating appreciation of the child's condition and distress. Expressions of frustration or anger will tend to exacerbate the child's difficulty. Information should be conveyed in a straightforward, calm manner at an appropriate level of understanding. The child should be given some choices to help him or her feel some sense of control. If the child does not respond to supportive but firm limits and his or her behavior poses a danger, physical restraints may be used. When a child or adolescent is put in restraints, a number of steps must be followed (Table 120-2). Sometimes containment in restraints makes children feel safe from their impulses and helps them regain control. If verbal interventions and physical restraints do not work, then medication becomes necessary. First, it is essential to rule out any organic causes of the behavior that would contraindicate sedation or respiratory depression. Then low doses of neuroleptics may be given (haloperidol 0.5 to 3 mg PO or IM).

Once a patient's safety has been ensured, the preliminary diagnosis and treatment plan are formulated. Patients usually present to the emergency department for a crisis, either as a first event or as an exacerbation of an ongoing illness. The treatment plan must address both immediate and long-term issues. As hospital stays are increasingly short, many psychiatric problems are man-

TABLE 120-3 Possible Indications for Hospitalization

Suicidal
Homicidal
Family unable to care for child
Physical and/or sexual abuse
Failure of outpatient treatment
Stabilization on or adjustment of medication

aged on an outpatient basis. The examining physician must be aware of both the determinants of an inpatient stay (Table 120-3) and the availability and capabilities of outpatient and community services.

SUICIDE

Youth suicide has increasingly become a major public health problem, the incidence having quadrupled in the past 40 years, with the sharpest rise in 14- to 18-year-olds. The presence of a firearm in the house increases the risk of a successful suicide more than twofold. A large percentage of suicidal adolescents have mood disorders, conduct disorders, substance abuse disorders, or antisocial personality traits. Depression and schizophrenia are known correlates of suicidal behavior. Social and environmental factors include interpersonal conflict, disrupted romances, legal or disciplinary problems, defective parent bonding, and racial difficulties. There is growing evidence that gay and lesbian adolescents may be at a greater risk for suicide.

Assessment

The assessment of suicidal behavior or ideation requires understanding of the presence and degree of suicidal intent. The general assessment format, described above and in Table 120-1, can be used as a basic outline. An in-depth evaluation of a child's social support is crucial. Following below are important areas of assessment.

Medical/Physical

The management consists first of a thorough physical examination and assessment and treatment of any ingestions or self-inflicted injuries. Victims of trauma, especially that involving drugs or alcohol, may have been engaging in risky behavior and must also be evaluated for suicidal traits.

Mental Status Examination

A mental status examination includes observation for such signs as depressed mood, crying, poor eye contact, flat or sad affect, poor concentration, and poor memory. Additionally, general observations about grooming and motor activity are useful. It is always important to ask direct questions about suicidal thoughts. Areas about which to question the child and parents are summarized in Table 120-1.

Past/Family History

Patients who have attempted suicide in the past are more likely to attempt suicide again. This information may be available only from a parent or other support figure. In addition, a family history of suicidal behavior or other psychiatric conditions increases the risk of suicide in offspring.

Support System

An emergency assessment of the youth's support system must be included in the decision on disposition. The support system includes other family members, friends, health care professionals, teachers, and counselors to whom the youth has access: people to whom he or she may turn if a crisis or suicidal ideation arises. Both the patient and the family should be questioned about available supports and the patient's ability to utilize them. Members of this support system may have to be taught, in the emergency department, how to handle another suicidal situation should it arise. Phone numbers of a crisis team, therapist, and other emergency services must be given to these caregivers. It is also important to educate the parents about the most lethal means of suicide, firearms. Should the family have firearms in the home, some action must be taken to eliminate the youth's access to them.

Management

If a patient denies having made a suicide attempt, it is still important to complete a thorough physical evaluation and toxicology screen. The child may not have been truthful. If the suicidal child is hospitalized on a medical unit immediately after a suicide attempt, constant monitoring must be in place, including a 24-h observer. Similar monitoring is necessary in the emergency department prior to transfer. Once the suicidal patient has been medically cleared, a decision must be made about whether the child can safely return home with subsequent outpatient care, or whether he or she must be hospitalized.

The criteria for admission to a psychiatric unit are increasingly stringent. Reasons for hospitalization include the following:

- Inability to maintain a no-suicide contract
- Active suicidal ideation (plan and intent)
- High intent or lethality of attempt
- Psychosis
- Severe depression
- Substance abuse
- Bipolar disorder
- Serious aggression
- Previous suicide attempts
- Previous noncompliance
- Sexual, physical, or emotional abuse
- Severe parental psychopathology
- Family unable or unwilling to monitor or protect patient

PSYCHOSIS

A psychotic patient may exhibit marked disruptions in cognition, perception, and reality testing. Patients may experience hallucinations or delusions or aberrations in behavior and thought processes. *Acute psychosis* refers to the development of a psychotic process over days to weeks.

Presentation and Differential Diagnosis

Psychosis may stem from either psychiatric or organic illness. The major functional causes of psychosis in childhood include pervasive developmental disorders, schizophrenia, posttraumatic stress disorder, and mood or personality disorders. In prepubertal children, organicity is a common cause of psychosis. Organic precipitants of psychosis include drug and alcohol intoxication, drug withdrawal, prescription medications, central nervous system insult (tumor, abscess, temporal lobe epilepsy, traumas), sepsis, and metabolic and endocrine disorders. A psychotic child will often present in a confused, agitated manner. Thoughts may be bizarre, distorted, and disconnected from reality. There may be disturbance in memory, concentration, and mood. The child may show little insight or judgment and may have hallucinations. Acute disorientation, change in consciousness, marked change in intellectual functioning, and visual hallucinations all point to organicity. The physical examination helps to differentiate organic and psychiatrically based psychosis. Basic laboratory evaluation includes a complete blood count, urinalysis, electrolytes, blood glucose, calcium, blood urea nitrogen, and drug and alcohol screens. Measurement of lead, medication, and lithium levels as well as other tests will be based on the history and physical. It may not be possible to rule out organic causes of psychosis in the emergency department.

It is important to alleviate a child's fear and anxiety. Children may develop psychotic symptoms when they are under stress. These episodes are often transient and nonrecurrent. Depressed children also develop psychotic symptoms. In this case the psychotic symptoms must be addressed and treated with neuroleptics in addition to the child's usual antidepressant medication.

Schizophrenia

Childhood schizophrenia is defined on the basis of characteristic psychotic symptoms, deficits in adaptive functioning, and duration of at least 6 months.

Symptoms

These include impairment of reality testing, perception, behavior, and capacity to relate socially. A patient may experience delusions, loose associations, catatonia, inappropriate or flattened affect, and hallucinations. Auditory hallucinations are the most frequently reported symptoms, exhibited by approximately 80 percent of schizophrenic patients. Auditory hallucinations are usually persecutory or commanding. Psychotic patients become dangerous when command hallucinations tell them to hurt themselves or someone else and when they exhibit poor impulse control, poor contact with reality, or poor decision making.

There are three patterns of illness. The onset most commonly appears to be insidious, with a gradual deterioration in functioning. In some instances the onset appears to be acute, without apparent premorbid signs of a disturbance. Last, some cases appear to have an insidious onset with an acute exacerbation. The differential diagnosis for schizophrenia includes mania, acute grief reactions, reactive psychosis, and organic psychosis.

Management

In the emergency department, treatment goals are focused on assessing the patient's safety, stabilizing acute symptoms, and either admission to the hospital or referral to appropriate outpatient services. First, the physician must determine whether there is a danger to the child or others and whether the family can provide care. If the patient is acutely agitated and medication must be given, low-dose neuroleptics are effective, safe, and fast-acting.

Haloperidol—2 to 10 mg for an adolescent or 0.5 to 3 mg for a child, PO or IM every 30 min, maximum dose of 40 mg—can be given until the patient calms down. Side effects of neuroleptics include dystonias, which respond to the anticholinergics Cogentin (1 to 2 mg PO or IM) or Benadryl (25 mg PO or IM); parkinsonian effects (which respond to Cogentin); and akathisias.

A child must be admitted if he or she is homicidal or suicidal. Inpatient treatment is also best if the patient or family is unable to provide adequate care and supervision, or if the patient needs to be stabilized on medication.

Mania

The essential feature of a manic episode is an expansive or irritable mood. The adolescent manic episode includes erratic and disinhibited behavior (excessive spending, gambling, promiscuity), low frustration tolerance, excessive energy, insomnia, anorexia and weight loss, and disruption of thought processes and content. There may be grandiose delusions, hallucinations, flights of ideas, and racing thoughts. Younger children (below 9 years of age) present with irritability and emotional lability. Both groups may show pressured speech, distractibility, and hyperactivity. Psychotic symptoms can be present in bipolar illness as part of a manic or depressive episode and tend to be mood-congruent. As with other causes of psychosis, an organic basis for manic behavior must be ruled out. Patients with mania secondary to bipolar illness frequently have a family history of mental illness. The differential diagnosis for mania includes drug reactions, organicity, attention deficit hyperactivity disorder, conduct disorder, drug and alcohol abuse, and schizophrenia.

Management

It is difficult to treat a full-blown manic episode on an outpatient basis. Manic patients tend to have poor impulse control and little insight. Because of their poor decision making, they put themselves or others at risk and may not be able to care for themselves. If this is the case, the patient must be hospitalized.

The first line of treatment for bipolar disorder is lithium. It is prophylactic in preventing mania but is not helpful in treating an acute episode. For this reason, lithium is started on the inpatient unit. Baseline laboratory tests ordered in the emergency department expedite starting the medication; these include a complete blood count, electrolytes, blood urea nitrogen, creatinine, creatinine clearance, urine osmolality, liver function, and thyroid func-

TABLE 120-4 Commonly Prescribed Antipsychotic Drugs and Dosages in Children and Adolescents

Generic name (trade name)	**Usual daily oral dose in milligrams** Children	Adolescents	Minimum age approved
Chlopromazine (Thorazine)	10–200	25–600	6 months
Haloperidol (Haldol)	0.25–6.0	1.0–16	3 years
Thioridazine (Mellaril)	10–200	50–500	2 years
Pimozide (Orap)	1–6	1–9	12 years
	(not to exceed 0.3 mg/kg)		
Clozapine (Clozaril)		100–900	16 years
Resperidone (Resperidol)		2–6	18 years

tion tests, as well as, for young women, a pregnancy test. If a patient is currently being treated with lithium, the lithium level should be checked. Therapeutic lithium levels are between 0.8 and 1.4, with toxicity occurring at levels of 2.0 and above. Lithium toxicity is potentially fatal. It is manifest by vomiting, diarrhea, severe tremor, seizures, and mental status changes. Manic patients who are management problems must be physically restrained. Once organic etiologies have been ruled out, neuroleptics or low-dose benzodiazepines (Tables 120-4 and 120-5) are given to help these patients regain control.

TABLE 120-5 Commonly Prescribed Benzodiazepines and Dosages in Children and Adolescents

Generic name (trade name)	Usual daily dosage for adults,[a] mg/kg/day	Minimum age approved
Chlordiazepoxide (Librium)	0.2–0.5	6 years
Diazepam (Valium)	0.07–0.5	6 months
Oxazepam (Serax)	0.014–1.7	6 years
Lorazepam (Ativan)	0.014–0.08	12 years
Alprazolam (Xanax)	0.014–0.08	18 years

[a] Dosages and indications not established for children and adolescents.

EMOTIONAL TRAUMA

A traumatized person has been exposed to a threat of death or serious injury to self or others and has responded to this event with intense fear, helplessness, or horror. This includes physically, sexually, or emotionally abused children; those who have witnessed violence in their neighborhoods or homes; and those who have been neglected and left without proper food or shelter. These children present as agitated, depressed, and dissociating (splitting off clusters of mental contents from conscious awareness) or hallucinating.

Children who experience trauma have both immediate and long-term psychological sequelae. These include recurrent nightmares and flashbacks and symptoms of increased arousal (problems falling asleep, irritability, difficulty concentrating, hypervigilance, or exaggerated startle response). They can exhibit avoidance behavior around stimuli connected with the traumatic experience. The impact of trauma on a child depends on the nature of the trauma, the child's developmental level, whether the trauma was an acute or chronic event (e.g., chronic sexual abuse), and if the child's environment is able to provide support and protection in dealing with the trauma.

Treatment

If a child presents acutely, medical intervention is the first priority. This should be explained as clearly as possible, as the child is already feeling overwhelmed and out of control. Emergency department personnel should be calm and provide reassurance. At times a traumatized child may present in an extremely agitated, dissociating, or psychotic manner. If the child is actively hallucinating or dissociating and does not respond to verbal or chemical interventions, hospitalization for stabilization in an inpatient setting is needed. As children begin to work through the trauma, they may need professional help in processing, understanding, and resolving the event.

THE RUNAWAY CHILD

Every year, close to a million adolescents in America run away from home, and many of them remain homeless for months or longer. Common causes include a difficult home situation, pursuit of excitement, and fleeing from physical, sexual, or psychological abuse. Such crises as divorce, parental discord, pregnancy, or homosexuality also lead a child to run away. This action is meant to call attention to a family's distress, to escape punishment, to demonstrate anger, or as a means of manipulation.

Runaway children often engage in prostitution and crime in order to survive. Sequelae include health problems, sexually transmitted diseases, and drug abuse. Psychologically, they are fearful, lonely, and unhappy.

Treatment

A runaway child who has presented to the emergency department represents a window of opportunity for intervention. The physician should try to uncover why the child ran away. Children who have been physically or sexually abused need to be assessed, treated, and provided with safe shelter. Child protection agencies must be notified. If hospitalization is not indicated for other reasons, and the parents are able and willing to care for the child safely, the child may be released. In the majority of cases, the child and family can benefit from family and individual therapy on an outpatient basis.

THE CHILD WHO IS VIOLENT OR ACTING OUT

Occasionally a child will present with violent or acting-out behavior, including threats, property destruction, stealing, fire-setting, or other disruptive acts. The parents are generally unable to cope or set appropriate limits. If a child or adolescent has committed a crime, the police must be notified.

Treatment

First, rule out any organic basis for erratic behavior. A violent child may need to be restrained either for safety or to prevent him or her from running away. Listening to the parents, supporting them, and helping them assess the situation realistically may be enough to get through the presenting crisis. If it is determined that there is no immediate danger, the child can be discharged home with outpatient referrals. If the family is unable or unwilling to take the child home, or if the child represents a danger, hospitalization is unavoidable.

INFANTILE AUTISM

Infantile autism has its onset before the patient reaches 30 months of age. The autistic child demonstrates poor social relations; gross deficits in language development, with abnormal speech patterns; and an idiosyncratic response to the environment (as illustrated by Dustin Hoffman in the movie *Rain Man*). Autism is frequently associated with congenital blindness, mental retardation (75 percent), and grand mal seizures (25 percent).

Management

Autistic children present with an acute exacerbation of behavior problems (agitation, anxiety, destructiveness). This could be caused by increased stress, change in the child's caregiver, or change in the child's routine. The treatment includes psychotherapy, behavioral therapy, and a structured educational program. Symptoms of agitation and destructiveness respond to neuroleptics. Autistic children may be more sensitive to medication and respond to smaller amounts than cohorts of similar age. The risk of extrapyramidal side effects with neuroleptics makes it mandatory to use the smallest effective dose for the minimum amount of time. If the child's behavior responds to medication acutely, he or she may be discharged home. If the child does not respond or the family is overwhelmed, short-term hospitalization may be necessary while appropriate placement is arranged.

DEATH OF A CHILD IN THE EMERGENCY DEPARTMENT

The physician must deal with resuscitation, notification, interviewing the family when abuse is suspected, addressing the issue of organ donation, supporting the next of kin, and facilitating the grieving process. The death of a child is often devastating to parents, family, and emergency department staff, making these tasks extremely difficult. While cultural differences, circumstances surrounding the death, and individual variations make each situation unique, having a protocol in place can ease the burden of the physician and staff while also ensuring that the family is properly attended.

Protocol for Addressing Death in the Emergency Department

1. The emergency department staff must contact the family. The news of a child's death should not be given over the phone. The parents should be asked to come to the hospital immediately. If possible, it is best to wait until both parents are present and tell them together.
2. The family should be placed in a quiet, secluded room. It should be a place where they can remain for some time, with access to a telephone.
3. While a child is being resuscitated and immediately after a death, a staff liaison should be available for consistent communication, to answer questions, and to help meet any of the family's immediate needs.
4. The emergency department staff should arrange support for

the family (other family members or friends, clergy, or the family physician).

5. The physician should let the family know about their child's death as soon as possible, as they are fearing the worst.
6. The physician should briefly review what is to be said before entering the room, outlining what measures were taken in trying to save the child. When possible, parents should be reassured that the child was not in pain and did not suffer. It is best to use kind, firm, and precise language.
7. The parents should be encouraged to view and touch the body after being warned about their child's condition, particularly if there is mutilation or disfigurement.
8. The physician must help the family make final decisions and arrangements. This includes discussing an autopsy and organ donation.
9. The family should be given, in writing, the name of the attending physician and the telephone number of the funeral home. It is important to arrange follow-up for the family with a family physician or mental health professional to help with any unresolved issues that may surface in the weeks immediately following the death.
10. The family should be told what a grief reaction entails, as this can help them to prepare for feelings and behaviors that may arise later.
11. The way in which the physician communicates is one of the most important aspects of helping a family in the time surrounding the death of a child. Families who have experienced the death of a child recall the manner in which they were told, as opposed to any specific information imparted. A compassionate, supportive, straightforward approach can go a long way toward helping a family accept the death of their child.

In a normal grief reaction in adults, the acute phase lasts a few weeks to months; the depressive phase can last up to a year. Acutely, parents experience feelings of shock, denial, anger, guilt, and being completely overwhelmed. Reactions may range from silence to hysterical crying. There may be anger, which is often directed at other family members or the hospital staff.

After the initial shock wears off, parents often feel powerless. They may withdraw into sadness and hopelessness. Fatigue and loss of appetite can persist for weeks to months.

In the final phase of a grief reaction, the mourner comes to terms with the reality of the loss. The total process often takes from 6 months to a year and includes periods of both anger and anxiety before resolution occurs.

A child's death has a profound impact on the siblings as well as the parents. Children are more likely to have difficulties with the comprehension of death and the processes of grief and mourning. Their response can range from apparent indifference to feelings of rage and desperation to sadness and yearning for the dead sibling. Children may also manifest their grief with hypochondriacal or regressive behavior, wetting or soiling themselves. With support and guidance, these behaviors usually resolve. Common concerns that must be addressed in almost all bereaved children are (1) feeling that they have caused the death, (2) worrying that the same thing will happen to them, and (3) worrying that the same thing will happen to their parents. An empathetic, concerned adult who can address a child's questions honestly at the appropriate developmental level can help the child begin to make sense of the loss.

It is difficult to draw the line between a normal reaction to the death of a family member and pathological grief. Pathological bereavement reactions are more common for families when the loss is sudden, unexpected, violent, or associated with other deaths, and when social supports are lacking. If there is continued denial that the death occurred, consider pathological grief if

- Regressive behavior persists
- Denial of the death persists
- Destructive behavior occurs
- Guilt, anxiety, or clinginess increase or persist

These children need professional evaluation. Many pathological grief reactions can be prevented or modified by early intervention, such as family meetings focused on sharing grief and mourning within the family.

In addition to periods of relief from grief-stricken parents, the child needs advice on how to cope with other children's questions and adults' expressions of condolence as well as factual information about the cause of death and the processes of death, burial, and cremation. The child needs advice about viewing the body, attending the funeral, returning to school, and promoting healthy mourning.

SUBSTANCE ABUSE

Many children begin drug use between 12 and 18 years of age. The earlier in life drug use begins, the greater the likelihood of serious abuse in adulthood. Up to 50 percent of the fatal accidents, disabling injuries, suicides, and homicides in adolescence are associated with substance abuse. A short emergency department assessment and intervention can make a difference in identifying potential problem users and directing them to a treatment program.

Assessment

Common presentations include acute intoxication, associated trauma, drug reaction, or parental requests for assessment. Assessment begins with a history of use patterns. Since patients minimize or deny their problems, substance abuse is probably the most commonly missed pediatric diagnosis.

Next, the parents are asked about their knowledge of drug use, changes in the child's behavior, and changes in school performance. Behaviors suggestive of drug use include acute mental status changes, aggression, delirium, lethargy, or a marked change in a child's normal behavior. A family history of substance abuse or evidence of parental substance abuse increases the chance that the youth is abusing drugs. Finally, blood or urine toxicology studies for illicit substances are done or, if the patient is acutely intoxicated, specific drug levels are checked.

Management

Any medical problems associated with drug use must be managed. Disposition may require admission for the medical complications of abuse, or the patient may be handled medically as an outpatient. In addition, the physician will need to have a list of the available community social services and their phone numbers. Arranging an intake from the emergency department for a drug abuse program increases the chances that the patient will follow up on the referral. Treatment options include hospital-based detoxification units, outpatient substance abuse programs, methadone maintenance programs, Narcotics Anonymous, Alcoholics Anonymous, or school-based support and treatment programs.

PSYCHIATRIC LEGAL ISSUES IN THE EMERGENCY DEPARTMENT

There are four areas of the law that are pertinent to treating problem children in the emergency department: dangerousness, commitment, duty to treat, and confidentiality. Every state has a mental health code establishing statutory standards and duties for the physician. Failure to follow the specific statutes of a state produces a presumption of negligence.

Children must be committed when they pose a danger to themselves or others. The parent or guardian of a child may give signed permission to hospitalize the child against his or her will. Whether or not a parent has a right to refuse services for a dangerous child will vary from state to state. This action may constitute an act of child neglect and mandate a referral to the state abuse agency.

Duty to treat in the emergency department is very explicit. Federal law requires that if a child is mentally unstable (i.e., the child might be seriously harmed by not being admitted), the physician must provide or arrange appropriate care independent of ability to pay. In most states the physician is liable for all the consequences of failure to admit a dangerous child, including liability to third persons injured by a mentally ill child. Detaining a child without adhering to appropriate legal procedures may be a violation of the child's civil rights or an illegal detention. Consulting a child psychiatrist who is familiar with the specific legal issues of the state helps to protect both the emergency physician and the child.

Psychiatric medication and treatment may be given against the will of an adolescent patient only when immediate serious harm to the patient or someone else would result from failure to do so. If this is not the case, most states require a court order for medication of an adolescent against his or her will. Reasons for use of medication and restraints must be documented.

Finally, most states have mental health confidentiality laws that require different forms of consent from the customary releases for medical information. If substance abuse is involved, additional federal confidentiality standards apply.

The physician is bound by all statutes to provide appropriate care, even when the care must be given involuntarily. There are statutes protecting patients' rights and freedoms. The emergency physician must be familiar with the particular laws in his or her state to meet the patient's needs while walking the fine line between protection and intrusion on a patient's rights.

PSYCHIATRIC EMERGENCIES ASSOCIATED WITH TREATMENT

Parkinsonian symptoms, which are associated with the use of neuroleptics, are characterized by muscular rigidity, finger and hand tremor, drooling, akinesia, and masklike facies. These symptoms respond to antiparkinsonian medication such as benztropine mesylate (Cogentin) 0.5 to 2 mg bid to tid or diphenhydramine (Benadryl) 12.5 to 50 mg tid. The period of maximum risk is 5 to 30 days after initiation of the neuroleptic.

Acute dystonic reactions are also often associated with the use of high-potency neuroleptics such as haloperidol or thiothixine. They are characterized by acute, painful muscle spasms, often in the face, mouth, or neck. The period of maximum risk is 1 to 5 days after initiating therapy. Treatment of these reactions consists of the administration of anticholinergic antiparkinsonian drugs (benztropine or diphenhydramine). There is usually a rapid response.

The neuroleptic malignant syndrome is a life-threatening condition most often described in adults but also seen in children and adolescents. It carries a 16 percent mortality rate. Cardinal features are exposure to neuroleptic, altered mental status (agitation, disorientation), fever, autonomic instability (fluctuating blood pressure and pulse), increased muscle tone or rigidity, elevated creatine phosphokinase (CPK), and abnormal liver function tests. Treatment is supportive, often in the intensive care unit. Those who recover from this syndrome do so completely. Reintroduction of neuroleptics is possible but should be done with caution. High-potency multiple neuroleptics are to be avoided.

For a more detailed discussion, see Schwarz E, Wright T: Psychiatric emergencies, chap. 120, p. 663, in *Pediatric Emergency Medicine: A Comprehensive Study Guide.*

APPENDIX A Contraindications and Precautions for Immunization

Contraindication/precaution

Anaphylactic reaction to vaccine
Anaphylactic reaction to a vaccine constituent
Moderate or severe illness with or without fever

Vaccine may be given

History of mild to moderate local reaction with previous vaccination, such as swelling or soreness in the area where the vaccine was given
Mild acute illness with or without fever or convalescent phase of illness
Recent exposure to an infectious disease
Current antimicrobial therapy or history of antimicrobial allergy in patients or relatives.
History of prematurity (same dosage and indications as for normal full-term infants)

Source: *Ann. Emer. Med.* 28:3, September 1996. Used with permission.

APPENDIX B Management of Hyperbilirubinemia in the Healthy Term Newborn

	TSB[a] Level, mg/dL (μmol/L)			
Age, hours	Consider Phototherapy[b]	Phototherapy	Exchange Transfusion if Intensive Phototherapy Fails[c]	Exchange Transfusion and Intensive Phototherapy
≤24[d]	...	...	...	...
25–48	≥12 (170)	≥15 (260)	≥20 (340)	≥25 (430)
49–72	≥15 (260)	≥18 (310)	≥25 (430)	≥30 (510)
>72	≥17 (290)	≥20 (340)	≥25 (430)	≥30 (510)

[a] TSB indicates total serum bilirubin.
[b] Phototherapy at these TSB levels is a clinical option, meaning that the intervention is available and may be used *on the basis of individual clinical judgment.*
[c] Intensive phototherapy should produce a decline of TSB of 1 to 2 mg/dL within 4 to 6 h and the TSB level should continue to fall and remain below the threshold level for exchange transfusion. If this does not occur, it is considered a failure of phototherapy.
[d] Term infants who are clinically jaundiced at ≤24 h old are not considered healthy and require further evaluation.

Index

Note: Page numbers in italics indicate figures; those followed by t indicate tables.